W9-BXV-689

las agruras (el ardor), acedía
la enfermedad del corazón
el fallo cardíaco
el soplo del corazón
la hemorragia
las almorranas, las hemorroides
la hepatitis
la hernia
el herpes
la presión alta
la urticaria
la ronquera
enfermo(a)
la enfermedad
la inmunización
el infarto
la infección
la inflamación
el daño la lastimadura, la herida
la picazón, la comezón
la piel amarilla, la ictericia
el cálculo en el riñón, la piedra en el riñón
la laringitis
la lesión, el daño
la leucemia
los piojos
el bulto
el tumor, la malignidad
maligno(a)
el sarampión
la meningitis
la menopausia
la metástasis
la migrañia, la jaqueca
la esclerosis múltiple
las paperas
la distrofia muscular
mudo(a)
obeso(a)
la sobredosis
el sobrepeso
el dolor
  el dolor de crecimiento
  el dolor de parto
  el dolor de miembro fantasma
  el dolor referido
  el dolor agudo

shooting pain	el dolor punzante
burning pain	el dolor que arde
intense pain	el dolor intenso
severe pain	el dolor severo
intermittent pain	el dolor intermitente
throbbing pain	el dolor palpitante
palpitation	la palpitación
paralysis	la parálisis
Parkinson's disease	la enfermedad de Parkinson
pneumonia	la pulmonía
psoriasis	la psoriasis
pus	el pus
rash	la roncha, el salpullido, la erupción
relapse	la recaída
renal	renal
rheumatic fever	la fiebre reumitáca
roseola	la roséola
rubella	la rubéola
rupture	la ruptura
scab	la costra
scar	la cicatriz
scratch	el rasguño
senile	senil
shock	el choque
sore	la llaga
spasm	el espasmo
sprain	la torcedura
stomachache	el dolor del estómago
stomach ulcer	la úlcera del estómago
suicide	el suicidio
swelling	la hinchazón
syphilis	la sífilis
tachycardia	la taquicardia
toothache	el dolor de muela
toxemia	la toxemia
trauma	el trauma
tuberculosis	la tuberculosis
tumor	el tumor
ulcer	la úlcera
unconsciousness	la pérdida del conocimiento
virus	el virus
vomit	el vómito, los vómitos
wart	la verruga
weakness	la debilidad
wheeze	el jadeo, la silba
wound	la herida
yellow fever	la fiebre amarilla

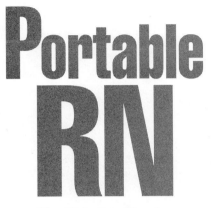

Portable RN

The All-in-One Nursing Reference

Portable
RN

The All-in-One Nursing Reference

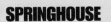

SPRINGHOUSE
Springhouse, Pennsylvania

Staff

Publisher
Judith A. Schilling McCann, RN, MSN

Creative Director
Jake Smith

Editorial Director
David Moreau

Clinical Director
Joan M. Robinson, RN, MSN, CCRN

Editors
Julie Munden (senior editor),
Stacey Ann Follin, Carol H. Munson

Clinical Editors
Joanne Bartelmo, RN, MSN;
Anita Lockhart, RN,C, MSN;

Copy Editors
Jaime L. Stockslager (supervisor),
Kimberly Bilotta, Heather Ditch,
Amy Furman, Shana Harrington,
Dona Hightower, Carolyn Petersen,
Marcia Ryan, Dorothy P. Terry,
Pamela Wingrod, Helen Winton

Designers
Arlene Putterman (associate design
director), Linda Franklin (book design),
Susan Hopkins Rodzewich (project
manager), Joseph John Clark,
Donna S. Morris, Jeffrey Sklarow

Projects Coordinator
Liz Schaeffer

Electronic Production Services
Diane Paluba (manager),
Joyce Rossi Biletz

Manufacturing
Patricia K. Dorshaw (manager),
Otto Mezei (book production manager)

Editorial Assistants
Beverly Lane, Beth Janae Orr,
Elfriede Young

Indexer
Manjit Sahai

The clinical procedures described and recommended in this publication are based on research and consultation with medical and nursing authorities. To the best of our knowledge, these procedures reflect currently accepted clinical practice; nevertheless, they can't be considered absolute and universal recommendations. For individual application, treatment recommendations must be considered in light of the patient's clinical condition and, before administration of new or infrequently used drugs, in light of the latest package-insert information. The authors and publisher disclaim responsibility for any adverse effects resulting directly or indirectly from the suggested procedures, from any undetected errors, or from the reader's misunderstanding of the text.

© 2002 by Springhouse Corporation. All rights reserved. No part of this publication may be used or reproduced in any manner whatsoever without written permission except for brief quotations embodied in critical articles and reviews. For information, write Springhouse Corporation, 1111 Bethlehem Pike, P.O. Box 908, Springhouse, PA 19477-0908. Authorization to photocopy items for internal or personal use, or for the internal or personal use of specific clients, is granted by Springhouse Corporation for users registered with the Copyright Clearance Center (CCC) Transactional Reporting Service, provided that the fee of $.75 per page is paid directly to CCC, 222 Rosewood Dr., Danvers, MA 01923. For those organizations that have been granted a photocopy license by CCC, a separate system of payment has been arranged. The fee code for users of the Transactional Reporting Service is 1582551421/01 $00.00 + .75.

Printed in the United States of America.

PRN – D N O S A J J
03 02   10 9 8 7 6 5 4 3 2

FOCUS CHARTING is a registered trademark of Creative Healthcare Management, Inc.

Library of Congress Cataloging-in-Publication Data
Portable RN : the all-in-one nursing reference.
   p. ; cm.
   Includes bibliographical references and index.
      ISBN 1-58255-142-1 (alk. paper)
      1. Nursing—Handbooks, manuals, etc. I. Lippincott Williams & Wilkins. Springhouse Division.
      [DNLM: 1. Nursing Process—Handbooks.
2. Nursing Care—methods—Handbooks.
WY 49 P839 2002]
RT51 .P676 2002
610.73—dc21   2001040099

Contents

Contributors and consultants

Cheryl L. Brady, RN, MSN
Adjunct Faculty
Kent State University
East Liverpool, Ohio

Claire Campbell, RN, MSN, CFNP
Family Nurse Practitioner
HealthSouth Medical Center, Outpatient
Clinic
Dallas

Ellen P. Digan, MA, MT(ASCP)
Professor of Biology
Coordinator, MLT Program
Manchester (Conn.) Community
College

Cynthia J. Fine, RN, MSN, CIC
Infection Control and Employee Health
Program Consultant
Catholic Healthcare West
Oakland, Calif.

Carol Ann Knauff, RN, MSN, CCRN
Clinical Educator
Grandview Hospital
Sellersville, Pa.

Jim Koestner, PHARMD
Clinical Pharmacist
Vanderbilt University Hospital
Nashville, Tenn.

**Vickie A. Miracle, RN, EdD, CCNS,
CCRN**
Director of Education
Jewish Hospital Heart and Lung
Institute
Louisville, Ky.

Christine Normile
Apheresis Specialist
Hospital of the University of
Pennsylvania
Philadelphia

**Linda Honan Pellico, RN,CS,
MSN, CCRN**
Director of Graduate Entry Prespecialty
in Nursing
Yale University School of Nursing
New Haven, Conn.

**Theresa A. Posani, RN, MS, CCNS,
CCRN, CNA, CS**
Critical Care Clinical Nurse Specialist
Presbyterian Hospital of Dallas

Marilyn Smith-Stoner, RN, PHD
Adjunct Faculty
University of Phoenix
Ontario, Calif.

Laura M. Waters, RN, MS
Professor of Nursing
East Stroudsburg (Pa.) University

Foreword

Registered nurses (RNs) everywhere tell the same story: We're doing more than ever and we're doing it with less help. If you care for patients in the acute care environment, you're profoundly aware of the frequency with which patients present with multisystem diseases and the complexities you face in treating them. You must be armed with knowledge yet be able to perform quickly under pressure. The scope of your work has expanded exponentially and, in this time of rapid change, you need to have resources that are timely and accurate, succinct yet comprehensive.

Welcome *Portable RN: The All-in-One Nursing Reference!* This unique book has it all — clear, useful information that can answer your complex clinical questions with ease. This book was especially designed for you, the RN.

With *Portable RN,* you'll get up-to-date information on everything from drug interactions to patient education. You'll discover how to troubleshoot problems with commonly used equipment, such as gastric tubes and respiratory monitors; interpret common laboratory test results with ease; and ensure effective drug therapy. You'll have the book in your pocket and at your fingertips, ready to provide you with concise, comprehensive answers to your questions.

This compact powerhouse of clinical information provides you with the latest on common procedures, laboratory findings, common disorders, life-threatening complications, and many other clinical issues. Chapters 1 and 2 review common physical assessment techniques and findings and common reasons for seeking care. Cues are given for abnormal findings so that you can assess for potential causes to prevent further complications. *Portable RN* gives you warning patterns so you can respond to patients and treat them accurately.

Chapter 3 covers interpreting cardiac rhythms using electrocardiogram and rhythm strips, and chapter 4 gives reference values for common laboratory tests, significant laboratory test results, and ways to interpret those results quickly and precisely. Organized alphabetically, chapter 5 covers common disorders and how to treat and prevent them. Each entry in this chapter begins with a brief description and follows with the major causes, possible complications, assessment findings, diagnostic tests, treatments, nursing diagnoses and interventions and, finally, patient teaching instructions. Chapter 6 reviews preoperative and postoperative patient care, including patient-teaching needs and discharge planning. Chapter 7 presents common procedures and how to perform them safely and accurately.

Chapter 8 covers prevention and control of contagious diseases. It reviews universal precautions, lists reportable diseases, and features an overview of basic procedures for disease prevention.

In chapter 9, you'll find extensive coverage on how to spot and correct everyday equipment problems with I.V. lines, respiratory monitors, ventilators, and more.

Chapters 10, 11, and 12 review drug administration, dosage calculations, and drug hazards, respectively. You'll find comprehensive coverage of the methods for safely administering medications, calculating dosages correctly, and avoiding common hazards of medication administration.

Chapter 13 explores how to detect and treat life-threatening complications. Such common complications as brain herniation, hypertensive crisis, septic shock, and tracheal erosion are covered. Each entry features a descriptive introduction followed by causes, signs and symptoms, treatments, and nursing interventions.

Chapter 14 examines today's latest alternative and complementary therapies. Find out about enhancing and healing techniques, such as aromatherapy, meditation, and therapeutic massage, and how to implement other therapies, including art, dance, and yoga.

Chapter 15 provides examples of commonly used documentation forms and how to complete them correctly and concisely. Chapter 16 offers you a survival guide to home health care, covering the ethical and legal aspects as well as how to ensure safe home care visits, work with home health aids, interpret reimbursement, and resolve case management issues.

Throughout the book you'll find helpful logos such as *Age alerts* that call your attention to considerations for young and elderly patients and *Patient teaching tips* that give you ways to ensure better learning and compliance.

Finally, five appendices cover cultural considerations in patient care, helpful medical abbreviations and terms, a list of the latest North American Nursing Diagnosis Association Tax-

onomy II codes, and two charts that highlight herb-drug interactions and how to monitor your patients that use herbs.

Given the limited resources, the shortage of care providers, and patient complexities, the reality of being an RN in today's health care system is that you must be able to multitask in the moment. Therefore, it's imperative that information is accurate and readily accessible. The nursing profession is continually faced with new developments. How can you arm yourself? Keep the best, most current resources at your fingertips.

Although a single resource can't substitute for a living, breathing RN, *Portable RN* may be the next best thing — knowledgeable, efficient, and always ready and able to help.

Linda Honan Pellico, MSN, APRN, CCRN

Director of Graduate Entry
 Prespecialty in Nursing
Yale University School of Nursing
New Haven, Conn.

1

Assessment
Reviewing the techniques

Reviewing assessment techniques

Performing a 10-minute assessment

You won't always want or need to assess a patient in 10 minutes. However, rapid assessment is crucial when you must intervene quickly — such as when a hospitalized patient complains of a change in his physical, mental, or emotional status.

You may also perform a rapid assessment to confirm a diagnostic finding. For example, if arterial blood gas analysis indicates a low oxygen content, you'll quickly assess the patient for other signs of oxygen deprivation, such as an increased respiratory rate and cyanosis.

General guidelines

Try to assess the patient not only quickly but also systematically. To save time, cover some of the assessment components simultaneously. For example, make your general observations while checking the patient's vital signs or asking history questions.

Be flexible. You won't necessarily use the same sequence each time. Let the patient's reason for seeking care and your initial observations guide your assessment. Sometimes, you may be unable to obtain a quick history and instead will have to rely on your observations and the information on the patient's chart.

Keep the patient calm and cooperative. If you don't know him, first introduce yourself by name and title. Remain calm, and reassure him that you can help. If your demeanor can reduce his anxiety, he'll be more likely to give you accurate information.

Avoid drawing quick conclusions. In particular, don't assume that the patient's current complaint is related to his admitting diagnosis.

When every minute counts, follow these steps.

Assess airway, breathing, and circulation

As your first priority, this assessment may consist of just a momentary observation. However, when a patient appears to be unconscious or has difficulty breathing, you'll assess him more thoroughly to detect the problem and intervene immediately.

Make general observations

Note the patient's mental status, general appearance, and level of consciousness for clues to the nature and severity of his condition.

Assess vital signs

Take the patient's body temperature, pulse, respiratory rate, and blood pressure. They provide a quick overview of physiologic condition as well as valuable information about the heart, lungs, and blood vessels. The seriousness of the patient's reason for seeking care and your general observations of his condition will determine how extensively you measure vital signs.

Age alert A patient's age, activity level, and physical and emotional condition may affect his vital signs. Compare with the patient's baseline, if available.

Conduct the health history

Use pointed questions to explore the patient's perception of his reason for seeking care. Find out what's bothering him the most. Ask him to quantify the problem. Does he, for instance, feel worse today than he did yesterday? Such questions will help you focus your assessment. If you're in a hurry or the patient can't respond, obtain information from other sources, such as family members, medical history, admission forms, and the patient's chart.

Perform the physical examination
Begin by concentrating on areas related to the patient's reason for seeking care — the abdomen, for example, if the patient complains of abdominal pain. Compare the results with baseline data, if available.

Sometimes, you may have to perform a complete head-to-toe or body systems assessment — for instance, if a patient is unresponsive (yet has no breathing or circulatory problems) or is confused and, thus, unreliable. However, in most cases, the patient's reason for seeking care, your general observations, and your findings regarding the patient's vital signs will guide your assessment.

Guidelines for an effective interview

When you have time for a full assessment, you'll begin by interviewing the patient. Developing an effective interviewing technique will help you collect pertinent health history information efficiently. Use these guidelines to enhance your interviewing skills.

Be prepared
■ Before the interview, review all available information. Read current clinical records and, if applicable, previous records. This will focus the interview, prevent the patient from tiring, and save you time.

■ Review with the patient what you've learned to ensure the information is correct. Keep in mind that the patient's current complaint may be unrelated to his history.

Create a pleasant interviewing atmosphere
■ Select a quiet, well-lighted, and relaxing setting. Keep in mind that extraneous noise and activity can interfere with concentration, as can excessive or insufficient light. A relaxing atmosphere eases the patient's anxiety, promotes comfort, and conveys your willingness to listen.
■ Ensure privacy. Some patients won't share personal information if they suspect that others can overhear. You may, however, let friends or family members remain if the patient requests it or if he needs their help.
■ Make sure the patient feels as comfortable as possible. If the patient is tired, short of breath, or frightened, you should provide care and reschedule the history taking.
■ Take your time. If you appear rushed, you may distract the patient. Give him your undivided attention. If you have little time, you should focus on specific areas of interest and return later instead of hurrying through the entire interview.

Establish a good rapport
■ Sit and chat with the patient for a few minutes before the interview. Standing may suggest that you're in a hurry, thus leading the patient to rush and omit important information.
■ Explain the interview's purpose. Emphasize how the patient benefits when the health care team has the in-

formation needed to diagnose and treat a disorder.

■ Show your concern for the patient's story. Maintain eye contact, and occasionally repeat what he tells you. If you seem preoccupied or disinterested, he may choose not to confide in you.

■ Encourage the patient to help you develop a realistic plan of care that will serve his perceived needs.

Set the tone and focus

■ Encourage the patient to talk about his reason for seeking care. This helps you focus on his most troublesome signs and symptoms and provides an opportunity to assess the patient's emotional state and level of understanding.

■ Keep the interview informal but professional. Allow the patient time to answer questions fully and to add his own perceptions.

■ Speak clearly and simply. Avoid using medical terms.

Age alert Make sure the patient understands you, especially if he's elderly. If you think he doesn't, ask him to restate what you've discussed.

■ Pay close attention to the patient's words and actions, interpreting not only what he says but also what he doesn't say.

Age alert If the patient is a child, direct as many questions as possible to him. Rely on the parents for information if the child is very young.

Choose your words carefully

■ Ask open-ended questions to encourage the patient to provide complete and pertinent information. Avoid yes-or-no-type questions.

■ Listen carefully to the patient's answers. Use his words in your subsequent questions to encourage him to elaborate on his signs, symptoms, and other problems.

Take notes

■ Avoid documenting everything during the interview, but make sure to jot down important information, such as dates, times, and key words or phrases. Use these to help you recall the complete history for the medical record.

■ If you're tape recording the interview, obtain written consent from the patient.

Assessing overall health

For a quick look at the patient's overall health, ask these questions.

■ Has your weight changed? Do your clothes, rings, and shoes fit?

■ Do you have nonspecific signs and symptoms, such as weakness, fatigue, night sweats, or fever?

■ Can you keep up with normal daily activities?

■ Have you had any unusual symptoms or problems recently?

■ How many colds or other minor illnesses have you had in the last year?

■ What prescription and over-the-counter drugs do you take?

Assessing activities of daily living

For a comprehensive look at the patient's health and health history, ask these questions.

Diet and elimination

■ How would you describe your appetite?

■ What do you normally eat in a 24-hour period?

■ What foods do you like and dislike? Is your diet restricted at all?

■ How much fluid do you drink during an average day?

■ Are you allergic to any food?

■ Do you prepare your meals, or does someone prepare them for you?

■ Do you go to the grocery store, or does someone else shop for you?

■ Do you snack and, if so, on what?

■ Do you eat a variety of foods?

■ Do you have enough money to purchase the groceries you need?

■ When do you usually go to the bathroom? Has this pattern recently changed?

■ Do you take any foods, fluids, or drugs to maintain your normal elimination patterns?

Exercise and sleep

■ Do you have a special exercise program? What is it? How long have you been following it? How do you feel after exercising?

■ How many hours do you sleep each day? When? Do you feel rested afterward?

■ Do you fall asleep easily?

■ Do you take any drugs or do anything special to help you fall asleep?

■ What do you do when you can't sleep?

■ Do you wake up during the night?

■ Do you have sleepy spells during the day? When?

■ Do you routinely take naps?

■ Do you have any recurrent and disturbing dreams?

■ Have you ever been diagnosed with a sleep disorder, such as narcolepsy or sleep apnea?

Recreation

■ What do you do when you aren't working?

■ What kind of nonpaid work do you do for enjoyment?

■ How much leisure time do you have?

■ Are you satisfied with what you can do in your leisure time?

■ Do you and your family share leisure time?

■ How do your weekends differ from your weekdays?

Tobacco, alcohol, and drugs

■ Do you use tobacco? If so, what kind? How much do you use each day? Each week? For how long have you used it? Have you ever tried to stop?

■ Do you drink alcoholic beverages? If so, what kind (beer, wine, whiskey)?

■ How much alcohol do you drink each day? Each week? What time of day do you usually drink?

■ Do you usually drink alone or with others?

■ Do you drink more when you're under stress?

■ Has drinking ever hampered your job performance?

■ Do you or your family worry about your drinking?

■ Do you feel dependent on alcohol?

■ Do you feel dependent on coffee, tea, or soft drinks? How much of these beverages do you drink in an average day?

■ Do you use drugs not prescribed by a doctor (marijuana, sleeping pills, tranquilizers)?

Assessing the family

When assessing how and to what extent the patient's family fulfills its functions, remember to assess both the family into which the patient was born (family of origin) and, if different, the current family.

Because the following questions target a nuclear family — that is, mother, father, and children — you may need to modify them somewhat for single-parent families, families that include grandparents, patients who live alone, or unrelated individuals who live as a family. Remember, you're assessing the *patient's perception* of family function.

Affective function
To assess how family members regard each other, ask these questions.
■ How do the members of your family treat each other?
■ How do they feel about each other?
■ How do they regard each other's needs and wants?
■ How are feelings expressed in your family?
■ Can family members safely express both positive and negative feelings?
■ What happens in the family when members disagree?
■ How do family members deal with conflict?

Socialization and social placement
To assess the flexibility of family responsibilities, which aids discharge planning, ask these questions.
■ How satisfied are you and your partner with your roles as a couple?
■ How did you decide to have (or not to have) children?
■ Do you and your partner agree about how to bring up the children? If not, how do you work out differences?
■ Who is responsible for taking care of the children? Is this mutually satisfactory?

■ How well do you feel your children are growing up?
■ Are family roles negotiable within the limits of age and ability?
■ Do you share cultural values and beliefs with the children?

Health care function
To identify the family caregiver and thus facilitate discharge planning, ask these questions.
■ Who takes care of family members when they're sick? Who makes doctor appointments?
■ Are your children learning personal hygiene, healthful eating habits, and the importance of sleep and rest?
■ How does your family adjust when a member is ill and unable to fulfill expected roles?

Family and social structure
To assess the value the patient places on family and other social structures, ask these questions.
■ How important is your family to you?
■ Do you have any friends you consider family?
■ Does anyone other than your immediate family (for example, grandparents) live with you?
■ Are you involved in community affairs? Do you enjoy the activities?

Economic function
To explore money issues and their relation to power roles within the family, ask these questions.
■ Does your family income meet the family's basic needs?
■ Who makes decisions about family money allocation?

(Text continues on page 12.)

Performing palpation techniques

Palpation uses pressure to assess structure size, placement, pulsation, and tenderness. Ballottement, a variation, involves bouncing tissues against the hand to assess rebound of floating structures.

Light palpation

To perform light palpation, press gently on the skin, indenting it ½″ to ¾″ (1 to 2 cm). Use the lightest touch possible; too much pressure blunts your sensitivity. Close your eyes to concentrate on feeling.

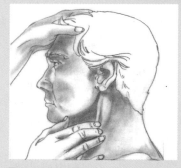

Deep palpation

To perform deep palpation, indent the skin about 1½″ (4 cm). Place your other hand on top of the palpating hand to control and guide your movements. To perform a variation of deep palpation that allows pinpointing an inflamed area, push down slowly and deeply, then lift your hand away quickly. If the patient complains of increased pain as you release the pressure, you have identified rebound tenderness.

Use both hands (bimanual palpation) to trap a deep, underlying hard-to-palpate organ (such as the kidney or spleen) or to fix or stabilize an organ (such as the uterus) while palpating with the other hand.

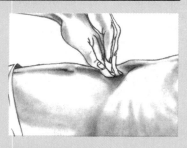

Light ballottement

To perform light ballottement, apply light, rapid pressure from quadrant to quadrant of the patient's abdomen. Keep your hand on the skin surface to detect tissue rebound.

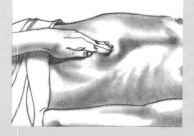

Deep ballottement

To perform deep ballottement, apply abrupt, deep pressure; then release, but maintain contact.

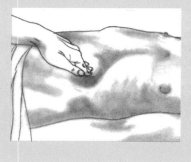

Performing percussion techniques

Percussion has two basic purposes; to produce percussion sounds and to elicit tenderness. It involves three types: indirect, direct, and blunt percussion.

Indirect percussion
The most commonly used method, indirect percussion produces clear, crisp sounds when performed correctly. To perform indirect percussion, use the second finger of your nondominant hand as the pleximeter (the mediating device used to receive the taps) and the middle finger of your dominant hand as the plexor (the device used to tap the pleximeter). Place the pleximeter finger firmly against a body surface, such as the upper back. With your wrist flexed loosely, use the tip of your plexor finger to deliver a crisp blow just beneath the distal joint of the pleximeter. Make sure you hold the plexor perpendicular to the pleximeter. Tap lightly and quickly, removing the plexor as soon as you have delivered each blow.

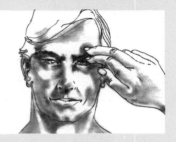

Blunt percussion
To perform blunt percussion, strike the ulnar surface of your fist against the body surface. Alternatively, you may use both hands by placing the palm of one hand over the area to be percussed and then making a fist with the other hand and using it to strike the back of the first hand. Both techniques aim to elicit tenderness — not to create a sound — over such organs as the kidneys, gallbladder, or liver. (Another blunt percussion method, used in the neurologic examination, involves tapping a rubber-tipped reflex hammer against a tendon to create a reflexive muscle contraction.)

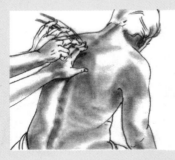

Direct percussion
To perform direct percussion, tap your hand or fingertip directly against the body surface as shown at the top of the next column. This method helps assess an adult's sinuses for tenderness.

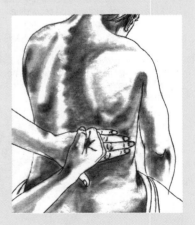

Identifying percussion sounds

Percussion produces sounds that vary according to the tissue being percussed. This chart shows important percussion sounds along with their characteristics and typical locations.

SOUND	INTENSITY	PITCH	DURATION
Resonance	Moderate to loud	Low	Moderate to long
Tympany	Loud	High	Moderate
Dullness	Soft to moderate	High	Long
Hyperresonance	Very loud	Very low	Long
Flatness	Soft .	High	Short

Performing auscultation

Auscultation of body sounds — particularly those that the heart, lungs, blood vessels, stomach, and intestines produce — detects both high-pitched and low-pitched sounds. Although you can perform auscultation directly over a body area using only your ears, you'll typically perform it indirectly, using a stethoscope.

Assessing high-pitched sounds
To properly assess high-pitched sounds, such as breath sounds and first and second heart sounds, use the diaphragm of the stethoscope. Make sure you place the diaphragm's entire surface firmly on the patient's skin. If the area is excessively hairy, improve diaphragm contact and reduce extraneous noise by applying water or water-soluble jelly to the skin before auscultating.

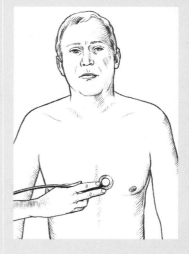

QUALITY	SOURCE
Hollow	Normal lung
Drumlike	Gastric air bubble; intestinal air
Thudlike	Liver; full bladder; pregnant uterus; spleen
Booming	Hyperinflated lung (as in emphysema)
Flat	Muscle; bone; or tumor

Assessing low-pitched sounds

To assess low-pitched sounds, such as heart murmurs and third and fourth heart sounds, lightly place the bell of the stethoscope on the appropriate area. Don't exert pressure. If you do, the patient's chest will act as a diaphragm and you'll miss low-pitched sounds. If the patient is extremely thin or emaciated, use a stethoscope with a pediatric chestpiece.

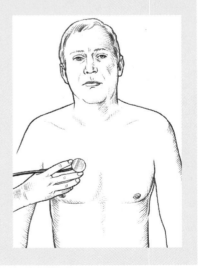

Assessing the cardiovascular system

Initial cardiovascular questions

■ Ask the patient about cardiac problems, such as palpitations, tachycardia or other irregular rhythms, chest pain, dyspnea on exertion, paroxysmal nocturnal dyspnea, and cough.

■ Explore vascular problems. Does the patient experience cyanosis, edema, ascites, intermittent claudication, cold extremities, or phlebitis?

■ Ask about postural hypotension, hypertension, rheumatic fever, varicose veins, and peripheral vascular diseases.

■ Ask when, if ever, the patient had his last electrocardiogram.

Inspecting the precordium

■ First, place the patient in a supine position, with his head flat or elevated for his respiratory comfort. If you're examining an obese patient or one with large breasts, have the patient sit upright. This will bring the heart closer to the anterior chest wall and make any pulsations more visible. If time allows, you can use tangential lighting to cast shadows across the chest. This makes it easier to see any abnormalities.

■ Standing to the patient's right (unless you're left-handed), remove the clothing covering his chest wall. Quickly identify the following anatomic sites, named for their underlying structures: the sternoclavicular, pulmonary, aortic, right ventricular, epigastric, and left ventricular areas.

■ Make a visual sweep of the chest wall, watching for movement, pulsations, and exaggerated lifts or heaves (strong outward thrusts seen at the sternal border or the apex during systole).

Measuring blood pressure

When you assess the patient's blood pressure, you're measuring the fluctuating force that blood exerts against arterial walls as the heart contracts and relaxes. To measure accurately, follow these steps.

Preparing the patient

Before beginning, make sure the patient is relaxed and hasn't eaten or exercised in the past 30 minutes. The patient can sit, stand, or lie down during blood pressure measurement.

Applying the cuff and stethoscope

■ To obtain a reading in an arm (the most common measurement site), wrap the sphygmomanometer cuff snugly around the upper arm above the antecubital area (the inner aspect of the elbow), with the cuff bladder centered over the brachial artery.

Age alert When taking an infant's or child's blood pressure, use the appropriate size cuff. Because blood pressure may be inaudible in children younger than age 2, consider using an electronic stethoscope or Doppler to get a more accurate measurement.

■ Most cuffs have arrows that should be placed over the brachial artery. Make sure you use the proper-sized cuff for the patient.

■ Keep the mercury manometer at eye level; if your sphygmomanometer has an aneroid gauge, place it level with the patient's arm. Keep the patient's arm level with the heart by placing it on a table or a chair arm or by supporting it with your hand. Rest a recumbent patient's arm at his side. Don't use the patient's muscle strength to hold up the arm; tension from muscle contraction can elevate systolic pressure and distort your findings.

■ Next, palpate the brachial pulse just below and slightly medial to the antecubital area. Place the earpieces of the stethoscope in your ears, and position the stethoscope head over the brachial artery, just distal to the cuff or slightly beneath it.

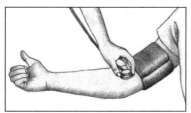

Generally, you'll use the easy-to-handle, flat diaphragm to auscultate the pulse; however, you may need to use the bell if the patient has a diminished or hard-to-locate pulse, because the bell detects the low-pitched sound of arterial blood flow more effectively.

Obtaining the blood pressure reading

■ Watching the manometer, pump the bulb until the mercury column or aneroid gauge reaches about 20 mm Hg above the point at which the pulse disappears. Then slowly open the air valve and watch the mercury drop or the gauge needle descend. Release the pressure at a rate of about 3 mm Hg/ second, and listen for pulse sounds (Korotkoff's sounds). These sounds, which determine the blood pressure measurement, are classified as follows:

Phase I
Onset of clear, faint tapping, with intensity that increases to a thud or louder tap.

Phase II
Tapping that changes to a soft, swishing sound.

Phase III
Return of clear, crisp tapping sound.

Phase IV
(first diastolic sound)
Sound becomes muffled and takes on a blowing quality.

Phase V
Sound disappears.

■ As soon as you hear blood begin to pulse through the brachial artery, note the reading on the aneroid dial or mercury column. Reflecting phase I (the first Korotkoff's sound), this sound coincides with the patient's systolic pressure. Continue deflating the cuff, noting the point at which pulsations diminish or become muffled — phase IV (the fourth Korotkoff's sound) — and then disappear — phase V (the fifth Korotkoff's sound). For children and highly active adults, many authorities consider phase IV the most accurate reflection of blood pressure.

The American Heart Association and the World Health Organization recommend documenting phases I, IV, and V. To avoid confusion and to make your measurements more useful, follow this format for recording blood pressure: systolic/muffling/disappearance (for example, 120/80/76).

Positioning the patient for cardiac auscultation

During auscultation, you'll typically stand to the right of the patient, who is in a supine position. The patient may lie flat or at a comfortable elevation.

If heart sounds seem faint or undetectable, try repositioning the patient. Alternate po-

Forward–leaning position

This position is best for hearing high-pitched sounds related to semilunar valve problems, such as aortic and pulmonic valve murmurs. To auscultate these sounds, help the patient to the forward-leaning position, and place the diaphragm of the stethoscope over the aortic and pulmonic areas in the right and left second intercostal space.

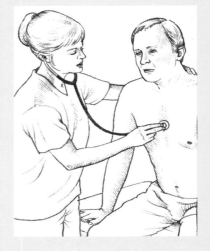

Auscultating heart sounds

Using a stethoscope with 10″ to 12″ (25- to 30-cm) tubing, follow these steps to auscultate heart sounds.

■ Locate the four different auscultation sites, as illustrated at right.

In the aortic area, blood moves from the left ventricle during systole, crossing the aortic valve and flowing through the aortic arch. In the pulmonic area, blood ejected from the right ventricle during systole crosses the pulmonic valve and flows through the main pulmonary artery. In the tricuspid area, sounds reflect blood movement from the right atrium across the tricuspid valve, filling the right ventricle during diastole. In the mitral, or apical, area, sounds represent blood flow across the mitral valve and the left ventricular filling during diastole.

■ Begin auscultation in the aortic area, placing the stethoscope in the second intercostal space along the right sternal border.

■ Then move to the pulmonic area, located in the second intercostal space at the left sternal border.

■ Next, assess the tricuspid area, which lies in the fifth intercostal space along the left sternal border.

■ Finally, listen in the mitral area, located in the fifth intercostal space near the midclavicular line.

Note: If the patient's heart is enlarged, the mitral area may be closer to the anterior axillary line.

sitioning may enhance the sounds or make them seem louder by bringing the heart closer to the surface of the chest. Common alternate positions include a seated, forward-leaning position and left-lateral decubitus position.

Left-lateral decubitus position

This position is best for hearing low-pitched sounds related to atrioventricular valve problems, such as mitral valve murmurs and extra heart sounds. To auscultate these sounds, help the patient to left-lateral decubitus position, and place the bell of the stethoscope over the apical area. If these positions don't enhance heart sounds, try auscultating with the patient standing or squatting.

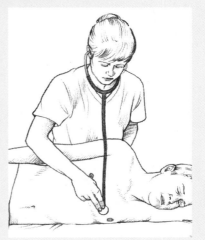

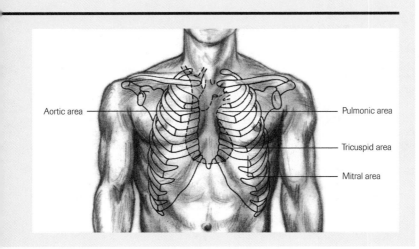

Aortic area

Pulmonic area

Tricuspid area

Mitral area

Palpating arterial pulses

To palpate arterial pulses, you'll apply pressure with your index and middle fingers positioned as shown here.

Carotid pulse
Lightly place your fingers just medial to the trachea and below the jaw angle.

Brachial pulse
Position your fingers medial to the biceps tendon.

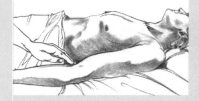

Radial pulse
Apply gentle pressure to the medial and ventral side of the wrist just below the thumb.

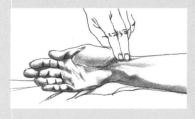

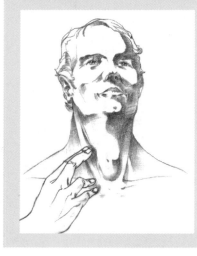

Assessing the respiratory system

Initial respiratory questions

■ Inquire about dyspnea or shortness of breath. Does your patient have breathing problems after physical exertion? Also ask him about pain, wheezing, paroxysmal nocturnal dyspnea, and orthopnea (number of pillows used).
■ Ask whether the patient experiences cough, sputum production, hemoptysis, or night sweats.
■ Find out if he has emphysema, pleurisy, bronchitis, tuberculosis, pneumonia, asthma, or frequent respiratory tract infections.

Inspecting the chest

Position the patient to allow access to his posterior and anterior chest. If his condition permits, have him sit on the edge of a bed or examining table or on a chair, leaning forward with his arms folded across his chest. If this isn't possible, place him in semi-Fowler's position for the anterior chest examination. Then ask him to lean forward slightly and use the side rails or mattress for support while you quickly examine his posterior chest. If he can't lean forward, place him in a lateral position or ask another staff member to help him sit up.

Systematically compare one side of the chest to the other.

Femoral pulse
Press relatively hard at a point inferior to the inguinal ligament. For an obese patient, palpate in the crease of the groin halfway between the pubic bone and the hip bone.

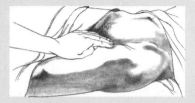

Popliteal pulse
Press firmly against the popliteal fossa at the back of the knee.

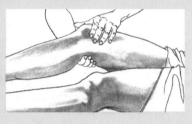

Posterior tibial pulse
Apply pressure behind and slightly below the malleolus of the ankle.

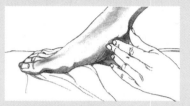

Dorsalis pedis pulse
Place your fingers on the medial dorsum of the foot while the patient points the toes down. In this site, the pulse is difficult to palpate and may seem to be absent in some healthy patients.

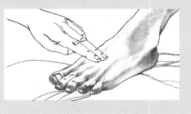

■ First, inspect the patient's chest for obvious problems, such as draining, open wounds, bruises, abrasions, scars, and cuts. Also look for less-obvious problems, such as rib deformities, fractures, lesions, or masses.

■ Examine the shape of the patient's chest wall. Observe the anteroposterior and transverse diameters.

■ Note the patient's respiratory pattern, watching for characteristics such as pursed-lip breathing.

■ Observe chest movement during respirations. The chest should move upward and outward symmetrically on inspiration. Factors that may affect movement include pain, poor positioning, and abdominal distention. Watch for paradoxical movement (possibly resulting from fractured ribs or flail chest) and asymmetrical expansion (atelectasis or underlying pulmonary disease).

■ Check for accessory muscle use and retraction of intercostal spaces during inspiration (possibly indicating respiratory distress). You may notice sudden, violent intercostal retraction (airway obstruction or tension pneumothorax); retraction of abdominal muscles during expiration (chronic obstructive pulmonary disease and other obstructive disorders); inspiratory intercostal bulging (cardiac enlargement or aneurysm); or localized expiratory bulging (rib fracture or flail chest).

Palpating the thorax

Palpation of the anterior and posterior thorax can detect structural and skin abnormalities, areas of pain, and chest asymmetry. To perform this technique, use the fingertips and palmar surfaces of one or both hands, palpating systematically and in a circular motion. Alternate palpation from one side of the thorax to the other.

Anterior thorax
Begin palpation in the supraclavicular area (#1 in the diagram at right). Then follow the sequence: infraclavicular, sternal, xiphoid, rib, and axillary areas.

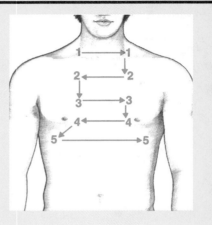

Palpating for tactile fremitus

Because sound travels more easily through solid structures than through air, assessing for tactile fremitus — which involves palpating for voice vibrations — provides valuable information about the contents of the lungs. Follow this procedure.

■ Place your open palm flat against the patient's chest without touching the chest with your fingers.

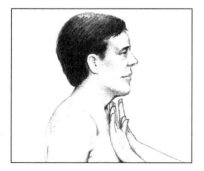

■ Ask the patient to repeat a resonant phrase like "ninety-nine" or "blue moon" as you systematically move your hands over his chest from the central airways to the lung periphery and back. Always proceed systematically from the top of the suprascapular area to the interscapular, infrascapular, and hypochondriac areas (found at the level of the 5th and 10th intercostal spaces to the right and left of midline).

■ Repeat this procedure on the posterior thorax. You should feel vibrations of equal intensity on either side of the chest. The fremitus normally occurs in the upper chest, close to the bronchi, and feels strongest at the second intercostal space on either side of the sternum. Little or no fremitus should occur in the lower chest. The intensity of the vibrations varies according to the thickness and structure of the patient's chest wall as well as the patient's voice intensity and pitch.

Percussing the thorax

Thorax percussion helps determine the boundaries of the lungs and the amount of gas, liquid, or solid in the lungs. Per-

Posterior thorax

Begin palpation in the supraclavicular area, move to the area between the scapulae (interscapular), then below the scapulae (infrascapular), and finally down to the lateral walls of the thorax.

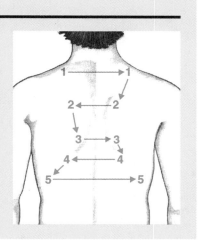

cussion can effectively assess structures as deep as 1³⁄₄″ to 3″ (4.5 to 7.5 cm).

To percuss a patient's thorax, always use indirect percussion, which involves striking one finger with another. Proceed systematically, percussing the anterior, lateral, and posterior chest over the intercostal spaces.

Avoid percussing over bones, such as over the manubrium, sternum, xiphoid, clavicles, ribs, vertebrae, or scapulae. Because of their denseness, bones produce a dull sound on percussion and, therefore, yield no useful information.

Always follow the same percussion sequence, comparing sound variations from one side to the other. This helps ensure consistency and prevents you from overlooking any important findings.

Anterior thorax

Place your hands over the lung apices in the supraclavicular area. Then proceed downward, moving from side to side at 1¹⁄₂″ to 2″ (4 to 5 cm) intervals as shown in the next column. Anterior chest percussion should produce res nance from below the clavicle to the

fifth intercostal space on the right (where dullness occurs close to the liver) and to the third intercostal space on the left (where dullness occurs near the heart).

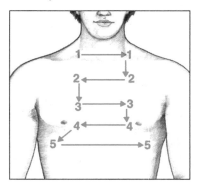

Posterior thorax

Progress in a zigzag fashion from the suprascapular to the interscapular to the infrascapular areas, avoiding the vertebral column and the scapulae, as shown at the top of the next page. Posterior percussion should sound resonant to the level of T10.

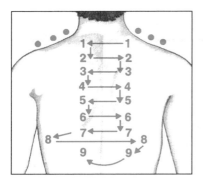

Lateral thorax

Starting at the axilla, move down the side of the rib cage, percussing between the ribs as shown below. Lateral chest percussion should produce resonance to the sixth or eighth intercostal space.

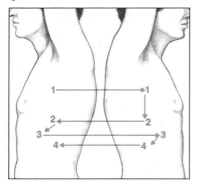

Auscultating breath sounds

Auscultating breath sounds, an important step in physical assessment, helps you detect abnormal fluid or mucus accumulation and obstructed air passages.

To detect breath sounds, auscultate the anterior, lateral, and posterior thorax, following the same sequence that you used for thorax percussion. Begin at the upper lobes, and move from side to side and down, comparing findings.

 Age alert If the patient is a child, begin just below the right

clavicle, moving to the mid-sternum, left clavicle, left nipple, and finally the right nipple. Assess one full breath (inspiration and expiration) at each point.

Auscultate the lungs for normal, abnormal, and absent breath sounds. Classify breath sounds by location, intensity, pitch, and duration during inspiratory and expiratory phases.

Assessing the neurologic system

Initial neurologic questions

■ Ask the patient his full name and the date, time, and place where he is now.
■ Investigate the character of any headaches (frequency, intensity, location, and duration).
■ Determine whether your patient has vertigo or syncope.
■ Ask about a history of seizures or use of anticonvulsants.
■ Explore any cognitive disturbances, including recent or remote memory loss, hallucinations, disorientation, speech and language dysfunction, or inability to concentrate.
■ Ask if the patient has a history of sensory disturbances, including tingling, numbness, and sensory loss.
■ Explore any motor problems, including problems with gait, balance, coordination, tremor, spasm, or paralysis.
■ Find out if cognitive, sensory, or motor symptoms have interfered with his activities of daily living.

Assessing neurologic vital signs

A supplement to routine measurement of temperature, pulse, and respirations, neurologic vital signs are used to evaluate the patient's level of consciousness (LOC), pupillary activity, and level of orientation to time, place, and person.

LOC reflects brain stem function and usually provides the first sign of central nervous system deterioration. Changes in pupillary activity may signal increased intracranial pressure (ICP). Level of orientation evaluates higher cerebral functions. Evaluating muscle strength and tone, reflexes, and posture also may help identify nervous system damage. Finally, respiratory rate and pattern can help locate brain lesions and determine their size.

Equipment

Penlight ◆ thermometer ◆ stethoscope ◆ sphygmomanometer ◆ pupil size chart

Implementation

■ Explain the procedure to the patient, even if he's unresponsive.
■ Assess LOC.
■ Ask the patient his full name. If he responds appropriately, assess his orientation to time, place, and person. Assess the quality of his replies.
■ Assess the patient's ability to understand and follow one-step commands that require a motor response. For example, ask him to open and close his eyes. Note whether he can maintain his LOC.
■ If the patient doesn't respond to commands, squeeze the nail beds on his fingers and toes with moderate pressure and note his response. Or, rub the upper portion of his sternum between the second and third intercostal space with your knuckles. Check motor responses bilaterally to rule out monoplegia and hemiplegia.

Examine pupils and eye movement

■ Ask the patient to open his eyes. If he's unresponsive, lift his upper eyelids. Inspect pupils for size and shape, and compare for equality. To evaluate more precisely, use a chart showing the various pupil sizes.

■ Test the patient's direct light response. First, darken the room. Hold each eyelid open in turn, keeping the other eye covered. Swing the penlight from the patient's ear toward the midline of the face. Shine the light directly into the eye. Normally, the pupil constricts immediately when exposed to light and then dilates immediately when the light is removed. Wait 20 seconds before testing the other pupil to allow it to recover from reflex stimulation.

■ Test consensual light response. Hold both eyelids open, but shine the light into one eye only. Watch for constriction in the other pupil, which indicates proper nerve function.

■ Brighten the room and have the conscious patient open his eyes. Observe eyelids for ptosis or drooping. Then check extraocular movements. Hold up one finger and ask the patient to follow it with his eyes as you move your finger up, down, laterally, and obliquely. See if the patient's eyes track together to follow your finger (conjugate gaze). Watch for involuntary jerking or oscillating eye movements (nystagmus).

■ Check accommodation. Hold up one finger midline to the patient's face and several feet away. Have the patient focus on your finger as you move it toward his nose. His eyes should converge, and his pupils should constrict equally.

■ Test the corneal reflex by rapidly moving the palm of your hand toward the patient's open eyes. This forces air against the corneas and normally causes a blink reflex.

■ If the patient is unconscious, test the oculocephalic (doll's eye) reflex. Hold the patient's eyelids open. Quickly but gently turn the patient's head to one side and then the other. If the patient's eyes move in the opposite direction from the side to which you turn the head, the reflex is intact.

Note: Never test this reflex if you know or suspect that the patient has a cervical spine injury.

Evaluate motor function

■ If the patient is conscious, test his grip strength in both hands at the same time. Extend your hands, ask the patient to squeeze your fingers as hard as he can, and compare the strength of each hand. Grip strength is usually slightly stronger in the dominant hand.

■ Test arm strength by having the patient close his eyes and hold his arms straight out in front of him with palms up. See if either arm drifts downward or pronates, which indicates weakness. Test leg strength by having the patient raise his legs, one at a time, against gentle downward pressure from your hand.

■ If the patient is unconscious, exert pressure on each fingernail bed. If the patient withdraws, compare the strength of each limb.

Note: If decorticate or decerebrate posturing develops in response to painful stimuli, notify the doctor immediately. (See *Comparing decerebrate and decorticate postures.*)

■ Flex and extend the extremities on both sides to evaluate muscle tone.

■ Test the plantar reflex in all patients. Stroke the lateral aspect of the sole of the patient's foot with your thumbnail. Normally, this elicits flexion of all toes. Watch for a positive Babinski's sign — dorsiflexion of the great toe with fanning of the other toes — which indicates an upper motor neuron lesion.

■ Test for Brudzinski's and Kernig's signs in patients suspected of having meningitis.

Complete the neurologic examination

■ Take the patient's temperature, pulse rate, respiration rate, and blood pressure. Especially note pulse pressure — the difference between systolic and diastolic pressure — because widening pulse pressure can indicate increasing ICP.

Special considerations

Note: If a patient's status was previously stable and he suddenly develops a change in neurologic or routine vital signs, assess his condition further, and notify the doctor immediately.

Comparing delirium, dementia, and depression

The chart below highlights distinguishing characteristics of delirium, dementia, and depression.

Clinical feature	Delirium
Onset	Acute, sudden
Course	Short, diurnal fluctuations in symptoms, worse at night, in darkness, and on awakening
Progression	Abrupt
Duration	Hours to less than 1 month, seldom longer

Comparing decerebrate and decorticate postures

Decerebrate posture results from damage to the upper brain stem. In this posture, the arms are adducted and extended, with the wrists pronated and the fingers flexed. The legs are stiffly extended, with plantar flexion of the feet.

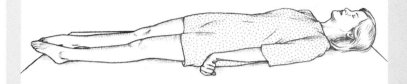

Decorticate posture results from damage to one or both corticospinal tracts. In this posture, the arms are adducted and flexed, with the wrists and fingers flexed on the chest. The legs are stiffly extended and internally rotated, with plantar flexion of the feet.

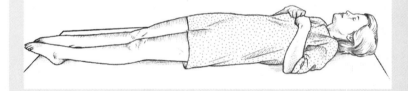

Dementia	Depression
Gradual	Sudden or brief onset
Lifelong; symptoms progressive and irreversible	Diurnal effects, typically worse in the morning; situational fluctuations but less than with acute confusion
Slow but uneven	Variable, rapid or slow but even
Months to years	At least 2 weeks, can be several months to years (Note: *Diagnostic and Statistical Manual of Mental Disorders,* 4th Edition, specifies at least 6 weeks in duration for diagnosis.)

(continued)

Comparing delirium, dementia, and depression *(continued)*

Clinical feature	Delirium
Awareness	Reduced
Alertness	Fluctuates, lethargic or hypervigilant
Attention	Decreased
Orientation	Generally impaired, but reversible
Memory	Recent and immediate impaired
Thinking	Disorganized, distorted, fragmented; incoherent speech, either slow or accelerated
Perception	Distorted, illusions, delusions, and hallucinations; difficulty distinguishing between reality and misperceptions
Speech	Incoherent
Psychomotor behavior	Variable, hypokinetic, hyperkinetic, and mixed
Sleep and wake cycle	Altered sleep and wake cycle
Affect	Variable affective anxiety, restlessness, irritability; reversible
Mental status testing	Distracted from task, numerous errors

Assessing cerebellar function

To evaluate cerebellar function, you'll test the patient's whole-body coordination and extremity coordination.

Heel-to-toe walking

To assess balance, ask the patient to walk heel to toe. Although he may be slightly unsteady, he should be able to walk and maintain his balance.

Dementia	Depression
Clear	Clear
Generally normal	Normal
Generally normal	May decrease temporarily
May be impaired as disease progresses	May be disoriented
Recent and remote impaired	Selective or patchy impairment
Difficulty with abstraction, thoughts impoverished, judgment impaired, words difficult to find	Intact but with themes of hopelessness, helplessness, or self-deprecation
Misperceptions usually absent	Intact, delusions and hallucinations absent except in severe cases
Dysphasia as disease progresses; aphasia	Normal, slow, or rapid
Normal, may have apraxia	Variable, psychomotor retardation or agitation
Fragmented	Insomnia or somnolence
Affect tends to be superficial, inappropriate, and labile; attempts to conceal deficits in intellect; personality changes, aphasia, agnosia may be present; lacks insight	Affect depressed, dysphoric mood, exaggerated and detailed complaints, preoccupied with personal thoughts, insight present, verbal elaboration
Failings highlighted by family, frequent "near miss" answers, struggles with test, great effort to find an appropriate reply, frequent requests for feedback on performance	Failings highlighted by patient, frequent "don't know," little effort, frequently gives up, indifferent toward examination, doesn't care or attempt to find answer

Romberg's test

To perform this test, ask the patient to stand with his feet together, his eyes open, and his arms at his side. Hold your outstretched arms on either side of him so you can support him if he sways to one side or the other. Observe his balance; then ask him to close his eyes. Note whether he loses his balance or sways. If he falls to one side, the Romberg test result is abnormal. Patients with cerebellar dysfunction have difficulty maintaining their balance with their eyes closed because they can't use the visual cues that orient them to the upright position.

Point-to-point movements

To evaluate the patient's extremity coordination, test point-to-point movements. Have the patient sit about 2′ (0.5 m) away from you. Hold your index finger up, and ask him to touch the tip of his index finger to the tip of yours and then to touch his nose. Now, move your finger and ask him to repeat the maneuver. Gradually, have him increase his speed as you repeat the test. Then test his other hand. Expect the patient to be more accurate with his dominant hand. A patient with cerebellar dysfunction will overshoot his target, and his movements will be jerky.

Rapid skilled movements

To further evaluate the patient's extremity coordination, test rapid skilled movements. Ask the patient to touch the thumb of his right hand to his right index finger and then to each of his remaining fingers. Then instruct him to increase his speed. Observe his movements for smoothness and accuracy. Repeat the test on his left hand.

Assessing reflexes

Assessment of deep tendon and superficial reflexes provides information about the intactness of the sensory receptor organ. It also evaluates how well the afferent nerve relays the sensory message to the spinal cord, the spinal cord or brain stem segment mediates the reflex, the lower motor neurons transmit messages to the muscles, and the muscles respond to the motor message.

To evaluate the patient's reflexes, test deep tendon and superficial reflexes and observe the patient for primitive reflexes.

Deep tendon reflexes

Before you test a deep tendon reflex, make sure the limb is relaxed and the joint is in midposition; for instance, the knee or elbow should be flexed at a 45-degree angle. Then distract the patient by asking him to focus on an object across the room. If he focuses on his performance, the cerebral cortex may dampen his response. You can also distract the patient by using Jendrassik's maneuver. Simply instruct him to clench his teeth or to squeeze his thigh. Document which technique you used to distract the patient.

Always move from head to toe in testing deep tendon reflexes, and compare contralateral reflexes. To elicit the reflex, tap the tendon lightly but firmly with the reflex hammer. Then grade the briskness of the response: 0 (no response), 1+ (diminished), 2+ (normal), 3+ (brisker than average), 4+ (hyperactive).

Biceps reflex

Position the patient's arm so his elbow is flexed at a 45-degree angle and his arm is relaxed. Place your thumb or index finger over the biceps tendon and your remaining fingers loosely over the triceps muscle. Strike your thumb or index finger with the pointed tip of the reflex hammer, and watch and feel for contraction of the biceps muscle and flexion of the forearm.

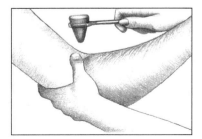

Triceps reflex

Have the patient abduct his arm and place his forearm across his chest. Strike the triceps tendon about 2″ (5 cm) above the olecranon process on the extensor surface of the upper arm. Watch for contraction of the triceps muscle and extension of the forearm.

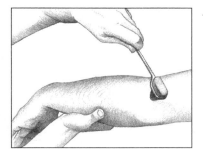

Brachioradialis reflex

Instruct the patient to rest the ulnar surface of his hand on his knee and to partially flex his elbow. With the tip of the hammer, strike the radius about 2″ proximal to the radial styloid. Watch for supination of the hand and flexion of the forearm at the elbow.

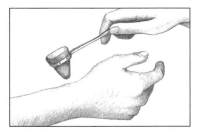

Patellar reflex

Have the patient sit on the side of the bed with his legs dangling freely. If he can't sit up, flex his knee at a 45-degree angle and place your nondominant hand behind it for support. Strike the patellar tendon just below the patella, and look for contraction of the quadriceps muscle in the anterior thigh and for extension of the leg.

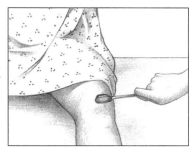

Achilles reflex

Slightly flex the foot and support the plantar surface. Using the pointed end of the reflex hammer, strike the Achilles tendon. Watch for plantar flexion of the foot and ankle.

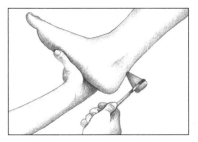

Superficial reflexes

These reflexes include the abdominal, cremasteric, and plantar reflexes. To elicit these reflexes, you'll stimulate that patient's skin or mucous membranes. To document your findings, use a plus sign (+) to indicate that a reflex is present and a minus sign (−) to indicate that it's absent.

Abdominal reflex

Place the patient in the supine position, with arms at his sides and his knees slightly flexed. Using the tip of the reflex hammer, a key, or an applicator stick, briskly stroke both sides of the abdomen above and below the umbilicus, moving from the periphery toward the midline. After each stroke, watch for abdominal muscle contraction and movement of the umbilicus toward the stimulus. If you're evaluating an obese patient, retract the umbilicus to the side opposite the stimulus and note whether it pulls toward the stimulus. Aging and disease of the upper and lower motor neurons cause an absent abdominal reflex.

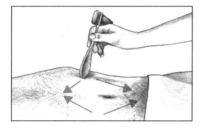

Cremasteric reflex
With a male patient, use an applicator stick to lightly stimulate the inner thigh. Watch for contraction of the cremaster muscle in the scrotum and prompt elevation of the testicle on the side of the stimulus. This reflex may be absent in patients with upper or lower motor neuron disease.

Plantar reflex
Using an applicator stick, a tongue blade, or a key, slowly stroke the lateral side of the patient's sole from the heel to the great toe. The normal response is plantar flexion of the toes. In an elderly patient, this normal response may be diminished because of arthritic deformities of the toe or foot.

In patients with disorders of the pyramidal tract (such as cerebrovascular accident), the Babinski's reflex, an abnormal response, is elicited. The patient responds to the stimulus with dorsiflexion of his great toe. You may also see a more pronounced response in which the other toes extend and abduct. In some cases, you may even see dorsiflexion of the ankle, knee, and hip.

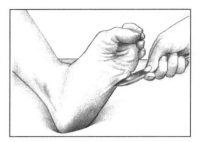

Primitive reflexes
Although normal in infants, primitive reflexes are pathologic in adults.

Grasp reflex
Apply gentle pressure to the patient's palm with your fingers. If he grasps your fingers between his thumb and index finger, suspect cortical (premotor cortex) damage.

Snout reflex
Tap lightly on the patient's upper lip. Lip pursing indicates frontal lobe damage.

Sucking reflex
If the patient begins sucking while you're feeding him or suctioning his mouth, you've elicited a reflex that indicates cortical damage characteristic of advanced dementia.

Glabellar reflex
Repeatedly tap the bridge of the patient's nose. A persistent blinking response indicates diffuse cortical dysfunction.

(Text continues on page 33.)

Assessing the cranial nerves

Cranial nerve assessment provides valuable information about the condition of the central nervous system, particularly the brain stem. Because a disorder can affect any cranial nerve, knowing how to test each nerve is important. The techniques vary according to the nerve being tested.

Cranial nerve and assessment technique	Normal findings
Olfactory (CN I) After checking the patency of the patient's nostrils, have him close both eyes. Then occlude one nostril, and hold a familiar, pungent substance — such as coffee, tobacco, soap, or peppermint — under the patient's nose, and ask him to identify it. Repeat this technique with the other nostril.	The patient should be able to detect and identify the smell correctly. If he reports detecting the smell but can't name it, offer a choice, such as, "Do you smell lemon, coffee, or peppermint?"
Optic (CN II) and oculomotor (CN III) To assess the optic nerve, check visual acuity, visual fields, and the retinal structures. To assess the oculomotor nerve, check pupil size, pupil shape, and pupillary response to light.	The pupils should be equal, round, and reactive to light. When assessing pupil size, look for trends. For example, watch for a gradual increase in the size of one pupil or the appearance of unequal pupils in a patient whose pupils were previously equal.
Oculomotor (CN III), trochlear (CN IV), and abducens (CN VI) To test the coordinated function of these three nerves, assess them simultaneously by evaluating the patient's extraocular eye movement.	The eyes should move smoothly and in a coordinated manner through all six directions of eye movement. Observe each eye for rapid oscillation (nystagmus), movement not in unison with that of the other eye, or inability to move in certain directions (ophthalmoplegia). Also note any complaint of double vision (diplopia).

(continued)

Cranial nerve and assessment technique	**Normal findings**

Trigeminal (CN V)

To assess the sensory portion of the trigeminal nerve, gently touch the right, then the left, side of the patient's forehead with a cotton ball while his eyes are closed. Instruct him to state the moment the cotton touches the area. Compare the patient's response on both sides. Repeat the technique on the right and the left cheek and on the right and left jaw. Next, repeat the entire procedure using a sharp object. The cap of a disposable ballpoint pen can be used to test light touch (dull end) and sharp stimuli (sharp end). (If an abnormality appears, also test for temperature sensation by touching the patient's skin with test tubes filled with hot and cold water and asking him to differentiate between them.)

The patient with a normal trigeminal nerve should report feeling both light touch and sharp stimuli in all three areas (forehead, cheek, and jaw) on both sides of his face.

To assess the motor portion of the trigeminal nerve, ask the patient to clench his jaws. Palpate the temporal and masseter muscles bilaterally, checking for symmetry. Try to open the patient's clenched jaws. Next, watch for symmetry as the patient opens and closes his mouth.

The jaws should clench symmetrically and remain closed against resistance.

Assess the corneal reflex.

The lids of both eyes should close when a wisp of cotton is lightly stroked across a cornea.

Facial (CN VII)

To test the motor portion of the facial nerve, ask the patient to wrinkle his forehead, raise and lower his eyebrows, smile to show teeth, and puff out his cheeks. Also, with the patient's eyes tightly closed, attempt to open the eyelids. With each of these movements, observe closely for symmetry.

Normal facial movements are symmetrical.

To test the sensory portion of the facial nerve, which supplies taste sensation to the anterior two-thirds of the tongue, first prepare four marked, closed containers: one containing salt; another, sugar; a third, vinegar (or lemon); and a fourth, quinine (or bitters). Then, with the patient's eyes closed, place salt on the anterior two-thirds of his tongue using a cotton swab or dropper. Ask him to identify the taste as sweet, salty, sour, or bitter. Rinse the patient's mouth with water. Repeat this procedure, alternating flavors and sides of the tongue until all four flavors have been tested on both sides. Taste sensations to the posterior third of the tongue are supplied by the glossopharyngeal nerve (CN IX) and are usually tested at the same time.

Normal taste sensations are symmetrical.

Assessing the cranial nerves *(continued)*

Cranial nerve and assessment technique	Normal findings

Acoustic (CN VIII)
To assess the acoustic portion of this nerve, test the patient's hearing acuity.

The patient should be able to hear a whispered voice or a watch tick.

To assess the vestibular portion of this nerve, observe the patient for nystagmus and disturbed balance and note reports of dizziness or vertigo.

The patient should display normal eye movement and balance and have no dizziness or vertigo.

Glossopharyngeal (CN IX) and vagus (CN X)
To assess these nerves, which have overlapping functions, first listen to the patient's voice for indications of a hoarse or nasal quality. Then watch the patient's soft palate when he says "ah." Next, test the gag reflex after warning the patient. To evoke this reflex, rough the posterior wall of the pharynx with a cotton swab or tongue blade.

The patient's voice should sound strong and clear. The soft palate and the uvula should rise when he says "ah," and the uvula should remain midline. The palatine arches should remain symmetrical during movement and at rest. The gag reflex should be intact. If it appears decreased or the pharynx moves asymmetrically, evaluate each side of the posterior wall of the pharynx to confirm integrity of both cranial nerves.

Spinal accessory (CN XI)
To assess this nerve, press down on the patient's shoulders as he attempts to shrug against this resistance. Note shoulder strength and symmetry while inspecting and palpating his trapezius muscle. Then apply resistance to his turned head while he attempts to return it to a midline position. Note neck strength while inspecting and palpating the sternocleidomastoid muscle. Repeat for the opposite side.

Normally, both shoulders should be able to overcome the resistance equally well. The neck should overcome resistance in both directions.

Hypoglossal (CN XII)
To assess this nerve, observe the patient's protruded tongue for deviation from midline, atrophy, or fasciculations (very fine muscle flickerings indicative of lower motor neuron disease). Next, have him move his tongue rapidly from side to side with his mouth open, then to curl his tongue up toward his nose, and then down toward his chin. Then use a tongue blade to apply resistance to his protruded tongue and ask him to try to push it to one side. Repeat on the other side and note tongue strength. Listen to the patient's speech for the sounds d, l, n, and t. If general speech suggests a problem, have the patient repeat a phrase or series of words containing these sounds.

Normally, the tongue should be midline and the patient should be able to move it right to left equally as well as up and down. The pressure that the tongue exerts on the tongue blade should be equal on both sides. Speech should be clear.

Assessing the pupils

Pupillary changes can signal different conditions. Use these illustrations and lists of causes to help you detect problems.

Bilaterally equal and reactive

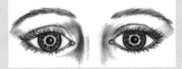

- Normal

Unilateral, dilated (4 mm), fixed, and nonreactive

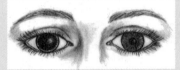

- Uncal herniation with oculomotor nerve damage
- Brain stem compression from an expanding lesion or an aneurysm
- Increased intracranial pressure
- Tentorial herniation
- Head trauma with subsequent subdural or epidural hematoma
- Normal in some people

Bilateral, dilated (4 mm), fixed, and nonreactive

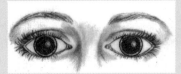

- Severe midbrain damage
- Cardiopulmonary arrest (hypoxia)
- Anticholinergic poisoning

Bilateral, midsized (2 mm), fixed and nonreactive

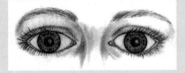

- Midbrain involvement caused by edema, hemorrhage, infarctions, lacerations, contusions

Unilateral, small (1.5 mm), and nonreactive

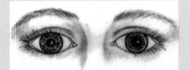

- Disruption of sympathetic nerve supply to the head caused by spinal cord lesion above T1

Bilateral, pinpoint (less than 1 mm), and usually nonreactive

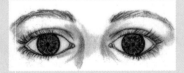

- Lesion of pons, usually after hemorrhage, leading to blocked sympathetic impulses
- Opiates, such as morphine (pupils may be reactive)

Using the Glasgow Coma Scale

The Glasgow Coma Scale provides an objective way to evaluate a patient's level of consciousness and to detect changes from the baseline. To use this scale, evaluate and score your patient's best eye-opening response, verbal response, and motor response. A total score of 15 indicates that he's alert; oriented to time, place, and person and can follow simple commands. A comatose patient will score 7 points or less. A score of 3 indicates deep coma and a poor prognosis.

Eye-opening response
■ Open spontaneously (Score: 4)
■ Open to verbal command (Score: 3)
■ Open to pain (Score: 2)
■ No response (Score: 1)

Verbal response
■ Oriented and converses (Score: 5)
■ Disoriented and converses (Score: 4)
■ Uses inappropriate words (Score: 3)
■ Makes incomprehensible sounds (Score: 2)
■ No response (Score: 1)

Motor response
■ Obeys verbal command (Score: 6)
■ Localizes painful stimulus (Score: 5)
■ Flexion, withdrawal (Score: 4)
■ Flexion, abnormal — decorticate rigidity (Score: 3)
■ Extension — decerebrate rigidity (Score: 2)
■ No response (Score: 1)

Assessing the GI system

Initial GI questions

■ Explore signs and symptoms, such as appetite and weight changes, dysphagia, nausea, vomiting, heartburn, stomach or abdominal pain, frequent belching or flatulence, hematemesis, and jaundice. Has the patient had ulcers?
■ Determine whether the patient frequently uses laxatives. Ask about hemorrhoids, rectal bleeding, character of stools (color, odor, and consistency), and changes in bowel habits. Does he have a history of diarrhea or constipation?
■ Ask if he has had hernias, gallbladder disease, or liver disease such as hepatitis.
■ Find out if he has experienced abdominal swelling or ascites.
■ If the patient is older than age 50, inquire about the date and results of his last Hemoccult test.

Inspecting the abdomen

Place the patient in the supine position with his arms at his sides and his head on a pillow to help relax the abdominal muscles.

Mentally divide the abdomen into quadrants or regions. Systematically inspect all areas, if time and the patient's condition permit, concluding with the symptomatic area.

Then examine the patient's entire abdomen, observing overall contour, color, and skin integrity. Look for rashes, scars, or incisions from past surgeries. Observe the umbilicus for protrusions or discoloration.

Note any visible abdominal asymmetry, masses, pulsations, or peristalsis. You can detect masses — especially hepatic and splenic — more easily by inspecting the areas while the patient takes a deep breath and holds it. This forces the diaphragm downward, increasing intra-abdominal pressure and reducing the size of the abdominal cavity.

Finally, examine the rectal area for redness, irritation, or hemorrhoids.

Note: If your patient is pregnant, vary the assessment position depending on the stage of pregnancy. For example, if the patient is in her final weeks, avoid the supine position because it may impair respiratory excursion and blood flow. To enhance comfort, have the patient lie on her side or assume semi-Fowler's position. Also during the assessment, remember the normal variations: increased pigmentation of the abdominal midline, purplish striae, and upward displacement of the abdominal organs and the umbilicus.

Auscultating bowel sounds

Auscultate the abdomen to detect sounds that provide information on bowel motility and the condition of abdominal vessels and organs.

To auscultate bowel sounds, which result from air and fluid movement through the bowel, press the diaphragm of the stethoscope against the abdomen and listen carefully. Auscultate the quadrants systematically.

Air and fluid moving through the bowel by peristalsis normally creates soft, bubbling sounds with no regular pattern, commonly with soft clicks and gurgles interspersed. A hungry patient may have the normal, familiar "stomach growl," a condition of hyperperistalsis called borborygmi. Rapid, high-pitched, loud, and gurgling bowel sounds are hyperactive and may occur normally in a hungry patient. Sounds occurring at a rate of one every minute or longer are hypoactive and normally occur after bowel surgery or after the colon has filled with feces.

When describing bowel sounds be specific — for example, indicate whether they're quiet or loud gurgles, occasional gurgles, fine tinkles, or loud tinkles.

In a routine complete assessment, auscultate for a full 5 minutes before determining that bowel sounds are absent. However, if you're pressed for time, perform a rapid assessment. If

you can't hear bowel sounds within 2 minutes, suspect a serious problem. Even if subsequent palpation stimulates peristalsis, still report a long silence in that quadrant.

Before reporting absent bowel sounds, make sure the patient has an empty bladder; a full bladder may obscure the sounds. Gently pressing on the abdominal surface may initiate peristalsis and audible bowel sounds, as will having the patient eat or drink something.

Next, lightly apply the bell of the stethoscope to each quadrant to auscultate for vascular sounds, such as bruits and venous hums, and for friction rubs. Normally, you shouldn't hear vascular sounds.

Percussing the abdomen

Abdominal percussion helps determine the size and location of abdominal organs and helps you identify areas of tenderness, gaseous distention, ascites, or solid masses.

To perform this technique, percuss in all four quadrants, moving clockwise to the percussion sites in each quadrant, as shown below. Keep appropriate organ locations in mind as you progress. However, if the patient complains of pain in a particular quadrant, adjust the percussion sequence to percuss that quadrant last. When tapping, move your right finger away quickly so you don't inhibit vibrations.

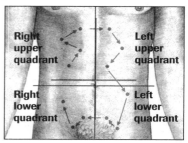

When assessing a tender abdomen, have the patient cough; then lightly percuss where the cough produced the pain, helping to localized the involved area. As you percuss, note areas of dullness, tympany, and flatness as well as any patient complaints of tenderness.

Percussion sounds vary depending on the density of underlying structures; usually, you'll detect dull notes over solids and tympanic notes over air. The predominant abdominal percussion sound is tympany, created by percussion over an air-filled stomach or intestine. Dull sounds normally occur over the liver and spleen, a lower intestine filled with feces, and a bladder filled with urine. Distinguishing abdominal percussion notes may be difficult in obese patients.

Note: Keep in mind that abdominal percussion or palpation is contraindicated in patients with abdominal organ transplants or suspected abdominal aortic aneurysm. Perform it cautiously in patients with suspected appendicitis.

Palpating the abdomen

Abdominal palpation provides useful clues about the character of the abdominal wall; the size, condition, and consistency of abdominal organs; the presence and nature of any abdominal masses; and the presence, degree, and location of abdominal pain. For a rapid assessment, palpate primarily to detect areas of pain and tenderness, guarding, rebound tenderness, and costovertebral-angle tenderness.

Age alert An abdominal mass in a child may be a nephroblastoma. Don't palpate it, to avoid spreading tumor cells.

Light palpation
Use light palpation to detect tenderness, areas of muscle spasm or rigidity, and superficial masses. To palpate for superficial masses in the abdominal wall, have the patient raise his head and shoulders to tighten the abdominal muscles. The tension obscures a deep mass, but a wall mass remains palpable.

This technique also may help you determine whether pain originates from the abdominal muscles or from deeper structures.

If you detect tenderness, check for involuntary guarding, or abdominal rigidity. As the patient exhales, palpate the abdominal rectus muscles. Normally, they should soften and relax on exhalation; note abnormal muscle tension or inflexibility. Involuntary guarding points to peritoneal irrigation. In generalized peritonitis, rigidity is severe and diffuse, commonly described as a "boardlike" abdomen.

A tense or ticklish patient may exhibit voluntary guarding. Help him relax with deep breathing, inhaling through his nose and exhaling through his mouth.

If a patient complains of abdominal pain, check for rebound tenderness. Because this maneuver can be painful, perform it near the end of your abdominal assessment. Press your fingertips into the site where the patient reports pain or tenderness. As you quickly release the pressure, the abdominal tissue will rebound. If the patient reports pain as the tissue springs back, you've elicited rebound tenderness.

Deep palpation
If time permits, perform deep abdominal palpation to detect deep tenderness or masses and to evaluate organ size. If you feel a mass, note its size, shape, consistency, and location. If the patient complains of pain or tenderness, note if the location is generalized or localized. Also note any guarding the patient exhibits during deep palpation. You may feel a tensing of a small or

large area of abdominal musculature directly below your fingers.

Eliciting abdominal pain

Rebound tenderness and the iliopsoas and obturator signs can indicate conditions such as appendicitis or peritonitis. During assessment, you can elicit these signs of abdominal pain.

Rebound tenderness
Place the patient in the supine position with the knees flexed to relax the abdominal muscles. Place your hands gently on the right lower quadrant at McBurney's point, located about midway between the umbilicus and the anterior superior iliac spine. Slowly and deeply dip your fingers into the area.

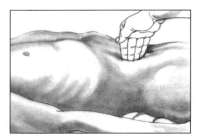

Now release the pressure in a quick, smooth motion. Pain on release — rebound tenderness — is a positive sign. The pain may radiate to the umbilicus. *Caution:* Don't repeat this maneuver, to minimize the risk of rupturing an inflamed appendix.

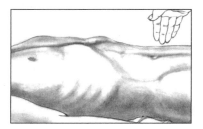

Iliopsoas sign
Place the patient in the supine position with the legs straight. Instruct the patient to raise the right leg upward as you exert slight downward pressure with your hand.

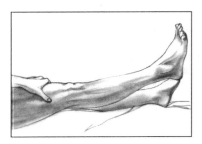

Repeat maneuver with the left leg. Increased abdominal pain, with testing on either leg, is a positive result, indicating irritation of the psoas muscle.

Obturator sign
Place the patient in the supine position with the right leg flexed 90 degrees at the hip and knee. Hold the patient's leg just above the knee and at the ankle; then rotate the leg laterally and medially. Pain in the hypogastric region is a positive sign, indicating irritation of the obturator muscle.

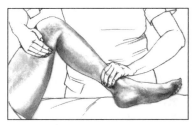

Percussing, palpating, and hooking the liver

You can estimate the size and position of the liver through percussion and palpation (or, in some cases, hooking).

The following illustrations show you the correct hand positions for these three techniques.

Liver percussion

Begin by percussing the abdomen along the right midclavicular line, starting below the level of the umbilicus. Move upward until the percussion notes change from tympany to dullness, usually at or slightly below the costal margin. Mark the point of change with a felt-tip pen.

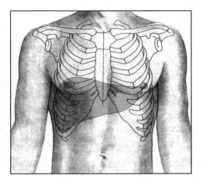

Percuss along the right midclavicular line, starting above the nipple. Move downward until percussion notes change from normal lung resonance to dullness, usually at the fifth to seventh intercostal space. Again, mark the point of change with a felt-tip pen. Estimate liver size by measuring the distance between the two marks.

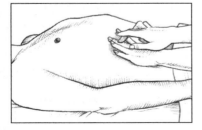

Liver palpation

Place one hand on the patient's back at the approximate height of the liver. Place your other hand below your mark of liver fullness on the right lateral abdomen. Point your fingers toward the right costal margin, and press gently in and up as the patient inhales deeply. This maneuver may bring the liver edge down to a palpable position.

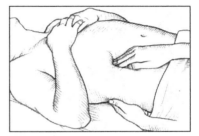

Liver hooking

If liver palpation is unsuccessful, try hooking the liver. To do so, stand on the patient's right side, below the area of liver dullness, as shown below. As the patient inhales deeply, press your fingers inward and upward, attempting to feel the liver with the fingertips of both hands.

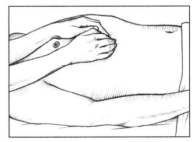

Palpating for indirect inguinal hernia

To check for an indirect inguinal hernia, examine the patient while he stands. Then examine him in a supine position with his knee flexed on the side you're examining. Place your gloved index finger on the neck of his scrotum and gently push upward into the inguinal canal, as shown below. When you've inserted your finger as far as possible, ask him to bear down and cough. A hernia will feel like a mass of tissue that withdraws when met by the finger.

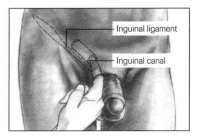

Inguinal ligament

Inguinal canal

Assessing the urinary system

Initial urinary questions

■ Ask about urine color, oliguria, and nocturia. Does your patient experience incontinence, dysuria, frequency, urgency, or difficulty with urinary stream (such as reduced flow or dribbling)?

■ Find out about pyuria, urine retention, and passage of calculi.

■ Ask about a history of bladder, kidney, or urinary tract infections.

Age alert If your patient is a child, ask his parents if they've had any problems with toilet training or bed-wetting.

Evaluating urine color

For important clues to your patient's current health status, ask about any urine color changes. Such changes can result from fluid intake, medications, and dietary factors as well as from various disorders.

Appearance	Indication
Amber or straw color	Normal
Cloudy	Infection, inflammation, glomerulonephritis, vegetarian diet
Colorless or pale straw color (dilute urine)	Excess fluid intake, anxiety, chronic renal disease, diabetes insipidus, diuretic therapy
Dark brown or black	Acute glomerulonephritis, drugs, (such as nitrofurantoin and chlorpromazine)
Dark yellow or amber (concentrated urine)	Low fluid intake, acute febrile disease, vomiting or diarrhea causing large fluid loss
Green-brown	Bile duct obstruction
Orange-red to orange-brown	Urobilinuria, drugs (such as phenazopyridine), obstructive jaundice (tea-colored urine)
Red or red-brown	Porphyria, hemorrhage, drugs (such as doxorubicin)

Inspecting the urethral meatus

Put on gloves before examining the urethral meatus.

To inspect a male patient's urethral meatus, have him lie in the supine position and drape him, exposing only his penis. Then compress the tip of the glans to open the urethral meatus, which should be located in the center of the glans. Check for swelling, discharge, signs of urethral infection, and ulcerations, which can signal a sexually transmitted disease (STD).

To inspect a female patient's urethral meatus, help her into the dorsal lithotomy position and drape her, exposing only the area to be assessed. Then spread the labia and look for the urethral meatus. It should be a pink, irregular, slitlike opening located at the midline just above the vagina. Check for swelling, discharge, signs of urethral infection, a cystocele, and ulcerations, a sign of an STD.

Percussing the urinary organs

Percuss the kidneys to elicit pain or tenderness, and percuss the bladder to elicit percussion sounds. Before you start, tell the patient what you're going to do. Otherwise, he may be startled, and you could mistake his reaction for a feeling of acute tenderness.

Kidney percussion

With the patient sitting upright, percuss each costovertebral angle (the angle over each kidney whose borders are formed by the lateral and downward curve of the lowest rib and the spinal column). To perform direct percussion, place your left palm over the costovertebral angle and gently strike it with your right fist, as shown in the next column. Use just enough force to cause a painless but perceptible thud. To perform indirect percussion, gently strike

your fist over each costovertebral angle. The normal patient will feel a thudding sensation or pressure during percussion. Make sure you percuss both sides of the body to assess both kidneys. Pain or tenderness suggests a kidney infection.

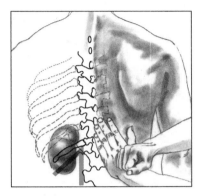

Bladder percussion

Before percussing the bladder, have the patient urinate. Then ask the patient to lie in the supine position. Next, using direct percussion, percuss the area over the bladder, beginning 2″ (5 cm) above the symphysis pubis, as shown below. To detect differences in sound, percuss toward the base of the bladder. Percussion normally produces a tympanic sound. (Over a urine-filled bladder, it produces a dull sound.)

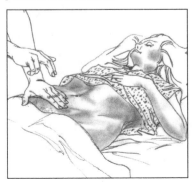

Palpating the urinary organs

Bimanual palpation of the kidneys and bladder may detect tenderness, lumps, and masses. In the normal adult, the kidneys usually can't be palpated because of their location deep within the abdomen. However, they may be palpable in a thin patient or in one with reduced abdominal muscle mass. (Because the right kidney is slightly lower than the left, it may be easier to palpate.) Keep in mind that both kidneys descend with deep inhalation.

If palpable, the bladder normally feels firm and relatively smooth. However, keep in mind that an adult's bladder may not be palpable.

Kidney palpation

Help the patient into the supine position, and expose the abdomen from the xiphoid process to the symphysis pubis. Standing at the patient's right side, place your left hand under the back, midway between the lower costal margin and the iliac crest, as shown below.

Next, place your right hand on the patient's abdomen, directly above your left hand. Angle this hand slightly toward the costal margin. To palpate the right lower edge of the right kidney, press your right fingertips about 1½″ (4 cm) above the right iliac crest at the midinguinal line; press your left fingertips upward into the right costovertebral angle, as shown below.

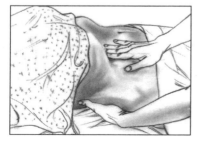

Instruct the patient to inhale deeply so that the lower portion of the right kidney can move down between your hands. If it does, note the shape and size of the kidney. Normally, it feels smooth, solid, and firm, yet elastic. Ask the patient if palpation causes tenderness.

Note: Avoid using excessive pressure to palpate the kidney because this may cause intense pain.

To assess the left kidney, move to the patient's left side and position your hands as described above, but with this change: Place your right hand 2″ (5 cm) above the left iliac crest. Then apply pressure with both hands as the patient inhales. If the left kidney can be palpated, compare it to the right kidney; it should be the same size.

Bladder palpation

Before palpating the bladder, make sure the patient has voided. Then locate the edge of the bladder by pressing deeply in the midline about 1″ to 2″ (2.5 to 5 cm) above the symphysis pubis, as shown below.

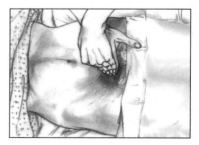

As the bladder is palpated, note its size and location and check for lumps, masses, and tenderness. The bladder normally feels firm and relatively smooth. (Keep in mind that an adult's bladder may not be palpable.) During deep palpation, the patient may report the urge to urinate — a normal response.

Assessing the male reproductive system

Initial questions for the male patient

■ Ask the patient about penile discharge or lesions and testicular pain or lumps.
■ Determine whether the patient performs testicular self-examinations. Has he had a vasectomy?
■ Ask about STDs and other infections. Assess his knowledge of how to prevent STDs, including acquired immunodeficiency syndrome.
■ Find out if the patient has a history of prostate problems.
■ Ask if he's satisfied with his sexual function. Does he have any concerns about impotence or sterility? Also inquire about his contraceptive practices.

Inspecting and palpating the male genitalia

First, ask the patient to disrobe from the waist down and to cover himself with a drape. Then put on gloves and examine his penis, scrotum and testicles, inguinal and femoral areas, and prostate gland.

Penis

Observe the penis. Its size will depend on the patient's age and overall development. The penile skin should be slightly wrinkled and pink to light brown in a white patient, and light brown to dark brown in a black patient. Check the penile shaft and glans for lesions, nodules, inflammation, and swelling. Also check the glans for smegma, a cheesy secretion. Then gently compress the glans and inspect the urethral meatus for discharge, inflammation, and lesions, specifically genital warts. If you note

any discharge, obtain a culture specimen.

Using your thumb and forefinger, palpate the entire penile shaft. It should be somewhat firm, and the skin should be smooth and movable. Note any swelling, nodules, or indurations.

Scrotum and testicles

Have the patient hold his penis away from his scrotum so that you can observe the scrotum's general size and appearance. The skin will be darker than the rest of the body. Spread the surface of the scrotum, and examine the skin for swelling, nodules, redness, ulceration, and distended veins. You'll probably notice some sebaceous cysts — firm, white to yellow, nontender cutaneous lesions. Also check for pitting edema, a sign of cardiovascular disease. Spread the pubic hair and check the skin for lesions and parasites.

Gently, palpate both testicles between your thumb and first two fingers. Assess their size, shape, and response to pressure (typically, a deep visceral pain). The testicles should be equal in size. They should feel firm, smooth, and rubbery and should move freely in the scrotal sac. If you note any hard, irregular areas or lumps, transilluminate the testicle by darkening the room and pressing the head of a flashlight against the scrotum, behind the lump. The testicle will appear as an opaque shadow, as will any lumps, masses, warts, or blood-filled areas. Transilluminate the other testicle to compare your findings.

Next, palpate the epididymis, normally located in the posterolateral area of the testicle. It should be smooth, discrete, nontender, and free from swelling or induration.

Finally, palpate each spermatic cord, located above each testicle. Begin palpating at the base of the epididymis and continue to the inguinal canal. The vas deferens is a smooth, movable cord inside the spermatic cord. If you feel any swelling, irregularity, or nodules, transilluminate the problem area, as described above. If serous fluid is present, you'll see a red glow; if tissue and blood are present, you won't see this glow.

Prostate gland

Usually, a doctor performs prostate palpation as part of a rectal assessment. However, if the patient hasn't scheduled a separate rectal assessment, you may palpate the prostate during the reproductive system assessment. Because palpation of the prostate usually is uncomfortable and may embarrass the patient, begin by explaining the procedure and reassuring the patient that the procedure shouldn't be painful.

Have the patient urinate to empty the bladder and reduce discomfort during the examination. Then ask him to stand at the end of the examination table, with his elbows flexed and his upper body resting on the table. If he can't assume this position because he's unable to stand, have him lie on his left side with his right knee and hip flexed or with both knees drawn up toward his chest.

Inspect the skin of the perineal, anal, and posterior scrotal surfaces. The skin should appear smooth and unbroken, with no protruding masses.

Apply water-soluble lubricant to your gloved index finger. Then introduce the finger, pad down, into the patient's rectum. Instruct the patient to relax to ease passage of the finger through the anal sphincter.

Using the pad of your index finger, palpate the prostate on the anterior rectal wall, located just past the anorectal ring. The prostate should feel smooth and rubbery. Normal size varies but usually is about that of a walnut. The prostate shouldn't protrude into the rec-

tum lumen. The proximal portions of the seminal vesicles sometimes may be palpated, as corrugated structures, above the superolateal to midpoint section of the gland.

Assessing the female reproductive system

Initial questions for the female patient

■ Ask your patient about her age at menarche and the character of her menses (frequency, regularity, and duration). What was the date of her last period? Does she have a history of menorrhagia, metrorrhagia, or amenorrhea? If she's postmenopausal, find out the date of menopause.
■ Ask if she has irregular or painful vaginal bleeding, dyspareunia, or frequent vaginal infections.
■ Ask about the character of any pregnancies (number, durations, deliveries, and abortions, either spontaneous or induced). Has she had any problems with infertility?
■ Find out what birth control method she uses.
■ Determine the dates of her last gynecologic examination and Papanicolaou (Pap) test.
■ Ask about STDs and other infections. Assess her knowledge of how to prevent STDs, including acquired immunodeficiency syndrome.
■ Explore the patient's satisfaction with her sexual function.

Inspecting the female genitalia

Before starting the examination, ask the patient to urinate. Next, help her into the dorsal lithotomy position and drape her. After putting on gloves, examine the patient's external and internal genitalia and her breasts, as appropriate.

Inspecting the external genitalia

Observe the skin and hair distribution of the mons pubis. Spread the hair with your fingers to check for lesions and parasites.

Next, inspect the skin of the labia majora, spreading the hair to examine for lesions, parasites, and genital warts. The skin should be slightly darker than the rest of the body, and the labia majora should be round and full. Examine the labia minora, which should be dark pink and moist. In nulliparous women, labia majora and minora are close together; in women who have experienced vaginal deliveries, they may gape open.

Closely, observe each vulvar structure for syphilitic chancres and cancerous lesions. Examine the area of Bartholin's and Skene's glands and ducts for swelling, erythema, ducts enlargement, or discharge. Next, inspect the urethral opening. It should be slitlike and the same color as the mucous membranes. Look for erythema, polyps, and discharge.

Inspecting the internal genitalia

First, select a speculum that's appropriate for the patient. In most cases, you'll use a Graves speculum. However, if the patient is a virgin or nulliparous or has a contracted introitus due to menopause, you should use a Pedersen speculum.

Hold the speculum's blades under warm running water. This warms the blades and helps to lubricate them, making insertion easier and more comfortable for the patient. Don't use commercial lubricants — they're bacteriostatic and will distort cells on Pap tests. Sit or stand at the foot of the examination table. Tell the patient that she'll feel some pressure, then insert the speculum.

While inserting and withdrawing the speculum, note the color, texture, and mucosal integrity of the vagina and any vaginal secretions. A white, odorless, thin discharge is normal.

With the speculum in place, examine the cervix for color, position, size, shape, mucosal integrity, and discharge. The cervix should be smooth, round, rosy pink, and free from ulcerations and nodules. A clear watery discharge is normal during ovulation; a slightly bloody discharge is normal just before menstruation. Obtain a culture specimen of any other discharge. After inspecting the cervix, obtain a specimen for a Pap test.

When you've completed your examination, unlock the speculum blades and close them slowly while you begin withdrawing the instrument. Close the blades completely before they reach the introitus. Then withdraw the speculum from the vagina.

Palpating the uterus

To palpate the uterus bimanually, insert the index and middle fingers of one gloved hand into the patient's vagina, and place your other hand on the abdomen between the umbilicus and symphysis pubis. Press the abdomen in and down while you elevate the cervix and uterus with your two fingers, as shown below. Try to grasp the uterus between your hands.

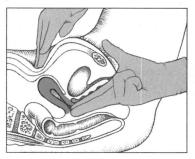

Then slide your fingers farther into the anterior fornix and palpate the body of the uterus between your hands. Note its size, shape, surface characteristics, consistency, and mobility. Note any tenderness of the uterine body and fundus. Also note fundal position.

Palpating the breasts and axillae

With the patient in a supine position, place a pillow under the shoulder on the side you're examining. Ask the patient to raise that arm above the head. Using your finger pads, palpate the breast in concentric circles from the center to the periphery.

Note the consistency of breast tissue. Check for nodules or unusual tenderness. In females, nodularity may increase before menstruation; tenderness may result from premenstrual fullness, cysts, or cancer. Any lump or mass that feels different from the rest of the breast may represent a pathologic change.

Palpate the areola and nipple, and compress the nipple between your thumb and index finger to detect discharge. If you see any, note the color, consistency, and quantity.

With the patient seated, palpate the axillae. Palpate the right axilla with the middle three fingers of one hand while supporting the patient's arm with your other hand. You can usually palpate one or more soft, small nontender, central nodes. If the nodes feel large or hard or are tender, or if the patient has a suspicious-looking lesion, try to palpate the other groups of lymph nodes.

Assessing the musculoskeletal system

Initial musculoskeletal questions

■ Ask if the patient experiences muscle pain, joint pain, swelling, tenderness, or difficulty with balance or gait. Does he have joint stiffness? If so, find out when it occurs and how long it lasts.
■ Inquire whether the patient has noticed noise with joint movement.
■ Find out if he has arthritis or gout.
■ Ask about a history of fractures, injuries, back problems, and deformities. Also ask about weakness and paralysis.
■ Explore any limitations on walking, running, or participation in sports. Do muscle or joint problems interfere with activities of daily living?

Age alert If the patient is a child, ask the parents if developmental milestones — such as sitting up, crawling, and walking — have been achieved.

Assessing range of motion

Assessment of joint range of motion (ROM) tests the joint function. To assess joint ROM, ask the patient to move specific joints through the normal ROM. If he can't do so, move the joints through passive ROM.

The following pages show each joint and illustrate the tests for ROM, including the expected degree of motion for each joint.

Shoulders
To assess forward flexion and backward extension, have the patient bring his straightened arm forward and up, then behind him.

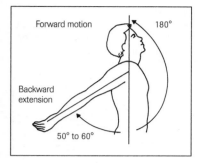

Assess abduction and adduction by asking the patient to bring his straightened arm to the side and up, then in front of him.

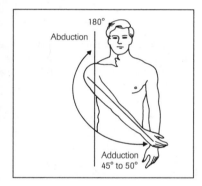

To assess external and internal rotation, have the patient abduct his arm with his elbow bent. Then ask him first to place his hand behind his head, then behind the small of his back.

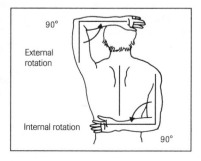

Elbows

Assess flexion by having the patient bend his arm and attempt to touch his shoulder. Assess extension by having him straighten his arm.

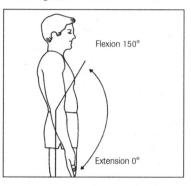

To assess pronation and supination, hold the patient's elbow in a flexed position, and ask him to rotate his arm until his palm faces the floor. Then rotate his hand back until his palm faces upward.

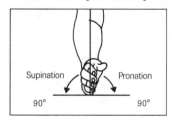

Wrists

To assess flexion, ask the patient to bend his wrist downward; assess extension by having him straighten his wrist. To assess hyperextension, ask him to bend his wrist upward.

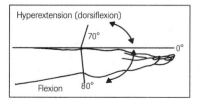

Assess radial and ulnar deviation by asking the patient to move his hand first toward the radial side, then toward the ulnar side.

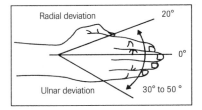

Fingers

To assess abduction and adduction, have the patient first spread his fingers and then bring them together. In abduction, there should be 20 degrees between the fingers; in adduction, the fingers should touch.

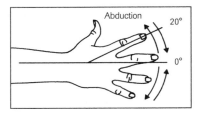

To assess extension and flexion, ask the patient first to straighten his fingers and then to make a fist with his thumb remaining straight.

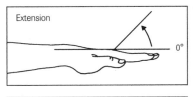

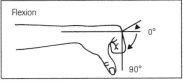

Thumbs

Assess extension by having the patient straighten his thumb. To assess flexion, have him bend his thumb at the top joint, then at the bottom.

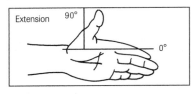

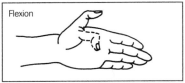

Assess adduction by having the patient extend his hand, bringing his thumb first to the index finger and then to the little finger.

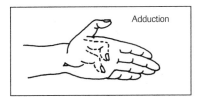

Hips

Assess flexion by asking the patient to bend his knee to his chest while keeping his back straight. If he has undergone total hip replacement, don't perform this movement without the surgeon's permission; motion can dislocate the prosthesis.

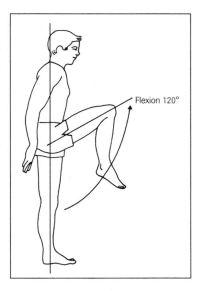

Flexion 120°

To assess abduction, have the patient move his straightened leg away from the midline.

To assess adduction, instruct the patient to move his straightened leg from the midline toward the opposite leg.

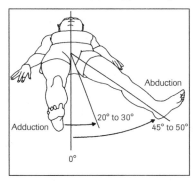

Abduction

Adduction
20° to 30°
45° to 50°
0°

Assess extension by having the patient straighten his knee. To assess hyperextension, ask him to extend his leg back straight. This motion can be performed with the patient in the prone or standing position.

To assess internal and external rotation, ask the patient to bend his knee and turn his leg inward. Then have him turn his leg outward.

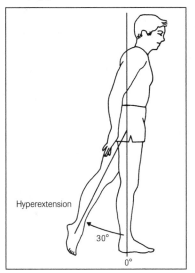

Hyperextension

30°

0°

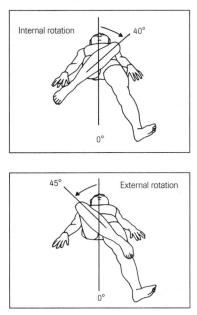

Internal rotation

40°

0°

45°

External rotation

0°

Knees

Ask the patient to straighten his leg at the knee to demonstrate extension; ask him to bend his knee and bring his foot up to touch his buttock to demonstrate flexion.

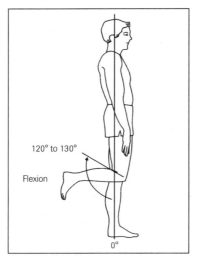

Toes

Assess extension and flexion by asking the patient to straighten and then curl his toes. Then check hyperextension by asking him to straighten his toes and point them upward.

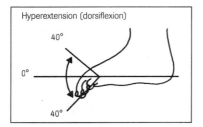

Ankles and feet

Have the patient demonstrate plantar flexion by bending his foot downward, and hyperextension by bending his foot upward.

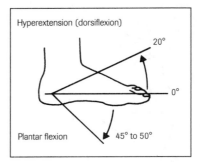

To assess eversion and inversion, ask the patient to point his toes. Have him turn his foot inward, then outward.

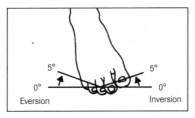

To assess forefoot adduction and abduction, stabilize the patient's heel while he turns his foot first inward, then outward.

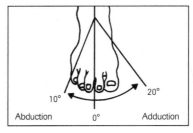

Testing muscle strength

Assess your patient's motor function by testing his strength in the affected limb. Have him attempt normal ROM movements against your resistance. (Before you begin muscle strength tests, find out whether the patient is right- or left-handed because the dominant arm is usually stronger.) Note the strength that the patient exerts against your resistance. If the muscle group is weak, you should lessen your resistance or provide no resistance to permit an accurate assessment. If necessary, position the patient so his limb doesn't have to resist gravity, and repeat the test.

Rate muscle strength on a scale from 0 to 5 (to minimize subjective interpretations of test findings), as follows:

0 = No visible or palpable contraction felt; paralysis
1 = Slight palpable contraction felt
2 = Passive ROM maneuvers when gravity is removed
3 = Active ROM against gravity
4 = Active ROM against gravity and light resistance
5 = Active ROM against full resistance; normal strength.

Deltoid

With your patient's arm fully extended, place on hand over his deltoid muscle and the other on his wrist. Have him abduct his arm to a horizontal position against your resistance; as he does, palpate for deltoid contraction.

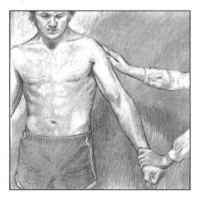

Biceps

With your hand on the patient's fist, have him flex his forearm against your resistance; observe for biceps contraction.

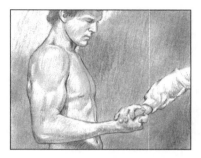

Triceps

Have the patient abduct and hold his arm midway between flexion and extension. Hold and support his arm at the wrist, and ask him to extend it against your resistance. Observe for triceps contraction.

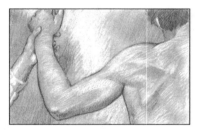

Dorsal interosseous

Have him extend and spread his fingers and resist your attempt to squeeze them together.

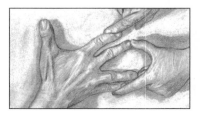

Forearm and hand (grip)
Have the patient grasp your middle and index fingers and squeeze them as hard as he can.

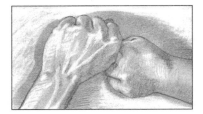

Psoas
While you support his leg, have the patient raise his knee and flex his hip against your resistance. Observe for psoas contraction.

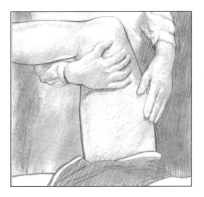

Quadriceps
Have the patient bend his knee slightly while you support his lower leg. Then ask him to extend his knee against your resistance; as he's doing so, palpate for quadriceps contraction.

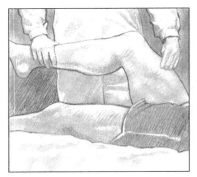

Gastrocnemius
With the patient in the prone position, support his foot and ask him to plantarflex his ankle against your resistance. Palpate for gastrocnemius contraction.

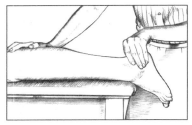

Anterior tibialis
With the patient sitting on the side of the examination table with his legs dangling, place your hand on his foot and ask him to dorsiflex his ankle against your resistance.

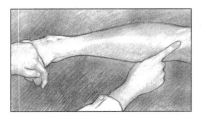

Extensor hallucis longus
With your fingers on his great toe, have him dorsiflex the toe against your

resistance. Palpate for extensor hallucis contraction.

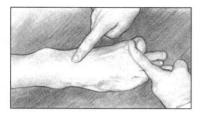

Assessing the skin

Initial skin questions

■ Determine if your patient has any known skin disease, such as psoriasis, eczema, or hives.

■ Ask him to describe any changes in skin pigmentation, temperature, moisture, or hair distribution.

■ Explore skin signs and symptoms, such as itching, rashes, or scaling. Is his skin excessively dry or oily?

■ Find out if the skin reacts to hot or cold weather. If so, how?

■ Ask if your patient has noticed easy bruising or bleeding, changes in warts or moles, or lumps. Ask about the presence and location of scars, sores, and ulcers.

Inspecting and palpating the skin

Before beginning your examination, make sure the lighting is adequate for inspection; then put on a pair of gloves. To examine the patient's skin, you'll use both inspection and palpation — sometimes simultaneously. During your examination, focus on such skin tissue characteristics as color, texture, turgor, moisture, and temperature. Also evaluate any skin lesions.

Color

Begin by systematically inspecting the skin's overall appearance. Remember,

skin color reflects the patient's nutritional, hematologic, cardiovascular, and pulmonary status.

Observe general coloring and pigmentation, keeping in mind racial differences as well as normal variations from one part of the body to another. Examine all exposed areas of the skin, including the face, ears, back of the neck, axillae, and backs of the hands and arms.

Note the location of any bruising, discoloration, or erythema. Look for pallor, a dusky appearance, jaundice, and cyanosis. Ask the patient if he has noticed any changes in skin color anywhere on his body.

Texture

Inspect and palpate the texture of the skin, noting thickness and mobility. Does the skin feel rough, smooth, thick, fragile, or thin? Changes can indicate local irritation or trauma, or they can be a result of problems in other body systems. For example, rough, dry skin is common in hypothyroidism; soft, smooth skin is common in hyperthyroidism. To determine if the skin over a joint is supple or taut, have the patient bend the joint as you palpate.

Turgor

Assessing the turgor, or elasticity, of the patient's skin helps you evaluate hydration. To assess turgor, gently squeeze the skin on the forearm. If it quickly returns to its original shape, the patient has normal turgor. If it resumes its original shape slowly or maintains a tented shape, the skin has poor turgor.

🌀 *Age alert* Decreased turgor occurs with dehydration as well as with aging. Increased turgor is associated with progressive systemic sclerosis.

To accurately assess skin turgor in an elderly patient, try squeezing the skin of the sternum or forehead instead of the forearm. In an elderly patient, the skin of the forearm tends to be flaccid, so it doesn't accurately represent the patient's hydration status.

Moisture
Observe the skin for excessive dryness or moisture. If the patient's skin is too dry, you may see reddened or flaking areas. Elderly patients commonly have dry, itchy skin. Moisture that appears shiny may result from oiliness.

If the patient is overhydrated, the skin may be edematous and spongy. Localized edema can occur in response to trauma or skin abnormalities such as ulcers. When you palpate local edema, make sure you document any associated discoloration or lesions.

Temperature
To assess skin temperature, touch the surface using the backs of your fingers. Inflamed skin will feel warm because of increased blood flow. Cool skin results from vasoconstriction. With hypovolemic shock, for instance, the skin feels cool and clammy.

Make sure you distinguish between generalized and localized warmth or coolness. Generalized warmth, or hyperthermia, is associated with fever stemming from a systemic infection or hyperthyroidism. Localized warmth occurs with a burn or localized infection. Generalized coolness occurs, with hypothyroidism; localized coolness, with arteriosclerosis.

Skin lesions
During your inspection, you may note vascular changes in the form of red, pigmented lesions. Among the most common are hemangiomas, telangiectases, petechiae, purpura, and ecchymoses. Keep in mind that these lesions may indicate disease. You'll see telangiectases, for instance, in pregnant patients as well as in those with hepatic cirrhosis.

Assessing dark skin

Be prepared for certain color variations when assessing dark-skinned patients. For example, some dark-skinned patients have a pigmented line, called Futcher's line, extending diagonally from the shoulder to the elbow. This is normal. Also normal are deeply pigmented ridges in the palms.

To detect color variations in dark-skinned and black patients, examine the sclerae, conjunctivae, buccal mucosa, tongue, lips, nail beds, palms, and soles. A yellowish brown color in dark-skinned patients or an ash-gray color in black patients indicates pallor, which results from a lack of the underlying pink and red tones normally present in dark skin.

Among dark-skinned blacks, yellowish pigmentation isn't necessarily an indication of jaundice. To detect jaundice in these patients, examine the hard palate and the slcerae.

Look for petechiae by examining areas with lighter pigmentation, such as the abdomen, gluteal areas, and the volar aspect of the forearm. To distinguish petechiae and ecchymoses from erythema in dark-skinned patients, apply pressure to the area. Erythematous areas will blanch, but petechiae or ecchymoses won't, because erythema is commonly associated with an increased skin for warmth.

When you assess edema in dark-skinned patients, remember that the affected area may have decreased color because fluid expands the distance between the pigmented layers and the external epithelium. When you palpate the affected area, it may feel tight.

Cyanosis can be difficult to identify in both white and black patients. Because certain factors, such as cold, affect the lips and nail beds, make sure you also assess the conjunctivae, palms, soles, buccal mucosa, and tongue.

Evaluating skin color variations

Color	Distribution	Possible cause
Absent	Small, circumscribed areas	Vitiligo
	Generalized	Albinism
Blue	Around lips (circumoral pallor) or generalized	Cyanosis. (*Note:* In black patients, bluish gingivae are normal.)
Deep red	Generalized	Polycythemia vera (increased red blood cell count)
Pink	Local or generalized	Erythema (superficial capillary dilation and congestion)
Tan to brown	Facial patches	Chloasma of pregnancy; butterfly rash of lupus erythematosus
Tan to brown bronze	Generalized (not related to sun exposure)	Addison's disease
Yellow	Sclera or generalized	Jaundice from liver dysfunction. (*Note:* In black patients, yellowish brown pigmentation of the sclera is normal.)
Yellow-orange	Palms, soles, and face; not sclera	Carotenemia (carotene in the blood)

To detect rashes in black or dark-skinned patients, you'll need to palpate the area for skin texture changes.

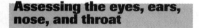

Assessing the eyes, ears, nose, and throat

Initial EENT questions

Eyes
■ Ask the patient about visual problems, such as myopia, hyperopia, blurred vision, or double vision. Does he wear corrective lenses?
■ Find out when his last eye examination was.

■ Ask if he has noticed any visual disturbances, such as rainbows around lights, blind spots, or flashing lights.
■ Ask if he experiences excessive tearing, dry eyes, itching, burning, pain, inflammation, swelling, color blindness, or photophobia.
■ Elicit any history of eye infections, eye trauma, glaucoma, cataracts, detached retina, or other eye disorders.
■ If he's older than age 50 or has a family history of glaucoma, inquire about the date and results of his last check for glaucoma.

Ears
■ Find out if the patient has hearing problems, such as deafness, poor hear-

ing, tinnitus, or vertigo. Is he abnormally sensitive to noise? Has he noticed any recent changes in his hearing?

■ Inquire about ear discharge, pain, or tenderness behind the ears.

■ Ask about frequent or recent ear infections or ear surgery.

■ Determine the date and result of his last hearing test.

■ Ask if he uses a hearing aid.

■ Determine his ear-care habits, including use of cotton-tipped swabs for ear wax removal.

Nose

■ Explore any nasal problems, including sinusitis, discharge, colds, coryza (more than four times a year), rhinitis, trauma, or frequent sneezing.

■ Determine whether your patient has an obstruction, breathing problems, or an inability to smell. Has he had nosebleeds?

■ Ask if he ever had surgery on his nose or sinuses. If so, explore when, why, and what type.

Mouth and throat

■ Investigate whether your patient has sores in the mouth or on the tongue. Does he have a history of oral herpes infection?

■ Find out if he has toothaches, bleeding gums, loss of taste, voice changes, dry mouth, or frequent sore throats.

■ If the patient has frequent sore throats, ask when they occur. Are they associated with fever or difficulty swallowing? How have the sore throats been treated medically?

■ Ask if the patient ever had a problem swallowing. If so, does he have trouble swallowing solids or liquids? Is the problem constant or intermittent? What precipitates the swallowing difficulty? What makes it go away?

■ Determine whether he has dental caries or tooth loss. Ask if he wears dentures or bridges.

■ Ask about the date and result of his last dental examination.

■ Explore his use of proper dental hygiene, including fluoride toothpaste.

Inspecting the conjunctivae

Bulbar conjunctiva

While wearing gloves, gently evert the patient's lower eyelid with the thumb of index finger, as shown below. Ask the patient to look up, down, left, and right as you examine the bulbar conjunctiva. It should be clear and shiny.

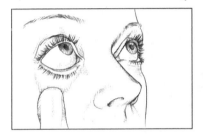

Palpebral conjunctiva

Check the palpebral conjunctiva only if you suspect a foreign body or if the patient complains of eyelid pain. To perform this examination, ask the patient to look down while you gently pull the medial eyelashes forward and upward with your thumb and index finger.

While holding the eyelashes, press on the tarsal border with a cotton-tipped applicator to evert the eyelid, as shown below. Hold the lashes against the brow and examine the conjunctiva, which should be pink with no swelling.

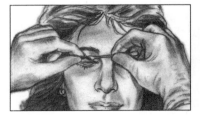

To return the eyelid to its normal position, release the eyelashes and ask the patient to look upward. If this doesn't invert the eyelid, grasp the eyelashes and gently pull them forward.

Testing the cardinal positions of gaze

This test of coordinated eye movements evaluates the oculomotor, trigeminal, and abducens nerves as well as the extraocular muscles. To perform the test, sit directly in front of the patient and ask him to remain still. Hold a small object, such as a pencil, directly in front of his nose at a distance of about 18″ (46 cm). Ask him to follow the object with his eyes without moving his head.

Then move the object to each of the six cardinal positions, returning it to midpoint after each movement. The patient's eyes should remain parallel as they move. Note any abnormal findings, such as nystagmus or the failure of one eye to follow the object.

Test each of the six cardinal positions of gaze; the left superior, the left lateral, the left inferior, the right inferior, the right lateral, and the right superior. These illustrations show testing of the three left positions.

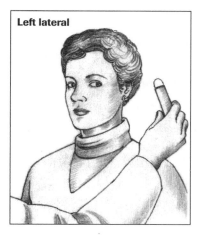

Left lateral

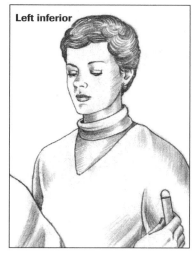

Left inferior

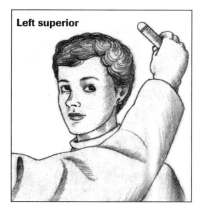

Left superior

Performing an ophthalmoscopic examination

To use an ophthalmoscope to help identify inner eye abnormalities, follow these steps.

■ Place the patient in a darkened or semidarkened room, with neither you nor the patient wearing glasses unless you're very myopic or astigmatic. However, either of you may wear contact lenses.

■ Sit or stand in front of the patient with your head about 18″ (46 cm) in front of and about 15 degrees to the right of the patient's line of vision in the right eye. Hold the ophthalmoscope in your right hand with the viewing aperture as close to your right eye as possible. Place your left thumb on the patient's right eyebrow to prevent hitting the patient with the ophthalmoscope as you move in close. Keep your right index finger on the lens selector to adjust the lens as necessary, as shown below. To examine the left eye, perform these steps on the patient's left side.

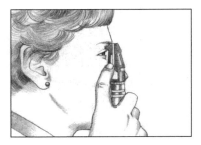

■ Instruct the patient to look straight ahead at a fixed point on the wall. Next, approaching from an oblique angle about 15″ (38 cm) out and with the diopter set at 0, focus a small circle of light on the pupil, as shown below.

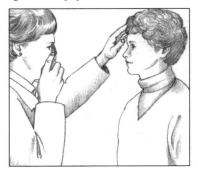

Look for the orange-red glow of the red reflex, which should be sharp and distinct through the pupil. The red reflex indicates that the lens is free from opacity and clouding.

■ Move closer to the patient, changing the lens selector with your forefinger to keep the retinal structures in focus, as shown below.

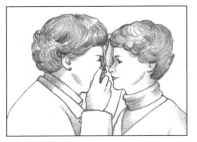

■ Change the lens selector to a positive diopter to view the vitreous humor, observing for any opacity.

■ Next, view the retina using a strong negative lens setting. Look for a retinal blood vessel, and follow that vessel toward the patient's nose, rotating the lens selector to keep the vessel in focus. Carefully examine all the retinal structures, including the retinal vessels, the optic disk, the retinal background, the macula, and the fovea centralis retinae.

■ Examine the vessels for their color, the size ratio of arterioles to veins, the arteriole light reflex, and the arteriovenous (AV) crossing. The crossing points should be smooth, without nicks or narrowings, and the vessels should be free from exudate, bleeding, and narrowing. Retinal vessels normally have an AV ratio of 2:3 or 4:5.

■ Evaluate the color of the retinal structures. The retina should be light yellow to orange and the background free from hemorrhages, aneurysms, and exudates. The optic disk, located on the nasal side of the retina, should be orange-red with distinct margins. The physiologic cup is normally yellow-white and readily visible.

■ Examine the macula last, and as briefly as possible, because it's very light-sensitive. The macula, which is darker than the rest of the retinal background, is free from vessels and located temporally to the optic disk. The fovea centralis retinae is a slight depression in the center of the macula.

Using the otoscope

Perform an otoscopic examination to assess the external auditory canal, tympanic membrane, and malleus. Before inserting the speculum into the patient's ear, check the canal opening for foreign particles or discharge. Palpate the tragus and pull up the auricle. If this area is tender, don't insert the speculum; the patient may have external otitis, and inserting the speculum could be painful.

If the ear canal is clear, straighten the canal by grasping the auricle and pulling it up and back, as shown below. Then insert the speculum.

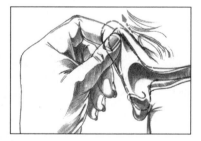

Age alert For an infant or a toddler, grasp the auricle and pull it down and back.

Hold the otoscope as shown at the top of the next column, with the hands parallel to the patient's head. Avoid hitting the ear canal with the speculum.

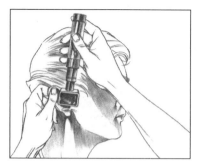

Inspecting the nostrils

For direct inspection of the nostrils, you'll need a nasal speculum and a small flashlight or penlight.

Have the patient sit in front of you and tilt his head back. Then insert the tip of the closed speculum into one of the nostrils until you reach the point where the blade widens. Slowly open the speculum as wide as you can without causing discomfort. Now shine the flashlight in the nostril to illuminate the area. The illustration below shows proper placement of the nasal speculum. The inset shows the structures that should be visible during an examination of the left nostril.

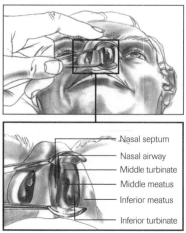

Nasal septum
Nasal airway
Middle turbinate
Middle meatus
Inferior meatus
Inferior turbinate

Note the color and patency of the nostril and the presence of any exudate. The mucosa should be moist, pink to red, and free from lesions and polyps. Normally, you wouldn't see any drainage, edema, or inflammation of the nasal mucosa, although some tissue enlargement is normal in a pregnant patient.

You should see the choana (posterior air passage), cilia, and the middle and inferior turbinates. Below each turbinate will be a groove, or meatus, where the paranasal sinuses drain.

When you've completed your inspection of one nostril, close the speculum and remove it. Then inspect the other nostril.

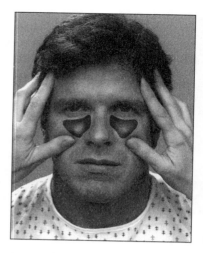

Inspecting and palpating the frontal and maxillary sinuses

During an inspection, you'll be able to examine the frontal and maxillary sinuses, but not the ethmoidal and sphenoidal sinuses. However, if the frontal and maxillary sinuses are infected, you can assume that the ethmoidal and sphenoidal are as well.

Begin by checking for swelling around the eyes, especially over the sinus area. Then palpate the frontal and maxillary sinuses for tenderness and warmth.

To palpate the frontal sinuses, place your thumb above the patient's eyes, just under the bony ridges of the upper orbits. Place your fingertips on his forehead and apply gently pressure.

To palpate the maxillary sinuses, place your thumbs as shown above right. Then apply gentle pressure by pressing your thumbs (or index and middle fingers) on each side of the nose just below the zygomatic bone (cheekbone).

Inspecting and palpating the thyroid gland

To locate the thyroid gland, observe the lower third of the patient's anterior neck. With the patient's neck extended slightly, look for masses or asymmetry in the gland. Ask him to sip water, with his neck still slightly extended. Watch the thyroid rise and fall with the trachea. You should see slight, symmetrical movement. A fixed thyroid lobe may indicate a mass.

Next, palpate the thyroid gland while standing in front of the patient. Locate the cricoid cartilage first; then move one hand to each side to palpate the thyroid lobes. The lobes can be difficult to feel because of their location and overlying tissues.

To evaluate the size and texture of the thyroid gland, ask the patient to tilt his head to the right. Then gently displace the thyroid toward the right. Have the patient swallow as you palpate the thyroid's lateral lobes, as shown at the top of the next page. Displace the thyroid toward the left to examine the left side.

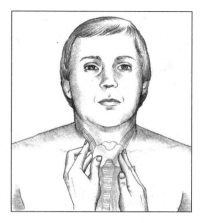

An enlarged thyroid may feel well defined and finely lobulated. Thyroid nodules feel like a knot, protuberance, or swelling; a firm, fixed nodule may be a tumor. Don't confuse thick neck muscles with an enlarged thyroid or goiter.

2 Assessment findings
Distinguishing health from disease

Normal findings

To distinguish between health and disease, you must be able to recognize normal assessment findings in each part of the body. When you perform a physical examination, use this head-to-toe roster of normal findings as a reference. It's designed to help you quickly zero in on physical abnormalities and evaluate your patient's overall condition.

Head and neck

Inspection
Head
■ a symmetrical, lesion-free skull
■ symmetrical facial structures with noncyanotic or vascular lesions
■ an ability to shrug the shoulders, a sign of an adequately functioning cranial nerve XI (accessory nerve).

Neck
■ unrestricted range of motion in the neck
■ no bulging of the thyroid
■ symmetrical, unswollen lymph nodes.

Palpation
Head
■ no lumps or tenderness on the head
■ symmetrical strength in the facial muscles, a sign of adequately functioning cranial nerves V and VII (trigeminal and facial nerves)
■ symmetrical sensation when you stroke a wisp of cotton on each cheek.

Neck
■ mobile, soft lymph nodes less than $1/2''$ (1 cm) with no tenderness
■ symmetrical pulses in the carotid arteries
■ a palpable, symmetrical, lesion-free thyroid and absence of thyroid tenderness

■ midline location of the trachea and absence of tracheal tenderness
■ no crepitus, tenderness, or lesions in the cervical spine
■ symmetrical muscle strength in the neck.

Eyes

Inspection
■ no edema, scaling, or lesion on eyelids
■ eyelids completely covering the corneas when closed
■ eyelid color the same as surrounding skin color
■ palpebral fissures of equal height
■ margin of upper lid falling between superior pupil margin and superior limbus
■ symmetrical, lesion-free upper eyelids that don't sag or droop when the patient opens his eyes
■ evenly distributed eyelashes that curve outward
■ globe of eye neither protruding from nor sunken into orbit
■ eyebrows with equal size, color, and distribution
■ absence of nystagmus
■ clear conjunctiva with visible small blood vessels and no signs of drainage
■ white sclera visible through conjunctiva
■ a transparent anterior chamber that contains no visible material when you shine a penlight into the side of the eye
■ transparent, smooth, and bright cornea with no visible irregularities or lesions
■ closing of the lids of both eyes when you stroke each cornea with a wisp of cotton, a test of cranial nerve V (trigeminal nerve)
■ round, equal-sized pupils that react normally to light and accommodation
■ constriction of both pupils when you shine a light on one

- lacrimal structures free from exudate, swelling, and excessive tearing
- proper eye alignment
- parallel eye movement in each of the six cardinal fields of gaze.

Palpation
- absence of eyelid swelling or tenderness
- globes that feel equally firm without feeling overly hard or spongy
- lacrimal sacs that don't regurgitate fluid.

Ears

Inspection
- bilaterally symmetrical, proportionately sized auricles with a vertical measurement of $1\frac{1}{2}''$ to $4''$ (4 to 10 cm)
- tip of ear crossing eye–occiput line (an imaginary line extending from the lateral aspect of the eye to the occipital protuberance)
- long axis of ear perpendicular to (or no more than 10 degrees from perpendicular to) the eye–occiput line
- color match between ears and facial skin
- no signs of inflammation, lesions, or nodules
- no cracking, thickening, scaling, or lesions behind the ear when you bend the auricle forward
- no visible discharge from auditory canal
- a patent external meatus
- skin color on the mastoid process that matches the skin color of the surrounding area
- no redness or swelling
- otoscopic examination reveals normal drum landmarks and bright reflex, with no canal inflammation or drainage.

Palpation
- no masses or tenderness on the auricle

- no tenderness on the auricle or tragus during manipulation
- either small, nonpalpable lymph nodes on the auricle or discrete, mobile lymph nodes with no signs of tenderness
- well-defined, bony edges on the mastoid process with no signs of tenderness.

Nose and mouth

Inspection
Nose
- a symmetrical, lesion-free nose with no deviation of the septum or discharge
- little or no nasal flaring
- nonedematous frontal and maxillary sinuses
- an ability to identify familiar odors
- pinkish red nasal mucosa with no visible lesions and no purulent drainage
- no evidence of foreign bodies or dried blood in the nose.

Mouth
- pink lips with no dryness, cracking, lesions, or cyanosis
- symmetrical facial structures
- an ability to purse the lips and puff out the cheeks, a sign of an adequately functioning cranial nerve VII (facial nerve)
- an ability to easily open and close the mouth
- light pink, moist oral mucosa with no ulcers or lesions
- visible salivary ducts with no inflammation
- a white hard palate
- a pink soft palate
- pink gums with no tartar, inflammation, or hemorrhage
- all teeth intact with no signs of occlusion, caries, or breakage
- a pink tongue with no swelling, coating, ulcers, or lesions

■ a tongue that moves easily and without tremor, a sign of a properly functioning cranial nerve XII (hypoglossal nerve)

■ no swelling or inflammation on anterior and posterior arches

■ no lesions or inflammation on posterior pharynx

■ lesion-free tonsils that are the right size for the patient's age

■ a uvula that moves upward when the patient says "ah" and a gag reflex that occurs when a tongue blade touches the posterior pharynx. These are signs or properly functioning cranial nerves IX and X.

Palpation
Nose

■ no structural deviation, tenderness, or selling in the external nose

■ no tenderness or edema on the frontal and maxillary sinuses.

Mouth

■ lips free from pain and induration

■ no lesions, unusual color, tenderness, or swelling on the posterior and lateral surfaces of the tongue

■ no tenderness, nodules, or swelling on the floor of the mouth.

Lungs

Inspection

■ side-to-side symmetrical chest configuration

■ anteroposterior diameter less than the transverse diameter, with a 1:2 to 5:7 ratio in an adult

■ normal chest shape, with no deformities, such as a barrel chest, kyphosis, retraction, sternal protrusion, or depressed sternum

■ costal angle less than 90 degrees, with the ribs joining the spine at a 45-degree angle

■ quiet, unlabored respirations with no use of accessory neck, shoulder, or abdominal muscles. You should also see no intercostal, substernal, or supraclavicular retractions.

■ symmetrically expanding chest wall during respirations

■ normal adult respiratory rate of 16 to 20 breaths/minute. Expect some variation depending on your patient's age.

■ regular respiratory rhythm, with expiration taking about twice as long as inspiration. Men and children breathe diaphragmatically, whereas women breathe thoracically.

■ skin color that matches the rest of the body's complexion.

Palpation

■ warm, dry skin

■ no tender spots or bulges in the chest.

Percussion

■ resonant percussion sounds over the lungs.

Auscultation

■ loud, high-pitched bronchial breath sounds over the trachea

■ intense, medium-pitched bronchovesicular breath sounds over the mainstem bronchi, between the scapulae, and below the clavicles

■ soft, breezy, low-pitched vesicular breath sounds over most of the peripheral lung fields.

Heart

Inspection

■ no visible pulsations, except at the point of maximal impulse (PMI)

■ no lifts (heaves) or retractions in the four valve areas of the chest wall.

Palpation

■ no detectable vibrations or thrills

■ no lifts (heaves)

■ no pulsations, except at the PMI and epigastric area. At the PMI, a localized (less than ½″ [1-cm] diameter area) tapping pulse may be felt at the start of systole. In the epigastric area, pulsation from the abdominal aorta may be palpable.

Auscultation

■ a first heart sound (S_1) — the *lub* sound heard best with the diaphragm of the stethoscope over the mitral area when the patient is in a left lateral position. It sounds longer, lower, and louder there than second heart sounds (S_2). S_1 splitting may be audible in the tricuspid area .

■ an S_2 sound — the *dub* sound heard best with the diaphragm of the stethoscope in the aortic area while the patient sits and leans over. It sounds shorter, sharper, higher, and louder there than S_1 sounds. Normal S_2 splitting may be audible in the pulmonic area on the inspiration.

■ a third heart sound (S_3) in children and slender, young adults with no cardiovascular disease is normal. It usually disappears when adults reach ages 25 to 35. In an older adult, it may signify ventricular failure. S_3 may be heard best with the bell of the stethoscope over the mitral area with the patient in a supine position and exhaling. It sounds short, dull, soft, and low.

■ murmurs may be functional in children and young adults, but are abnormal in older adults. Innocent murmurs are soft, short, and vary with respirations and patient position. They occur in early systole and are heard best in pulmonic or mitral areas with the patient in a supine position.

Abdomen

Inspection

■ skin free from vascular lesions, jaundice, surgical scars, and rashes

■ faint venous patterns (except in thin patients)

■ flat, round, or scaphoid abdominal contour

■ symmetrical abdomen

■ umbilicus positioned midway between the xiphoid process and the symphysis pubis, with a flat or concave hemisphere

■ no variations in the color of the patient's skin

■ no apparent bulges

■ abdominal movement apparent with respirations

■ pink or silver-white striae from pregnancy or weight loss.

Auscultation

■ high-pitched, gurgling bowel sounds, heard every 5 to 15 seconds through the diaphragm of the stethoscope in all four quadrants of the abdomen

■ vascular sounds heard through the bell of the stethoscope

■ venous hum over the inferior vena cava

■ no bruits, murmurs, friction rubs, or other venous hums.

Percussion

■ tympany predominantly over hollow organs including the stomach, intestines, bladder, abdominal aorta, and gallbladder

■ dullness over solid masses including the liver, spleen, pancreas, kidneys, uterus, and a full bladder.

Palpation

■ no tenderness or masses

■ abdominal musculature free from tenderness and rigidity

■ no guarding, rebound tenderness, distention, or ascites

■ unpalpable liver except in children. (If palpable, liver edge is regular, sharp, and nontender and is felt no more than ¾″ [2 cm] below the right costal margin.)

■ unpalpable spleen
■ unpalpable kidneys except in thin patients or those with a flaccid abdominal wall. (Right kidney is felt more commonly than left.)

Arms and legs

Inspection
■ no gross deformities
■ symmetrical body parts
■ good body alignment
■ no involuntary movements
■ a smooth gait
■ active range of motion in all muscles and joints
■ no pain with active range of motion
■ no visible swelling or inflammation of joints or muscles
■ equal bilateral limb length and symmetrical muscle mass.

Palpation
■ a normal shape with no swelling or tenderness
■ equal bilateral muscle tone, texture, and strength
■ no involuntary contractions or twitching
■ equally strong bilateral pulses.

Exploring the most common reasons for seeking care

A patient's reason for seeking care is the starting point for almost every initial assessment. You may be the patient's first contact, so you need to recognize the condition and determine the need for medical or nursing intervention. To thoroughly evaluate the patient's reason for seeking care, you need to ask the right health history questions, conduct a physical examination based on the history data you collect, and analyze possible causes of the problem.

This alphabetical list examines the most common reasons for seeking care encountered in nursing practice. For each one, you'll find a concise description, detailed questions to ask during the history, areas to focus on during the physical examination, and common causes to consider.

Anxiety

A subjective reaction to a real or imagined threat, anxiety is a nonspecific feeling of uneasiness or dread. It may be mild to moderate or severe. Mild to moderate anxiety may cause slight physical or psychological discomfort. Severe anxiety may be incapacitating or even life-threatening.

Anxiety is a normal response to actual danger, prompting the body (through stimulation of the sympathetic and parasympathetic nervous systems) to purposeful action. It's also a normal response to physical and emotional stress, which virtually any illness can produce. Anxiety can also be precipitated or exacerbated by many nonpathologic factors, including lack of sleep, poor diet, and excessive intake of caffeine or other stimulants. However, excessive, unwarranted anxiety may indicate an underlying psychological problem.

Health history
■ What are you anxious about? When did the anxiety first occur? What were the circumstances? What do you think caused it?
■ Is the anxiety constant or sporadic? Do you notice any precipitating factors?
■ How intense is the anxiety? What decreases it?
■ Do you smoke? Do you use caffeine? Alcohol? Drugs? What medications do you take?

Physical examination

Perform a complete physical examination, focusing on any complaints that the anxiety may trigger or aggravate.

Causes

■ *Asthma.* In allergic asthma attacks, acute anxiety occurs with dyspnea, wheezing, productive cough, accessory muscle use, hyperresonant lung fields, diminished breath sounds, coarse crackles, cyanosis, tachycardia, and diaphoresis.

■ *Conversion disorder.* Chronic anxiety is characteristic along with one or two somatic complaints that have no physiologic basis. Common complaints are dizziness, chest pain, palpitations, a lump in the throat, and choking.

■ *Hyperthyroidism.* Acute anxiety may be an early sign of this disorder. Classic signs include heat intolerance, weight loss despite increased appetite, nervousness, tremor, palpitations, sweating, an enlarged thyroid, and diarrhea. Exophthalmos may occur.

■ *Hyperventilation syndrome.* This disorder produces acute anxiety, pallor, circumoral and peripheral paresthesia and, occasionally, carpopedal spasms.

■ *Mitral valve prolapse.* Panic may occur in patients with this valvular disorder, which is referred to as the click-murmur syndrome. The disorder also may cause paroxysmal palpitations accompanied by sharp, stabbing, or aching precordial pain. Its hallmark is a midsystolic click, followed by an apical systolic murmur.

■ *Mood disorder.* In the depressive form of this disorder, chronic anxiety occurs with varying severity. The hallmark is depression upon awakening, which abates during the day. Associated findings include dysphoria; anger; insomnia or hypersomnia; decreased libido, interest, energy, and concentration; appetite disturbance; multiple somatic complaints; and suicidal thoughts.

■ *Obsessive-compulsive disorder.* Chronic anxiety occurs in this disorder, along with recurrent, unshakable thoughts or impulses to perform ritualistic acts. The patient recognizes these acts as irrational but can't control them. Anxiety builds if he can't perform these acts and diminishes after he does.

■ *Phobias.* In these disorders, chronic anxiety occurs along with persistent fear of an object, activity, or situation that results in a compelling desire to avoid it. The patient recognizes the fear as irrational but can't suppress it.

■ *Postconcussion syndrome.* This syndrome may produce chronic anxiety or periodic attacks of acute anxiety. Associated symptoms include irritability, insomnia, dizziness, and mild headache. The anxiety is usually most pronounced in situations demanding attention, judgment, or comprehension.

■ *Posttraumatic stress disorder.* This disorder produces chronic anxiety of varying severity and is accompanied by intrusive, vivid memories and thoughts of the traumatic event. The patient also relives the event in dreams and nightmares. Insomnia, depression, and feelings of numbness and detachment are common.

■ *Somatoform disorder.* Most common in adolescents and young adults, this disorder is characterized by chronic anxiety and various somatic complaints that have no physiologic basis. Anxiety and depression may be prominent or hidden by dramatic, flamboyant, or seductive behavior.

■ *Other causes.* Angina pectoris, chronic obstructive pulmonary disease, heart failure, hypochondrial neurosis, hypoglycemia, myocardial infarction, pheochromocytoma, pneumothorax, and pulmonary embolism can cause anxiety. Certain drugs cause anxiety, especially sympathomimetics and central nervous system stimulants. Also, many antidepressants can cause paradoxical anxiety.

Cough, nonproductive

A nonproductive cough is a noisy, forceful expulsion of air from the lungs that doesn't yield sputum or blood. One of the most common signs of a respiratory disorder, a nonproductive cough can be ineffective and cause damage, such as airway collapse, rupture of the alveoli, or blebs.

A nonproductive cough that later becomes productive is a classic sign of a progressive respiratory disease. An acute nonproductive cough has a sudden onset and may be self-limiting. A nonproductive cough that persists beyond 1 month is considered chronic; such a cough commonly results from cigarette smoking.

Health history
■ When did the cough begin? Does a certain body position or specific activity relieve or exacerbate it? Does it get better or worse at certain times of the day? How does the cough sound? Does it occur often? Is it paroxysmal?
■ Does pain accompany the cough?
■ Have you noticed any recent changes in your appetite, energy level, exercise tolerance, or weight? Have you had surgery recently? Do you have any allergies? Do you smoke? Have you been exposed recently to fumes or chemicals?
■ What medications are you taking?

Physical examination
Note whether the patient appears agitated, anxious, confused, diaphoretic, flushed, lethargic, nervous, pale, or restless. Is his skin cold or warm, clammy or dry?

Observe the rate and depth of his respirations, noting any abnormal patterns. Then examine his chest configuration and chest wall motion.

Check the patient's nose and mouth for congestion, drainage inflammation, and signs of infection. Then inspect his neck for vein distention and tracheal deviation.

As you palpate the patient's neck, note any enlarged lymph nodes or masses. Next, percuss his chest while listening for dullness, flatness, and tympany. Finally, auscultate his lungs for crackles, decreased or absent breath sounds, pleural friction rubs, rhonchi, and wheezes.

Causes
Asthma
Typically, an asthma attack occurs at night, starting with a nonproductive cough and mild wheezing. Then it progresses to audible wheezing, chest tightness, a cough that produces thick mucus, and severe dyspnea. Other signs include accessory muscle use, cyanosis, diaphoresis, flaring nostrils, flushing, intercostal and supraclavicular retractions on inspiration, prolonged expirations, tachycardia, and tachypnea.

Interstitial lung disease
With this disorder, the patient has a nonproductive cough and progressive dyspnea. He may also be cyanotic and fatigued, and have fine crackles, finger clubbing, chest pain, and a recent weight loss.

Other causes
A nonproductive cough may stem from an airway occlusion, atelectasis, common cold, hypersensitivity pneumonitis, pericardial effusion, pleural effusion, pulmonary embolism, *Hantavirus* infection, and sinusitis. Also, incentive spirometry, intermittent positive-pressure breathing, and suctioning can bring on a nonproductive cough.

Age alert Acute otitis media, which commonly occurs in infants and young children because of their short eustachian tubes, also produces nonproductive coughing.

Cough, productive

With productive coughing, the airway passages are cleared of accumulated secretions that normal mucociliary action doesn't remove. The sudden, forceful, noisy expulsion contains sputum, blood, or both.

Usually caused by a cardiopulmonary disorder, productive coughing typically stems from an acute or chronic infection that causes inflammation, edema, and increased mucus production in the airways. Such coughing can also result from inhaling antigenic or irritating substances; in fact, the most common cause is cigarette smoking.

Health history
■ When did the cough begin? How much sputum do you cough up daily? Is sputum production associated with time of day, meals, activities, or environment? Has it increased since coughing began? What are the color, odor, and consistency of the sputum? How does the cough sound and feel? Have you ever had a productive cough before?
■ Have you noticed any recent changes in your appetite or weight?
■ Do you have a history of recent surgery or allergies? Do you smoke or drink alcohol? If so, how much? Do you work around chemicals or respiratory irritants?
■ What medications are you taking?

Physical examination
As you examine the patient's mouth and nose for congestion, drainage, and inflammation, note his breath odor. Then inspect his neck for vein distention. As he breathes, observe the chest for accessory muscle use, intercostal and supraclavicular retractions, and uneven expansion.

Palpate his neck for enlarged lymph nodes, masses, and tenderness. Next, percuss his chest, listening for dullness, flatness, and tympany. Finally, auscultate for abnormal breath sounds, crackles, pleural friction rubs, rhonchi, and wheezes.

Causes
Bacterial pneumonia
With this disorder, an initially dry cough becomes productive. Rust-colored sputum appears in pneumococcal pneumonia; brick red or currant-jelly sputum, in *Klebsiella* pneumonia; salmon-colored sputum, in staphylococcal pneumonia; and mucopurulent sputum, in streptococcal pneumonia.

Lung abscess
The cardinal sign of a ruptured lung abscess is coughing that produces copious amounts of purulent, foul-smelling and, possibly, blood-tinged sputum. A ruptured abscess can also cause anorexia, diaphoresis, dyspnea, fatigue, fever with chills, halitosis, headache, inspiratory crackles, plueritic chest pain, tubular or amphoric breath sounds, and weight loss.

Other causes
A productive cough can result from acute bronchiolitis, aspiration and chemical pneumonitis, bronchiectasis, the common cold, cystic fibrosis, lung cancer, pertussis, pulmonary embolism, pulmonary edema, and tracheobronchitis. Also, expectorants, incentive spirometry, and intermittent positive-pressure breathing can cause a productive cough.

Diplopia

Also called double vision, diplopia occurs when the extraocular muscles fail to work together, causing images to fall on noncorresponding parts of the retina. Diplopia can result from orbital lesions, eye surgery, or impaired function of the cranial nerves that supply the extraocular muscles.

Classified as binocular or monocular, diplopia is usually intermittent at first or affects near or far vision exclusively. Binocular diplopia usually results from ocular deviation or displacement, or retinal surgery. Monocular diplopia may result from an early cataract, retinal edema or scarring, or poorly fitting contact lenses.

Health history

■ When did you first notice your double vision? Are the images side by side (horizontal), one above the other (vertical), or both? Is the diplopia intermittent or constant? Are both eyes affected or just one? Is near or far vision affected? Does the diplopia occur only when you gaze in certain directions? Has the problem worsened, remained the same, or subsided? Does it worsen as the day progresses? Can you correct the problem by tilting your head? If so, ask the patient to show you, and note the direction of the tilt.
■ Do you have eye pain?
■ Have you had recent eye surgery? Do you wear contact lenses?
■ Have you had any previous vision problems? Has anyone in your family?
■ What medications are you taking?

Physical examination

Observe the patient for conjunctival infection, exophthalmos, lid edema, ocular deviation, and ptosis. Have him occlude one eye at a time; if he sees double with only one eye, he has monocular diplopia. Test his visual acuity and extraocular muscle function.

Causes
Botulism
Hallmark signs and symptoms of botulism are diplopia, dysarthria, dysphagia, and ptosis. Early findings include diarrhea, dry mouth, sore throat, and vomiting. Later, descending weakness or paralysis of extremity and trunk muscles causes dyspnea and hyporeflexia.

Intracranial aneurysm
A life-threatening disorder, intracranial aneurysm initially produces diplopia and eye deviation, perhaps accompanied by a dilated pupil on the affected side and ptosis. Other findings include a decreased level of consciousness; dizziness; neck and spinal pain and rigidity; a severe, unilateral, frontal headache, which becomes violent after rupture of the aneurysm; tinnitus; unilateral muscle weakness or paralysis; and vomiting.

Other causes
Alcohol intoxication, brain tumors, diabetes mellitus, encephalitis, eye surgery, head injury, migraine, multiple sclerosis, and orbital tumors may also cause diplopia.

Dizziness

A common symptom, dizziness is a sensation of imbalance or faintness sometimes associated with blurred or double vision, confusion, and weakness. Dizziness may be mild or severe, have an abrupt or gradual onset, and be aggravated by standing up quickly and alleviated by lying down. Episodes are usually brief.

Dizziness typically results from inadequate blood flow and oxygen supply to the cerebrum and spinal cord. It may occur with anxiety, respiratory and cardiovascular disorders, and postconcussion syndrome. Dizziness is also a key symptom of certain serious disorders, such as hypertension and vertebrobasilar artery insufficiency.

Health history
■ When did the dizziness start? How severe is it? How often does it occur, and how long does each episode last?

Does the dizziness abate spontaneously? Is it triggered by standing up suddenly or bending over?

■ Do you have blurred vision, chest pain, a chronic cough, diaphoresis, a headache, or shortness of breath?

■ Have you ever had hypertension or another cardiovascular disorder? What about diabetes mellitus, anemia, respiratory or anxiety disorders, or head injury?

■ What medications are you taking?

🌀 *Age alert* Many children have difficulty describing dizziness and instead complain of tiredness, stomach ache, and feeling sick.

Physical examination

Assess the patient's level of consciousness, respirations, and body temperature. As you observe his breathing, look for accessory muscle use or barrel chest. Look also for finger clubbing, cyanosis, dry mucous membranes, and poor skin turgor. Evaluate the patient's motor and sensory functions and reflexes.

Palpate the extremities for peripheral edema and capillary refill. Auscultate the patient's heart rate and rhythm and his breath sounds. Take his blood pressure while he's lying down, sitting, and standing. If the diastolic pressure exceeds 100 mm Hg, notify the doctor immediately and have the patient lie down.

Causes

Cardiac arrhythmias

Dizziness lasts for several minutes or longer and may precede fainting. Other signs and symptoms include blurred vision, confusion, hypotension, palpitations, paresthesia, weakness, and an irregular, rapid, or thready pulse.

Hypertension

Dizziness may precede fainting but may be relieved by rest. Other findings include blurred vision, elevated blood pressure, headache, and retinal changes, such as hemorrhage and papilledema.

Transient ischemic attack

Dizziness of varying severity occurs during a transient ischemic attack. Lasting from a few seconds to 24 hours, an attack may be triggered by turning the head to the side and typically signals an impending cerebrovascular accident. During an attack, blindness, or visual field deficits, diplopia, hearing loss, numbness, paresis, ptosis, and tinnitus may also occur.

Other causes

Dizziness may result from anemia, generalized anxiety disorder, orthostatic hypotension, panic disorder, or post-concussion syndrome. Also, dizziness may be an adverse reaction to certain drugs, such as anxiolytics, central nervous system depressants, narcotic analgesics, decongestants, antihistamines, antihypertensives, or vasodilators.

Some herbal medications, such as St. John's wort, can produce dizziness.

Dysphagia

Difficulty swallowing, or dysphagia, is the most common — and sometimes the only — symptom of an esophageal disorder. This symptom may also result from oropharyngeal, respiratory, and neurologic disorders, and from exposure to toxins. Patients with dysphagia have an increased risk of aspiration and choking, and of malnutrition and dehydration.

Health history

■ When did your trouble swallowing start? Is swallowing painful? If so, is the pain constant or intermittent? Can you point to the spot where you have the most trouble swallowing? Does eating alleviate or aggravate the problem? Do you have more trouble swallowing solids or liquids? Does the problem disappear after you try to swallow a few times? Is swallowing easier if you change position?

■ Have you or anyone in your family ever had an esophageal, oropharyngeal, respiratory, or neurologic disorder? Have you recently had a tracheotomy or been exposed to a toxin?

Physical examination

Evaluate the patient's swallowing and his cough and gag reflexes. As you listen to his speech, note any signs of muscle, tongue, or facial weakness; aphasia; or dysarthria. Is this voice nasal or hoarse? Check his mouth for dry mucous membranes and thick secretions.

Causes

Airway obstruction

A life-threatening condition, upper-airway obstruction is marked by mild to severe wheezing and respiratory distress. Dysphagia occurs along with gagging and dysphonia.

Esophageal carcinoma

Painless dysphagia typically accompanies rapid weight loss. As the carcinoma advances, dysphagia becomes painful and constant. The patient complains of a cough with hemoptysis, hoarseness, sore throat, and steady chest pain.

 Age alert For patients older than age 50 with head or neck cancer, dysphagia is commonly the initial reason for seeking care.

Esophagitis

A patient with corrosive esophagitis has dysphagia accompanied by excessive salivation, fever, hematemesis, intense pain in the mouth and anterior chest, and tachypnea. *Candida* esophagitis produces dysphagia and sore throat. In reflux esophagitis, dysphagia is a late symptom that usually accompanies stricture.

Hiatal hernia

The patient with a hiatal hernia may complain of belching, dysphagia, dyspepsia, flatulence, heartburn, regurgitation, and retrosternal or substernal chest pain aggravated by lying down or bending over.

Other causes

Dysphagia results from botulism, esophageal diverticula, external esophageal compression, hypocalcemia, laryngeal nerve damage, and Parkinson's disease. Radiation therapy and a tracheotomy may also cause dysphagia.

Dyspnea

Patients typically describe dyspnea as shortness of breath, but this symptom also refers to difficult or uncomfortable breathing. Its severity varies greatly and is generally unrelated to the seriousness of the underlying cause. Dyspnea may arise suddenly or slowly and may subside rapidly or persist for years.

Health history

■ When did the dyspnea first occur? Did it begin suddenly or gradually? Is it constant or intermittent? Does it occur during activity or while you're resting? Does anything seem to trigger, exacerbate, or relieve it? Have you ever had dyspnea before?

■ Do you have a productive or nonproductive cough or chest pain?

■ Have you recently had an upper respiratory tract infection or experienced trauma? Do you smoke? If so, how much and for how long? Have you been exposed to any allergens? Do you have any known allergies?

■ What medications are you taking?

Physical examination

Observe the patient's respirations, noting their rate and depth, and any breathing difficulties or abnormal respiratory patterns. Check for flaring nostrils, grunting respirations, inspiratory stridor, intercostal retractions during inspirations, and pursed-lip expirations.

Also, examine the patient for barrel chest, diaphoresis, neck vein distention, finger clubbing, and peripheral edema. Note the color, consistency, and odor of any sputum.

Palpate his chest for asymmetrical expansion, decreased diaphragmatic excursion, tactile fremitus, and subcutaneous crepitation. Also check the rate, rhythm, and intensity of his peripheral pulses.

As you percuss the lung fields, note dull, hyperresonant, or tympanic percussion sounds. Auscultate the lungs for bronchophony, crackles, decreased or absent unilateral breath sounds, egophony, pleural friction rubs, rhonchi, whispered pectoriloquy, and wheezing. Then auscultate the heart for abnormal sounds or rhythms, such as ventricular or atrial gallop, and for pericardial friction rubs and tachycardia. Also monitor the patient's blood pressure and pulse pressure.

Causes

Adult respiratory distress syndrome
In adult respiratory distress syndrome (ARDS), acute dyspnea is followed by accessory muscle use, crackles, grunting respirations, progressive respiratory distress, rhonchi, and wheezes. In the late stages, anxiety, cyanosis, decreased mental acuity, and tachycardia occur. Severe ARDS can produce signs of shock, such as cool, clammy skin and hypotension. The typical patient has no history of underlying cardiac or pulmonary disease but has sustained a recent pulmonary or systemic insult.

Airway obstruction (partial)
Inspiratory stridor and acute dyspnea occur as the patient tries to overcome the obstruction. Related findings include accessory muscle use, anxiety, asymmetrical chest expansion, cyanosis, decreased or absent breath sounds, diaphoresis, hypotension, and tachypnea. The patient may have aspirated vomitus or a foreign body, or been exposed to an allergen.

Asthma
Acute dyspneic attacks occur along with accessory muscle use, apprehension, dry cough, flushing or cyanosis, intercostal retractions, tachypnea, and tachycardia. On palpation, you'll detect decreased tactile fremitus. Hyperresonance occurs on chest percussion. On auscultation, you'll note wheezing and rhonchi or, during a severe episode, decreased breath sounds.

Heart failure
Dyspnea usually develops gradually or occurs as chronic paroxysmal nocturnal dyspnea. In ventricular failure, dyspnea occurs with basilar crackles, dependent peripheral edema, distended neck veins, fatigue, orthopnea, tachycardia, ventricular or atrial gallop, and weight gain. The patient may have a history of cardiovascular disease, or he may be taking a drug — such as amiodarone (Cordarone), a beta-adrenergic blocker, or a corticosteroid — that can precipitate heart failure.

Myocardial infarction
Sudden dyspnea occurs with crushing substernal chest pain that may radiate to the back, neck, jaw, and arms. The patient's history may include heart disease, hypertension, hypercholesterolemia, or use of a drug — such as cocaine, dextrothyroxine sodium (Choloxin), estramustine phosphate sodium (Emcyt), or aldesleukin (Proleukin) — that can precipitate a myocardial infarction (MI).

Pneumonia

Dyspnea occurs suddenly, usually accompanied by fever, pleuritic chest pain that worsens with deep inspiration, and shaking chills. The patient also has a dry or productive cough, depending on the stage and type of pneumonia. Sputum may be discolored and foul smelling. Crackles, decreased breath sounds, dullness on percussion, and rhonchi may also be present. The history may include exposure to a contagious organism, hazardous fumes, or air pollution.

Pulmonary edema

In pulmonary edema, severe dyspnea is commonly preceded by signs of heart failure, such as crackles in both lung fields, cyanosis, tachycardia, tachypnea, and marked anxiety. The patient may have a dry cough or one that produces copious amounts of pink, frothy sputum. The history may reveal cardiovascular disease, cyanosis, fatigue, and pallor.

Pulmonary embolism

Severe dyspnea occurs with intense angina-like or pleuritic pain aggravated by deep breathing and thoracic movement. Other findings include crackles, cyanosis, diffuse wheezing, dull percussion sounds, low-grade fever, nonproductive cough, pleural friction rubs, restlessness, tachypnea, and tachycardia. The patient's history may include acute MI, heart failure, hip or leg fractures, oral contraceptive use, pregnancy, thrombophlebitis, or varicose veins.

Other causes

Dyspnea may also result from anemia, anxiety, cardiac arrhythmias, cor pulmonale, inhalation injury, lung cancer, pleural effusion, and sepsis.

Fatigue

A common symptom, fatigue is a feeling of excessive tiredness, lack of energy, or exhaustion, accompanied by a strong desire to rest or sleep. Fatigue differs from weakness, which involves the muscles, but may accompany it.

A normal response to physical overexertion, emotional stress, and sleep deprivation, fatigue can also result from psychological and physiologic disorders, especially viral infections and endocrine, cardiovascular, or neurologic disorders.

Health history

■ When did the fatigue begin? Is it constant or intermittent? If it's intermittent, when does it occur? Does the fatigue worsen with activity and improve with rest, or vice versa? (The former usually signals a physiologic disorder; the latter, a psychological disorder.)

■ Have you experienced any recent stressful changes at home or at work?

■ Have you changed your eating habits? Have you recently lost or gained weight?

■ Have you or anyone in your family been diagnosed with any cardiovascular, endocrine, or neurologic disorders? What about viral infections or psychological disorders?

■ What medications are you taking?

Age alert Always ask older patients about fatigue because this symptom may be insidious and mask a more serious underlying condition.

Physical examination

Observe the patient's general appearance for signs of depression or organic illness. Is he unkempt? Expressionless? Tired or unhealthy looking? Is he slumped over? Assess his mental status, noting especially any agitation, attention deficits, mental clouding, or psychomotor impairment.

Causes

Anemia

Fatigue after mild activity is generally the first symptom of anemia. Other signs and symptoms typically include dyspnea, pallor, and tachycardia.

Cancer

Unexplained fatigue is commonly the earliest indication of cancer. Related signs and symptoms reflect the type, location, and stage of the tumor, and usually include abnormal bleeding, anorexia, nausea, pain, a palpable mass, vomiting, and weight loss.

Chronic infection

In a patient with a chronic infection, fatigue is usually the most prominent symptom — and sometimes the only one.

Depression

Chronic depression is almost always accompanied by persistent fatigue unrelated to exertion. The patient may also complain of anorexia, constipation, headache, and sexual dysfunction.

Diabetes mellitus

The most common symptom in this disorder, fatigue may begin insidiously or abruptly. Related findings include polydipsia, polyphagia, polyuria, and weight loss.

Heart failure

Persistent fatigue and lethargy are characteristic symptoms of heart failure. Left-sided heart failure produces exertional and paroxysmal nocturnal dyspnea, orthopnea, and tachycardia. Right-sided heart failure causes neck vein distention and, sometimes, a slight but persistent nonproductive cough.

Hypothyroidism

Fatigue occurs early in this disorder, along with forgetfulness, cold intolerance, weight gain, metrorrhagia, and constipation.

Myasthenia gravis

The cardinal symptoms of this disorder are easy fatigability and muscle weakness that worsen with exertion and abate with rest. These symptoms are related to the specific muscle groups affected.

Other causes

Anxiety, myocardial infarction, rheumatoid arthritis, systemic lupus erythematosus, and malnutrition can cause fatigue, as can certain drugs — notably antihypertensives and sedatives — and most types of surgery.

Fever

An abnormal elevation of body temperature above 98.6° F (37° C), fever (or pyrexia) is a common sign arising from disorders that affect virtually every body system. As a result, fever alone has little diagnostic value. However, persistently high fever is a medical emergency.

Fever can be classified as low (oral reading of 99° to 100.4° F [37.2° to 38° C]), moderate (100.5° to 104° F [38° to 40° C]), or high (above 104° F [40° C]). Fever above 108° F (42.2° C) causes unconsciousness and, if prolonged, brain damage.

Age alert Infants and young children experience higher and more prolonged fevers, more rapid temperature increases, and greater temperature fluctuations than older children or adults.

Health history

■ When did the fever begin? How high did it reach? Is the fever constant,

or does it disappear and then reappear later?
■ Do you also have chills, fatigue, or pain?
■ Have you had any immunodeficiency disorders, infections, recent trauma or surgery, or diagnostic tests? Have you traveled recently?
■ What medications are you taking? Have you recently had anesthesia?

Causes
Infectious and inflammatory disorders
Fever may be low, as in Crohn's disease and ulcerative colitis, or extremely high, as in bacterial pneumonia. It may be remittent, as in infectious mononucleosis; sustained, as in meningitis; or relapsing, as in malaria. Fever may arise abruptly, as in Rocky Mountain spotted fever, or insidiously, as in mycoplasmal pneumonia. Typically, it accompanies a self-limiting disorder such as the common cold.

Medications
Fever and rash commonly result from hypersensitivity to quinidine, methyldopa (Aldomet), procainamide hydrochloride (Pronestyl), phenytoin (Dilantin), anti-infectives, barbiturates, iodides, and some antitoxins. Fever can also result from the use of chemotherapeutic agents and medications that decrease sweating such as anticholinergics. Toxic doses of salicylates, amphetamines, and tricyclic antidepressants can cause fever.

Other causes
Fever may also result from an injection of contrast media used in diagnostic tests, from surgery, and from blood transfusion reactions.

Headache

The most common neurologic symptom, a headache may be mild to severe, localized or generalized, constant or intermittent. About 90% of all headaches are benign and can be described as vascular, muscle contracting, or a combination of both.

Occasionally, this symptom indicates a severe neurologic disorder. A generalized, pathologic headache may result from disorders associated with intracranial inflammation, increased intracranial pressure (ICP), meningeal irritation, or a vascular disturbance. A headache may also result from eye and sinus disorders and from the effects of drugs, tests, and treatments.

Health history
■ When did the headache first occur? Is the pain mild, moderate, or severe? Is it localized or generalized? If it's localized, where does it occur? Is it constant or intermittent? If it's intermittent, what's the duration? How would you describe the pain; for example, is it stabbing, dull, throbbing, or viselike? Does anything seem to trigger it, exacerbate it, or relieve it?
■ Have you also experienced confusion, dizziness, drowsiness, eye pain, fever, muscle twitching, nausea, photophobia, seizures, speaking or walking difficulties, neck stiffness, visual disturbances, vomiting, or weakness?
■ Have you been under unusual stress at home or at work? For family members: Have you noticed any changes in the patient's behavior or personality?
■ Do you have a history of blood dyscrasia, cardiovascular disease, glaucoma, hemorrhagic disorders, hypertension, poor vision, seizures, or smoking? Have you had any recent traumatic injuries, dental work, or sinus, ear, or systemic infections?
■ What medications are you taking?

Physical examination
Observe the rate and depth of the patient's respirations, noting any breathing difficulty or abnormal patterns. Then inspect his head for bruising,

swelling, and sinus bleeding. Check also for Battle's sign, neck stiffness, otorrhea, and rhinorrhea.

Assess the patient's level of consciousness (LOC). Is he drowsy, lethargic, or comatose? Examine his eyes, noting pupil size, equality, and response to light. With the patient both at rest and active, note any tremors.

Gently palpate the skull and sinuses for tenderness. Unless head trauma has occurred, slowly move the neck to check for nuchal rigidity or pain. Then assess the patient's motor strength. Palpate his peripheral pulses, noting their rate, rhythm, and intensity.

Check for a positive Babinski's reflex. As you percuss for other reflexes, note any hyperreflexia. Then auscultate over the temporal artery, listening for bruits. Also monitor the patient's blood pressure and pulse pressure.

Causes
Brain abscess
A headache stemming from a brain abscess typically intensifies over a few days, localizes to a particular spot, and is aggravated by straining. The headache may be accompanied by a decreased LOC (drowsiness to deep stupor), focal or generalized seizures, nausea, and vomiting. Depending on the abscess site, the patient may also have aphasia, ataxia, impaired visual acuity, hemiparesis, personality changes, or tremors. Signs of an infection may or may not appear. The patient's history may include systemic, chronic middle ear, mastoid, or sinus infection; osteomyelitis of the skull or a compound fracture; or a penetrating head wound.

Brain tumor
Initially, the headache develops near the tumor site and becomes generalized as the tumor grows. Pain is usually intermittent, deep-seated, dull, and most intense in the morning. It's aggravated by

coughing, stooping, Valsalva's maneuver, and changes in head position.

Cerebral aneurysm (ruptured)
This headache is sudden and excruciating. It may be unilateral and usually peaks within minutes of the rupture. The headache may be accompanied by nausea, vomiting, and signs of meningeal irritation. The patient may lose consciousness. His history may include hypertension or other cardiovascular disorders, a stressful lifestyle, or smoking.

Encephalitis
This headache is severe and generalized and is accompanied by a deteriorating LOC over a 48-hour period. Fever, focal neurologic deficits, irritability, nausea, nuchal rigidity, photophobia, seizures, and vomiting may also develop. The patient's history may reveal exposure to the viruses that commonly cause encephalitis, such as mumps or herpes simplex.

Epidural hemorrhage (acute)
A progressively severe headache immediately follows a brief loss of consciousness. Then the patient's LOC rapidly and steadily declines. Accompanying signs and symptoms include increasing ICP, ipsilateral pupil dilation, nausea, and vomiting. The patient's history usually reveals head trauma within the past 24 hours.

Glaucoma (acute angle-closure)
An ophthalmic emergency, glaucoma may cause an excruciating headache. Other signs and symptoms include blurred vision, cloudy cornea, halo vision, moderately dilated and fixed pupil, photophobia, nausea, and vomiting.

Hypertension
Patients with hypertension may have a slightly throbbing occipital headache on awakening. Then, during the day,

the severity may decrease. But if the patient's diastolic blood pressure exceeds 120 mm Hg, the headache remains the constant and is considered a medical emergency because of the potential for cerebral vascular accident.

Meningitis

The patient experiences a severe constant, generalized headache that starts suddenly and worsens with movement. He may also have chills, fever, hyperreflexia, nuchal rigidity, and positive Kernig's and Brudzinski's signs. His history may include recent systemic or sinus infection, dental work, or exposure to bacteria or viruses that commonly cause meningitis, such as *Haemophilus influenzae, Streptococcus pneumoniae,* enteroviruses, and mumps.

Migraine

A severe, throbbing headache, migraine may follow a 5- to 15-minute prodrome of dizziness; tingling of the face, lips or hands; unsteady gait; and visual disturbances. Other signs and symptoms include anorexia, nausea, photophobia, and vomiting.

Sinusitis (acute)

Patients with sinusitis have a dull, periorbital headache that's typically aggravated by bending over or touching the face. They may also have fever, malaise, nasal discharge, nasal turbinate edema, sinus tenderness, and sore throat. Sinus drainage relieves the sinusitis.

Subarachnoid hemorrhage

The hallmarks of this disorder are a sudden, violent headache along with dizziness, hypertension, ipsilateral pupil dilation, nausea, nuchal rigidity, seizures, vomiting, and an altered LOC that may rapidly progress to coma. The patient's history may include congenital vascular defects, arteriovenous malformation, cardiovascular disease, smoking, or excessive stress.

Subdural hematoma

A severe, localized headache usually follows head trauma that causes an immediate loss of consciousness, a latent period of drowsiness, confusion or personality changes, and agitation. Later, signs of increased ICP may develop. If the head trauma occurred within 3 days of the onset of signs and symptoms, the hematoma is acute; within 3 weeks, subacute; after more than 3 weeks, chronic. About 50% of patients with this disorder have no history of head trauma.

Other causes

Cervical traction, lumbar puncture, myelography, withdrawal from a vasopressor or a sympathomimetic, or use of indomethacin (Indocin), digoxin (Lanoxin), nitroglycerin (Nitrostat), isosorbide dinitrate (Isordil), or another vasodilator can cause headaches. Also, use of certain herbal medicines — such as St. John's wort, ginseng, and ephedra — can cause headaches.

Heartburn

A substernal burning sensation that rises in the chest and may radiate to the neck or throat, heartburn (also known as pyrosis) results from the reflux of gastric contents into the esophagus. Usually, it's accompanied by regurgitation. Because increased intra-abdominal pressure contributes to reflux, heartburn commonly occurs with pregnancy, ascites, or obesity, but it may also be caused by GI disorders, connective tissue disease, and certain drugs.

In most cases, heartburn develops after meals or when a person lies down, bends over, lifts heavy objects, or exercises vigorously. It usually worsens with swallowing and improves when the person sits upright or takes antacids. Some patients confuse heartburn with a myocardial infarction (MI), but a patient who is having a MI typically has other symptoms besides a burning sensation.

Health history
■ When did the heartburn start? Do certain foods or beverages seem to trigger it? Does stress or fatigue seem to aggravate it? Do movement, certain body positions, or very hot or cold liquids worsen or relieve it? Where exactly is the burning sensation? Does it radiate to other areas? Does it cause you to regurgitate sour- or bitter-tasting fluids? Have you ever had heartburn before?
■ Do you have a history of GI problems or connective tissue disease? For women of child-bearing age: Are you pregnant?
■ What medication are you taking?

Physical examination
Auscultate the heart and lungs to rule out a heart or lung disorder. Palpate the abdomen for abdominal pain.

Causes
Esophageal cancer
Heartburn may indicate esophageal cancer. The first symptom is usually painless dysphagia that progressively worsens. Eventually, partial obstruction and rapid weight loss occur. The patient may complain of a feeling of substernal fullness, hoarseness, nausea, sore throat, steady pain in the posterior and anterior chest, and vomiting.

Gastroesophageal reflux
Severe, chronic heartburn is the most common symptom of this disorder. The heartburn usually occurs within 1 hour after eating and may be triggered by certain foods or beverages. It worsens when the person lies down or bends over and abates when he sits, stands, or ingests antacids. Other findings include a dull retrosternal pain that may radiate, dysphagia, flatulent dyspepsia, and postural regurgitation.

Peptic ulcer
Heartburn and indigestion usually signal the onset of a peptic ulcer attack. Most patients experience a gnawing, burning pain in the left epigastrium, although some report sharp pain. The pain typically occurs when the stomach is empty and is generally relieved by taking antacids. The pain may also occur after the patient ingests coffee, aspirin, or alcohol.

Scleroderma
A connective tissue disease, scleroderma may cause esophageal dysfunction resulting in heartburn, bloating after meals, odynophagia, the sensation of food sticking behind the sternum, and weight loss. Other GI effects include abdominal distention, constipation or diarrhea, and malodorous, floating stools.

Other causes
Heartburn may also be caused by esophageal diverticula, obesity, and use of certain drugs, including aspirin, nonsteroidal anti-inflammatory drugs, anticholinergics, inhaled corticosteroids, inhaled beta-adrenergic blockers, and drugs having anticholinergic effects.

Hematuria

A cardinal sign of renal and urinary tract disorders, hematuria is the presence of blood in the urine. Hematuria may be evident or a urine test for occult blood may confirm it.

The bleeding may be continuous or intermittent, is commonly accompanied by pain, and may be aggravated by prolonged standing or walking. Dark or brownish blood indicates renal or upper urinary tract bleeding; bright red blood, lower urinary tract bleeding.

Health history
■ When did you first notice blood in your urine? Does it occur every time you urinate? Are you passing any clots?

Have you ever had this problem before?

■ Do you have any pain? If so, does the pain occur only when you urinate, or is it continuous?

■ Do you have bleeding hemorrhoids? Have you had any recent trauma or performed any strenuous exercise? Do you have a history of renal, urinary, prostatic, or coagulation disorders? For female patients, are you menstruating?

■ What medications are you taking?

Physical examination

Check the urinary meatus for any bleeding or abnormalities. Then, palpate the abdomen and flanks, noting any pain or tenderness. Finally, percuss the abdomen and flanks, especially the costovertebral angle, to elicit any tenderness.

Causes

Bladder cancer

A primary cause of gross hematuria in men, bladder cancer may produce pain in the bladder, rectum, pelvis, flank, back, or legs. You may also note signs of urinary tract infection.

Calculi

Both bladder and renal calculi produce hematuria, which may be accompanied by signs and symptoms of urinary tract infection. Bladder calculi usually produce gross hematuria, pain referred to the penile or vulvar areas and, in some patients, bladder distention. Renal calculi may produce either microscopic or gross hematuria.

Glomerulonephritis

Usually, acute glomerulonephritis begins with gross hematuria. It may also produce anuria or oliguria, flank and abdominal pain, and increased blood pressure. Chronic glomerulonephritis typically causes microscopic hematuria accompanied by generalized edema, increased blood pressure, and proteinuria.

Nephritis

Acute nephritis causes fever, a maculopapular rash, and microscopic hematuria. In chronic interstitial nephritis, the patient may have dilute, almost colorless urine along with polyuria.

Pyelonephritis (acute)

A typical sign of pyelonephritis is microscopic or macroscopic hematuria that progresses to grossly bloody hematuria. After the infection resolves, microscopic hematuria may persist for a few months. Other finds include flank pain, high fever, and signs and symptoms of a urinary tract infection.

Renal infarction

Patients with renal infarction usually have gross hematuria. Other symptoms include anorexia, costovertebral angle tenderness, and constant, severe flank and upper abdominal pain.

Other causes

Hematuria may result from benign prostatic hyperplasia, bladder trauma, obstructive nephropathy, polycystic kidney disease, renal trauma, and urethral trauma. It may result from a diagnostic test, such as cystoscopy or renal biopsy, or use of a drug, such as an anticoagulant; a chemotherapeutic agent, such as aldesleukin (Proleukin), BCG intravesical (TheraCys), ifosfamide (Ifex), or leuprolide (Lupron); etretinate (Tegison); or thiabendazole (Mintezol). Also, certain herbal medicines, such as garlic and gingko biloba, may cause hematuria when taken with an anticoagulant.

Hemoptysis

The expectoration of blood or bloody sputum from the lungs or tracheobronchial tree is known as hemoptysis. Usually resulting from a tracheobronchial tree abnormality, hemoptysis is associated with inflammatory conditions or lesions that cause erosion and necrosis of bronchial tissues and blood vessels.

Hemoptysis is sometimes confused with bleeding from the mouth, throat, nasopharynx, or GI tract. Severe hemoptysis requires emergency endotracheal intubation and suctioning.

Health history
■ When did you begin expectorating blood? How much blood or sputum are you expectorating? How often?
■ Did you recently have a flulike syndrome? Have you had any recent invasive pulmonary procedures or chest trauma?
■ Do you smoke? Did you ever smoke? If so, how much? Have you ever been diagnosed with a cardiac, respiratory, or bleeding disorder?
■ What medications are you taking? Are you taking an anticoagulant?

Physical examination
After assessing the patient's level of consciousness, examine his nose, mouth, and pharynx for sources of bleeding. Observe the rate and depth of his respirations, noting any breathing difficulty or abnormal breathing patterns. Also, as he breathes, look for abnormal chest movement, accessory muscle use, and retractions. Inspect the skin for central and peripheral cyanosis, diaphoresis, lesions, and pallor.

Palpate the rate, rhythm, and intensity of the peripheral pulses. Then feel the chest, noting abnormal pulsations, diaphragmatic tenderness, and fremitus. Check for respiratory excursion. If the patient has a history of trauma, carefully check the position of the trachea and note any edema.

As you percuss over the lung fields, note any dullness, flatness, hyperresonance, or tympany. Then auscultate the lungs for crackles, rhonchi, and wheezes, and the heart for bruits, gallops, murmurs, and pleural friction rubs. Also, monitor the patient's blood pressure and pulse pressure.

Causes
Bronchitis (chronic)
With this disorder, the patient usually has a productive cough that lasts at least 3 months and leads to expectoration of blood-streaked sputum. Other respiratory signs include dyspnea, prolonged expiration, scattered rhonchi, and wheezing.

Lung abscess
A patient with a lung abscess expectorates copious amounts of bloody, purulent, foul-smelling sputum. He also has anorexia, chills, diaphoresis, fever, headache, and pleuritic or dull chest pain. Lung auscultation may reveal tubular breath sounds or crackles. Percussion reveals dullness on the affected side. The patient may have a history of a recent pulmonary infection or evidence of poor oral hygiene with dental or gingival disease.

Lung cancer
Ulceration of the bronchus commonly causes recurring hemoptysis (an early sign), which can vary from blood-streaked sputum to blood. Related findings include anorexia, chest pain, dyspnea, fever, a productive cough, weight loss, and wheezing.

Pulmonary edema
A patient with pulmonary edema may expectorate copious amounts of frothy, blood-tinged, pink sputum. He may also complain of dyspnea and orthopnea. On examination, you may detect diffuse crackles in both lung fields and a ventricular gallop.

Tracheal trauma
With tracheal trauma, the bleeding appears to come from the back of the throat. Accompanying signs and symp-

toms include airway occlusion, dysphagia, hoarseness, neck pain, and respiratory distress.

Other causes
Hemoptysis may also result from bronchiectasis, coagulation disorders, cystic fibrosis, lung or airway injuries from diagnostic procedures, and primary pulmonary hypertension.

Hoarseness

A rough or harsh-sounding voice, hoarseness can be acute or chronic. It may result from infections or inflammatory lesions or exudates in the larynx, from laryngeal edema, from compression or disruption of the vocal cords or recurrent laryngeal nerve damage, or from irritating polyps on the vocal cords. Hoarseness can also occur with aging because the laryngeal muscles and mucosa atrophy, leading to diminished control of the vocal cords. Hoarseness may be exacerbated by excessive alcohol intake, smoking, inhalation of noxious fumes, excessive talking, and shouting.

Health history
■ When did the hoarseness start? Is it constant or intermittent? Does anything relieve or exacerbate it? Have you been overusing your voice?
■ Have you also had a cough, a dry mouth, difficulty swallowing dry food, shortness of breath, or a sore throat?
■ Have you ever had cancer or other disorders? Do you regularly drink alcohol or smoke? If so, how much?

Physical examination
Inspect the patient's mouth and throat for redness or exudate, possibly indicating an upper respiratory tract infection. Ask him to stick out his tongue: If he can't, the hypoglossal nerve (cranial nerve XII) may be impaired.

As the patient breathes, observe for asymmetrical chest expansion, intercostal retractions, nasal flaring, stridor, and other signs of respiratory distress.

Palpate the patient's neck for masses and the cervical lymph nodes and thyroid gland for enlargement. Then palpate the trachea to check for deviation.

As you percuss the chest wall, note any dullness. Then auscultate the lungs for crackles, rhonchi, tubular sounds, or wheezes. To detect bradycardia, auscultate the heart.

Causes
Inhalation injury
Exposure to a fire or an explosion can cause an inhalation injury, which produces coughing, hoarseness, orofacial burns, singed nasal hair, and soot-stained sputum. Subsequent signs and symptoms include crackles, rhonchi, wheezes, and respiratory distress.

Laryngitis
Persistent hoarseness may be the only sign of chronic laryngitis. In acute laryngitis, hoarseness or a complete loss of voice develops suddenly. Related findings include cough, fever, pain (especially during swallowing or speaking), profuse diaphoresis, rhinorrhea, and sore throat.

Vocal cord polyps
With this disorder, a raspy hoarseness will be the reason for seeking care. The patient may also have a chronic cough and a crackling voice.

Other causes
Hoarseness may result from hypothyroidism, pulmonary tuberculosis, rheumatoid arthritis, and laryngeal cancer (most common in men ages 50 to 70). Prolonged intubation, surgical severing of the recurrent laryngeal

nerve, and a tracheostomy may also produce hoarseness.

🌀 *Age alert* In infants and young children, hoarseness commonly stems from acute laryngotracheobronchitis (croup).

Nausea

A profound feeling of revulsion to food, or a signal of impending vomiting, nausea is usually accompanied by anorexia, diaphoresis, hypersalivation, pallor, tachycardia, tachypnea, and vomiting. A common symptom of GI disorders, nausea may also result from electrolyte imbalances; infections; metabolic, endocrine, and cardiac disorders; early months of pregnancy; drug therapy; surgery; and radiation therapy. Also, severe pain, anxiety, alcohol intoxication, overeating, and ingestion of something distasteful can trigger nausea.

Health history
■ When did the nausea begin? Is it intermittent or constant? How severe is it?
■ Do you have any other signs and symptoms, such as abdominal pain, loss of appetite, changes in bowel habits, excessive belching or gas, weight loss or vomiting?
■ For female patients: Are you pregnant or could you be? Have you ever had a GI, endocrine, or metabolic disorder? Have you had any recent infections? Have you ever had cancer or radiation therapy or chemotherapy?
■ What medications are you taking? Do you drink alcohol and, if so, how much?

Physical examination
Examine the patient's skin for bruises, jaundice, poor turgor, and spider angiomas. Then inspect his abdomen for distention.

Because palpation and percussion can affect the frequency and intensity of bowel sounds, you should auscultate the abdomen first. Listen for bowel sounds in each quadrant. Then, using the bell of the stethoscope, listen for abdominal bruits.

As you palpate the abdomen, note any rigidity, tenderness, or rebound tenderness. Next, palpate the size of the liver. Then percuss the abdomen and liver for any abnormalities.

Causes
Appendicitis
The patient with appendicitis will feel nauseated and may vomit. He'll also have vague epigastric or periumbilical discomfort that localizes in the right lower quadrant.

Cholecystitis (acute)
In this disorder, nausea commonly follows severe right upper quadrant pain that may radiate to the back or shoulders. Associated finding include abdominal tenderness, vomiting and, possibly, abdominal rigidity and distention, diaphoresis, and fever with chills.

Gastritis
Patients with gastritis often experience nausea, especially after ingestion of alcohol, aspirin, spicy foods, or caffeine. Belching, epigastric pain, fever, malaise, and vomiting of mucus or blood may also occur.

Other causes
Nausea may result from cirrhosis, an electrolyte imbalance, labyrinthitis, metabolic acidosis, myocardial infarction, a renal or urologic disorder, or ulcerative colitis. Use of an anesthetic, an antibiotic, an antineoplastic, ferrous sulfate, oral potassium, or quinidine, or an overdose of a digitalis glycoside or theophylline may also trigger nausea, as may radiation therapy or surgery —

especially abdominal surgery. Certain herbal medicines, such as gingko biloba and St. John's wort, may also cause nausea.

Pain, abdominal

Usually, abdominal pain results from GI disorders, but it can also stem from reproductive, genitourinary, musculoskeletal, or vascular disorders; from drug use; or from the effect of toxins. Abdominal pain may originate in the abdominopelvic viscera, the parietal peritoneum, or the capsules of the liver, kidneys, or spleen. The pain may be acute or chronic, diffuse or localized.

Health history

■ When did the pain begin? What does it feel like? How long does it last? Where exactly is it? Does it radiate to other areas, such as the chest or back? Does it get better or worse when you change position, move, exert yourself, cough, eat, or have a bowel movement?
■ Does fever occur during episodes of pain? Do you have appetite changes, constipation, diarrhea, nausea, pain with urination, pink or cloudy urine, vomiting, or urinary frequency or urgency?
■ Do you have a history of adrenal disease, heart disease, recent infection, or recent blunt trauma to the abdomen, flank, or chest? Have you had any condition that could predispose you to emboli or that could narrow an arterial lumen? Have you recently undergone a urinary tract procedure or surgery? Have you traveled to a foreign country recently?
■ For women of childbearing age: What was the date of your last menses? Has your menstrual pattern changed? Could you be pregnant?
■ Have you ever used I.V. drugs? Do you drink alcohol? If so, how much and how often? What prescription drugs do you take?

Physical examination

After assessing the patient's level of consciousness, observe his skin for diaphoresis, jaundice, and turgor. Then check for coolness, discoloration, and edema of the arms and legs. Inspect the abdomen and chest for signs of trauma: A bluish discoloration around the umbilicus (Cullen's sign) and around the flank area (Turner's sign) can indicate blunt trauma. Obtain a record a baseline measurement of abdominal girth at the umbilicus.

After inspecting for neck vein distention, observe the rate and depth of respirations, noting any abnormal patterns. Observe the color and odor of the patient's urine.

Because palpation and percussion can affect the frequency and intensity of bowel sounds, you should auscultate the abdomen first. Listen for bowel sounds in each quadrant, noting whether the sounds are high-pitched and tinkling, hyperactive, or absent.

Listen to the patient's heart and breath sounds for abnormalities. Also, monitor his blood pressure and pulse pressure.

As you systematically palpate the abdominal, pelvic, flank, and epigastric areas, note any enlarged organs, masses, rigidity, tenderness, rebound tenderness, or tenderness with guarding. Check the patient's peripheral pulses for rate, rhythm, and intensity.

Percuss each abdominal quadrant, noting tenderness, increased pain, and percussion sounds. Dull percussion sounds indicate free fluid; hollow sounds, air.

Causes

Abdominal aortic aneurysm (dissecting)
Constant, dull upper abdominal pain radiating to the lower back typically accompanies rapid aneurysm enlargement and may indicate a rupture. Palpation may reveal an epigastric mass

that pulsates before rupture. On auscultation, you may detect a systolic bruit over the aneurysm. You may also note abdominal rigidity, increasing abdominal girth, and signs of hypovolemic shock.

Abdominal trauma

The patient may have generalized or localized abdominal pain along with abdominal ecchymosis, abdominal tenderness, or vomiting. If he's hemorrhaging into the peritoneal cavity, you may note abdominal rigidity, dullness on percussion, and increasing abdominal girth. You may hear hollow bowel sounds if an abdominal organ has been perforated, or bowel sounds may be absent. Bowel sounds heard in the chest cavity usually signal a diaphragmatic tear.

Appendicitis

The patient with appendicitis may have sudden pain in the epigastric or umbilical region that increases over a few hours or days, along with flulike symptoms. Anorexia, constipation or diarrhea, nausea, and vomiting precede the pain, which may be dull or severe. Pain localizes at McBurney's point in the right lower quadrant. Abdominal rigidity and rebound tenderness may also occur.

Ectopic pregnancy

Lower abdominal pain may be sharp, dull, or cramping, and either constant or intermittent. The pain may be accompanied by breast tenderness, nausea, vaginal bleeding, vomiting, and urinary frequency. The patient typically has a 1- to 2-month history of amenorrhea. Rupture of the fallopian tube produces sharp lower abdominal pain, which may radiate to the shoulders and neck and become extreme on cervical or adnexal palpation.

Hepatitis

Liver enlargement from any type of hepatitis causes discomfort or dull pain and tenderness in the right upper quadrant.

Intestinal obstruction

With an intestinal obstruction, short episodes of intense, colicky, cramping pain alternate with pain-free periods.

Pancreatitis

The characteristic symptom of pancreatitis is fulminating, continuous upper abdominal pain that may radiate to both flanks and to the back.

Renal calculi

Depending on the location of the calculi, the patient may feel severe abdominal or back pain. However, the classic symptom of renal calculi is colicky pain that travels from the costovertebral angle to the flank, the suprapubic region, and the external genitalia.

Other causes

Abdominal pain may result from adrenal crisis, cholecystitis, heart failure, diabetic ketoacidosis, diverticulitis, hepatic abscess, mesenteric artery ischemia, myocardial infarction, an ovarian cyst, a perforated ulcer, peritonitis, pneumonia, pneumothorax, pyelonephritis, renal infarction, or splenic infarction. Also, salicylates and nonsteroidal antiinflammatory drugs can produce abdominal pain.

Pain, back

Back pain may be acute, chronic, constant, or intermittent. It also may remain localized in the back or radiate along the spine or down one or both legs. A patient's pain may be exacerbated by activity (most commonly, stooping or lifting) and alleviated by rest. Or it may be unaffected by either.

Intrinsic back pain results from muscle spasm, nerve root irritation, fracture, or a combination of these causes. It usually occurs in the lower back or lumbosacral area. Back pain may also be referred from the abdomen, possibly signaling a life-threatening disorder.

Health history

■ When did the pain first occur? What does it feel like? Is it mild, moderate, or severe? Is it constant or intermittent? Where exactly is it? Is it associated with activity? What relieves or exacerbates it? For women of childbearing age: Does the pain occur before or during your menses?
■ Have you had recent episodes of abdominal tenderness or rigidity, fever, nausea, or vomiting? Do you feel any unusual sensations in your legs? Have you had urinary frequency or urgency or painful urination?
■ Do you have a history of trauma, back surgery, or urinary tract surgery, procedures, obstructions, or infections?
■ What medications are you taking?

Physical examination

Observe the rate and depth of respirations, noting any breathing difficulty or abnormal breathing patterns. Check the skin for diaphoresis, discoloration, edema, mottling, and pallor. Then inspect the back, legs, and abdomen for signs of trauma. After checking for abdominal distention, take a baseline abdominal girth measurement.

Because palpation and percussion can affect the frequency and intensity of bowel sounds, you should auscultate the abdomen first. Listen for bowel sounds in each quadrant. Then listen over the abdominal aorta for bruits and over the lungs for crackles. Also monitor the patient's blood pressure and pulse pressure.

Palpate the abdominal, epigastric, and pelvic areas for abdominal rigidity, enlarged organs, masses, and tenderness. If you feel any pulsations, don't palpate deeply. Check the peripheral pulses for rate, rhythm, and intensity. Then gently palpate the painful area, noting contractions, excessive muscle tone, or spasm.

Finally, percuss each abdominal quadrant. Noting any abnormal sounds, increased pain, or tenderness.

Causes

Abdominal aortic aneurysm (dissecting)
Low back pain and dull upper abdominal pain commonly accompany a rapidly enlarging aneurysm and may indicate the early stages of rupture. On palpation, you may detect tenderness over the aneurysm area and a pulsating epigastric mass. Other signs include absent femoral and pedal pulses, mottling of the skin below the waist, and signs of hypovolemic shock.

Pancreatitis
Fulminating, continuous abdominal pain that may radiate to the back and both flanks characterizes pancreatitis. You may also note abdominal tenderness, rigidity, and distention; fever; hypoactive bowel sounds; pallor; tachycardia; and vomiting. The history may include alcohol abuse, use of a thiazide diuretic, gallbladder disease, and trauma.

Pyelonephritis (acute)
The patient with acute pyelonephritis has progressive back pain or tenderness in the flank area, accompanied by costovertebral angle pain and abdominal pain in one or two quadrants. Associated signs and symptoms include dysuria, high fever, hematuria, nocturia, shaking chills, vomiting, and urinary frequency and urgency. The history may reveal a recent urinary tract procedure, urinary tract infection or

obstruction, compromised renal function, or neurogenic bladder.

Other causes
Back pain may also result from appendicitis, cholecystitis, a herniated disk, a lumbosacral sprain, osteoporosis, a perforated ulcer, renal calculi, a tumor, or vertebral osteomyelitis.

Pain, chest

Patients describe chest pain in many ways. They may report a dull ache, a sensation of heaviness or fullness, a feeling of indigestion, or a sharp, shooting pain. The pain may be constant or intermittent, may radiate to other body parts, and may arise suddenly or gradually. Patients may say that stress, anxiety, exertion, deep breathing, or certain foods seem to trigger the pain.

Chest pain may indicate several acute and life-threatening cardiopulmonary and GI conditions. But it can also result from musculoskeletal and hematologic disorders, anxiety, and certain drugs.

Health history
■ When did the chest pain begin? Did it develop suddenly or gradually? Is the pain localized or diffuse? Does it radiate to the neck, jaw, arms, or back? Is the pain sharp and stabbing or dull and aching? Is it constant or intermittent? Does breathing, changing positions, or eating certain foods exacerbate or relieve the pain?
■ Do you have other signs and symptoms, such as coughing, shortness of breath, headache, nausea, palpitations, vomiting, or weakness?
■ Have you ever had cardiac or respiratory disease, cardiac surgery, chest trauma, or intestinal disease? Do you have a family history of cardiac disease?

■ Do you drink alcohol or use illicit drugs? What medications are you taking?

Physical examination
Assess the patient's skin temperature, color, and general appearance, noting coolness, cyanosis, diaphoresis, mottling below the waist, pallor, peripheral edema, and prolonged capillary refill time. Also look for facial edema, jugular vein distention, and tracheal deviation. Note any signs of altered level of consciousness, anxiety, dizziness, or restlessness.

Observe the rate and depth of the patient's respirations, noting any abnormal patterns or breathing difficulty. If the patient has a productive cough, examine the sputum.

Palpate the patient's neck, chest, and abdomen. Note any asymmetrical chest expansion, masses, subcutaneous (S.C.) crepitation, tender areas, tracheal deviation, or tactile fremitus. Also palpate his peripheral pulses, and record their rate, rhythm, and intensity.

As you percuss over an affected lung, note any dullness. Then auscultate the lungs to identify crackles, diminished or absent breath sounds, pleural friction rubs, rhonchi, or wheezes. Auscultate the heart for clicks, gallops, murmurs, and pericardial friction rub. To check for abdominal bruits, apply the bell of the stethoscope over the abdominal aorta. Also monitor the patient's blood pressure closely.

Causes
Angina
Angina usually begins gradually, builds to a peak, and then slowly subsides. The pain can last from 2 to 10 minutes. It occurs in the retrosternal region and radiates to the neck, jaw, and arms. Associated signs and symptoms include diaphoresis, dyspnea, nausea, vomiting, palpitations, and tachycardia. On

auscultation, you may detect an atrial gallop (or fourth heart sound [S_4]), or a murmur. Attacks may occur at rest or be provoked by exertion, emotional stress, or a heavy meal.

Aortic aneurysm (dissecting)
A patient with a dissecting aortic aneurysm complains of sudden, excruciating, tearing pain in the chest and neck, radiating to the upper back, lower back, and abdomen. Other signs and symptoms include abdominal tenderness; heart murmurs; jugular vein distention; systolic bruits; tachycardia; weak or absent femoral or pedal pulses; and pale, cool, diaphoretic, mottled skin below the waist.

Cholecystitis
With this disorder, the patient has sudden epigastric or right upper quadrant pain, which may be steady or intermittent, radiate to the back, and be sharp or intense. Other signs and symptoms include chills, diaphoresis, nausea, and vomiting. Palpation of the right upper quadrant may reveal distention, rigidity, tenderness, and a mass.

Myocardial infarction
Usually, the patient has severe crushing substernal pain that radiates to the left arm, jaw, or neck. The pain may be accompanied by anxiety, clammy skin, diaphoresis, dyspnea, a feeling of impending doom, nausea, vomiting, pallor, and restlessness. The patient may have an atrial gallop (or an S_4), crackles, hypotension, or hypertension, murmurs, and a pericardial friction rub. A history of heart disease, hypertension, hypercholesterolemia, or cocaine abuse is common.

Peptic ulcer
A sharp, burning pain arising in the epigastric region, usually hours after eating, characterizes peptic ulcer. Other signs and symptoms include epigastric tenderness, nausea, and vomiting. Food or antacids usually relieve the pain.

Pneumothorax
A collapsed lung produces a sudden, sharp, severe chest pain that's commonly unilateral and that increases with chest movement. You may detect decreased breath sounds, hyperresonant or tympanic percussion sounds, and S.C. crepitation. Other signs and symptoms include accessory muscle use, anxiety, asymmetrical chest expansion, nonproductive cough, tachycardia, and tachypnea. The history may include chronic obstructive pulmonary disease, lung cancer, diagnostic or therapeutic procedures involving the thorax, or thoracic trauma.

Pulmonary embolism
Typically, the patient experiences sudden dyspnea with an intense anginalike or pleuritic ischemic pain that's aggravated by deep breathing and thoracic movement. Other findings include anxiety, cough with blood-tinged sputum, crackles, dull percussion sounds, restlessness, and tachycardia. If the embolism is large, the cardiovascular, pulmonary, and neurologic systems may be compromised. The patient's history may reveal thrombophlebitis, a hip or leg fracture, acute myocardial infarction, heart failure, pregnancy, or the use of oral contraceptives.

Other causes
Chest pain may also result from abrupt withdrawal of beta-adrenergic blockers, acute bronchitis, anxiety, esophageal spasm, esophageal reflux, lung abscess, muscle strain, pancreatitis, pneumonia, a rib fracture, or tuberculosis.

Palpitations

Defined as a person's conscious awareness of his own heartbeat, palpitations are usually felt over the precordium or in the throat or neck. The patient may describe his heart as pounding, jumping, turning, fluttering, flopping, or missing or skipping beats. Palpitations may be regular or irregular, fast or slow, and paroxysmal or sustained. Besides cardiac causes, palpitations may stem from anxiety, drug reactions, hypertension, thyroid hormone deficiency, and several other problems.

Health history
■ When did the palpitations start? Where do you feel them? How would you describe them? What were you doing when they started? How long did they last? Have you ever had palpitations before?
■ Do you have chest pain, dizziness, or weakness along with the palpitations?
■ Are you under unusual stress at home or at work? Have you recently undergone multiple blood transfusions or an infusion of phosphate?
■ Have you ever had thyroid disease, calcium or vitamin D deficiency, malabsorption syndrome, bone cancer, renal disease, hypoglycemia, or cardiovascular or pulmonary disorders that may produce arrhythmias or hypertension?
■ What medications are you taking? Are you taking an over-the-counter drug that contains caffeine or a sympathomimetic, such as a cough, cold, or allergy preparation? Do you smoke or drink alcohol? If so, how much?

Physical examination
Assess the patient's level of consciousness, noting any anxiety, confusion, or irrational behavior. Check his skin for pallor and diaphoresis. Then observe the eyes for exophthalmos.

Note the rate and depth of his respirations, checking for abnormal patterns and breathing difficulty. Also inspect the fingertips for capillary nail bed pulsations.

To check for thyroid gland enlargement, gently palpate the patient's neck. Then palpate his muscles for weakness and twitching. Evaluate his peripheral pulses, noting the rate, rhythm, and intensity. Assess his reflexes for hyperreflexia.

Auscultate the heart for gallops and murmurs, and the lungs for abnormal breath sounds. Also monitor blood pressure and pulse pressure.

Causes
Acute anxiety attack
Palpations may be accompanied by diaphoresis, facial flushing, and trembling. The patient usually hyperventilates, which may lead to dizziness, syncope, and weakness.

Cardiac arrhythmias
Paroxysmal or sustained palpitations may occur with dizziness, fatigue, and weakness. Other signs and symptoms include chest pain, confusion, decreased blood pressure, diaphoresis, pallor, and an irregular, rapid, or slow pulse rate. The patient may be taking a drug that can cause cardiac arrhythmias — for instance, an antihypertensive, a sympathomimetic, a ganglionic blocker, an anticholinergic, or a methylxanthine.

Thyrotoxicosis
In this disorder, sustained palpitations may accompany diaphoresis, diarrhea, dyspnea, heat intolerance, nervousness, tachycardia, tremors, and weight loss despite increased appetite. Exophthalmos and an enlarged thyroid gland may also develop.

Other causes

Palpitations may also arise from anemia, aortic insufficiency, hypocalcemia, hypertension, hypoglycemia, mitral valve stenosis or prolapse, and pheochromocytoma. Also, certain herbal medicines, such as ginseng and ephedra, may cause palpitations.

Paresthesia

Paresthesia is an abnormal sensation, commonly described as a numbness, prickling, or tingling, that's felt along peripheral nerve pathways. It may develop suddenly or gradually and be transient or permanent. A common symptom of many neurologic disorders, paresthesia may also occur in certain systemic disorders and with the use of certain drugs.

Health history

■ When did the paresthesia begin? What does if feel like? Where does it occur? Is it transient, or constant?
■ Have you had recent trauma, surgery, or an invasive procedure that may have injured peripheral nerves? Have you been exposed to industrial solvents or heavy metals? Have you had long-term radiation therapy? Do you have any neurologic, cardiovascular, metabolic, renal, or chronic inflammatory disorders, such as arthritis or lupus erythematosus?
■ What medications are you taking?

Physical examination

Focus on the patient's neurologic status, assessing his level of consciousness and cranial nerve function. Also note this skin color and temperature.

Test muscle strength and deep tendon reflexes in the extremities that paresthesia has affected. Systematically evaluate light touch, pain, temperature, vibration, and position sensation. Then palpate his pulses.

Causes

Arterial occlusion (acute)

A patient with a saddle embolus may complain of sudden paresthesia and coldness in one or both legs. Aching pain at rest, intermittent claudication, and paresis are also characteristic. The leg becomes mottled, and a line of temperature and color demarcation develops at the level of the occlusion. Pulses are absent below the occlusion and capillary refill time is diminished.

Brain tumor

Tumors that affect the parietal lobe may cause progressive contralateral paresthesia accompanied by agnosia, agraphia, apraxia, homonymous hemianopia, and loss of proprioception.

Herniated disk

Herniation of a lumbar or cervical disk may cause acute or gradual paresthesia along the distribution pathways of the affected spinal nerves. Other neuromuscular effects include muscle spasms, severe pain, and weakness.

Herpes zoster

Paresthesia, an early symptom of herpes zoster, occurs in the dermatome that the affected spinal nerve supplies. Within several days, this dermatome is marked by a pruritic, erythematous, vesicular rash accompanied by sharp, shooting pain.

Spinal cord injury

Paresthesia may occur in a partial spinal cord transection after spinal shock resolves. The paresthesia may be unilateral or bilateral and occur at or below in the level of the lesion.

Other disorders

Paresthesia may result from arthritis, a cerebrovascular accident, migraine headache, multiple sclerosis, peripheral neuropathies, vitamin B_{12} deficiency, hypocalcemia, and heavy metal or solvent poisoning. Also, long-term radiation therapy, parenteral gold therapy, and certain drugs — such as chemotherapeutic agents, guanadrel (Hylorel), interferons, and isoniazid (Laniazid) — may cause paresthesia.

Rash, papular

Consisting of small, raised, circumscribed and, possibly, discolored lesions, a papular rash can erupt anywhere on the body and in various configurations. A characteristic sign of many cutaneous disorders, a papular rash may also result from allergies or from infectious, neoplastic, or systemic disorders.

Age alert In bedridden elderly patients, the first sign of a pressure ulcer is commonly an erythematous area, sometimes with firm papules.

Health history
■ When and where did the rash erupt? What did it look like? Has it spread or changed in any way? If so, when and how did it spread?
■ Does the rash itch or burn? Is it painful or tender?
■ Have you had a fever, GI distress, or a headache? Do you have any allergies? Have you had any previous skin disorders, infections, sexually transmitted diseases, or tumors? What childhood diseases have you had?
■ Have you recently been bitten by an insect or a rodent or exposed to anyone with an infectious disease?
■ What medications are you taking? Have you applied any topical agents to the rash and, if so, when was the last application?

Physical examination
Observe the color, configuration, and location of the rash.

Causes
Acne vulgaris
The rupture of enlarged comedones produces inflamed and, possibly, painful and pruritic papules, pustules, nodules, or cysts. They may appear on the face, shoulders, chest, and back.

Insect bites
Venom from insect bites — especially those of ticks, lice, flies, and mosquitoes — may cause an allergic reaction that produces a papular, macular, or petechial rash. Associated findings include fever, headache, lymphadenopathy, myalgia, nausea, and vomiting.

Kaposi's sarcoma
A neoplastic disorder most commonly found in patients with acquired immunodeficiency syndrome, Kaposi's sarcoma produces purple or blue papules or macules on the extremities, ears, and nose. Firm pressure causes these lesions to decrease in size, but they return to their original size within 10 to 15 seconds. The lesions may become scaly, ulcerate, and bleed.

Psoriasis
In this disorder, small, erythematous, pruritic papules appear on the scalp, chest, elbows, knees, back, buttocks, and genitalia. The papules may be painful. They enlarge and coalesce, forming elevated, red, plaques covered by silver scales, except in moist areas, such as the genitalia. The scales may flake off easily or thicken, covering the plaque. Other common findings include pitted fingernails and arthralgia.

Other causes
Infectious mononucleosis or sarcoidosis may produce a papular rash. Such a rash may also be caused by nonsteroidal anti-inflammatory drugs, succimer (Chemet), and interferons.

Rash, pustular

Crops of pustules (small, elevated, circumscribed lesions), vesicles (small blisters), and bullae (large blisters) filled with purulent exudate make up a pustular rash. The lesions vary in size and shape and may be generalized or localized (limited to the hair follicles or sweat glands).

Pustules may result from skin disorders, systemic disorders, ingestion of certain drugs, and exposure to skin irritants. Although many pustular lesions are sterile, a pustular rash usually indicates infection.

Health history
■ When and where did the rash erupt? Did another type of skin lesion precede the pustules?
■ What does the rash look like? Has it spread or changed in any way? If so, how and where did it spread?
■ Have you or a family member ever had a skin disorder or allergies?
■ What medications are you taking? Have you applied any topical medication to the rash and, if so, when did you last apply it?

Physical examination
Examine the entire skin surface, noting if it's dry, oily, moist, or greasy. Record the exact location, distribution, color, shape, and size of the lesions.

Causes
Folliculitis
A bacterial infection of the hair follicles, folliculitis produces individual pustules, each pierced by a hair. The patient may also suffer from pruritus. Hot-tub folliculitis is characterized by pustules on the area that a bathing suit covers.

Scabies
Threadlike channels or burrows under the skin characterize scabies, a disorder that can also produce pustules, vesicles, and excoriations. The lesions are 1 to 10 cm long, with a swollen nodule or red papule containing the itch mite. In men, crusted lesions commonly develop on the glans and shaft of the penis and on the scrotum. In women, lesions may form on the nipples. Other common sites include the wrists, elbows, axillae, and waist.

Other causes
A pustular rash may result from acne vulgaris, blastomycosis, furunculosis, and pustular psoriasis. Also, certain drugs — such as bromides, iodides, corticotropin, corticosteroids, lithium (Eskalith), phenytoin (Dilantin), phenobarbital (Luminal), isoniazid (Laniazid), and oral contraceptives — can cause a pustular rash.

Rash, vesicular

The lesions in a vesicular rash are scattered or linear vesicles that are sharply circumscribed and usually less than 0.5 cm in diameter. They may be filled with clear, cloudy, or bloody fluid. Lesions larger than 0.5 cm in diameter are called bullae. A vesicular rash may be mild or severe, transient, or permanent.

Health history
■ When and where did the rash erupt? Did other skin lesions precede the vesicles?
■ What does the rash look like? Has it spread or changed in any way? If so, how and where did it spread?
■ Do you or your family have a history of allergies or skin disorders?
■ Have you recently had an infection or been bitten by an insect?

Physical examination
Examine the patient's skin and note the location, general distribution, color, shape, and size of the lesions. Check

for crusts, macules, papules, scales, scars, and wheals. Note whether the outer layer of epidermis separates easily from the basal layer.

Palpate the vesicles or bullae to determine whether they're flaccid or tense.

Causes
Burns
Thermal burns that affect the epidermis and part of the dermis commonly cause vesicles and bullae, along with erythema, moistness, pain, and swelling.

Herpes zoster
First, fever and malaise occur. Then the vesicular rash appears along a dermatome. This rash is accompanied by pruritis, deep pain, and paresthesia or hyperesthesia, usually of the trunk and sometimes of the arms and legs. The vesicles erupt, dry up, and form scabs in about 10 days. Occasionally, herpes zoster involves the cranial nerves; such involvement produces dizziness, eye pain, facial palsy, hearing loss, impaired vision, and loss of taste.

Other causes
Other causes of vesicular rashes include dermatitis, herpes simplex, insect bites, pemphigus, scabies, tinea pedis, and toxic epidermal necrolysis.

Vision loss

Vision loss can occur suddenly or gradually, be temporary or permanent, and may range from a slight impairment to total blindness. It may result from eye, neurologic, and systemic disorders as well as from trauma and reactions to certain drugs.

Health history
■ When did the loss first occur? Did it occur suddenly or gradually? Does it affect one or both eyes? Does it affect all or part of the visual field?
■ Are you experiencing blurred vision, halo vision, nausea, pain, photosensitivity, or vomiting with the vision loss?
■ Have you had a recent facial or eye injury?
■ Have you ever had a cardiovascular or endocrine disorder, an infection, or allergies? Does anyone in your family have a history of vision loss or other eye problems?
■ What medications are you taking?

Physical examination
Observe the patient's eyes for conjunctival or scleral redness, drainage, edema, foreign bodies, and signs of trauma. With a flashlight, examine the cornea and iris. Observe the size, shape, and color of the pupils. Then test direct and consensual light reflexes and visual accommodation, extraocular muscle function, and visual acuity. Gently palpate each eye, noting any hardness. Then auscultate over the neck and temple for carotid bruits.

Causes
Glaucoma
Acute angle-closure glaucoma may cause rapid blindness. Findings include halo vision, nonreactive pupillary response, photophobia, rapid onset of unilateral inflammation and pain, and reduced visual acuity. By contrast, chronic open-angle glaucoma progresses slowly. Usually bilateral, it causes aching eyes, halo vision, peripheral vision loss, and reduced visual acuity.

Eye trauma
Sudden unilateral or bilateral vision loss may occur after eye injury. The loss may be total or partial, permanent or temporary. The eyelids may be reddened, edematous, and lacerated.

Other causes
Vision loss may also be caused by congenital rubella or syphilis, herpes zoster, Marfan's syndrome, a pituitary tumor, retrolental fibroplasia, and drugs such as digitalis glycosides, indomethacin (Indocin), ethambutol hydrochloride (Myambutol), and methanol.

Visual floaters

Particles of blood or cellular debris that move about in the vitreous humor appear as spots or dots when they enter the visual field. Chronic floaters commonly occur in elderly or myopic patients. But the sudden onset of visual floaters commonly signals retinal detachment, an ocular emergency.

Health history
■ When did the floaters first appear? What do they look like? Did they appear suddenly or gradually? If they appeared suddenly, did you also see flashing lights and have a curtainlike loss of vision?
■ Are you nearsighted, and do you wear corrective lenses?
■ Do you have a history of eye trauma or other eye disorders, allergies, granulomatous disease, diabetes mellitus, or hypertension?
■ What medications are you taking?

Physical examination
Inspect the eyes for signs of injury, such as bruising or edema. Then assess the patient's visual acuity, using the Snellen alphabet or "E" chart.

Causes
Retinal detachment
Floaters and light flashes appear suddenly in the portion of the visual field where the retina has detached. As retinal detachment progresses (a painless process), gradual vision loss occurs, with the patient seeing a "curtain"

falling in front of his eyes. Ophthalmoscopic examination reveals a gray, opaque, detached retina with an indefinite margin. Retinal vessels appear almost black.

Vitreous hemorrhage
Rupture of retinal vessels produces a shower of red or black dots or a red haze across the visual field. Vision blurs suddenly in the affected eye, and visual acuity may be greatly reduced.

Other causes
Visual floaters may also result from posterior uveitis.

Weight loss

Weight loss can reflect decreased food intake, increased metabolic requirements, or a combination of the two. Its causes include endocrine, neoplastic, GI, and psychological disorders; nutritional deficiencies; infections; and neurologic lesions that cause paralysis and dysphagia. Weight loss may also accompany conditions that prevent sufficient food intake, such as painful oral lesions, ill-fitting dentures, and the loss of teeth. Weight loss may stem from poverty, adherence to fad diets, excessive exercise, or drug use.

Health history
■ When did you first notice you were losing weight? How much weight have you lost? Was the loss intentional? If not, can you think of any reason for it?
■ What do you usually eat in a day? Have your eating habits changed recently? Why?
■ Have your stools changed recently? For instance, have you noticed bulky, floating stools or have you had diarrhea? What about abdominal pain, excessive thirst, excessive urination, heat intolerance, nausea, or vomiting?

■ Have you felt anxious or depressed? If so, why?

■ What medications are you taking? Do you take diet pills or laxatives to lose weight?

Physical examination
Record the patient's height and weight. As you take his vital signs, note his general appearance. Does he appear well nourished? Do his clothes fit? Is muscle wasting evident?

Next, examine his skin for turgor and abnormal pigmentation, especially around the joints. Does he have jaundice or pallor? Examine his mouth, including the condition of his teeth or dentures. Also check his eyes for exophthalmos and his neck for swelling.

Finally, palpate the patient's abdomen for liver enlargement, masses, and tenderness.

Causes
Anorexia nervosa
A psychogenic disorder, anorexia nervosa is most common in young women and is characterized by a severe, self-imposed weight loss. This may be accompanied by amenorrhea, blotchy or sallow skin, cold intolerance, constipation, frequent infections, loss of fatty tissue, loss of scalp hair, and skeletal muscle atrophy.

Cancer
Weight loss is a common sign of cancer. Associated signs and symptoms reflect the type, location, and stage of the tumor, and typically include abnormal bleeding, anorexia, fatigue, nausea, pain, a palpable mass, and vomiting.

Crohn's disease
Weight loss occurs with abdominal pain, anorexia, and chronic cramping. Other findings include abdominal distention, tenderness, and guarding; diarrhea; hyperactive bowel sounds; pain; and tachycardia.

Depression
Patients with severe depression may experience weight loss, along with anorexia, apathy, fatigue, feelings of worthlessness, and insomnia or hypersomnia. Other signs and symptoms include incoherence, indecisiveness, and suicidal thoughts or behavior.

Leukemia
Acute leukemia causes a progressive weight loss accompanied by bleeding tendencies, high fever, and severe prostration. Chronic leukemia causes a progressive weight loss with anemia, anorexia, bleeding tendencies, an enlarged spleen, fatigue, fever, pallor, and skin eruptions.

Other causes
Weight loss may result from adrenal insufficiency, diabetes mellitus, gastroenteritis, cryptosporidiosis, lymphoma, ulcerative colitis, and thyrotoxicosis. Drugs such as amphetamines, chemotherapeutic agents, laxatives, and thyroid preparations can also cause weight loss.

3

ECGs
Interpreting them with ease and accuracy

Normal ECG

How to read any ECG: An 8-step guide

An electrocardiogram (ECG) waveform has three basic elements: a P wave, a QRS complex, and a T wave. They're joined by five other useful diagnostic elements: the PR interval, the U wave, the ST segment, the J point, and the QT interval. The diagram below shows how these elements are related.

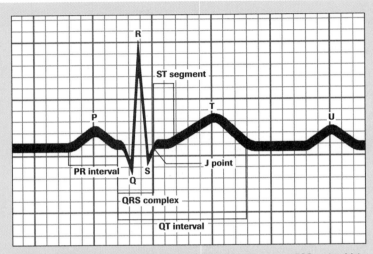

The following 8-step guide will enable you to read any electrocardiogram (ECG).

Step 1: Evaluate the P wave

Observe the P wave's size, shape, and location in the waveform. If the P wave consistently precedes the QRS complex, the sinoatrial (SA) node is initiating the electrical impulse, as it should be.

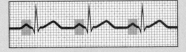

Step 2: Evaluate the atrial rhythm

The P wave should occur at regular intervals, with only small variations associated with respiration. Using a pair of calipers, you can easily measure the interval between P waves—the P-P interval. Compare the

P-P intervals in several ECG cycles. Make sure the calipers are set at the same point—at the beginning of the wave or on its peak. Instead of lifting the calipers, rotate one of its legs to the next P wave, to ensure accurate measurements.

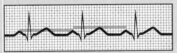

Step 3: Determine the atrial rate

To determine the atrial rate quickly, count the number of P waves in two 3-second segments. Multiply this number by 10. For a more accurate determination, count the number of small squares between two P waves, using either the apex of the wave or the initial upstroke of the wave. Each small square equals 0.04 second; 1,500 squares equal 1 minute ($0.04 \times 1,500 = 60$ seconds). So, divide 1,500 by the number of squares you counted between the P waves. This gives you the atrial rate — the number of contractions per minute.

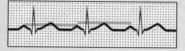

Step 4: Calculate duration of the PR interval

Count the number of small squares between the beginning of the P wave and the beginning of the QRS complex. Multiply the number of squares by 0.04 second. The normal interval is between 0.12 and 0.20 second, or between 3 and 5 small squares wide. A wider interval indicates delayed conduction of the impulse through the atrioventricular node to the ventricles. A short PR interval indicates the impulse originated in an area other than the SA node.

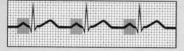

Step 5: Evaluate the ventricular rhythm

Use the calipers to measure the R-R intervals. Remember to place the calipers on the same point of the QRS complex. If the R-R intervals remain consistent, the ventricular rhythm is regular.

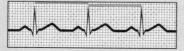

Step 6: Determine the ventricular rate

To determine the ventricular rate, use the same formula as in Step 3. In this case, however, count the number of small squares between two R waves to do the calculation. Also check that the QRS complex is shaped appropriately for the lead you're monitoring.

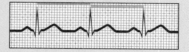

Step 7: Calculate the duration of the QRS complex

Count the number of squares between the beginning and the end of the QRS complex and multiply by 0.04 second. A normal QRS complex is less than 0.12 second, or less than 3 small squares wide. Some references specify 0.06 to 0.10 second as the normal duration for the QRS complex.

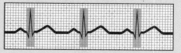

Step 8: Calculate the duration of the QT interval

Count the number of squares from the beginning of the QRS complex to the end of the T wave. Multiply this number by 0.04 second. The normal range is 0.36 to 0.44 second, or 9 to 11 small squares wide.

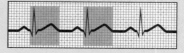

Normal sinus rhythm

When the heart functions normally, the sinoatrial (SA) node acts as the primary pacemaker, initiating the electrical impulses that set the rhythm for cardiac contractions. The SA node assumes this role because its automatic firing rate exceeds that of the heart's other pacemakers, allowing cells to depolarize spontaneously. Two factors account for increased automaticity. First, during the resting phase of the depolarization-repolarization cycle, SA node cells have the least negative charge. Second, depolarization actually begins during the resting phase.

Based on the location of the electrical disturbance, an arrhythmia can be classified as a sinus, atrial, junctional, or ventricular arrhythmia or an atrioventricular (AV) block. Functional disturbances in the SA node produce sinus arrhythmias. Enhanced automaticity of atrial tissue or reentry may produce atrial arrhythmias, the most common arrhythmias.

Junctional arrhythmias originate in the area around the AV node and the bundle of His. These arrhythmias usually result from a suppressed higher pacemaker or blocked impulses at the AV node.

Ventricular arrhythmias originate in ventricular tissue below the bifurcation of the bundle of His. These rhythms may result from reentry or enhanced automaticity or after depolarization.

An AV block results from an abnormal interruption or delay of atrial impulse conduction to the ventricles. It may be partial or total and may occur in the AV node, bundle of His, or Purkinje system.

Characteristics and interpretation

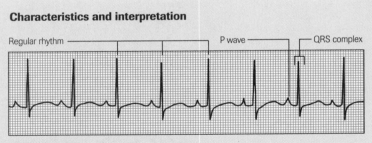

LEAD II

Atrial rhythm: regular
Ventricular rhythm: regular
Atrial rate: 60 to 100 beats/minute (80 beats/minute shown)
Ventricular rate: 60 to 100 beats/minute (80 beats/minute shown)
P wave: normally shaped (All P waves have a similar size and shape; a P wave precedes each QRS complex.)
PR interval: within normal limits (0.12 to 0.20 second) and constant (0.20-second duration shown)

QRS complex: within normal limits (0.06 to 0.10 second) (All QRS complexes have the same configuration. The duration shown here is 0.12 second.)
T wave: normally shaped; upright and rounded (Each QRS complex is followed by a T wave.)
QT interval: within normal limits (0.36 to 0.44 second) and constant (0.44-second duration shown)

Arrhythmias

Sinus arrhythmia

In sinus arrhythmia, the heart rate stays within normal limits but the rhythm is irregular and corresponds to the respiratory cycle and variations in vagal tone. During inspiration, an increased volume of blood returns to the heart, reducing vagal tone and increasing sinus rate. During expiration, venous return decreases, vagal tone increases, and sinus rate slows.

Conditions unrelated to respiration may also produce sinus arrhythmia. These conditions include an inferior-

wall myocardial infarction, digoxin toxicity, and increased intracranial pressure.

Sinus arrhythmia is easily recognized in elderly, pediatric, and sedated patients. The patient's pulse rate increases with inspiration and decreases with expiration. Usually, the patient is asymptomatic.

Intervention

Treatment usually isn't necessary, unless the patient is symptomatic or the sinus arrhythmia stems from an underlying cause. If the patient is symptomatic and his heart rate falls below 40 beats/minute, atropine may be administered.

Characteristics and interpretation

Cyclic irregular rhythm

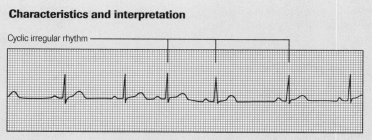

LEAD II

Atrial rhythm: irregular, corresponding to the respiratory cycle
Ventricular rhythm: irregular, corresponding to the respiratory cycle
Atrial rate: within normal limits; varies with respiration (60 beats/minute shown)
Ventricular rate: within normal limits; varies with respiration (60 beats/minute shown)
P wave: normal size and configuration (One P wave precedes each QRS complex.)

PR interval: within normal limits (0.16-second, constant interval shown)
QRS complex: normal duration and configuration (0.06-second duration shown)
T wave: normal size and configuration
QT interval: within normal limits (0.36-second interval shown)
Other: phasic slowing and quickening of the rhythm

Sinus bradycardia

Characterized by a sinus rate of less than 60 beats/minute, sinus bradycardia usually occurs as the normal response to a reduced demand for blood flow. It's common among athletes, whose well-conditioned hearts can maintain stroke volume with reduced effort. Certain drugs — such as cardiac glycosides, calcium channel blockers, and beta-adrenergic blockers — may cause sinus bradycardia. It may occur after an inferior-wall myocardial infarction involving the right coronary artery, which provides the blood supply to the sinoatrial node. The rhythm may develop during sleep and in patients with increased intracranial pressure. It may also result from vagal stimulation during vomiting or defecation. Pathologi-cal sinus bradycardia may occur with sick sinus syndrome.

A patient with sinus bradycardia is asymptomatic if he's able to compensate for the drop in heart rate by increasing stroke volume. If not, he may have signs and symptoms of decreased cardiac output, such as hypotension, syncope, confusion, and blurred vision.

Intervention
If the patient is asymptomatic, treatment isn't necessary. If he has signs and symptoms, treatment aims to identify and correct the underlying cause. The heart rate may be increased with such drugs as atropine and isoproterenol (Isuprel). A temporary or permanent pacemaker may be inserted if the bradycardia persists.

Characteristics and interpretation

Regular rhythm with rate less than 60 beats/minute

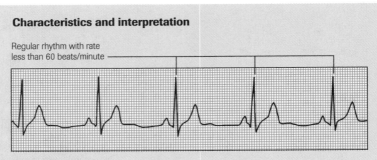

LEAD II

Atrial rhythm: regular
Ventricular rhythm: regular
Atrial rate: less than 60 beats/minute (50 beats/minute shown)
Ventricular rate: less than 60 beats/minute (50 beats/minute shown)
P wave: normal size and configuration (One P wave precedes each QRS complex.)

PR interval: within normal limits and constant (0.14-second duration shown)
QRS complex: normal duration and configuration (0.08-second duration shown)
T wave: normal size and configuration
QT interval: within normal limits (0.40-second interval shown)

Sinus tachycardia

Sinus tachycardia is a normal response to cellular demands for increased oxygen delivery and blood flow. Conditions that cause such a demand include heart failure, shock, anemia, exercise, fever, hypoxia, pain, and stress. Drugs that stimulate the beta receptors in the heart also cause sinus tachycardia. They include isoproterenol (Isuprel), aminophylline (Aminophylline), and inotropic agents such as dobutamine. Alcohol, caffeine, and nicotine may also produce sinus tachycardia.

An elevated heart rate increases myocardial oxygen demands. If the patient can't meet these demands (for example, because of coronary artery disease), ischemia and further myocardial damage may occur. If tachycardia exceeds 140 beats/minute for longer than 30 minutes, the electrocardiogram may show ST-segment and T-wave changes, indicating ischemia.

Intervention

Treatment focuses on finding the primary cause. If it's high catecholamine levels, a beta-adrenergic blocker may slow the heart rate. After myocardial infarction, persistent sinus tachycardia may precede heart failure or cardiogenic shock.

Characteristics and interpretation

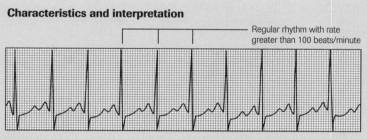

Regular rhythm with rate greater than 100 beats/minute

LEAD II

Atrial rhythm: regular
Ventricular rhythm: regular
Atrial rate: 100 to 160 beats/minute (110 beats/minute shown)
Ventricular rate: 100 to 160 beats/minute (110 beats/minute shown)
P wave: normal size and configuration (One P wave precedes each QRS complex. As the sinus rate reaches about 150 beats/minute, the P wave merges with the preceding T wave and may be difficult to identify. Examine the descending slope of the preceding T wave closely for notches, indicating the presence of the P wave. The P wave shown is normal.)
PR interval: within normal limits and constant (0.16-second duration shown)
QRS complex: normal duration and configuration (0.10-second shown)
T wave: normal size and configuration
QT interval: within normal limits and constant (0.36-second duration shown)
Other: gradual onset and cessation

Sinus arrest

Failure of the sinoatrial node to generate an impulse interrupts the sinus rhythm, producing "sinus pause" when one or two beats are dropped or "sinus arrest" when three or more beats are dropped. Such failure may result from an acute inferior-wall myocardial infarction, increased vagal tone, or use of certain drugs (cardiac glycosides, calcium channel blockers, and beta-adrenergic blockers). The arrhythmia may also be linked to sick sinus syndrome. The patient has an irregular pulse rate associated with the sinus rhythm pauses. If the pauses are infrequent, the patient is asymptomatic. If they occur frequently and last for several seconds, the patient may have signs of decreased cardiac output (CO).

Intervention
For a symptomatic patient, treatment focuses on maintaining CO and discovering the cause of the sinus arrest. If indicated, atropine may be given or a temporary or permanent pacemaker may be inserted.

Characteristics and interpretation

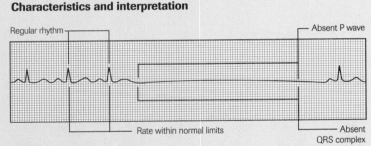

LEAD II

Atrial rhythm: regular, except for the missing complex
Ventricular rhythm: regular, except for the missing complex
Atrial rate: within normal limits but varies because of the pauses (94 beats/minute shown)
Ventricular rate: within normal limits but varies because of pauses (94 beats/minute shown)
P wave: normal size and configuration (One P wave precedes each QRS complex but is absent during a pause.)

PR interval: within normal limits and constant when the P wave is present; not measurable when the P wave is absent (0.20-second duration shown on all complexes surrounding the arrest)
QRS complex: normal duration and configuration; absent during a pause (0.08-second duration shown)
T wave: normal size and configuration; absent during a pause
QT interval: within normal limits; not measurable during pause (0.40-second, constant interval shown)

Premature atrial contractions

Premature atrial contractions (PACs) usually result from an irritable focus in the atria that supersedes the sinoatrial node as the pacemaker for one or two beats. Although PACs commonly occur in normal hearts, they're also associated with coronary artery disease and valvular heart disease. In an inferior-wall myocardial infarction (MI), PACs may indicate a concomitant right atrial infarct. In an anterior-wall MI, PACs are an early sign of left-sided heart failure. They also may warn of a more severe atrial arrhythmia, such as atrial flutter or fibrillation.

Possible causes include digoxin toxicity, hyperthyroidism, elevated catecholamine levels, acute respiratory failure, and chronic obstructive pulmonary disease.

Intervention
Symptomatic patients may be treated with propranolol (Inderal) and disopyramide (Norpace).

Characteristics and interpretation

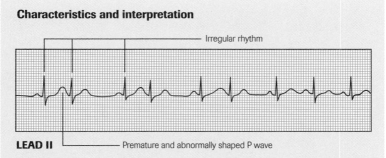

LEAD II — Premature and abnormally shaped P wave
— Irregular rhythm

Atrial rhythm: irregular (Incomplete compensatory pause follows PAC. Underlying rhythm may be regular.)
Ventricular rhythm: irregular (Incomplete compensatory pause follows PAC. Underlying rhythm may be regular.)
Atrial rate: varies with underlying rhythm (90 beats/minute shown)
Ventricular rate: varies with underlying rhythm (90 beats/minute shown)
P wave: premature and abnormally shaped; possibly lost in previous T wave (Varying configurations indicate multiform PACs.)

PR interval: usually normal but may be shortened or slightly prolonged, depending on the origin of ectopic focus (0.16-second, constant interval shown)
QRS complex: usually normal duration and configuration (0.08-second, constant duration shown)
T wave: usually normal configuration; may be distorted if the P wave is hidden in the previous T wave
QT interval: usually normal (0.36-second, constant interval shown)
Other: may occur in bigeminy or couplets

Atrial tachycardia

In atrial tachycardia, the atrial rhythm is ectopic and the atrial rate is rapid, shortening diastole. This results in a loss of atrial kick, reduced cardiac output, reduced coronary perfusion, and ischemic myocardial changes.

Although atrial tachycardia occurs in healthy patients, it's usually associated with high catecholamine levels, digoxin toxicity, myocardial infarction, cardiomyopathy, hyperthyroidism, hypertension, and valvular heart disease. Three types of atrial tachycardia exist:

atrial tachycardia with block, multifocal atrial tachycardia, and paroxysmal atrial tachycardia.

Intervention

If the patient is symptomatic, prepare for immediate cardioversion. If the patient's condition is stable, the doctor may perform carotid sinus massage (if no bruits are present) or prescribe a drug, such as adenosine (Adenocard), verapamil (Calan), digoxin (Lanoxin); a beta-adrenergic blocker; or diltiazem (Cardizem). If these measures fail, cardioversion may be necessary.

Characteristics and interpretation

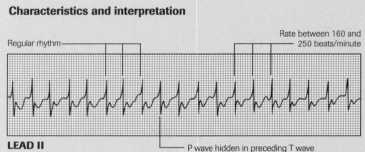

Regular rhythm

Rate between 160 and 250 beats/minute

LEAD II

P wave hidden in preceding T wave

Atrial rhythm: regular
Ventricular rhythm: regular
Atrial rate: three or more successive ectopic atrial beats at a rate of 160 to 250 beats/minute (210 beats/minute shown)
Ventricular rate: varies with atrioventricular conduction ratio (210 beats/minute shown)
P wave: 1:1 ratio with QRS complex, though generally indiscernible because of rapid rate; may be hidden in previous ST segment or T wave
PR interval: may be unmeasurable if P wave can't be distinguished from preceding T wave (If P wave is present, PR

interval is short when conduction through the AV node is 1:1. On this strip, the PR interval is indiscernible.)
QRS complex: usually normal unless aberrant intraventricular conduction is present (0.10-second duration shown)
T wave: may be normal or inverted if ischemia is present (inverted T waves shown)
QT interval: usually normal but may be shorter because of rapid rate (0.20-second interval shown)
Other: appearance of ST-segment and T-wave changes if tachyarrhythmia persists longer than 30 minutes

Atrial flutter

Characterized by an atrial rate of 300 beats/minute or more, atrial flutter results from multiple reentry circuits within the atrial tissue. Causes include conditions that enlarge atrial tissue and elevate atrial pressures. Atrial flutter is associated with myocardial infarction, increased catecholamine levels, hyperthyroidism, and digoxin toxicity. A ventricular rate of 300 beats/minute suggests the presence of an anomalous pathway.

If the patient's pulse rate is normal, he probably has no symptoms. If his pulse rate is high, he probably has signs and symptoms of decreased cardiac output, such as hypotension and syncope.

Intervention

The doctor may perform vagal stimulation to slow the ventricular response and demonstrate the presence of flutter waves. This intervention is contraindicated if a carotid bruit is present. If the patient is symptomatic, prepare for immediate cardioversion. A drug — such as a calcium channel blocker (diltiazem, verapamil) or a beta-adrenergic blocker (esmolol, metoprolol) — may be ordered to slow atrioventricular conduction. Digoxin may be ordered, but some experts question its use for urgent treatment. After the rate slows, if conversion to a normal rhythm hasn't occurred, procainamide (Pronestyl) or quinidine (Quinidex) may be ordered.

Characteristics and interpretation

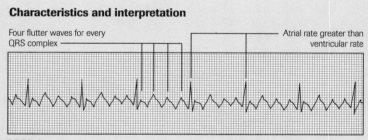

Four flutter waves for every QRS complex

Atrial rate greater than ventricular rate

LEAD II

Atrial rhythm: regular
Ventricular rhythm: may be regular or irregular, depending on the conduction ratio (regular rhythm shown)
Atrial rate: 300 to 350 beats/minute (300 beats/minute shown)
Ventricular rate: variable (70 beats/minute shown)
P wave: atrial activity seen as flutter waves, commonly with a saw-toothed appearance

PR interval: not measurable
QRS complex: usually normal but can be distorted by the underlying flutter waves (0.10-second, normal duration shown)
T wave: unidentifiable
QT interval: not measurable

Atrial fibrillation

Atrial fibrillation is defined as chaotic, asynchronous electrical activity in the atrial tissue. It results from multiple, multidirectional impulses (that is, in many reentry pathways) that cause the atria to quiver instead of contract regularly.

With this arrhythmia, blood may pool in the left atrial appendage and form thrombi that can be ejected into the systemic circulation. An associated rapid ventricular rate can decrease cardiac output.

Possible causes include valvular disorders, hypertension, coronary artery disease, myocardial infarction, chronic lung disease, ischemia, thyroid disorders, and Wolff-Parkinson-White syndrome. Atrial fibrillation may also result from high adrenergic tone secondary to physical exertion, sepsis or alcohol withdrawal, or the use of such drugs as aminophylline (Aminophylline) and cardiac glycosides.

Intervention

If the patient is symptomatic, synchronized cardioversion should be used immediately. Vagal stimulation may be used to slow the ventricular response, but it won't convert the arrhythmia. Drugs that may be ordered to slow atrioventricular conduction include calcium channel blockers (diltiazem) and beta-adrenergic blockers (metoprolol). Digoxin may be ordered if the patient's condition is stable. After the rate slows, if conversion to a normal sinus rhythm hasn't occurred, amiodarone (Cordarone), procainamide (Pronestyl), or quinidine (Quinidex) may be ordered. If atrial fibrillation lasts several days, anticoagulant therapy is recommended before pharmacologic or electrical conversion. If atrial fibrillation is of recent onset, ibutilide (Corvert) may be used to convert the rhythm.

Characteristics and interpretation

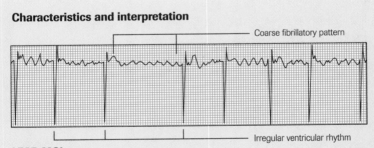

Coarse fibrillatory pattern

Irregular ventricular rhythm

LEAD MCL₁

Atrial rhythm: grossly irregular
Ventricular rhythm: grossly irregular
Atrial rate: greater than 400 beats/minute
Ventricular rate: 60 to 150 beats/minute, depending on treatment (80 beats/minute shown)
P wave: absent; appearance of erratic baseline fibrillatory waves (f waves) (When the f waves are pronounced, the arrhythmia is called coarse atrial fibrilla-

tion. When the f waves aren't pronounced, the arrhythmia is known as fine atrial fibrillation. On this strip, the f waves are pronounced.)
PR interval: indiscernible
QRS complex: duration usually within normal limits, with aberrant intraventricular conduction (0.08-second duration shown)
T wave: indiscernible
QT interval: not measurable

Junctional rhythm

Junctional rhythm occurs in the atrio-ventricular junctional tissue, producing retrograde depolarization of the atrial tissue and antegrade depolarization of the ventricular tissue. It results from conditions that depress sinoatrial node function, such as an inferior-wall myocardial infarction (MI), digoxin toxicity, and vagal stimulation. The arrhythmia may also stem from increased automaticity of the junctional tissue, which either digoxin toxicity or ischemia associated with an inferior-wall MI can cause.

A junctional rhythm with a ventricular rate of 60 to 100 beats/minute is known as an accelerated junctional rhythm. If the ventricular rate exceeds 100 beats/minute, the arrhythmia is called junctional tachycardia.

Intervention
Treatment aims to identify and manage the arrhythmia's primary cause. If the patient is symptomatic, treatment may include atropine to increase the sinus or junctional rate. Alternatively, the doctor may insert a pacemaker to maintain an effective heart rate.

Characteristics and interpretation

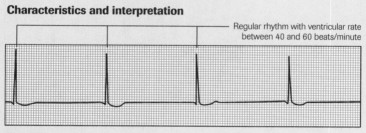

Regular rhythm with ventricular rate between 40 and 60 beats/minute

LEAD II

Atrial rhythm: regular
Ventricular rhythm: regular
Atrial rate: if discernible, 40 to 60 beats/minute (On this strip, the rate isn't discernible.)
Ventricular rate: 40 to 60 beats/minute (40 beats/minute shown)
P wave: usually inverted; may precede, follow, or fall within the QRS complex; may be absent (On this strip, the P wave is absent.)

PR interval: less than 0.12 second and constant if the P wave precedes the QRS complex; otherwise, not measurable (not measurable on this strip)
QRS complex: duration normal; configuration usually normal (0.08-second duration shown)
T wave: usually normal configuration
QT interval: usually normal (0.32-second duration shown)

Premature junctional contractions

In premature junctional contractions (PJCs), a junctional beat occurs before the next normal sinus beat. PJCs, which are ectopic beats, commonly result from increased automaticity in the bundle of His or the surrounding junctional tissue, which interrupts the underlying rhythm. The patient may complain of palpitations if PJCs are frequent.

PJCs most commonly result from digoxin toxicity. Other causes include ischemia associated with an inferior-wall myocardial infarction, excessive caffeine ingestion, and high levels of amphetamines in the body.

Intervention

In most cases, treatment is directed at the underlying cause.

Characteristics and interpretation

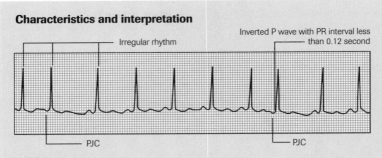

LEAD II

Atrial rhythm: irregular with PJC, but underlying rhythm may be regular
Ventricular rhythm: irregular with PJC, but underlying rhythm may be regular
Atrial rate: follows the underlying rhythm (100 beats/minute shown)
Ventricular rate: follows the underlying rhythm (100 beats/minute shown)
P wave: usually inverted; may precede, follow, or fall within the QRS complex; may be absent (shown preceding the QRS complex)

PR interval: less than 0.12 second on the PJC if P wave precedes the QRS complex; otherwise, not measurable (On this strip, the PR interval is 0.14 second and constant on the underlying rhythm and 0.06 second on the PJC.)
QRS complex: normal duration and configuration (0.06-second duration shown)
T wave: usually normal configuration
QT interval: usually within normal limits (0.30-second interval shown)

Premature ventricular contractions

Among the most common arrhythmias, premature ventricular contractions (PVCs) occur in healthy and diseased hearts. These ectopic beats occur singly, in bigeminy, trigeminy, quadrigeminy, or clusters and may result from certain drugs, electrolyte imbalance, or stress.

When you detect PVCs, you must determine whether the pattern indicates danger. Paired PVCs can produce ventricular tachycardia because the second PVC usually meets refractory tissue. Three or more in a row is a run of ventricular tachycardia. Multiform PVCs look different from one another and may arise from different ventricu-lar sites or be abnormally conducted. In R-on-T phenomenon, the PVC occurs so early that it falls on the T wave of the preceding beat. Because the cells haven't fully depolarized, ventricular tachycardia or fibrillation can result.

Intervention
If the PVCs are thought to result from a serious cardiac problem, lidocaine (Xylocaine) or another antiarrhythmic may be given to suppress ventricular irritability. When the PVCs are thought to result from a noncardiac problem, treatment aims at correcting the underlying cause — an acid-base or electrolyte imbalance, antiarrhythmic therapy, hypothermia, or high catecholamine levels.

Characteristics and interpretation

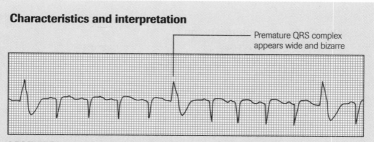

Premature QRS complex appears wide and bizarre

LEAD MCL₁

Atrial rhythm: irregular during PVC; underlying rhythm may be regular
Ventricular rhythm: irregular during PVC; underlying rhythm may be regular
Atrial rate: follows underlying rhythm (120 beats/minute shown)
Ventricular rate: follows underlying rhythm (120 beats/minute shown)
P wave: atrial activity independent of the PVC (If retrograde atrial depolarization exists, a retrograde P wave will distort the ST segment of the PVC. On this strip, no P wave appears before the PVC, but one occurs with each QRS complex.)
PR interval: determined by underlying rhythm; not associated with the PVC (0.12-second, constant interval shown)

QRS complex: occurs earlier than expected; duration exceeds 0.12 second and complex has a bizarre configuration; may be normal in the underlying rhythm (On this strip, it's 0.08 second in the normal beats; it's bizarre and 0.12 second in the PVC.)
T wave: occurs in the direction opposite that of the QRS complex; normal in the underlying complexes
QT interval: not usually measured in the PVC but may be within normal limits in the underlying rhythm (On this strip, the QT interval is 0.28 second in the underlying rhythm.)

Ventricular tachycardia

The life-threatening arrhythmia ventricular tachycardia develops when three or more premature ventricular contractions occur in a row and the rate exceeds 100 beats/minute. It may result from enhanced automaticity or reentry within the Purkinje system. The rapid ventricular rate reduces ventricular filling time; because atrial kick is lost, cardiac output drops. This puts the patient at risk for ventricular fibrillation.

Ventricular tachycardia usually results from acute myocardial infarction, coronary artery disease, valvular heart disease, heart failure, or cardiomyopathy. The arrhythmia can also stem from an electrolyte imbalance or from toxic levels of a drug, such as a cardiac glycoside, procainamide (Pronestyl), or quinidine. You may detect two variations of this arrhythmia: R-on-T phenomenon and torsades de pointes.

Intervention
This rhythm commonly degenerates into ventricular fibrillation and cardiovascular collapse, requiring immediate cardiopulmonary resuscitation and defibrillation. If the patient is symptomatic, prepare for immediate cardioversion, followed by antiarrhythmic therapy. Lidocaine (Xylocaine) or amiodarone (Cordarone) is usually administered immediately. If it proves ineffective, procainamide (Pronestyl) or sotalol (Betapace) is used.

Characteristics and interpretation

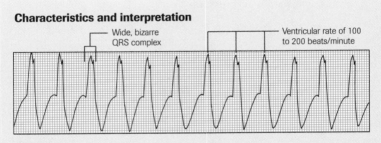

Wide, bizarre QRS complex

Ventricular rate of 100 to 200 beats/minute

LEAD MCL₁

Atrial rhythm: independent P waves possibly discernible with slower ventricular rates (On this strip, the P waves aren't visible.)
Ventricular rhythm: usually regular but may be slightly irregular (On this strip, it's regular.)
Atrial rate: can't be determined
Ventricular rate: usually 100 to 200 beats/minute (120 beats/minute shown)

P wave: usually absent; possibly obscured by the QRS complex; retrograde P waves possible presence
PR interval: not measurable
QRS complex: duration greater than 0.12 second; bizarre appearance, usually with increased amplitude (0.16 second-duration shown)
T wave: opposite the terminal forces of the QRS complex
QT interval: not measurable

Ventricular fibrillation

Defined as chaotic, asynchronous electrical activity within the ventricular tissue, ventricular fibrillation is a life-threatening arrhythmia that results in death if the rhythm isn't stopped immediately. Conditions leading to ventricular fibrillation include myocardial ischemia, hypokalemia, cocaine toxicity, hypoxia, hypothermia, severe acidosis, and severe alkalosis.

Patients with a myocardial infarction are at greatest risk for ventricular fibrillation during the initial 2 hours after the onset of chest pain. Those who experience ventricular fibrillation have a reduced risk of recurrence as healing progresses and scar tissue forms.

In ventricular fibrillation, a lack of cardiac output results in a loss of consciousness, pulselessness, and respiratory arrest. Initially, you may see coarse fibrillatory waves on the electrocardiogram strip. As the acidosis develops, the waves become fine and progress to asystole, unless defibrillation restores cardiac rhythm.

Intervention

Perform cardiopulmonary resuscitation until the patient can receive defibrillation. Administer epinephrine if initial defibrillation series is unsuccessful. Other drugs that may be used include lidocaine (Xylocaine), vasopressin (Pitressin), and procainamide (Pronestyl). Magnesium sulfate may be used for torsades de pointes or refractory ventricular fibrillation.

Characteristics and interpretation

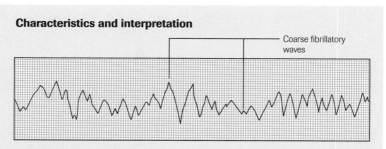

Coarse fibrillatory waves

LEAD MCL₁

Atrial rhythm: can't be determined
Ventricular rhythm: irregular
Atrial rate: can't be determined
Ventricular rate: can't be determined
P wave: indiscernible

PR interval: not measurable
QRS complex: replaced with fibrillatory waves; duration not discernible
T wave: can't be determined
QT interval: not measurable

Idioventricular rhythm

A life-threatening arrhythmia, idioventricular rhythm acts as a safety mechanism when all potential pacemakers above the ventricles fail to discharge or when a block prevents supraventricular impulses from reaching the ventricles.

The slow ventricular rate and loss of atrial kick associated with this life-threatening arrhythmia markedly reduce cardiac output, which in turn causes hypotension, confusion, vertigo, and syncope.

Intervention
Treatment aims to identify and manage the primary problem that triggered this safety mechanism.

Atropine or dopamine (Intropin) may be given to increase the atrial rate. A pacemaker may also be inserted to increase the heart rate and thereby improve cardiac output.

Characteristics and interpretation

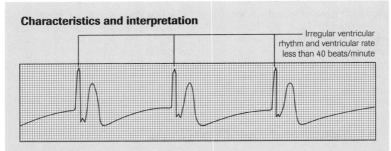

Irregular ventricular rhythm and ventricular rate less than 40 beats/minute

LEAD II

Atrial rhythm: can't be determined
Ventricular rhythm: usually regular, except with isolated escape beats (irregular rhythm shown)
Atrial rate: can't be determined
Ventricular rate: less than 40 beats/minute (30 beats/minute shown)
P wave: absent
PR interval: usually not measurable

QRS complex: duration greater than 0.12 second; complex is wide and has a bizarre configuration (On this strip, the complex is 0.20 second and bizarre.)
T wave: directed opposite terminal forces of QRS complex
QT interval: usually greater than 0.44 second (0.46-second interval shown)

Accelerated idioventricular rhythm

When the pacemaker cells above the ventricles fail to generate an impulse or when a block prevents supraventricular impulses from reaching the ventricles, idioventricular rhythms result. When the rate of an idioventricular rhythm ranges from 40 to 100 beats/minute, it's considered accelerated idioventricular rhythm, denoting a rate greater than the inherent pacemaker.

In this life-threatening arrhythmia, the cells of the His-Purkinje system operate as pacemaker cells. The characteristic waveform results from an area of enhanced automaticity within the ventricles, which may be associated with myocardial infarction, digoxin toxicity, or metabolic imbalances. Also, the arrhythmia commonly occurs during myo-

cardial reperfusion after thrombolytic therapy.

The patient may be symptomatic, depending on his heart rate and ability to compensate for the loss of the atrial kick. If symptomatic, he may experience signs and symptoms of decreased cardiac output (CO), including hypotension, confusion, syncope, and blurred vision.

Intervention

An asymptomatic patient needs no treatment. For a symptomatic patient, treatment focuses on maintaining CO and identifying the cause of the arrhythmia. The patient may require an atrial pacemaker to enhance CO. Remember, this rhythm protects the heart from ventricular standstill and shouldn't be treated with lidocaine (Xylocaine) or other antiarrhythmics.

Characteristics and interpretation

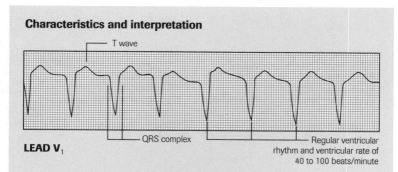

LEAD V₁

Atrial rhythm: can't be determined
Ventricular rhythm: usually regular
Atrial rate: can't be determined
Ventricular rate: 40 to 100 beats/minute
P wave: absent
PR interval: not measurable

QRS complex: duration greater than 0.12 second; wide and bizarre configuration
T wave: deflection usually opposite that of QRS complex
QT interval: may be within normal limits or prolonged

First-degree atrioventricular block

Defined as delayed conduction velocity through the atrioventricular (AV) node or His-Purkinje system, first-degree AV block is associated with an inferior-wall myocardial infarction and the effects of cardiac glycosides or amiodarone (Cordarone). The arrhythmia is also associated with chronic degeneration of the conduction system.

Most patients with first-degree AV block are asymptomatic.

Intervention
Management of first-degree AV block includes identifying and treating the underlying cause as well as monitoring the patient for signs of progressive AV block.

Characteristics and interpretation

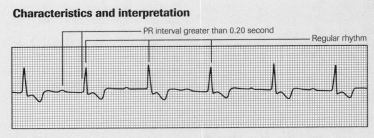

PR interval greater than 0.20 second

Regular rhythm

LEAD II

Atrial rhythm: regular
Ventricular rhythm: regular
Atrial rate: usually within normal limits (60 beats/minute shown)
Ventricular rate: usually within normal limits (60 beats/minute shown)
P wave: normal size and configuration (One P wave precedes each QRS complex.)

PR interval: greater than 0.20 second and constant (0.32-second duration shown)
QRS complex: usually normal duration and configuration (0.08-second duration and normal configuration shown)
T wave: normal size and configuration
QT interval: usually within normal limits (0.32-second interval shown)

Second-degree atrioventricular block, type I

In type I (Wenckebach or Mobitz I) second-degree atrioventricular (AV) block, diseased AV node tissues conduct impulses to the ventricles increasingly later, until one of the atrial impulses fails to be conducted or is blocked. Type I block most commonly occurs at the level of the AV node and is caused by an inferior-wall myocardial infarction, vagal stimulation, or digoxin toxicity.

The arrhythmia usually doesn't cause symptoms. However, a patient may have signs and symptoms of decreased cardiac output (CO), such as hypotension, confusion, and syncope. These effects occur especially if the patient's ventricular rate is slow.

Intervention

If the patient is asymptomatic, no intervention is required other than monitoring the electrocardiogram results frequently to see if a more serious form of AV block develops.

If the patient is symptomatic, the doctor may order atropine to increase the rate and to stop the decremental conduction through the AV node. Occasionally, the doctor may insert a temporary pacemaker to maintain an effective CO.

Characteristics and interpretation

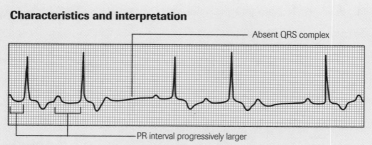

Absent QRS complex

PR interval progressively larger

LEAD II

Atrial rhythm: regular
Ventricular rhythm: irregular
Atrial rate: determined by the underlying rhythm (80 beats/minute shown)
Ventricular rate: slower than the atrial rate (50 beats/minute shown)
P wave: normal size and configuration
PR interval: progressively prolonged with each beat until a P wave appears without a QRS complex

QRS complex: normal duration and configuration; periodically absent (0.08-second duration shown)
T wave: normal size and configuration
QT interval: usually within normal limits (0.46-second, constant interval shown)
Other: usually distinguished by a pattern of group beating, referred to as the footprints of Wenckebach

Second-degree atrioventricular block, type II

A life-threatening arrhythmia produced by a conduction disturbance in the His-Purkinje system, a type II (Mobitz II) second-degree atrioventricular block causes an intermittent absence of conduction. In type II block, two or more atrial impulses are conducted to the ventricles with constant PR intervals, when suddenly, without warning, the atrial impulse is blocked. This type of block occurs in an anterior-wall myocardial infarction (MI), severe coronary artery disease, and chronic degeneration of the conduction system.

Intervention

If the patient is hypotensive, treatment aims at increasing his heart rate to improve cardiac output. Because the conduction block occurs in the His-Purkinje system, drugs that act directly on the myocardium usually prove more effective than those that increase the atrial rate. As a result, dopamine (Intropin) instead of atropine may be ordered to increase the ventricular rate.

If the patient has an anterior-wall MI, the doctor will immediately insert a temporary pacemaker to prevent ventricular asystole. For long-term management, the patient usually needs a permanent pacemaker.

Characteristics and interpretation

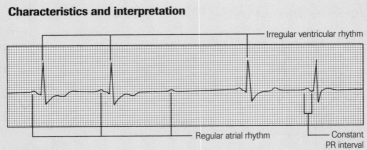

LEAD II

Atrial rhythm: regular
Ventricular rhythm: regular or irregular
Atrial rate: usually within normal limits (60 beats/minute shown)
Ventricular rate: may be within normal limits but less than the atrial rate (40 beats/minute shown)
P wave: normal size and configuration (Not all P waves are followed by a QRS complex.)

PR interval: constant and generally within normal limits for all conducted beats
QRS complex: usually greater than 0.16 second because of the presence of a preexisting bundle-branch block (0.12-second complex shown)
T wave: usually normal size and configuration
QT interval: usually within normal limits (0.44-second interval shown)

Third-degree atrioventricular block

Also called complete heart block, life-threatening third-degree atrioventricular (AV) block occurs when all supraventricular impulses are prevented from reaching the ventricles. If this type of block originates at the AV node, a junctional escape rhythm occurs; if it originates below the AV node, an idioventricular escape rhythm occurs.

Third-degree AV block involving the AV node may result from an inferior wall myocardial infarction (MI) or a toxic reaction to a drug, such as digox-

in, a beta-adrenergic blocker, or a calcium channel blocker. Third-degree AV block below the AV node may result from an anterior-wall MI or chronic degeneration of the conduction system.

Intervention

If cardiac output (CO) is inadequate or if the patient's condition is deteriorating, the doctor will order therapy to improve the ventricular rhythm. Initially, atropine may be ordered to increase the ventricular rate and improve CO until a pacemaker is available.

Characteristics and interpretation

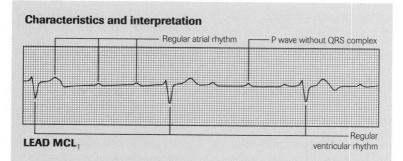

Regular atrial rhythm — P wave without QRS complex

Regular ventricular rhythm

LEAD MCL₁

Atrial rhythm: usually regular
Ventricular rhythm: usually regular
Atrial rate: usually within normal limits (90 beats/minute shown)
Ventricular rate: slow (30 beats/minute shown)
P wave: normal size and configuration
PR interval: not measurable because the atria and ventricles beat independently of each other
QRS complex: determined by the site of the escape rhythm (With a junctional

escape rhythm, the duration and configuration are normal; with an idioventricular escape rhythm, the duration is greater than 0.12 second and the complex is distorted. In the complex shown, the duration is 0.16 second, the configuration is abnormal, and the complex is distorted.)
T wave: normal size and configuration
QT interval: may be within normal limits (0.56-second interval shown)

12-lead ECGs

Basic components and principles

Whereas rhythm strips are used to detect arrhythmias, the 12-lead, or standard, electrocardiogram (ECG) has a different purpose. The most common test for evaluating cardiac status, the 12-lead ECG helps identify various pathologic conditions — most commonly, acute myocardial infarction.

The 12-lead ECG provides 12 views of the heart's electrical activity. (See *12 views of the heart.*) The 12 leads include:

■ three bipolar limb leads (I, II, and III)
■ three unipolar augmented limb leads (aV$_R$, aV$_L$, and aV$_F$)
■ six unipolar precordial, or chest, leads (V$_1$, V$_2$, V$_3$, V$_4$, V$_5$, and V$_6$).

Leads

The six limb leads record electrical potential from the frontal plane, and the six precordial leads record electrical potential from the horizontal plane. Each waveform reflects the orientation of a lead to the wave of depolarization passing through the myocardium. Normally, this wave moves through the heart from right to left and from top to bottom.

Bipolar leads
Bipolar leads record the electrical potential difference between two points on the patient's body, where you place electrodes.

■ Lead I goes from the right arm (–) to the left arm (+).
■ Lead II goes from the right arm (–) to the left leg (+).
■ Lead III goes from the left arm (–) to the left leg (+).

Because of the orientation of these leads to the wave of depolarization, the QRS complexes typically appear upright. In lead II, these complexes are usually the tallest because this lead parallels the wave of depolarization.

Unipolar leads
Unipolar leads (the augmented limb leads and the precordial leads) have only one electrode, which represents the positive pole. The ECG computes the negative pole. Lead aV$_R$ typically records negative QRS complex deflections because the wave of depolarization moves away from it. In the aV$_F$ lead, QRS complexes are positive; in the aV$_L$ lead, they're biphasic.

Unipolar precordial leads V$_1$ and V$_2$ usually have a small R wave because the direction of ventricular activation is left to right initially. That's because conduction time is normally faster down the left bundle branch than it is down the right. However, the wave of depolarization moves toward the left ventricle and away from these leads, causing a low S wave.

In leads V$_3$ and V$_4$, the R and S waves may have the same amplitude, and you won't see a Q wave. In leads V$_5$ and V$_6$, the initial ventricular activation appears as a small Q wave; the following tall R wave represents the strong wave of depolarization moving toward the left ventricle. These leads record a small or absent S wave.

Determining electrical axis

As electrical impulses travel through the heart, they generate small electrical forces called instant-to-instant vectors. The mean of these vectors represents the direction and force of the wave of depolarization, also known as the heart's electrical axis.

In a healthy heart, the wave of depolarization (or the direction of the electrical axis) originates in the sinoatrial node and travels through the atria and the atrioventricular node and on to the ventricles. So the normal

12 views of the heart

The electrocardiogram's six limb leads view the heart from six different angles. This chart shows the direction of each lead relative to the wave of depolarization and lists the six views of the heart revealed by these leads.

Planes of the heart	**Leads**	**View of the heart**
	STANDARD LIMB LEADS (BIPOLAR)	
	I	Lateral wall
	II	Inferior wall
	III	Inferior wall
	AUGMENTED LIMB LEADS (UNIPOLAR)	
	aV_R	Provides no specific view
	aV_L	Lateral wall
	aV_F	Inferior wall
	PRECORDIAL, OR CHEST, LEADS (UNIPOLAR)	
	V_1	Anteroseptal wall
	V_2	Anteroseptal wall
	V_3	Anterior and anteroseptal walls
	V_4	Anterior wall
	V_5	Anterolateral wall
	V_6	Anterolateral wall

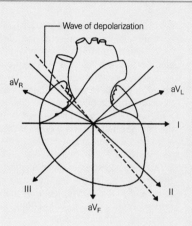

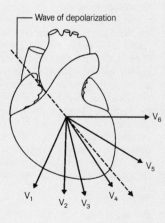

movement is downward and to the left — the direction of a normal electrical axis.

In an unhealthy heart, the wave of depolarization varies. That's because the direction of electrical activity swings away from areas of damage or necrosis.

A simple method for determining the direction of your patient's electrical axis is the quadrant method. Before you use this method, you need to understand the hexaxial reference system — a schematic view of the heart that uses the six limb leads.

As you know, these leads include the three standard limb leads (I, II, and III), which are bipolar, and the three augmented limb leads (aV_R, aV_L, and aV_F), which are unipolar. Combined, these leads give a view of the wave of depolarization in the frontal plane, including the right, left, inferior, and superior portions of the heart.

Hexaxial reference system

The axes of the six limb leads also make up the hexaxial reference system, which divides the heart into six equal areas. To use the hexaxial reference system, picture in your mind the position of each lead: lead I connects the right arm (negative pole) with the left arm (positive pole); lead II connects the right arm (negative pole) with the left leg (positive pole); and lead III connects the left arm (negative pole) with the left leg (positive pole). The augmented limb leads have only one electrode, which represents the positive pole. As a result, lead aV_R goes from the heart toward the right arm (positive pole); aV_L goes from the heart toward the left arm (positive pole); and aV_F goes from the heart to the left leg (positive pole).

Now, take this mental picture one step further and draw an imaginary line to illustrate the axis of each lead. For example, for lead I, you would draw a horizontal line between the right and left arms; for lead II, between the right arm and left leg; and so on. All the lines should intersect near the center, somewhere over the heart. If you draw a circle to represent the heart, you would end up with a rough pie shape, with each wedge representing a portion of the heart monitored by each lead. (See *Understanding the hexaxial reference system*.)

This schematic representation of the heart allows you to plot your patient's electrical axis. If his axis falls in the right lower quadrant, between 0 degrees and + 90 degrees, it's considered normal. An axis between + 90 degrees and + 180 degrees indicates right axis deviation; one between 0 degrees and − 90 degrees, left axis deviation; and one between − 180 degrees and − 90 degrees, extreme axis deviation (sometimes called the northwest axis). Some experts, however, feel that the portion from 0 degrees to − 30 degrees has no clinical significance.

Quadrant method

A simple, rapid method for determining the heart's axis is the quadrant method, in which you observe the main deflection of the QRS complex in leads I and aV_F. The QRS complex serves as the traditional marker for determining the electrical axis because the ventricles produce the greatest amount of electrical force when they contract. Lead I indicates whether impulses are moving to the right or left; lead aV_F, whether they're moving up or down. (See *Using the quadrant method,* page 122.)

On the waveform for lead I, a positive main deflection of the QRS complex indicates that the electrical impulses are moving to the right, toward the positive pole of the lead, which is at the 0-degree position on the hexaxial reference system. Conversely, a negative deflection indicates that the impulses are moving to the left, toward the negative pole of the lead, which is at the +180-degree position on the hexaxial reference system. On the waveform for lead aV$_F$, a positive deflection of the QRS complex indicates that the electrical impulses are traveling downward, toward the positive pole of the lead, which is at the +90-degree position of the hexaxial reference system. A negative deflection indicates that impulses are traveling upward, toward the negative pole of the lead, which is at the +90-degree position of the hexaxial reference system.

Plotting this information on the hexaxial reference system (with the horizontal axis representing lead I and the vertical axis representing lead aV$_F$) will reveal the patient's electrical axis. For example, if lead I shows a positive deflection of the QRS complex, darken the horizontal axis between the center of the hexaxial reference system and the 0-degree position. If lead aV$_F$ also shows a positive deflection of the QRS complex, darken the vertical axis between the center of reference system and the +90-degree position. The quadrant between the two axes you have darkened indicates the patient's electrical axis. In this case, it's the left lower quadrant, which indicates a normal electrical axis.

Causes of axis deviation

Determining a patient's electrical axis can help confirm a diagnosis or narrow the range of clinical possibilities. Many factors influence the electrical axis, including the position of the heart within the chest, the size of the heart, the conduction pathways, and the force of electrical generation.

As you know, cardiac electrical activity swings away from areas of damage or necrosis. More specifically, electrical forces in the healthy portion of the heart take over for weak, or even absent, electrical forces in the damaged

> ### Understanding the hexaxial reference system
>
> The hexaxial reference system consists of six bisecting lines, each representing one of the six limb leads, and a circle, representing the heart. The intersection of these lines divides the circle into equal 30-degree segments.
>
> Note that 0 degrees appears at the 3 o'clock position. Moving counterclockwise, the degrees become increasingly negative, until reaching ±180 degrees at the 9 o'clock position. The bottom half of the circle contains the corresponding positive degrees. A positive-degree designation doesn't necessarily mean that the pole is positive.

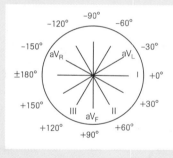

portion. For instance, after an inferior-wall myocardial infarction, portions of the inferior wall can no longer conduct electricity. As a result, the major electrical vectors shift to the left, resulting in a left axis deviation.

Typically, the damaged portion of the heart is the last area to be depolarized. For example, in a left anterior hemiblock, the left anterior fascicle of the left bundle branch can no longer conduct electricity. Therefore, the portion normally served by the left bundle branch is the last portion of the heart to be depolarized. This shifts electrical forces to the left; consequently, the ECG shows left axis deviation.

Using the quadrant method

This chart can help you quickly determine the direction of a patient's electrical axis, which is indicated by the gray arrow. First, observe the deflections of the QRS complexes in leads I and aV$_F$. Next, plot the deflections on the diagram. (Positive deflections are on the side that has positive degrees for that lead, and negative deflections are on the side that has negative degrees.) Then check the chart to determine if the patient's axis is normal or whether it has a left, right, or extreme deviation.

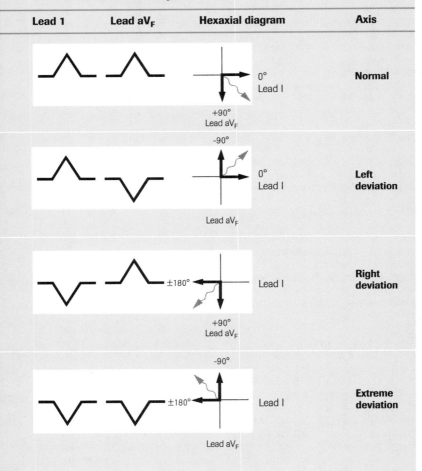

Lead 1	Lead aV$_F$	Hexaxial diagram	Axis
		0° Lead I / +90° Lead aV$_F$	Normal
		-90° / 0° Lead I / Lead aV$_F$	Left deviation
		±180° Lead I / +90° Lead aV$_F$	Right deviation
		-90° / ±180° Lead I / Lead aV$_F$	Extreme deviation

An opposite shift occurs with right bundle-branch block. In this condition, the wave of impulse travels quickly down the normal left side but much more slowly down the damaged right side. This shifts the electrical forces to the right, causing a right axis deviation.

An axis shift also takes place when the right or left ventricle is artificially paced. It likewise takes place when the ventricles are depolarizing abnormally, such as occurs in ventricular tachycardia. Both of these conditions can cause a left axis deviation or, occasionally, an extreme axis deviation.

Axis deviation may also result from ventricular hypertrophy. For example, an enlarged right ventricle generates greater electrical forces than normal and would consequently shift the electrical axis to the right. Wolff-Parkinson-White syndrome may produce a right, left, or extreme axis deviation, depending on which part of the ventricle is activated early.

Sometimes axis deviation may be a normal variation, as in infants and children, who normally experience right axis deviation. It may also stem from noncardiac causes. For example, if the heart is shifted in the chest cavity because of a high diaphragm from pregnancy, expect to find a left axis deviation. Also, if a patient's heart is situated on the right side of the chest instead of the left (a condition called dextrocardia), expect to find right axis deviation.

How to interpret a 12-lead ECG

You can use various methods to interpret a 12-lead electrocardiogram (ECG). Here's a logical, easy-to-follow, seven-step method that will help ensure that you're interpreting it accurately.

1. Find the lead markers and note the leads.

2. Note whether there are full or half standardization marks.

3. Using the four-quadrant method, observe the waveforms for leads I and aV_F, and determine the heart's axis. This can provide an early clue to a possible problem.

4. Note the R-wave progression through the six precordial leads. Normally, in the precordial leads, the R wave (the first positive deflection of the QRS complex) appears progressively taller from lead V_1 to lead V_6. Conversely, the S wave (the negative deflection after an R wave) appears extremely deep in lead V_1 and becomes progressively smaller through lead V_6. (See *Normal findings,* pages 125 to 127.)

5. Next, look at the T wave, which normally goes in the same direction as the QRS complex. If the main deflection of the QRS complex is positive, the T wave should be positive, too. If the main deflection of the QRS complex is negative, the T wave should be negative. The two exceptions to this are leads V_1 and V_2, in which a negative QRS complex with a positive T wave is normal.

If a T wave deflects in the opposite direction from the QRS complex, it's considered abnormal (except, as mentioned, in leads V_1 and V_2). Such a deflection is commonly referred to as an *inverted T wave* — a term that can be confusing when the QRS complex is negative and the T wave is actually positive. Keep in mind that in this case, inversion signifies that the T wave deflects in the direction opposite the QRS complex. It doesn't necessarily mean that the T wave is negative, as the word *inverted* suggests.

6. If you suspect a myocardial infarction (MI), start with lead I and continue through to lead V_6, observing the waveforms for changes in ECG characteristics that can indicate an acute MI, such as T-wave inversion, ST-segment elevation, and pathologic Q waves. Note the leads in which you see such changes and describe the changes. When first learning to interpret the 12-lead ECG, ignore lead

Locating myocardial damage

Wall affected	Leads	ECG changes	Artery involved	Reciprocal changes
Inferior (diaphragmatic)	II, III, aV_F	Q, ST, T	Right coronary artery (RCA)	I, aV_L and, possibly, V_4 through V_6
Posterolateral	I, aV_L, V_5, V_6	Q, ST, T	Circumflex or branch of left anterior descending (LAD) artery	V_1, V_2, or II, III, and aV_F
Anterior	V_1, V_2, V_3, V_4	Q, ST, T, loss of R-wave progression across precordial leads	Left coronary artery	II, III, aV_F
Posterior	V_1, V_2	None	RCA or circumflex, either of which supplies posterior descending artery	R greater than S in V_1 and V_2, ST-segment depression, T-wave elevation
Right ventricular	V_{4R}, V_{5R}, V_{6R}	Q, ST, T	RCA	None
Anterolateral	I, aV_L, V_4, V_5, V_6	Q, ST, T	LAD and diagonal branches, circumflex and obtuse marginal branches	II, III, aV_F
Anteroseptal	V_1, V_2, V_3	Q, ST, T, loss of R wave in V_1	LAD	None

aV_R, because it won't provide clues to left ventricular infarction or injury.

7. Determine the site and extent of myocardial damage. To do so, use the above chart *Locating myocardial damage,* and follow these steps:

■ Identify the leads recording pathologic Q waves. Look at the second column of the chart for those leads. Then look at the first column to find the corresponding myocardial wall, where infarction has occurred. Keep in mind that this chart serves as a guideline only. Actual areas of infarction may overlap or be larger or smaller than listed.

■ Identify the leads recording ST-segment elevation (or depression for reciprocal leads), and use the chart to locate the corresponding areas of myocardial injury.

■ Identify the leads recording T-wave inversion, and locate the corresponding areas of ischemia.

Normal findings

LEAD I

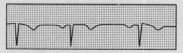

P wave: upright
Q wave: small or none
R wave: largest wave
S wave: none present, or smaller than R wave
T wave: upright
U wave: none present
ST segment: may vary from + 1 to − 0.5 mm

LEAD II

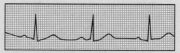

P wave: upright
Q wave: small or none
R wave: large (vertical heart)
S wave: none present, or smaller than R wave
T wave: upright
U wave: none present
ST segment: may vary from + 1 to − 0.5 mm

LEAD III

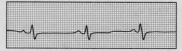

P wave: upright, diphasic, or inverted
Q wave: usually small or none (a Q wave must also be present in aV$_F$ to be considered diagnostic.)
R wave: none present to large wave
S wave: none present to large wave, indicating horizontal heart

T wave: upright, diphasic, or inverted
U wave: none present
ST segment: may vary from + 1 to − 0.5 mm

LEAD aV$_R$

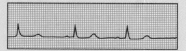

P wave: inverted
Q wave: none, small wave, or large wave present
R wave: none or small wave present
S wave: large wave (may be QS)
T wave: inverted
U wave: none present
ST segment: may vary from + 1 to − 0.5 mm

LEAD aV$_L$

P wave: upright, diphasic, or inverted
Q wave: none, small wave, or large wave present (A Q wave must also be present in lead I or precordial leads to be considered diagnostic.)
R wave: none, small wave, or large wave present (A large wave indicates horizontal heart.)
S wave: none present to large wave (A large wave indicates vertical heart.)
T wave: upright, diphasic, or inverted
U wave: none present
ST segment: may vary from + 1 to − 0.5 mm

(continued)

Normal findings *(continued)*

LEAD aV_F

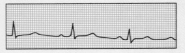

P wave: upright
Q wave: none, or small wave present
R wave: none, small wave, or large wave present (A large wave suggests vertical heart.)
S wave: none to large wave present (A large wave suggests horizontal heart.)
T wave: Upright, diphasic, or inverted
U wave: none present
ST segment: may vary from +1 to −0.5 mm

LEAD V₁

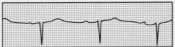

P wave: upright, diphasic, or inverted
Q wave: deep QS pattern may be present
R wave: none present or less than S wave
S wave: large (part of QS pattern)
T wave: usually inverted but may be upright and diphasic
U wave: none present
ST segment: may vary from 0 to +1 mm

LEAD V₂

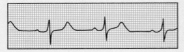

P wave: upright
Q wave: deep QS pattern may be present

R wave: none present or less than S wave (wave may become progressively larger)
S wave: large (part of QS pattern)
T wave: upright
U wave: upright, lower amplitude than T wave
ST segment: may vary from 0 to +1 mm

LEAD V₃

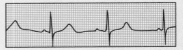

P wave: upright
Q wave: none or small wave present
R wave: less than, greater than, or equal to S wave (Wave may become progressively larger.)
S wave: large (greater than, less than, or equal to R wave)
T wave: upright
U wave: upright, lower amplitude than T wave
ST segment: may vary from 0 to +1 mm

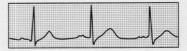

LEAD V₄
P wave: upright
Q wave: none or small wave present
R wave: progressively larger wave; R wave greater than S wave
S wave: progressively smaller (less than R wave)
T wave: upright
U wave: upright, lower amplitude than T wave
ST segment: may vary from +1 to −0.5 mm

Normal findings *(continued)*

LEAD V₅

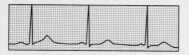

P wave: upright
Q wave: small
R wave: progressively larger but less than 26 mm
S wave: progressively smaller; less than the S wave in V₄
T wave: upright
U wave: none present
ST segment: may vary from +1 to −0.5 mm

LEAD V₆

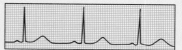

P wave: upright
Q wave: small
R wave: largest wave but less than 26 mm
S wave: smallest; less than the S wave in V₅
T wave: upright
U wave: none present
ST segment: may vary from +1 to −0.5 mm

Acute myocardial infarction

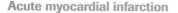

An acute myocardial infarction (MI) can arise from any condition in which myocardial oxygen supply can't meet oxygen demand. Starved of oxygen, the myocardium suffers progressive ischemia, leading to injury and, eventually, to infarction.

In most cases, an acute MI involves the left ventricle, although it can also involve the right ventricle or the atria, and is classified as either Q wave or non–Q wave.

In an acute transmural MI, the characteristic electrocardiogram (ECG) changes result from the three I's — ischemia, injury, and infarction.

■ Ischemia results from a temporary interruption of the myocardial blood supply. Its characteristic ECG change is T-wave inversion, a result of altered tissue repolarization. ST-segment depression also may occur.

ISCHEMIA

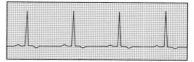

Ischemia produces T-wave inversion

■ Injury to myocardial cells results from a prolonged interruption of blood flow. Its characteristic ECG change, ST-segment elevation, reflects altered depolarization. Usually, an elevation greater than 0.1 mV is considered significant.

INJURY

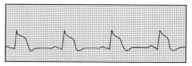

Injury produces ST-segment elevation

■ Infarction results from an absence of blood flow to myocardial tissue, leading to necrosis. The ECG shows pathologic Q waves, reflecting abnormal depolarization in damaged tissue or absent depolarization in scar tissue. The characteristic of a pathologic Q wave is a duration of 0.04 second or an amplitude measuring at least one-third the height of the entire QRS complex.

INFARCTION

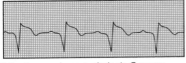

Infarction produces pathologic Q waves

Besides these three characteristic ECG changes, you may see reciprocal (or mirror image) changes. Reciprocal changes — most commonly, ST-segment depression or tall R waves — occur in the leads opposite those reflecting the area of ischemia, injury, or infarction.

Acute MI phases

To detect an acute MI, look for ST-segment elevation first, followed by T-wave inversion and pathologic Q waves.

Serial ECG recordings yield the best evidence of an MI. Normally, an acute MI progresses through the following phases.

Hyperacute phase

This phase begins a few hours after the onset of an acute MI. You'll see ST-segment elevation and upright (usually peaked) T waves.

Fully evolved phase

This phase starts several hours after MI onset. You'll see deep T-wave inversion and pathologic Q waves.

Resolution phase

This appears within a few weeks of an acute MI. You'll see normal T waves.

Stabilized chronic phase

After the resolution phase, you'll see permanent pathologic Q-waves revealing an old infarction.

With an acute non–Q-wave MI, you may see persistent ST-segment depression, T-wave inversion, or both. However, pathologic Q waves may not appear. To differentiate an acute non–Q-wave MI from myocardial ischemia, cardiac enzyme tests must be performed.

It's important to remember that for a true clinical diagnosis of an acute MI, a patient must have symptoms, ECG changes, and elevated cardiac enzyme levels. If the patient shows such signs and symptoms as chest pain, left arm pain, diaphoresis, and nausea, proceed as if he has had an acute MI until this possibility has been ruled out.

Right-sided ECG, leads V$_{1R}$ to V$_{6R}$

A right-sided electrocardiogram (ECG) provides information about the extent of damage to the right ventricle, especially during the first 12 hours of a myocardial infarction (MI). Right-sided ECG leads, placed over the right side of the chest in similar but reversed positions from the left precordial leads, are called unipolar right-sided chest leads.

Placing electrodes

Right-sided ECG leads are precordial leads designated by the letter V, a number representing the electrode position, and the letter R, indicating lead placement on the right side of the chest. Lead positions are:

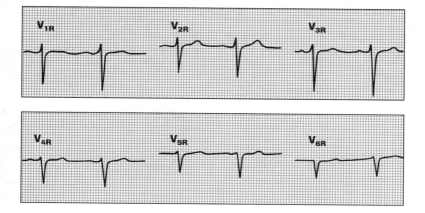

- V_{1R}: fourth intercostal space, left sternal border
- V_{2R}: fourth intercostal space, right sternal border
- V_{3R}: midway between V_{2R} and V_{4R}, on a line joining these two locations
- V_{4R}: fifth intercostal space, right midclavicular line
- V_{5R}: fifth intercostal space, right anterior axillary line
- V_{6R}: fifth intercostal space, right midaxillary line.

Understanding polarity

The right-sided chest ECG leads measure the difference in electrical potential between a right-sided chest electrode and a central terminal. The chest electrode used in each of the right V leads is positive. The negative electrode is obtained by adding together leads I, II, and III, whose algebraic sum equals zero.

Viewing the heart

Chest leads, whether on the left or the right side of the chest, view the horizontal plane of the heart. The placement of left precordial leads gives a good picture of the electrical activity within the left ventricle. Because the right ventricle lies behind the left ventricle, the ability to evaluate right ventricular electrical activity when using only left precordial leads is limited. Right-sided ECG leads provide a better picture of the right ventricular wall. This may be especially useful when evaluating a patient for a right ventricular MI.

Leads V_{1R} and V_{2R} provide limited visualization of the right ventricle. Leads V_{3R} through V_{6R} are the most useful right ventricular leads. A decrease in the R wave with an increase in the S wave is normally seen from V_{1R} through V_{6R}, the reverse of the standard left precordial leads. V_{3R} to V_{6R} (particularly V_{4R}) are the most commonly used and the most helpful leads when looking for ECG changes indicating right ventricular ischemia and infarction.

Left bundle-branch block

In left bundle-branch block, a conduction delay or block occurs in both the left posterior and the left anterior fascicles of the left bundle. This delay or block disrupts the normal left-to-right direction of depolarization. As a result, normal septal Q waves are absent. Because of the block, the wave of depolarization must move down the right bundle first and then spread from right to left.

This arrhythmia may indicate underlying heart disease such as coronary artery disease. It carries a more serious prognosis than right bundle-branch block because of its close correlation with organic heart disease, and it requires a large lesion to block the thick, broad left bundle branch.

Intervention
When left bundle-branch block occurs along with an anterior-wall myocardial infarction, it usually signals complete heart block, which requires insertion of a pacemaker.

Characteristics and interpretation

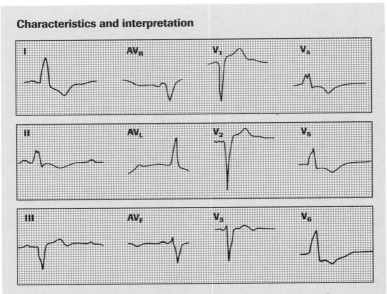

Rhythm: regular atrial and ventricular rhythms
Rate: atrial and ventricular rates within normal limits
P wave: normal size and configuration
PR interval: within normal limits
QRS complex: duration that varies from 0.10 to 0.12 second in incomplete left bundle-branch block (It's at least 0.12 second in complete block. Lead V_1 shows a wide, entirely negative rS complex [rarely a wide rS complex]. Leads I, aV_L, and V_6 show a wide, tall R wave without a Q or S wave.)
T wave: deflection opposite that of the QRS complex in most leads
QT interval: may be prolonged or within normal limits
Other: several of changes paralleling the magnitude of the QRS complex aberration, with normal axis or left axis deviation; delayed intrinsicoid deflection over the left ventricle (lead V_6)

Right bundle-branch block

In the conduction delay or block associated with right bundle-branch block, the initial left-to-right direction of depolarization isn't affected. The left ventricle depolarizes on time, so the intrinsicoid deflection in leads V_5 and V_6 (the left precordial leads) takes place on time as well. However, the right ventricle depolarizes late, causing a late intrinsicoid deflection in leads V_1 and V_2 (the right precordial leads). This late depolarization also causes the axis to deviate to the right.

Intervention

One potential complication of a myocardial infarction is a bundle-branch block. Some blocks require treatment with a temporary pacemaker. Others are monitored only to detect progression to a more complete block.

Characteristics and interpretation

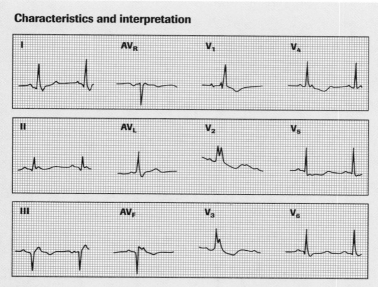

Rhythm: regular atrial and ventricular rhythms

Rate: atrial and ventricular rates within normal limits

P wave: normal size and configuration

PR interval: within normal limits

QRS complex: duration of at least 0.12 second in complete block and 0.10 to 0.12 second in incomplete block (In lead V_1, the QRS complex is wide and can appear in one of several patterns: an rSR' complex with a wide S and R' wave; an rS complex with a wide R wave; and a wide R wave with an M-shaped pattern. The complex is mainly positive, with the R wave occurring late. In leads I, aV$_L$, and V_6, a broad S wave can be seen.)

T wave: in most leads, deflection opposite that of the QRS-complex deflection

QT interval: may be prolonged or within normal limits

Other: in the precordial leads, occurrence of triphasic complexes because the right ventricle continues to depolarize after the left ventricle depolarizes, thereby producing a third phase of ventricular stimulation

Pericarditis

An inflammation of the pericardium, the fibroserous sac that envelops the heart, pericarditis can be acute or chronic. The acute form may be fibrinous or effusive, with a purulent serous or hemorrhagic exudate. Chronic constrictive pericarditis causes dense fibrous pericardial thickening. Regardless of the form, pericarditis can cause cardiac tamponade if fluid accumulates too quickly. It can also cause heart failure if constriction occurs.

In pericarditis, electrocardiogram changes occur in four stages. Stage 1 coincides with the onset of chest pain. Stage 2 begins within several days. Stage 3 starts several days after stage 2. Stage 4 occurs weeks later.

Intervention
Pericarditis is usually treated with aspirin or nonsteroidal anti-inflammatory drugs. A last resort is prednisone, quickly tapered over 3 days.

Characteristics and interpretation

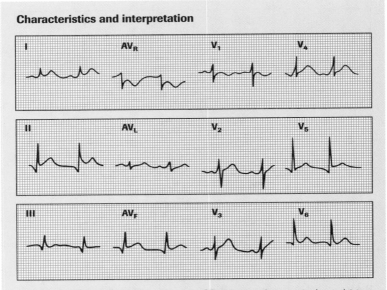

Rhythm: usually regular atrial and ventricular rhythms

Rate: atrial and ventricular rates usually within normal limits

P wave: normal size and configuration

PR interval: usually depressed in all leads except V_1 and aV_R, in which it may be elevated

QRS complex: within normal limits, but with a possible decrease in amplitude

ST segment: in stage 1, elevated 1 to 2 mm in a concave pattern in leads I, II, and III and the precordial leads

T wave: flattened in stage 2, inverted in stage 3 (lasting for weeks or months), and returning to normal in stage 4 (although sometimes becoming deeply inverted)

QT interval: within normal limits

Other: possible atrial fibrillation or tachycardia from sinoatrial node irritation

Digoxin: ECG effects

Digoxin increases the force of myocardial contraction, decreases conduction velocity through the atrioventricular (AV) node to slow the heart rate, and prolongs the effective refractory period of the AV node by direct and sympatholytic effects on the sinoatrial node. Excess amounts of this drug can slow conduction through the AV node and cause irritable ectopic foci in the ventricles.

Electrocardiogram (ECG) changes only indicate that the patient is receiving a form of digoxin. If an arrhythmia

develops, these ECG changes can help identify the cause of the arrhythmia as digoxin toxicity.

Virtually any type of arrhythmia can be caused by an excess of digoxin. The most common ones include premature ventricular contractions (especially bigeminy), paroxysmal atrial tachycardias with or without a block, second-degree heart block, and sinus arrest.

Intervention
Monitor the patient for noncardiac symptoms of digoxin toxicity. Withhold digoxin for 1 to 2 days before performing electrical cardioversion.

Characteristics and interpretation

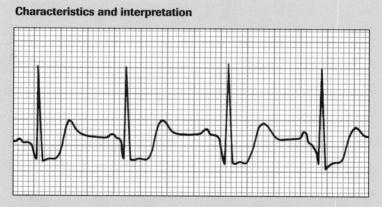

Rhythm: regular atrial and ventricular rhythms
Rate: atrial and ventricular rates are usually within normal limits, but bradycardia is possible
P wave: decreased voltage; may be notched
PR interval: within normal limits or prolonged
QRS complex: within normal limits
ST segment: gradual sloping, causing ST-segment depression in the direction opposite that of the QRS deflection

T wave: may be flattened and inverted in a direction opposite that of the QRS-complex deflection
Other: QT interval commonly shortened; ST-segment sloping and depression and QT-interval shortening from digoxin use but not necessarily signs of digoxin toxicity; ST-segment depression and T-wave inversion in leads with negatively deflected QRS complexes, possibly indicating a need to reduce the digoxin dose

Quinidine: ECG effects

An antiarrhythmic that decreases sodium transport through cardiac tissues, quinidine slows conduction through the atrioventricular (AV) node. It also prolongs the effective refractory period and decreases automaticity.

Although electrocardiogram changes occur as a result of quinidine use, they aren't necessarily a sign of quinidine toxicity. At toxic levels, however, quinidine can cause sinoatrial and AV block and ventricular arrhythmias.

Intervention

Prolongation of the QT interval is a sign that the patient is predisposed to developing polymorphic ventricular tachycardia. Preventing ventricular tachyarrhythmias involves administering a cardiac glycoside for atrial tachyarrhythmias before quinidine.

Characteristics and interpretation

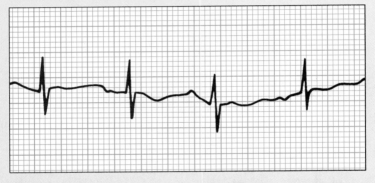

Rhythm: regular atrial and ventricular rhythms
Rate: atrial and ventricular rates within normal limits
P wave: may be widened and notched, especially in leads I and II
PR interval: within normal limits

QRS complex: widens slightly (Abnormal widening may be an early sign of developing quinidine toxicity.)
ST segment: commonly depressed
T wave: may be flattened or inverted
QT interval: may be prolonged
U wave: may be visible

4 Common laboratory tests
Giving care and interpreting results

Specimen identification

Guide to color-top collection tubes

The color of the specimen collection tube you use indicates the type of test to be performed, as shown below.

Color and draw volume	Additive	Test purpose
Red (2 to 20 ml)	None	Serum studies
Lavender (2 to 10 ml)	EDTA	Whole blood studies
Green (2 to 15 ml)	Heparin (sodium, lithium, or ammonium)	Plasma studies
Blue (2.7 or 4.5 ml)	Sodium citrate and citric acid	Coagulation studies on plasma
Black (2.7 or 4.5 ml)	Sodium oxalate	Coagulation studies on plasma
Gray (3 to 10 ml)	Glycolytic inhibitor, such as sodium fluoride, powdered oxalate salt, or glycolytic-microbial inhibitor	Glucose determinations on serum or plasma
Marble-top	Silicone gel	Serum separation

Laboratory tests

Alanine aminotransferase

Alanine aminotransferase (ALT) is one of two specialized enzymes called aminotransferases that catalyze a reversible amino group transfer in the Krebs cycle and that can accumulate in the bloodstream when liver cells are injured. ALT serves as an indicator of hepatic disease. It appears primarily in the cytoplasm of liver cells with smaller amounts in the kidneys, heart, and skeletal muscles. When damage occurs, ALT is released from the cytoplasm into the bloodstream, in many cases before jaundice appears. This test is also referred to as alanine transaminase.

Purpose
■ To help detect and evaluate treatment of hepatic disease — especially hepatitis, and cirrhosis without jaundice
■ To help distinguish between myocardial and hepatic tissue damage (when used with the aspartate aminotransferase test)
■ To assess hepatoxicity of certain drugs

Procedure-related nursing care
Explain the purpose of the test to the patient, and tell him you'll need to

take a blood sample. Withhold hepatotoxic cholestatic drugs, if possible, before the test is performed.

Perform a venipuncture, collecting the sample in a 7-ml red-top tube. If necessary, you can store serum samples for up to 3 days at room temperature.

Reference values
Serum ALT levels range from 10 to 35 units/L in males and 9 to 24 units/L in females.

Abnormal results
Extremely high levels of ALT (up to 50 times normal) suggest viral or severe drug-induced hepatitis, or another hepatic disease with extensive necrosis.

Moderate to high elevations may indicate infectious mononucleosis, chronic hepatitis, intrahepatic cholestasis or cholecystitis, or early or severe hepatic congestion caused by heart failure.

Slight to moderate elevations may appear with any condition that produces acute hepatocellular injury, such as active cirrhosis and drug-induced or alcoholic hepatitis. Marginal elevations occasionally occur with acute myocardial infarction, reflecting secondary hepatic congestion or release of some ALT from myocardial tissue.

Aldosterone, serum

This test measures serum levels of aldosterone, the principal mineralocorticoid secreted by the zona glomerulosa of the adrenal cortex. Aldosterone regulates ion transport across cell membranes in the renal tubules, helping to maintain blood pressure and volume and to regulate fluid and electrolyte balance.

Aldosterone secretion is controlled primarily by the renin-angiotensin-aldosterone system, serum potassium level, and corticotropin. Hyponatremia, hypovolemia, and other disorders that provoke renin release stimulate aldosterone secretion. Similarly, high potassium levels trigger aldosterone secretion through a potent feedback system.

Purpose
■ To help diagnose primary and secondary aldosteronism, hypoaldosteronism, salt-losing syndrome, and adrenal hyperplasia

Procedure-related nursing care
Explain the purpose of the test to the patient, and tell him the test requires two blood samples. Instruct him to maintain a low-carbohydrate, normal-sodium (3 g/day or 135µ/mol) diet for at least 2 weeks (preferably 30 days) before the test.

If the patient is premenopausal, specify the phase of her menstrual cycle on the laboratory slip. (Aldosterone levels may fluctuate during the menstrual cycle.) If aldosterone levels will be measured using radioimmunoassay, make sure the patient hasn't undergone a radioactive scan during the week preceding the test.

Perform a venipuncture in the morning while the patient is still in a supine position after a night's rest. Collect the sample in a 7-ml red-top tube. Note the time and the patient's position during venipuncture on the laboratory request.

Draw another sample 4 hours later after the patient has been up and about and while he stands. Use another 7-ml red-top tube, noting the time and the patient's position on the laboratory slip. Tell the patient he can resume his normal diet.

Reference values
Normally, serum aldosterone levels (in a standing, nonpregnant patient) range from 1 to 16 ng/dl. The range for an adult who has been standing for at least 2 hours is 4 to 31 ng/dl. Values in females vary.

*Abnormal resu_*

Excessive aldoste
to primary or sec
Primary aldoster(
may result from ;
ma, bilateral adre
commonly, cance
ronism can result
increase renin-an;
as sodium depleti
renovascular hyp(
cirrhosis, nephrot
pathic edema. Otl
ticotropin treatme
(third trimester).

Depressed ald
indicate primary hypoaldosteronism,
salt-losing syndrome, toxemia of pregnancy, Addison's disease, renin deficiency, or hypokalemia.

Alkaline phosphatase

This test measures serum levels of alkaline phosphatase (ALP), which are particularly sensitive to mild biliary obstruction.

An enzyme that's most active at a pH of about 9.0, ALP influences bone calcification and lipid and metabolite transport. Total serum levels reflect the combined activity of several ALP isoenzymes found in the liver, bones, kidneys, intestinal lining, and placenta.

Purpose
■ To detect focal hepatic lesions causing biliary obstruction, such as tumors or abscesses
■ To supplement information from other liver function studies and GI enzyme tests
■ To detect skeletal diseases primarily characterized by marked osteoblastic activity
■ To assess the effectiveness of vitamin D therapy used for deficiency-induced rickets

the laboratory method used. Total serum ALP levels, as measured by chemical inhibition, range from 30 to 90 units/L for men. For women younger than age 45, total ALP levels range from 76 to 196 units/L; for women older than age 45, the range widens to 87 to 250 units/L.

Pregnant women have elevated ALP levels.

Abnormal results
Significant elevations in ALP levels usually indicate skeletal disease or an extrahepatic or intrahepatic biliary obstruction that causes cholestasis. Many acute hepatic diseases also cause ALP levels to rise before serum bilirubin levels change.

A moderate increase may reflect acute biliary obstruction from hepatocellular inflammation in active cirrhosis, mononucleosis, or viral hepatitis. Alternatively, it may reflect osteomalacia or deficiency-induced rickets.

A sharp increase in ALP levels may indicate complete biliary obstruction by malignant or infectious infiltrations or fibrosis. Such markedly high levels are most common in patients with Paget's disease and occur occasionally in patients with extensive bone metastasis or hyperparathyroidism.

Rarely, low ALP levels can signal hypophosphatasia or protein or magnesium deficiency.

Ammonia, plasma

Used to help determine the severity of hepatocellular damage, this test measures plasma levels of ammonia. Normally, the body uses ammonia to rebuild amino acids. The liver then converts the ammonia to urea for excretion by the kidneys. In liver diseases, however, ammonia can bypass the liver and accumulate in the blood.

Purpose
■ To help monitor the progression of severe hepatic disease and the effectiveness of therapy
■ To recognize impending or established hepatic coma

Procedure-related nursing care
If the patient is conscious, explain the purpose of the test and tell him it requires a blood sample. Tell him to fast overnight, because protein intake may alter the test results.

Before performing the venipuncture, notify laboratory personnel so that they can start their preparations. They'll have only 20 minutes from the time you draw the sample to perform the test.

Perform the venipuncture, collecting the sample in a 10-ml green marble-top tube. Handle the sample gently to prevent hemolysis. Pack the container in ice, and send it to the laboratory immediately. (Don't use a chilled container.)

Before removing pressure from the venipuncture site, make sure the bleeding has stopped. Hepatic disease can prolong bleeding time.

Reference values
Plasma ammonia levels are normally less than 50 µg/dl.

Abnormal results
Severe hepatic disease and hepatic coma caused by cirrhosis or acute hepatic necrosis commonly cause elevated plasma ammonia levels. High levels also occur in patients with Reye's syndrome, GI hemorrhage, severe heart failure, pericarditis, hemolytic disease of the neonate, or leukemia.

Amylase, serum

An enzyme synthesized primarily in the pancreas and the salivary glands and secreted into the GI tract, amylase helps digest starch and glycogen in the mouth, stomach, and intestines. Changes in serum amylase levels can indicate acute pancreatic disease.

Purpose
■ To diagnose acute pancreatitis
■ To distinguish acute pancreatitis from causes of abdominal pain that require immediate surgery
■ To assess pancreatic injury caused by abdominal trauma or surgery

Procedure-related nursing care
Explain the purpose of the test to the patient, and tell him you'll need a blood sample. Instruct him to avoid consuming alcohol before the test.

This blood test should be done before either diagnostic or therapeutic interventions. If the patient reports severe pain in his left upper abdominal quadrant, collect the sample in a 7-ml red-top tube immediately.

Reference values
More than 20 methods of measuring serum amylase levels exist, with different ranges of normal values. Test values can't always be converted to a standard measurement. Serum levels normally range from 60 to 180 units/L.

Abnormal results

The highest serum amylase levels occur 4 to 12 hours after the onset of acute pancreatitis. In 48 to 72 hours, the levels drop to normal. If the doctor suspects pancreatitis but the patient has normal serum levels, a urine test should be ordered.

Moderate serum elevations may result from an obstruction of the common bile duct, the pancreatic duct, or the ampulla of Vater; pancreatic injury from a perforated peptic ulcer; pancreatic cancer; acute salivary gland disease; ectopic pregnancy; peritonitis; ovarian or lung cancer; or impaired renal function.

Slight elevations may occur in an asymptomatic patient. An amylase fractionation test may help determine the source of the amylase and aid in the selection of further tests.

Depressed levels can result from chronic pancreatitis, pancreatic cancer, cirrhosis, hepatitis, and toxemia of pregnancy.

Anion gap

The anion gap test measures the difference between serum levels of two anions, chloride (Cl^-) and bicarbonate (HCO_3^-), on the one hand, and serum levels of two cations, sodium (Na^+) and potassium (K^+), on the other hand. Calculation of the anion gap is based on this physical principle: *Total* concentrations of cations and anions are normally equal, accounting for the electrical neutrality of serum. Thus, any gap between the measured anions and cations reflects the serum concentration of unmeasured anions; sulfates, phosphates, organic acids (such as ketone bodies and lactic acid), and proteins.

An increased anion gap indicates a rise in one or more of these unmeasured anions. This may occur in patients with metabolic acidosis that is

characterized by excessive organic or inorganic acids, including lactic acidosis and ketoacidosis.

A normal anion gap, however, doesn't rule out metabolic acidosis. When acidosis results from a loss of HCO_3^- in urine or other body fluids, renal reabsorption of Na^+ promotes Cl^- retention, and the anion gap remains unchanged. Thus, metabolic acidosis resulting from excessive Cl^- levels is known as normal anion gap acidosis.

Purpose

■ To distinguish types of metabolic acidosis
■ To monitor renal function in a patient receiving total parenteral nutrition

Procedure-related nursing care

Explain the purpose of the test to the patient, and tell him the test requires a blood sample. Then perform a venipuncture, and collect the sample in a 7- to 10-ml red-top tube. Handle the specimen carefully to prevent hemolysis.

Reference values

The anion gap should range from 8 to 14 mEq/L.

Abnormal results

An anion gap above 14 mEq/L results from the buildup of metabolic acids and occurs with conditions that cause organic acids, sulfates, or phosphates to accumulate. Such conditions include renal failure; ketoacidosis from starvation, diabetes mellitus, or alcohol ingestion; lactic acidosis; and salicylate, methanol, ethylene glycol (antifreeze), or paraldehyde toxicity.

Although rare, an anion gap below 8 mEq/L may occur in patients with hypermagnesemia or paraproteinemic states, such as multiple myeloma and Waldenström's macroglobulinemia.

Arterial blood gas analysis

Arterial blood gas (ABG) analysis evaluates gas exchange in the lungs by measuring the partial pressures of oxygen (PaO_2) and carbon dioxide ($PaCO_2$) in arterial blood. PaO_2 indicates how much oxygen the lungs are delivering to the blood. $PaCO_2$ indicates how efficiently the lungs eliminate carbon dioxide.

The test also measures the arterial sample's pH, which indicates the acid-base balance, or the hydrogen ion (H^+) concentration. Acidity indicates an H^+ excess; alkalinity, an H^+ deficit. Other ABG measurements include oxygen (O_2) content, oxygen saturation (SaO_2), and bicarbonate (HCO_3^-) levels.

You may draw blood for ABG analysis by percutaneous arterial puncture or from an arterial line.

Purpose
■ To evaluate the efficiency of pulmonary gas exchange
■ To determine the blood's acid-base balance
■ To monitor respiratory therapy
■ To assess the efficiency of mechanical ventilation

Procedure-related nursing care
Before the procedure
Explain the purpose of the test to the patient, and tell him it requires a blood sample. Instruct him to breathe normally while you draw the sample. If you need to perform an arterial puncture, warn him that he may feel brief cramping or throbbing pain at the puncture site.

If the patient has started receiving mechanical ventilation, wait at least 15 minutes before drawing the sample. In that way, you'll get an accurate measurement of the patient's response to mechanical ventilation. If a patient is receiving oxygen therapy, discontinue it for 15 to 20 minutes, if ordered, before drawing a sample. With a patient receiving intermittent positive-pressure breathing, wait at least 20 minutes after treatment stops before drawing the sample; such treatment alters ABG values. For the same reason, don't suction a patient right before drawing an arterial sample.

During the procedure
Perform an arterial puncture or collect the sample from the arterial line, drawing the blood into a heparinized syringe. Put the sample into a bag of ice.

After the procedure
If you performed an arterial puncture, apply pressure to the puncture site for at least 5 minutes — 10 minutes if you used the femoral artery — and tape a gauze pad firmly over it. Avoid taping around the entire limb.

Note on the laboratory request whether the patient was receiving oxygen therapy or breathing room air when you drew the sample. If appropriate, note the oxygen flow rate. For a patient receiving mechanical ventilation, note the fraction of inspired oxygen and tidal volume. For any patient, note the rectal temperature and respiratory rate. Send the sample and the laboratory request to the laboratory.

Monitor the patient's vital signs. Observe a patient who received an arterial puncture for signs and symptoms of circulatory impairment — including swelling, discoloration, pain, numbness, and tingling in the bandaged arm or leg — and check the puncture site for bleeding.

Reference values
ABG values should fall within these ranges:
■ O_2 content — 15% to 23%
■ PaO_2 — 75 to 100 mm Hg
■ $PaCO_2$ — 35 to 45 mm Hg
■ pH — 7.35 to 7.45
■ SaO_2 — 94% to 100%
■ HCO_3^- — 22 to 26 mEq/L.

Abnormal results

A PaO_2 level below 50 mm Hg usually indicates hypoxia. A value between 50 and 75 mm Hg may indicate hypoxia, depending on the patient's age and the oxygen concentration he's receiving. After age 60, patient's normal PaO_2 may fall below 75 mm Hg.

A $PaCO_2$ above 45 mm Hg indicates hypoventilation or hypercapnia; below 35 mm Hg, hyperventilation or hypocapnia. The $PaCO_2$ value can also signal a respiratory acid-base imbalance. A level above 45 mm Hg points to respiratory acidosis; below 35 mm Hg, respiratory alkalosis.

A pH greater than 7.42 indicates alkalosis; pH less than 7.35, acidosis.

A patient with a PaO_2 between 60 and 100 mm Hg should have an SaO_2 above 85%. If his SaO_2 drops sharply, his PaO_2 has probably fallen below 50 mm Hg.

An HCO_3^- value above 26 mEq/L points to metabolic, or kidney-related, alkalosis; below 22 mEq/L, metabolic acidosis.

Recognizing acid–base disorders

Disorder	ABG Findings	Possible causes
Respiratory acidosis (excess CO_2 retention)	■ pH < 7.35 ■ HCO_3^- > 26 mEq/L (if compensating) ■ $PaCO_2$ > 45 mm Hg	■ Central nervous system depression from drugs, injury, or disease ■ Hypoventilation from respiratory, cardiac, musculoskeletal, or neuromuscular disease
Respiratory alkalosis (excess CO_2 loss)	■ pH > 7.45 ■ HCO_3^- < 22 mEq/L (if compensating) ■ $PaCO_2$ < 35 mm Hg	■ Hyperventilation due to anxiety, pain, or improper ventilator settings ■ Respiratory stimulation from drugs, disease, hypoxia, fever, or high room temperature ■ Gram-negative bacteremia
Metabolic acidosis (HCO_3^- loss or acid retention)	■ pH < 7.35 ■ HCO_3^- < 22 mEq/L ■ $PaCO_2$ < 35 mm Hg (if compensating)	■ Depletion of HCO_3^- from renal disease, diarrhea, or small-bowel fistulas ■ Excessive production of organic acids from hepatic disease, endocrine disorders, such as diabetes mellitus, hypoxia, shock, or drug toxicity ■ Inadequate excretion of acids due to renal disease
Metabolic alkalosis (HCO_3^- retention or acid loss)	■ pH > 7.45 ■ HCO_3^- > 26 mEq/L ■ PaO_2 > 45 mm Hg (if compensating)	■ Loss of hydrochloric acid from prolonged vomiting or gastric suctioning ■ Loss of potassium from increased renal excretion (as in diuretic therapy) or corticosteroid overdose ■ Excessive alkali ingestion

Aspartate aminotransferase

Aspartate aminotransferase (AST) serves as an indicator of hepatic and cardiac diseases. A hepatic enzyme, AST is found in the cytoplasma and mitochondria of many cells — mainly in the liver, heart, skeletal muscles, kidneys, pancreas and, to a lesser extent, the red blood cells. When cellular damage occurs, AST is released into serum. You also may hear this test referred to as aspartate transaminase.

Purpos

■ To ai
tial diag
■ To m
cardiac
■ To d
tion (MI
and lact

Proced
Explain
patient
quires
admissi
next 2 c

Perform the venipuncture, collecting the sample in a 7-ml red-top tube. To obtain the most reliable results, draw serum samples at the same time each day.

Reference values
AST levels should range from 8 to 20 units/L in males and 5 to 40 units/L in females.

Abnormal results
AST levels fluctuate according to the extent of cellular necrosis. Thus, levels may rise slightly and transiently early in the disorder and peak during the most acute phase. Depending on when the initial sample is drawn, subsequent AST levels may rise — indicating in-

creasing tissue damage — or fall — indicating tissue repair. These relative changes provide a reliable way to monitor cellular damage.

Extremely high elevations (more than 20 times normal) may indicate acute viral hepatitis, severe skeletal muscle trauma, extensive surgery, drug-induced hepatic injury, or severe passive hepatic congestion.

High elevations (from 10 to 20 times normal) can result from a severe MI, severe infectious mononucleosis, or al... ls may also ... or resolu- ... at cause ex-

... ions (from 5 ... oint to Du- ... hy, dermato- ... tis. These ... g the pro- ... es of dis- ... ations.

... ions (from 2 ... dicate he- ... hepatic tu- ... ulmonary ... l syndrome, or fatty liver.

AST levels rise slightly after the first few days of a biliary duct obstruction. Relatively low elevations also occur at some time during all of the preceding conditions.

Bilirubin, serum

This test measures serum levels of bilirubin, the predominant pigment in bile. The major product of hemoglobin catabolism, bilirubin is formed in the reticuloendothelial system. It's then bound to albumin, a plasma protein, and transported to the liver as unconjugated (indirect or prehepatic) bilirubin. There it joins with glucuronide acid to form bilirubin diglucuronide, and is excreted into bile as conjugated (direct or posthepatic) bilirubin.

Effective bilirubin conjugation and excretion depend on a properly functioning hepatobiliary system and a normal turnover rate of red blood cells (RBCs). Thus, measuring levels of indirect and direct bilirubin can help evaluate hepatobiliary function and RBC production.

Purpose
■ To evaluate liver function
■ To help detect jaundice and monitor its progression
■ To help diagnose biliary obstruction and hemolytic anemia
■ To determine if a neonate requires an exchange transfusion or phototherapy

Procedure-related nursing care
Explain the purpose of the test to the patient, and tell him you'll need a blood sample. Instruct him to fast for at least 4 hours before the test.

Perform the venipuncture, collecting the sample in a 10- to 15-ml red-top tube. Protect the sample from strong sunlight and ultraviolet light. Tell the patient he can resume his normal diet.

A heelstick may be performed on a neonate.

Reference values
Indirect serum bilirubin levels should measure at or below 1.1 mg/dl; direct serum bilirubin levels, less than 0.5 mg/dl. In neonates, total bilirubin levels should measure 1 to 12 mg/dl.

Abnormal results
Elevated indirect serum bilirubin levels can result from hemolysis, a transfusion reaction, hemolytic or pernicious anemia, hemorrhage, or hepatocellular dysfunction (possibly resulting from viral hepatitis or congenital enzyme deficiencies, such as Gilbert syndrome and Crigler-Najjar syndrome).

Elevated direct serum bilirubin levels usually indicate biliary obstruction. In this disorder, direct bilirubin, blocked from its normal pathway through the liver into the biliary tree, overflows into the bloodstream. Such obstruction may be intrahepatic (from viral hepatitis, cirrhosis, or a chlorpromazine reaction) or extrahepatic (from gallstones or gallbladder or pancreatic cancer). An obstruction also may result from bile duct disease.

If the biliary obstruction continues, indirect bilirubin levels may also rise because of hepatic damage. In patients with severe chronic hepatic damage, direct bilirubin levels may return to normal or near-normal levels eventually, but indirect bilirubin levels remain elevated.

In a neonate, if bilirubin levels reach or exceed 18 mg/dl, an exchange transfusion is needed.

Blood urea nitrogen

This test measures the nitrogen fraction of urea, the chief end product of protein metabolism. Formed in the liver from ammonia and excreted by the kidneys, urea accounts for 40% to 50% of the blood's nonprotein nitrogen.

The blood urea nitrogen (BUN) level reflects protein intake and renal excretory capacity. The serum creatinine test, however, is a more reliable indicator of uremia.

Purpose
■ To evaluate renal function and aid in the diagnosis of renal disease
■ To help assess hydration

Procedure-related nursing care
Explain the purpose of the test to the patient, and tell him you'll need a

blood sample. Then perform a venipuncture, collecting the sample in a 10-ml to 15-ml red-top tube.

Reference values

BUN levels should range from 8 to 20 mg/dl, but they can be slightly higher in elderly patients.

Abnormal results

Elevated BUN levels occur in patients with renal disease, reduced renal blood flow (caused by dehydration, for example), urinary tract obstruction, or a condition that increases protein catabolism (such as burns).

Depressed BUN levels occur in patients with severe hepatic damage, malnutrition, or overhydration.

Calcium, serum

Used to detect several disorders, this test measures serum levels of calcium — a cation that helps regulate and promote neuromuscular and enzyme activity, skeletal development, and blood coagulation. The body absorbs calcium from the GI tract, provided that it contains sufficient vitamin D, and excretes calcium in urine and feces. More than 98% of the body's calcium is found in the bones and teeth; calcium can, however, shift in and out of these structures. For example, when calcium levels in the blood drop below normal, calcium can move out of the bones and teeth to help restore blood levels.

Purpose

■ To help diagnose neuromuscular, skeletal, and endocrine disorders; arrhythmias; blood-clotting deficiencies; and acid-base imbalance

Procedure-related nursing care

Explain the purpose of the test to the patient, and tell him it requires a blood sample. Then perform a venipuncture, collecting the sample in a 10- to 15-ml red-top tube.

Reference values

Serum calcium levels should range from 8.9 to 10.1 mg/dl.

Abnormal results

Abnormally high serum calcium levels (hypercalcemia) may result from hyperparathyroidism and parathyroid tumors (caused by oversecretion of parathyroid hormone), Paget's disease of the bone, multiple myeloma, metastatic cancer, multiple fractures, or prolonged immobilization. Elevated serum calcium levels may also result from inadequate excretion of calcium, as in adrenal insufficiency and renal disease; excessive calcium ingestion; or overuse of antacids such as calcium carbonate.

Low calcium levels (hypocalcemia) may result from insufficient calcium intake, hypoparathyroidism, total parathyroidectomy, malabsorption, Cushing's syndrome, renal failure, acute pancreatitis, and peritonitis.

Carcinoembryonic antigen

Carcinoembryonic antigen (CEA) is a protein normally found in embryonic endodermal epithelium and fetal GI tissue. Production of CEA stops before birth, but it may begin again later if a neoplasm develops. Because biliary obstruction, alcoholic hepatitis, chronic heavy smoking, and other conditions also raise CEA levels, this test can't be used as a general indicator of cancer. However, measurement of enzyme CEA levels by immunoassay is useful for staging and monitoring treatment of certain cancers.

Purpose

■ To monitor the effectiveness of cancer therapy

■ To help stage colorectal cancer preoperatively and to test for its recurrence

Procedure-related nursing care

Explain the purpose of the test to the patient and, if appropriate, inform him that the test will be repeated to monitor the effectiveness of therapy. Tell him that you'll need to take a blood sample.

Perform a venipuncture, and collect the sample in a 7-ml red-top tube. Handle the sample gently to prevent hemolysis, and send it to the laboratory immediately.

Reference values

Normal serum CEA values are less than 5 ng/ml in nonsmokers.

Abnormal results

If CEA levels are higher than normal before surgical resection, chemotherapy, or radiation therapy, their return to normal within 6 weeks suggests successful treatment. However, persistently elevated CEA levels suggest residual or recurrent tumor.

High CEA levels are characteristic in various malignant conditions, particularly endodermally derived neoplasms of the GI organs and the lungs, and in certain nonmalignant conditions, such as benign hepatic disease, hepatic cirrhosis, alcoholic pancreatitis, and inflammatory bowel disease.

Elevated CEA levels may also result from nonendodermal carcinomas, such as breast cancer and ovarian cancer.

Cerebrospinal fluid analysis

A clear substance circulating in the subarachnoid space, cerebrospinal fluid (CSF) has several vital functions. It protects the brain and spinal cord from injury and transports products of neurosecretion, cellular biosynthesis, and cellular metabolism through the central nervous system (CNS).

A doctor usually obtains three CSF samples by lumbar puncture between the third and fourth lumbar vertebrae. If a patient has an infection at this site, lumbar puncture is contraindicated, and the doctor may instead perform a cisternal puncture. If a patient has increased intracranial pressure, the doctor must remove the CSF with extreme caution because the removal of fluid causes a rapid reduction in pressure, which could trigger brain stem herniation. The doctor may instead perform a ventricular puncture on this patient. CSF samples may also be obtained during other neurologic tests, such as myelography or pneumoencephalography.

Purpose

■ To measure CSF pressure to help detect an obstruction of CSF circulation

■ To aid in diagnosing viral or bacterial meningitis, and subarachnoid or intracranial hemorrhage, tumors, and abscesses

■ To aid in diagnosing neurosyphilis and chronic CNS infections

Procedure-related nursing care

Before the procedure

Explain the purpose of the test to the patient, and describe the procedure. Make sure the patient has signed a consent form. Tell him to remain still and breathe normally during the procedure because movement and hyperventilation can alter pressure readings and cause injury. Following these instructions will also reduce his risk of headache — the most common adverse effect of a lumbar puncture.

Just before the procedure, obtain a lumbar puncture tray. Place the labeled tubes at the bedside, making sure the labels are numbered sequentially, and include the patient's name, the date, and his room number as well as any laboratory instructions.

During the procedure

If you're assisting with the procedure, position the patient as directed — usually on his side at the edge of the bed with his knees drawn up as far as possible. This position allows full flexion of the spine and easy access to the lumbar subarachnoid space. Place a small pillow under the patient's head, and bend his head forward so that his chin touches his chest. Help him hold this position during the procedure. Stand in front of him, and place one hand around his neck and the other around his knees.

If the doctor wants the patient sitting, have him sit on the edge of the bed and lower his chest and head toward his knees. Help the patient maintain this position throughout the procedure.

Monitor the patient for signs of adverse reactions, such as elevated pulse rate, pallor, or clammy skin.

Make sure the samples are placed in the appropriately labeled tubes. Record the collection time on the test request form; then send the form and the labeled samples to the laboratory immediately.

After the procedure

After a lumbar puncture, the patient usually lies flat for 8 hours. Some doctors, however, allow a 30-degree elevation of the head of the bed. Encourage the patient to drink plenty of fluids, and remind him that raising his head may cause a headache. If he develops a headache, administer an analgesic as ordered.

Check the puncture site for redness, swelling, drainage, CSF leakage, and hematoma every hour for the first 4 hours, then every 4 hours for the next 20 hours. Monitor the patient's level of consciousness, pupillary reaction, and vital signs. Also observe him for signs and symptoms of complications of the lumbar puncture, such as meningitis, cerebellar tonsillar herniation, and medullary compression.

Reference values

Normal CSF pressure ranges from 50 to 180 mm H_2O. The CSF should appear clear and colorless. Normal protein content ranges between 15 and 45 mg/dl; normal gamma globulin levels, between 3% and 12% of total protein. Glucose levels range between 45 and 85 mg/dl, which is two-thirds of the blood glucose level. CSF should contain 0 to 5 white blood cells per microliter and no red blood cells. All serologic tests should be nonreactive.

The chloride level should be 118 to 120 mEq/L. The Gram stain should reveal no organisms.

Abnormal results

For a listing of abnormal results and their possible causes, see *CSF analysis: Abnormal results.*

CSF analysis: Abnormal results

Element	Abnormal result	Possible causes
Cerebrospinal fluid (CSF) pressure	■ Increase	■ Increased intracranial pressure from hemorrhage, tumor, or edema caused by trauma
	■ Decrease	■ Spinal subarachnoid obstruction above puncture site
Appearance	■ Cloudy	■ Infection
	■ Xanthochromic	■ Elevated protein level or red blood cell (RBC) breakdown
	■ Bloody	■ Subarachnoid, intracerebral, or intraventricular hemorrhage; spinal cord obstruction; traumatic puncture
	■ Brown	■ Meningeal melanoma
	■ Orange	■ Systemic carotenemia
Protein	■ Marked increase	■ Tumor, trauma, hemorrhage, diabetes mellitus, polyneuritis, blood in CSF
	■ Marked decrease	■ Rapid CSF production
Gamma globulin	■ Increase	■ Demyelinating disease (such as multiple sclerosis), neurosyphilis, Guillain-Barré syndrome
Glucose	■ Increase	■ Systemic hyperglycemia
	■ Decrease	■ Systemic hypoglycemia, bacterial or fungal infection, meningitis, mumps, postsubarachnoid hemorrhage
Cell count	■ Increase in white blood cell count	■ Meningitis, acute infection, onset of chronic illness, tumor, abscess, infarction, demyelinating disease (such as multiple sclerosis)
	■ RBCs present	■ Hemorrhage or traumatic puncture
Serologic tests	■ Reactive	■ Neurosyphilis
Chloride	■ Decrease	■ Infected meninges (tuberculosis or meningitis)
Gram stain	■ Gram-positive or gram-negative organisms	■ Bacterial meningitis

Chloride, serum

This test measures serum levels of chloride, the major extracellular fluid anion. Interacting with sodium, the major extracellular cation, chloride helps regulate blood volume and arterial pressure by helping to maintain the osmotic pressure of blood.

Chloride levels affect acid-base balance, varying inversely with bicarbonate levels. Excessive chloride loss in gastric juices or other secretions can cause hypochloremic metabolic alkalosis; excessive chloride retention or ingestion can lead to hyperchloremic metabolic acidosis.

Purpose
■ To detect acid-base imbalance
■ To help evaluate fluid status and extracellular cation-anion balance

Procedure–related nursing care
Explain the purpose of the test to the patient, and tell him it requires a blood sample. Then perform a venipuncture, collecting the sample in a 10- to 15-ml red-top tube.

Reference values
Serum chloride levels should range from 100 to 108 mEq/L.

Abnormal results
Elevated chloride levels (hyperchloremia) can result from severe dehydration, complete renal shutdown, head injury (producing neurogenic hyperventilation), and primary aldosteronism.

Usually associated with low sodium and potassium levels, low chloride levels (hypochloremia) can stem from prolonged vomiting, gastric suctioning, intestinal fistula, chronic renal failure, or Addison's disease. Dilutional hypochloremia can result from heart failure or edema that leads to excess extracellular fluid.

Cholesterol, total

This test measures the circulating levels of free cholesterol and cholesterol esters — the two forms in which this biochemical compound appears in the body.

A structural component in cell membranes and plasma lipoproteins, cholesterol is absorbed from the diet and synthesized in the liver and other body tissues. It helps form adrenocorticoid steroids, bile salts, androgens, and estrogens.

A diet high in saturated fat raises cholesterol levels by stimulating the absorption of lipids, including cholesterol, from the intestine; a diet low in saturated fat lowers cholesterol levels.

Purpose
■ To assess the risk of coronary artery disease (CAD)
■ To evaluate fat metabolism
■ To help diagnose nephrotic syndrome, pancreatitis, hepatic disease, hypothyroidism, and hyperthyroidism

Procedure–related nursing care
Explain the purpose of the test to the patient, and tell him it requires a blood sample. Make sure he fasts overnight and refrains from drinking alcohol for 24 hours before the procedure.

Perform a venipuncture, collecting the sample in a 7-ml red-top tube. Send it to the laboratory immediately.

Tell the patient he may resume his normal diet.

Reference values
Total cholesterol levels vary with age and sex, normally ranging from 150 to 200 mg/dl.

Abnormal results

Cholesterol levels above 250 mg/dl generally indicate a high risk of CAD and the need for treatment. A patient with a level between 200 and 240 mg/dl has a moderate risk. If he has other risk factors — if he smokes or has high blood pressure, for instance — his risk of CAD is considered high. Elevated cholesterol levels (hypercholesterolemia) can also indicate incipient hepatitis, lipid disorders, bile duct blockage, nephrotic syndrome, obstructive jaundice, pancreatitis, or hypothyroidism. Abnormally high levels usually require further testing to determine the causative disorder.

Low serum cholesterol levels (hypocholesterolemia) can result from malnutrition, cellular necrosis of the liver, or hyperthyroidism.

Complete blood count

A common test, the complete blood count (CBC) provides a fairly comprehensive picture of all the blood's formed elements. Typically, the CBC includes these components: hemoglobin levels, hematocrit, red blood cell (RBC) and white blood cell (WBC) counts, as well as the WBC differential and stained RBC examination, which are commonly done together.

A CBC is especially useful for evaluating conditions in which the hematocrit doesn't parallel the RBC count, such as microcytic or macrocytic anemia.

After the WBC differential, the same stained slide is evaluated for RBC distribution and morphology — including changes in cell contents, color, size, and shape. This examination provides more information for detecting leukemia, anemia, and thalassemia.

Purpose

■ To compare the status of specific blood elements
■ To help detect and evaluate anemias and leukemia
■ To indicate the need for further definitive studies

Procedure-related nursing care

Explain the purpose of the test to the patient, and tell him it requires a blood sample. Then perform a venipuncture, collecting at least a 5-ml sample in a lavender-top tube.

Reference values

(See the entries for the individual tests that make up the CBC.)

Abnormal results

Variations in the size and shape of RBCs are reported as occasional, slight, moderate, marked, or very marked; structural variations are reported as the number of immature or nucleated RBCs per 100 WBCs. Cell inclusions are also noted.

(For implications of specific abnormal results, see the entries for the individual tests that make up the CBC.)

Creatine kinase

An enzyme found mainly in muscle cells and brain tissue, creatine kinase (CK) catalyzes the transfer of a phosphate group from adenosine triphosphate to creatine, releasing energy in the process. Because of this key role in energy production, CK reflects tissue catabolism. An increase in serum CK levels indicates cellular trauma.

CK occurs as three distinct isoenzymes: CK-BB, found mainly in brain tissue; CK-MB, located in cardiac muscle (although a small amount also appears in skeletal muscle); and CK-MM, found in skeletal muscle. Because each isoenzyme is associated with a specific location, fractionation and measurement can help pinpoint the site of tissue destruction. Total CK levels help diagnose skeletal muscle disorders, but CK-MM, which constitutes more than 99% of the total CK normally present in serum, acts as a more specific indicator.

Purpose
■ To diagnose acute myocardial infarction (MI) and reinfarction
■ To evaluate possible causes of chest pain and to monitor the severity of myocardial ischemia after cardiac surgery or catheterization or cardioversion
■ To detect skeletal muscle disorders that don't have a neurogenic origin, such as Duchenne's muscular dystrophy and early dermatomyositis

Procedure-related nursing care
Explain the purpose of the test to the patient, and tell him you'll need to collect several blood samples. If he's being tested for a skeletal muscle disorder, instruct him to avoid exercising for 24 hours before the test.

Perform a venipuncture, collecting the sample in a 7-ml red-top tube. If the patient needs an I.M. injection, draw the sample either before the injection or at least 1 hour after it — otherwise, the test results may be altered. Send the sample to the laboratory at once.

Always collect the sample on schedule, and note the time on the laboratory request. For a patient with chest pain, note how many hours have elapsed since the patient started having chest pain.

Reference values
Total CK levels determined by the most commonly performed assay in North America range from 55 to 170 units/L

for men and from 30 to 135 units/L for women. Typical ranges for isoenzyme levels are as follows: CK-BB, 0% of total CK; CK-MB, 0% to 3% of total CK; CK-MM, 97% to 100% of total CK.

Abnormal results
Detectable CK-BB levels may indicate brain tissue injury, certain widespread malignant tumors, severe shock, or renal failure. However, such elevations don't confirm a specific diagnosis.

CK-MB levels greater than 5% of total CK (more than 10 units/L) are usually considered positive for an MI. With an acute MI or cardiac surgery, CK-MB levels begin rising in 2 to 4 hours, peak in 12 to 24 hours, and return to normal in 24 to 48 hours. Persistent elevations or increasing levels indicate ongoing myocardial damage. (See *Serum enzyme and isoenzyme levels after an MI.*) Total CK levels follow roughly the same pattern but rise slightly later. Serious skeletal muscle injury (as occurs in patients with certain muscular dystrophies), polymyositis, and severe myoglobinuria may slightly elevate CK-MB levels.

Rising CK-MM values follow skeletal muscle damage from trauma, such as surgery and I.M. injection. Extremely high levels (50 to 100 times normal) may occur in patients with such diseases as dermatomyositis or muscular dystrophy. Sharp elevations also occur with muscular activity caused by agitation such as an acute psychotic episode. A moderate rise develops in patients with hypothyroidism.

Elevated total CK levels may occur in patients with severe hypokalemia, carbon monoxide poisoning, malignant hyperthermia, or alcoholic cardiomyopathy. CK levels also increase after seizures. Occasionally, total CK levels rise after a pulmonary or cerebral infarction.

Serum enzyme and isoenzyme levels after an MI

Because they're released by damaged tissue, serum enzymes and isoenzymes (cat-alytic proteins that vary in concentration in specific organs) can help identify the compromised organ and assess the extent of damage. The serum enzyme and isoen-zyme determinations listed below are most significant in myocardial infarction (MI).

Isoenzymes

■ Creatine kinase-MB (CK-MB): in the heart muscle and a small amount in skeletal muscle
■ Lactate dehydrogenase 1 and 2 (LD_1, LD_2): in the heart, brain, kidneys, liver, skeletal muscles, and red blood cells

Enzymes

■ Troponin-I and troponin-T (the cardiac contractile proteins): greater sensitivity than CK-MB in detecting myocardial injury

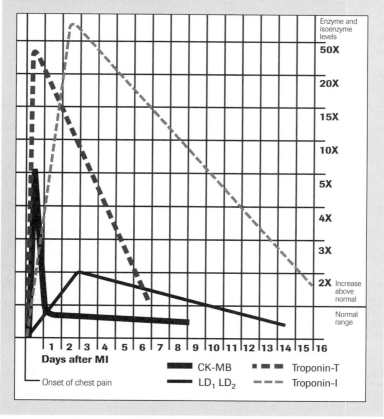

Creatinine, serum

A quantitative analysis of serum creatinine levels, this test provides a more sensitive measure of renal damage than blood urea nitrogen levels do. That's because renal impairment is virtually the only cause of elevated serum creatinine levels.

Creatinine, a nonprotein end product of creatine metabolism, appears in serum in amounts proportional to the body's muscle mass. The kidneys easily excrete creatinine, with little or no tubular reabsorption, so creatinine levels are directly related to the glomerular filtration rate.

Purpose
■ To assess renal glomerular filtration
■ To screen for renal damage

Procedure-related nursing care
Explain the purpose of the test to the patient, and tell him you'll need a blood sample. Instruct him to restrict food and fluid intake for about 8 hours before the test.

Perform a venipuncture, using a 10- to 15-ml red-top tube.

Reference values
Serum creatinine levels in men range from 0.8 to 1.2 mg/dl; in women, from 0.6 to 0.9 mg/dl.

Abnormal results
Elevated serum creatinine levels generally indicate renal disease that has damaged at least 50% of the nephrons. Elevated levels are also associated with gigantism and acromegaly. Decreased levels may result from a loss of muscle mass in advanced muscular dystrophy.

Creatinine clearance

This test determines how efficiently the kidneys clear creatinine from the blood. The clearance rate is expressed in terms of the volume of blood (in milliliters) that the kidneys can clear of creatinine in 1 minute. The test requires a blood sample and a timed urine specimen.

Creatinine, the chief metabolite of creatine, is produced and excreted in constant amounts that are proportional total muscle mass. Normal physical activity, diet, and urine volume have little effect on this production, although strenuous exercise and a high-protein diet can affect it.

Purpose
■ To asses renal function (primarily glomerular filtration)
■ To monitor the progression of renal insufficiency

Procedure-related nursing care
Explain the purpose of the test to the patient. Tell him that you'll need a timed urine specimen and at least one blood sample. Describe the urine collection procedure. Also tell him to avoid eating an excessive amount of meat before the procedure and to avoid strenuous exercise during the urine collection period.

Collect a time urine specimen for a 2-, 6-, 12-, or 24-hour period, as ordered. During the collection period, perform a venipuncture, collecting the blood sample in a 7-ml red-top tube.

Collect the urine specimen in a bottle containing a preservative to prevent creatinine degradation. Refrigerate it or keep it on ice during the collection period. At the end of the period, send the specimen to the laboratory. Then tell the patient he may resume his normal diet and activities.

Reference values
For men, the normal creatinine clearance ranges from 97 to 137 ml/minute. For women, the creatinine clearance ranges from 88 to 128 ml/minute. For older patients, creatinine clearance de-

clines by 6 ml/minute for each succeeding decade of life.

Abnormal results

A low creatinine clearance rate may result from reduced renal blood flow (from shock or renal artery obstruction), acute tubular necrosis, acute or chronic glomerulonephritis, advanced bilateral renal lesions (as occur in patients with polycystic kidney disease, renal tuberculosis, or cancer), or nephrosclerosis. Heart failure and severe dehydration may also cause the creatinine clearance rate to drop.

An elevated creatinine clearance rate usually has little diagnostic significance.

Erythrocyte sedimentation rate

A sensitive but nonspecific test, the erythrocyte sedimentation rate (ESR) measures the time needed for erythrocytes (red blood cells) in a whole blood sample to settle to the bottom of a vertical tube. It commonly provides the earliest indication of disease when other chemical or physical signs are still normal. The rate typically rises significantly in widespread inflammatory disorders caused by infection or autoimmune mechanisms. Localized inflammation and cancer may prolong the ESR elevation.

Purpose

■ To aid in diagnosing occult disease, such as tuberculosis, tissue necrosis, and connective tissue disease
■ To monitor inflammatory and malignant disease

Procedure-related nursing care

Explain the purpose of the test to the patient, and tell him you'll need a blood sample. Then perform a venipuncture, collecting the sample in a 7-ml lavender-top tube. Mix the specimen and anticoagulant well.

Examine the sample for clots and clumps, and then send it to the laboratory immediately.

Reference values

The ESR normally ranges from 0 to 15 mm/hour in men, and from 0 to 20 mm/hour in women. Values gradually increase with age.

Abnormal results

The ESR rises with most anemias, pregnancy, acute or chronic inflammation, tuberculosis, paraproteinemias (especially multiple myeloma and Waldenström's macroglobulinemia), rheumatic fever, rheumatoid arthritis, and some types of cancer.

Polycythemia, sickle cell anemia, hyperviscosity, and low plasma protein levels tend to depress the ESR.

Glucose, fasting plasma

Also known as the fasting blood sugar test, the fasting plasma glucose test measures the patient's plasma glucose levels after a 12- to 14-hour fast.

When a patient fasts, his plasma glucose levels decrease, stimulating the release of the hormone glucagon. This hormone raises plasma glucose levels by accelerating glycogenolysis, stimulating gluconeogenesis, and inhibiting glycogen synthesis. Normally, the secretion of insulin stops the rise in glucose levels. In patients with diabetes, however, the absence or deficiency of insulin allows glucose levels to remain persistently elevated.

Purpose

■ To screen for diabetes mellitus and other glucose metabolism disorders
■ To monitor drug or dietary therapy in patients with diabetes mellitus
■ To help determine the insulin requirements of patients who have uncontrolled diabetes mellitus and those

who require parenteral or enteral nutritional support

■ To help evaluate patients with known or suspected hypoglycemia

Procedure-related nursing care

Explain the purpose of the test to the patient. Tell him that it requires a blood sample and that he must fast (taking only water) for 12 to 14 hours before the test.

If the patient is known to have diabetes, you should draw his blood before he receives insulin or an oral antidiabetic. Tell him to watch for signs and symptoms of hypoglycemia, such as weakness, restlessness, nervousness, hunger, and sweating. Stress that he should report such signs and symptoms immediately.

Note the time of the patient's last pretest meal and pretest medication on the laboratory request. Also record the time the sample is collected.

Perform a venipuncture, collecting the sample in a 5-ml gray-top tube. If the sample can't be sent to the laboratory immediately, refrigerate it and transport it as soon as possible.

Give the patient a balanced meal or a snack after the procedure. Assure him that he can now eat and take medications withheld before the procedure.

Reference values

The normal range for fasting plasma glucose levels varies according to the length of the fast. Generally, after a 12- to 14-hour fast, normal values are between 70 and 100 mg/dl.

Abnormal results

Fasting plasma glucose levels greater than 100 mg/dl but less than 140 mg/dl may suggest impaired glucose tolerance. A 2-hour glucose tolerance test that yields a plasma glucose level between 140 and 200 mg/dl, and an intervening oral glucose tolerance test that yields a plasma glucose level

greater than or equal to 200 mg/dl confirm the diagnosis.

Levels greater than or equal to 140 mg/dl (obtained on two or more occasions) may indicate diabetes mellitus if other causes of the patient's hyperglycemia have been ruled out. Such a patient will also have a random plasma glucose level greater than or equal to 200 mg/dl along with the classic signs and symptoms of diabetes mellitus — polydipsia, polyuria, ketonuria, polyphagia, and rapid weight loss.

Elevated levels can also result from pancreatitis, recent acute illness (such as myocardial infarction), Cushing's syndrome, pituitary adenoma, pancreatitis, hyperthyroidism, or pheochromocytoma. Hyperglycemia may also stem from chronic hepatic disease, brain trauma, chronic illness, or chronic malnutrition and is typical in patients with eclampsia, anoxia, or a seizure disorder.

Depressed plasma glucose levels can result from hyperinsulinism (overdose of insulin being the most common cause), insulinoma, von Gierke's disease, functional or reactive hypoglycemia, hypothyroidism, adrenocortical insufficiency, congenital adrenal hyperplasia, hypopituitarism, islet cell carcinoma of the pancreas, hepatic necrosis, or glycogen storage disease.

Glucose, 2-hour postprandial plasma

This test requires a blood sample drawn 2 hours after the patient eats a meal. The results reflect the metabolic response to a carbohydrate challenge. Normally, the blood glucose level returns to the fasting level within 2 hours.

Purpose

■ To monitor the effectiveness of drug or diet therapy in patients with diabetes mellitus

■ To identify disorders associated with abnormal glucose metabolism
■ To confirm diabetes mellitus in patients with the classic signs and symptoms of the disorder

Procedure-related nursing care

Explain the purpose of the test to the patient. Tell him it requires a blood sample drawn 2 hours after a meal. Instruct him to fast overnight (except for water) and then to eat a breakfast that includes 100 g of carbohydrates. Stress that he should avoid smoking and strenuous exercise after the meal.

Note the time of the patient's meal, the sample collection time, and the time that last pretest insulin or antidiabetic dose was given on the laboratory request, if appropriate.

Perform a venipuncture, collecting the sample in a 5-ml gray-top tube. If you can't send the sample to the laboratory immediately, place the sample in the refrigerator and transport it as soon as possible.

Tell the patient he may resume eating and other activities that he discontinued before the test.

Reference values

For a person who doesn't have diabetes, postprandial glucose values are usually less than 145 mg/dl; levels may be slightly higher in older patients, increasing an average of 5 mg/dl for each decade.

Abnormal results

Values greater than 140 mg/dl are abnormal in adults younger than age 50; values greater than 160 ml/dl are abnormal in adults older than age 60. A value greater than or equal to 200 mg/dl, along with the classic signs and symptoms of diabetes mellitus, confirms a diagnosis of diabetes mellitus.

Other causes of elevated glucose levels include pancreatitis, Cushing's syndrome, acromegaly, pheochromocy-

toma, chronic hepatic disease, nephrotic syndrome, gastrectomy with dumping syndrome, and seizure disorders.

Depressed glucose levels occur in patients with hyperinsulinism, insulinoma, von Gierke's disease, functional or reactive hypoglycemia, hypothyroidism, adrenocortical insufficiency, congenital adrenal hyperplasia, hypopituitarism, islet cell carcinoma of the pancreas, hepatic necrosis, or glycogen storage disease.

Glucose tolerance test, oral

The most sensitive method of evaluating borderline diabetes mellitus, the oral glucose tolerance test measures carbohydrate metabolism after ingestion of a challenge dose of glucose.

With this test, the body rapidly absorbs the glucose, causing plasma glucose levels to rise and peak 30 minutes to 1 hour after ingestion. The pancreas responds by secreting more insulin, causing glucose levels to return to normal within 2 hours. During this period, plasma glucose levels are monitored to assess insulin secretion and the body's ability to metabolize glucose. Occasionally, levels are monitored for an additional 2 to 3 hours to aid diagnosis of hypoglycemia and malabsorption syndrome.

If the oral glucose tolerance test is performed on a patient with type 2 diabetes, his fasting plasma glucose levels may be within the normal range. However, insufficient secretions of insulin after ingestion of carbohydrates will cause his plasma glucose levels to rise sharply and return to normal slowly. This decreased tolerance for glucose helps confirm type 2 diabetes.

The oral glucose tolerance test shouldn't be performed on a person who's suspected of having insulinoma because prolonged fasting by such a patient can lead to fainting and coma. It also shouldn't be used for patients with fasting plasma glucose values greater than 140 mg/dl or postprandial plasma glucose values greater than 200 mg/dl.

Purpose
■ To confirm diabetes mellitus in selected patients
■ To aid in diagnosing hypoglycemia and malabsorption syndrome

Procedure-related nursing care
Before the procedure
Explain the purpose of the test to the patient, and tell him that it requires several blood samples and a urine specimen. Instruct him to maintain a high-carbohydrate diet, not to smoke, and to avoid caffeine and alcohol for 3 days before the test. Tell him to fast for 10 to 16 hours before the test and to avoid strenuous exercise for 8 hours before and during the test. Suggest that he bring a book or other quiet diversionary material with him because the procedure usually takes several hours.

Alert the patient to the signs and symptoms of hypoglycemia — weakness, restlessness, nervousness, hunger, and sweating — and tell him to report such signs and symptoms immediately.

Prepare the laboratory request, specifying the time of the patient's last meal and the times of the blood sample collections. Also note the time of the patient's last pretest insulin or oral antidiabetic dose, if appropriate.

During the procedure
Obtain a fasting blood sample by performing a venipuncture — usually between 7 a.m. and 9 a.m. Draw the sample into a 7-ml gray-top tube. Collect a urine specimen at the same time, if appropriate.

After collecting these samples, administer the test load of oral glucose. Record the time when the patient starts

drinking the solution. Encourage him to drink it all within 5 minutes.

You'll need to draw blood samples 30 minutes, 1 hour, 1½ hours, 2 hours, and 3 hours after the loading dose, as ordered. Use a 7-ml gray-top tube for each sample.

Tell the patient to lie down if he feels faint. If he develops severe hypoglycemia, draw a blood sample, record the time on the laboratory request, and discontinue the test. Administer I.V. glucose or have the patient drink a glass of orange juice to reverse the reaction.

Send all blood and urine samples to the laboratory immediately. If that isn't possible, refrigerate them and transport them as soon as possible.

After the procedure
Provide a balanced meal or snack, observing the patient for signs of a hypoglycemic reaction. Tell the patient to resume his normal diet and activities.

Reference values
Normally, plasma glucose levels peak at 160 to 180 mg/dl 30 minutes to 1 hour after administration of an oral glucose test dose and return to fasting levels (or lower) within 2 hours. Normal levels are less than 140 mg/dl after 2 hours.

Abnormal results
If the 2-hour sample and at least one other sample (taken up to 2 hours after a 75-g or greater glucose dose) show a glucose level greater than or equal to 200 mg/dl, the test confirms diabetes in a nonpregnant adult.

After an oral glucose dose of 100 g, gestational diabetes mellitus is confirmed in a pregnant patient if two plasma glucose levels equal or exceed a fasting value of 105 mg/dl, a 1-hour value of 190 mg/dl, a 2-hour value of 165 mg/dl, or a 3-hour value of 145 mg/dl.

Increased glucose levels are associated with other serious conditions — such as Cushing's syndrome, pheochromocytoma, central nervous system lesions, cirrhosis of the liver, myocardial or cerebral infarction, and hyperthyroidism — as well as with anxiety states and pregnancy.

Decreased glucose levels occur in patients with hyperinsulinism, malabsorption syndrome, adrenocortical insufficiency (Addison's disease), hypothyroidism, or hypopituitarism.

Hematocrit

A common test, hematocrit (HCT) measures the percentage of packed red blood cells (RBCs) in a whole blood sample. Thus, an HCT of 40% means that a 100-ml sample contains 40 ml of packed RBCs. The HCT value depends mainly on the number of RBCs but is also influenced by the size of the average RBC. Therefore, conditions that result in elevated levels of blood glucose and sodium (which cause swelling of RBCs) may produce elevated HCT. This test may be automatically performed as part of the complete blood count.

Purpose
■ To aid diagnosis of polycythemia, anemia, and abnormal states of hydration
■ To aid in calculating RBC indices
■ To monitor fluid imbalance
■ To monitor blood loss and evaluate blood replacement

Procedure-related nursing care
Explain the purpose of the test to the patient, and tell him it requires a blood sample drawn from his finger. Then perform a fingerstick on an adult, using a heparinized capillary tube with a red band on the anticoagulant end. Fill the capillary tube from the red-banded end to about two-thirds' capacity, and seal this end with clay.

A hematocrit can also be obtained from a specimen collected by venipuncture in a 7-ml lavender-top tube.

Reference values
HCT values vary, depending on the patient's sex and age, the type of sample, and the laboratory performing the test. Reference values range from 40% to 54% for men and from 37% to 47% for women.

Abnormal results
A high HCT value suggests polycythemia or hemoconcentration caused by blood loss; a low HCT value, anemia or hemodilution.

Hemoglobin, glycosylated

This test measures three minor hemoglobins (Hb): A_{1a}, A_{1b}, and A_{1c}. These three hemoglobins are variants of Hb A formed by glycosylation — a nearly irreversible molecular process in which glucose becomes chemically incorporated in Hb A. Because glycosylation occurs at a constant rate during the 120-day life span of a red blood cell (RBC), glycosylated Hb levels reflect the average blood glucose level during the preceding 6 to 10 weeks. This makes the test most appropriate for evaluating the long-term effectiveness of a patient's diabetes therapy.

Purpose
■ To monitor control of diabetes mellitus

Procedure-related nursing care
Explain the purpose of the test to the patient, and tell him it requires a blood sample. Instruct him to maintain his prescribed medication or diet regimen before the procedure.

Perform a venipuncture, collecting the sample in a 5-ml lavender-top tube. Fill the collection tube completely, and then invert it gently several times to mix the sample and the anticoagulant adequately.

After the test, schedule the patient for appropriate follow-up testing in 6 to 8 weeks.

Reference values
Glycosylated Hb values are reported as a percentage of the total Hb level within an RBC. Because Hb A_{1c} is present in a larger quantity than the other minor Hbs, it's the variant commonly measured. Reference values for Hb A_{1c} are usually 4.5% to 8% of the total Hb level within an RBC.

Abnormal results
If Hb A_{1c} accounts for more than 8% of the total Hb level within an RBC, the patient's diabetes mellitus isn't considered under control.

Hemoglobin, total

Usually done as part of the complete blood count, this test measures the grams of hemoglobin (Hb) found in a deciliter (dl, or 100 ml) of whole blood. Hb concentration correlates closely with the red blood cell (RBC) count and is affected by the Hb-RBC ratio and free plasma Hb levels.

Purpose
■ To measure the severity of anemia or polycythemia
■ To monitor the patient's response to therapy for anemia

Procedure-related nursing care
Explain the purpose of the test to the patient, and tell him it requires a blood sample. Then perform a venipuncture, collecting the sample in a 7-ml lavender-top tube.

Reference values
Normal Hb levels for a man range from 14 to 18 g/dl; for a women, from 12 to 16 g/dl.

Abnormal results
An elevated total Hb level suggests hemoconcentration from polycythemia or dehydration. A low concentration of Hb may indicate anemia, recent hemorrhage, or fluid retention that's causing hemodilution.

Hepatitis B surface antigen

The earliest and most reliable serologic marker of viral hepatitis infection, the hepatitis B surface antigen (HBsAg) appears in the serum of a patient with hepatitis B virus (HBV) as early as 14 days after exposure and throughout the acute stage of illness. The antigen can also be detected in a carrier's blood.

After donation, all blood is screened for HBV before it's stored. However, the test doesn't screen for any other form of hepatitis. (See *Hepatitis panel.*)

Purpose
■ To screen blood for HBV
■ To screen persons at high risk for contracting HBV, such as hemodialysis nurses
■ To aid differential diagnosis of viral hepatitis

Procedure-related nursing care
Explain the purpose of the test to the patient, and tell him that it requires a blood sample. Then perform a venipuncture, using a 10-ml red-top tube to collect the sample. Because HBV is a blood-borne infection, follow standard precautions. Make sure you wear gloves, avoid accidental needle puncture, wash your hands after the procedure, and properly dispose of the needle.

If you accidentally stick yourself with a used needle, report the incident immediately. Expect to receive gamma globulin to help prevent the disease.

Reference values
Serum is normally negative for HBsAg.

Abnormal results

The presence of HBsAg in a patient with hepatitis confirms HBV. In chronic carriers and persons with chronic active hepatitis, HBsAg may be present in serum several months after the onset of acute infection. HBsAg may also occur in more than 5% of patients with certain diseases other than hepatitis, such as hemophilia, Hodgkin's disease, and leukemia.

Hepatitis panel

These tests are performed on patients with symptoms of hepatitis. Positive results not only confirm diagnosis of hepatitis but also differentiate the type and status of the infection as well.

Test	Purpose	Implication of positive result
Anti-HAV (antibody to hepatitis A virus [HAV] antigen; also called HAV-Ab)	■ To rule out HAV infection ■ To determine immune status to HAV	■ Indicates need for supportive care and education ■ Can test for anti-HAV immunoglobulin M (IgM) and anti-HAV IgG ■ Presence of IgG: indicates unlikely cause of current symptoms and immunity to HAV
Anti-HBc (IgG and IgM) (antibody to hepatitis B virus [HBV] core antigen)	■ To differentiate acute from chronic HBV infection	■ Is occasional falsely positive ■ Must be interpreted in context of other tests ■ Indicates HBV infection as this marker doesn't appear after vaccination ■ If primarily anti-HBc IgM result: reveals acute hepatitis B (infected usually <6 months) and needs follow-up ■ If primarily anti-HBc IgG result: reveals chronic hepatitis B and needs follow-up
Anti-HBeAg (antibody to hepatitis Be antigen)	■ To select patients for interferon therapy ■ To select patients for liver transplantation	■ If anti-HBeAg is present: indicates favorable prognosis because body has mounted a defensive attack against HBV ■ Usually appears 8 to 16 weeks after exposure to HBV antigen; indicates an immune response has occurred
Anti-HbsAg (antibody to hepatitis B surface antigen; also called anti-HBs)	■ To check immune status to HBV	■ Indicates immune response to HBV due to HBV infection or HBV Ig or HBV vaccination ■ In acute infection, detectable after HbsAg disappears

(continued)

Hepatitis panel *(continued)*

Test	Purpose	Implication of positive result
Anti-HCV (antibody to hepatitis C virus [HCV]) enzyme-linked immunosorbent assay (ELISA)	■ To aid differential diagnosis of HCV ■ To screen blood donors (ELISA-1 and ELISA-2 are inexpensive, simple to perform, and highly sensitive; however, ELISA-2 is more sensitive.)	■ Does NOT indicate immunity ■ Appears 2 to 6 months after acute HCV infection, but may take up to 1 year ■ In the presence of elevated liver function tests (LFTs): indicates hepatitis C and needs follow-up ■ Low specificity compared with ribonucleic acid (RNA) testing*
Anti-HDV (antibody to hepatitis D virus [HDV])	■ To detect antibodies to hepatitis delta virus (HDV) RNA by polymerase chain reaction (HDV is a defective RNA virus that replicates efficiently only in the presence of HbsAg.)	■ If positive for HDV: indicates poor prognosis ■ 50% of patients with fulminant HBV also have HDV
HBeAg (hepatitis Be antigen)	■ To measure viral replication	■ High levels: very infectious patient
HbsAg (also called hepatitis-associated antigen, Australia antigen)	■ To screen blood donors and high-risk populations ■ To aid prenatal testing ■ To establish differential diagnosis of viral hepatitis	■ Needs follow-up ■ Elevation for >6 months indicative of chronic hepatitis B infection
HBV deoxyribonucleic acid	■ To measure viral presence (not antibodies) ■ To confirm HBV if HBV screen is positive result but LFTs are normal	■ Confirms HBV status and requires careful follow-up
HCV RNA (also called enzyme immunoassay 2 [EIA-2], HCV RNA RT-PCR [reverse transcriptase-polymerase chain reaction])	■ To measure viral presence (not antibodies) ■ To confirm hepatitis C virus (HCV) status (gold standard because it's the most sensitive, but it's expensive and requires technical skill) ■ To confirm HCV if HCV screen is positive but LFTs are normal	■ Confirms HCV status and requires careful follow-up

*A second-generation recombinant immunoblot assay (also called RIBA) is a commonly used supplemental assay, particularly in patients with normal ALT levels. The reactivity of antibodies toward each antigen band is reported as 1+ to 4+. If two or more bands react with an intensity of at least 1+, the result is indeterminate; however, the bands c22-3 and c33c are strongly associated with HCV RNA, and even an indeterminate result that includes one of them may indicate positive HCV infection.

Human chorionic gonadotropin, serum

This serum immunoassay provides a quantitative analysis of the human chorionic gonadotropin (HCG) beta-subunit level. Although it's more costly than the routine urine test ordered to confirm pregnancy, it's also much more sensitive.

Purpose

■ To detect early pregnancy or to determine the adequacy of hormone production in high-risk pregnancies
■ To aid in diagnosing trophoblastic tumors, such as hydatidiform mole or choriocarcinoma, and tumors that secrete HCG ectopically
■ To monitor treatment for induction of ovulation and conception

Procedure-related nursing care

Explain the purpose of the test to the patient, and tell her it requires a blood sample. Then perform a venipuncture, and collect at least a 7-ml sample in a red-top tube.

Reference values

Values for serum HCG should be less than 5 IU/ml.

Abnormal results

Elevated serum HCG levels may indicate pregnancy; sharply elevated levels may indicate a multiple pregnancy. Increased levels may also indicate a tumor, such as a hydatidiform mole, a trophoblastic neoplasm of the placenta, or nontrophoblastic carcinomas that secrete HCG. However, the HCG beta-subunit levels can't differentiate between pregnancy and tumor recurrence.

Low serum HCG beta-subunit levels can occur in ectopic pregnancy or pregnancy of less than 9 days.

Human chorionic gonadotropin, urine

Human chorionic gonadotropin (HCG) is a glycopeptide hormone produced by the trophoblastic cells of the placenta. Although its precise function is unclear, HCG, along with progesterone, apparently maintains the corpus luteum during early pregnancy.

Production of HCG increases steadily during the first trimester, peaking around the 10th week of gestation. Levels then fall to less than 10% of first trimester peak levels.

The qualitative analysis of HCG in the urine can detect pregnancy as early as 10 days after a missed menstrual period. Quantitative measurements may be used to evaluate a suspected hydatidiform mole or HCG-secreting tumors.

Purpose

■ To detect and confirm pregnancy
■ To aid the diagnosis of hydatidiform mole or HCG-secreting tumors

Procedure-related nursing care

Explain the purpose of the test to the patient, and inform her that it requires a first-voided morning specimen for a qualitative analysis or a 24-hour urine collection for a quantitative analysis.

Indicate on the laboratory request the date of the patient's last menstrual period.

Collect the appropriate urine specimen. If you're collecting a 24-hour specimen, you must either refrigerate it or keep it on ice during the entire collection period.

Reference values

In qualitative analysis, test results are positive, indicating that the patient is pregnant.

In quantitative analysis, urine HCG levels in the first trimester of a normal pregnancy may be as high as

500,000 IU/day; in the second trimester, they range from 10,000 to 25,000 IU/day; and in the third trimester, from 5,000 to 15,000 IU/day. After delivery, HCG levels decline rapidly, becoming undetectable within a few days.

You won't normally find measurable levels of HCG in the urine of men or nonpregnant women.

Abnormal results
After the first trimester, elevated urine HCG levels may indicate multiple pregnancy or hemolytic disease of the neonate. Depressed urine HCG levels may indicate threatened spontaneous abortion or ectopic pregnancy.

Measurable levels of HCG in men or nonpregnant women may indicate choriocarcinoma, testicular or ovarian tumors, melanoma, multiple myeloma, or gastric, hepatic, pancreatic, or breast cancer.

Human immunodeficiency virus

These tests detect antibodies, antigens, or ribonucleic acid caused by human immunodeficiency virus (HIV) in serum. HIV is the virus that causes acquired immunodeficiency syndrome (AIDS). Transmission occurs when a person's blood is directly exposed to body fluids containing the virus. The virus may be transmitted from one person to another through exchange of contaminated blood or blood products, during sexual intercourse with an infected partner, through sharing of I.V. drugs and syringes, or during pregnancy or breast-feeding (that is, from an infected mother to her child).

Initial identification of HIV is usually achieved through enzyme-linked immunosorbent assay. Positive findings are confirmed by Western blot test and immunofluorescence. (See *HIV testing.*)

Purpose
■ To screen for HIV in high-risk patients
■ To screen donated blood for HIV

Procedure-related nursing care
Explain the purpose of the test to the patient, and tell him it requires a blood sample.

Perform a venipuncture, collecting the sample in a 10-ml red-top tube. Because HIV is a blood-borne infection, following standard precautions. Make sure you wear gloves, avoid accidental needle puncture, wash your hands after the procedure, and properly dispose of the needle. If you accidentally stick yourself with a used needle, report the incident immediately.

Normal findings
Test results are normally negative. However, HIV-1 or HIV-2 antibodies may fall to undetectable levels in the final stages of AIDS. A positive result, indicating the presence of antibodies, necessitates further investigation. Immunocompromised patients may not produce these antibodies.

Abnormal findings
The test detects previous exposure to HIV-1 and HIV-2 1 to 6 months after infection occurs; antibody to p24 is typically the first HIV-1 antibody that's detectable. However, the test doesn't identify patients who have been exposed to the virus but haven't yet made antibodies. Most patients with AIDS have antibodies to HIV. A positive test for the HIV antibody can't determine whether a patient harbors actively replicating virus or when the patient will experience signs and symptoms of AIDS.

Many apparently healthy people have been exposed to HIV and have circulating antibodies. The test results for such people aren't false-positives.

HIV testing

Test and purpose	Implication	Sensitivity and specificity	Seroconversion time
Enzyme-linked immunosorbent assay (ELISA) or enzyme immunoassay (EIA) HIV-1/HIV-2 *Screening test*	Positive result needs a test to confirm diagnosis. Negative result needs no follow-up.	99.9% when combined with Western blot test	1 to 6 months
p24 antigen ELISA *Screening test*	Additional confirmatory test required for both negative and positive results.	Moderately low sensitivity; high specificity	Typically the first detectable level ($<$ 6 weeks)
Western blot *Confirmatory test*	Two or more bands indicates HIV. Absence of bands rules out HIV. Indeterminate result (1 band associated with HIV present) needs a retest in 1 month or a p24 or HIV RNA test.	99.9% when combined with ELISA/EIA test; 99.9% specificity	1 to 6 months
HIV ribonucleic acid (RNA) by reverse transcriptase-polymerase chain reaction (detects RNA after infection but before seroconversion) *Prognosis determination aid*	Positive result rules in HIV. Negative result needs no follow-up.	98% high specificity	1 to 6 months
HIV RNA by b deoxyribonucleic acid *Antiviral agent activity quantifier*	Lower result shows progress of antiviral therapy; indicates that therapy is working.	90% high specificity	1 to 6 months
Oral mucosal transudate *Screening test*	Positive result needs a test to confirm diagnosis. Negative result needs no follow-up.	As accurate as blood tests	1 to 6 months
CD4+ (which indicates immune competence) *Treatment decisions aid*	CD4+ count $<$ 200 confirms a diagnosis of AIDS.	High sensitivity and high specificity for prognosis	Not applicable
Reactive rapid test (detects HIV-1 in 5 to 30 minutes) *Rapid result screening test*	Positive result needs a test to confirm diagnosis. Negative result needs no follow-up.	99.9% high specificity	1 to 6 months

Human leukocyte antigen typing

The human leukocyte antigen (HLA) test identifies a group of antigens present on the surfaces of all nucleated cells but most easily detected on lymphocytes. There are four types of HLA: HLA-A, HLA-B, HLA-C, and HLA-D.

Purpose
■ To provide histocompatibility typing of tissue recipients and donors
■ To aid genetic counseling
■ To aid paternity testing

Procedure-related nursing care
Explain the purpose of the test to the patient, and tell him it requires a blood sample.

Check the patient's history for recent blood transfusions. HLA testing may be postponed if he has recently received a transfusion.

Perform a venipuncture, and collect the sample in a collection tube containing acid citrate dextrose solution, an anticoagulant.

Reference values
In HLA-A, HLA-B, and HLA-C testing, lymphocytes that react with the test antiserum undergo lysis; they're detected by phase microscopy. In HLA-D testing, leukocyte incompatibility is marked by blast formation, deoxyribonucleic acid synthesis, and proliferation.

Abnormal results
Incompatible HLA-A, HLA-B, HLA-C, or HLA-D groups may cause unsuccessful tissue transplantation.

International Normalized Ratio

The International Normalized Ratio (INR) system is viewed as the best means of standardizing measurement of prothrombin time to monitor oral anticoagulant therapy. It isn't used as a screening test for coagulopathies.

Purpose
■ To evaluate effectiveness of oral anticoagulant therapy

Procedure-related nursing care
Explain the purpose of the test to the patient, and tell him that the test requires a blood sample. Inform a patient who's receiving warfarin therapy that the test may be repeated at regular intervals to assess his response to treatment.

Perform a venipuncture and collect the sample in a 4.5-ml blue-top tube. Completely fill the collection tube; otherwise, an excess of citrate will appear in the sample. Gently invert the tube several times to thoroughly mix the sample and the anticoagulant.

Reference values
Normal INR for those receiving warfarin therapy is 2.0 to 3.0. For those with mechanical prosthetic heart valves, an INR of 2.5 to 3.5 is suggested.

Abnormal results
Increased INR values may indicate disseminated intravascular coagulation, cirrhosis, hepatitis, vitamin K deficiency, salicylate intoxication, or massive blood transfusion.

Lactate dehydrogenase

An enzyme, lactate dehydrogenase (LD) catalyzes the reversible conversion of muscle pyruvic acid into lactic acid. Because LD appears in almost all body tissues, cellular damage causes an elevation of total serum LD levels, thus limiting its diagnostic usefulness.

However, five tissue-specific isoenzymes can be identified and measured:

LD isoenzyme values: Abnormal results

This table shows the correlation between elevated isoenzyme levels (color boxes) and probable diagnoses.

DISEASE	LD_1	LD_2	LD_3	LD_4	LD_5
Cardiopulmonary					
Myocardial infarction	■	■			
Myocardial infarction with hepatic congestion	■	■			■
Rheumatic carditis	■	■			
Myocarditis	■				
Heart failure (decompensated)				■	■
Shock	■	■	■	■	■
Pulmonary infarction			■		■

DISEASE	LD_1	LD_2	LD_3	LD_4	LD_5
Hematologic					
Pernicious anemia	■	■			
Hemolytic anemia	■	■			
Sickle cell anemia	■	■			
Gastrointestinal					
Hepatobiliary disorder					■
Hepatitis					■
Active cirrhosis					■
Hepatic congestion					■

LD_1 and LD_2 appear primarily in the heart, red blood cells, and kidneys; LD_3, primarily in the lungs; and LD_4 and LD_5, in the liver and skeletal muscles. The fractionation of LD isoenzymes is widely used to detect myocardial infarction (MI) because LD_1 and LD_2 levels rise 12 to 48 hours after an MI begins, peak in 2 to 5 days, and drop to normal in 7 to 14 days if tissue necrosis doesn't persist.

Purpose

■ To aid differential diagnosis of MI, pulmonary infarction, anemias, and hepatic disease

■ To support creatine kinase (CK) isoenzyme test results in diagnosing an MI or to help in diagnosing an MI when CK-MB samples are drawn too late (more than 24 hours after the onset of an acute MI)

■ To monitor patient response to some forms of chemotherapy

Procedure-related nursing care

Explain the purpose of the test to the patient, and tell him it requires a blood sample. If the patient is suspected of having experienced an MI, tell him that the test will be repeated on the next two mornings to monitor progressive changes.

Perform a venipuncture, collecting the sample in a 7-ml red-top tube. Draw each sample on schedule to avoid missing peak levels and mark the collection time on the laboratory request.

Send the sample to the laboratory immediately. If transport is delayed, keep the sample at room temperature.

Reference values

Total LD levels should range from 100 to 225 units/L. Distribution of isoenzymes should be as follows:
- LD_1 — 14% to 26% of total
- LD_2 — 29% to 39% of total
- LD_3 — 20% to 26% of total
- LD_4 — 8% to 16% of total
- LD_5 — 6% to 16% of total.

Abnormal results

Because many common disorders raise total LD levels, isoenzyme electrophoresis is usually required for diagnosis. With some disorders, total LD levels may be within normal limits, but abnormal proportions of the isoenzymes indicate specific organ tissue damage. (See *LD isoenzyme values: Abnormal results,* page 167.) For instance, in patients with an acute MI, LD_1 levels are greater than LD_2 levels within 12 to 48 hours after the onset of symptoms. This reversal of the normal isoenzyme pattern typifies myocardial damage and is referred to as flipped LD.

Lipoprotein–cholesterol fractionation

Cholesterol fractionation tests isolate and measure the cholesterol in serum low-density lipoproteins (LDLs) and high-density lipoproteins (HDLs). LDL and HDL levels are considered significant because the Framingham Heart Study showed that the higher the HDL level, the lower the risk of coronary artery disease (CAD), and the higher the LDL level, the higher the risk of CAD.

Purpose

- To assess the risk of CAD

Procedure-related nursing care

Explain the purpose of the test to the patient, and tell him it requires a blood sample. Tell him to maintain his normal diet for 2 weeks before the test, to abstain from alcohol for 24 hours before the test, and to fast and avoid exercise for 12 to 24 hours before the test.

Perform a venipuncture, collecting the sample in a 7-ml red-top tube. Send the sample to the laboratory immediately, or place it in the refrigerator until you can transport it.

After the test, the patient may resume his diet and any activities restricted by the test.

Reference values

Normal HDL cholesterol levels range from 29 to 77 mg/dl, and normal LDL cholesterol levels range from 62 to 185 mg/dl. These values vary according to age, sex, geographic region, and ethnic group, so check with your laboratory for appropriate normal values.

Abnormal results

High LDL levels increase the risk of CAD. High HDL levels generally reflect a healthy state but also can indicate chronic hepatitis, early-stage primary biliary cirrhosis, or alcohol consumption. Rarely, a sharp rise (one as high as 100 mg/dl) in a second type of HDL ($alpha_2$-HDL) may signal CAD.

Magnesium, serum

This quantitative analysis measures serum levels of magnesium. Vital to neuromuscular function, this electrolyte helps regulate intracellular metabolism, activates many essential enzymes, and affects the metabolism of nucleic acids and proteins. Magnesium also helps transport sodium and potassium across cell membranes and, through its effect on the secretion of parathyroid hormone, influences intracellular calcium levels.

Most magnesium is found in bone and in intracellular fluid; a small amount is found in extracellular fluid. Absorbed by the small intestine, magnesium is excreted in the urine and feces.

Purpose
■ To evaluate electrolyte status
■ To assess neuromuscular or renal function

Procedure-related nursing care
Explain the purpose of the test to the patient, and tell him it requires a blood sample. Then perform a venipuncture, collecting the sample in a 7-ml red-top tube. Handle the sample gently to prevent hemolysis.

Reference values
Serum magnesium levels normally range from 1.7 to 2.1 mg/dl.

Abnormal results
Elevated serum magnesium levels (hypermagnesemia) most commonly occur in patients with renal failure, when the kidneys excrete inadequate amounts of magnesium. Adrenocortical insufficiency (Addison's disease) can also elevate serum magnesium levels.

Decreased serum magnesium levels (hypomagnesemia) most commonly result from chronic alcoholism. Other causes include diarrhea, malabsorption syndrome, faulty absorption after bowel resection, prolonged bowel or gastric aspiration, acute pancreatitis, primary aldosteronism, severe burns, hypercalcemic conditions (including hyperparathyroidism), and certain diuretic therapies.

Occult blood, fecal

Invisible because of its minute quantity, fecal occult blood can be detected by microscopic analysis or chemical test for hemoglobin, such as the guaiac or orthotoluidine tests. Small amounts of blood (2 to 2.5 ml/day) normally appear in the feces; these tests are designed to detect greater-than-normal quantities.

Purpose
■ To detect GI bleeding
■ To aid early diagnosis of colorectal cancer

Procedure-related nursing care
Explain the purpose of the test to the patient. Tell him it requires three stool specimens. (Occasionally only one random specimen will be used.) Instruct him to avoid contaminating the stool specimen with toilet tissue or urine. Tell him to maintain a high-fiber diet and to avoid eating red meats, poultry, fish, turnips, and horseradish for 48 to 72 hours before the test and throughout the collection period.

Collect three consecutive stool specimens or a random specimen, as appropriate. Send the specimen to the laboratory, or perform the test yourself, as ordered.

To perform the test yourself, obtain a small specimen from two different areas of each stool to allow for any variation in the distribution of blood. Use a commercially prepared Hemoccult card and developer. Apply two drops of the chemical developer to the paper covering the sample. Note the color after 1 minute. Typically, patients are given the card to take home with instructions to place a stool specimen on the card, close the window, and return the card. Later, the clinician applies the developer and watches for the color reaction.

Tell the patient he may resume his normal diet after the test.

Reference values
Normally, less than 2 ml of blood is present, and the test results in a green reaction.

Abnormal results
A blue reaction that occurs within 30 to 60 seconds is a positive indicator of fecal occult blood. If the blue color appears within this period, consider it strongly positive. However, a faint blue reaction is weakly positive and not necessarily abnormal.

A positive test result indicates GI bleeding that can result from several disorders, including varices, peptic ulcer, cancer, ulcerative colitis, dysentery, and hemorrhagic disease.

Partial thromboplastin time

The activated partial thromboplastin time (APTT) test evaluates all the clotting factors of the intrinsic pathway except platelets. Relying on an activator, such as kaolin, to shorten clotting time, this test measures the time needed to form a fibrin clot after calcium and phospholipid emulsion are added to a plasma sample.

Purpose
■ To screen for clotting factor deficiencies in the intrinsic pathway
■ To monitor heparin therapy

Procedure-related nursing care
Explain the purpose of the test to the patient, and tell him the test requires a blood sample. Inform a patient who's receiving heparin therapy that the test may be repeated at regular intervals to assess his response to treatment.

Perform a venipuncture, collecting a blood sample in a 4.5-ml blue-top tube.

Reference values
A fibrin clot should form 25 to 36 seconds after a reagent is added.

Abnormal results
A prolonged APTT may indicate a deficiency of certain plasma clotting factors or the presence of heparin, fibrin split products, fibrinolysin, or circulating anticoagulants that act as antibodies to specific clotting factors.

Phosphate, serum

This test measures serum levels of phosphate, the dominant cellular anion. Phosphate helps store and use body energy; helps regulate calcium levels, carbohydrate and lipid metabolism, and acid-base balance; and is essential to bone formation (about 85% of the body's phosphate is found in bone).

Phosphate is absorbed in the small intestine and excreted by the kidneys. Because calcium and phosphate interact in a reciprocal relationship, urinary excretion of phosphate increases or decreases in inverse proportion to serum calcium levels. Abnormal levels of phosphate result more commonly from improper excretion than they do from abnormal ingestion or absorption from dietary sources.

Purpose
■ To aid the diagnosis of renal disorders and acid-base imbalance
■ To detect endocrine, skeletal, and calcium disorders

Procedure-related nursing care

Explain the purpose of the test to the patient, and tell him it requires a blood sample. Then perform a venipuncture, collecting the sample in a 7-ml red-top tube. Handle the sample gently to prevent hemolysis.

Reference values

Serum phosphate levels normally range from 2.5 to 4.5 mg/dl (or from 1.8 to 2.6 mEq/L).

Abnormal results

Because serum phosphate levels alone have limited diagnostic value (only a few rare conditions directly affect phosphate metabolism), they should be interpreted in light of serum calcium levels. Although rarely clinically significant, elevated phosphate levels may result from skeletal disease, healing fractures, hypoparathyroidism, acromegaly, diabetic acidosis, high intestinal obstruction, or renal failure. Depressed phosphate levels may result from malnutrition, malabsorption syndrome, hyperparathyroidism, renal tubular acidosis, or treatment of diabetic acidosis.

Platelet count

Platelets, or thrombocytes, are the smallest formed elements in the blood. Vital to the formation of the homeostatic plug in vascular injury, platelets promote coagulation by supplying phospholipids to the intrinsic coagulation pathway. The platelet count is one of the most important screening tests for platelet function.

Purpose

■ To evaluate platelet production
■ To assess the effects of chemotherapy or radiation therapy on platelet production

■ To aid the diagnosis of thrombocytopenia or thrombocytosis
■ To confirm a visual estimate of platelet number and morphology from a stained blood film

Procedure-related nursing care

Explain the purpose of the test to the patient, and tell him it requires a blood sample. Then perform a venipuncture, collecting the sample in a 7-ml lavender-top tube. Gently mix the sample and the anticoagulant, and send the sample to the laboratory immediately.

Reference values

Normal platelet counts range from 150,000 to 400,000/µl.

Abnormal results

An increased platelet count (thrombocytosis) can result from hemorrhage; infectious disorders; cancer; ion deficiency anemia; recent surgery, pregnancy, or splenectomy; and inflammatory disorders such as collagen vascular disease. In such cases, the platelet count will return to normal after the patient recovers. However, the platelet count will remain elevated in patients with primary thrombocytosis, myelofibrosis with myeloid metaplasia, polycythemia vera, or chronic myelogenous leukemia.

A decreased platelet count (thrombocytopenia) can result from aplastic or hypoplastic bone marrow disease; infiltrative bone marrow disease, such as carcinoma, leukemia, or disseminated infection; megakaryocytic hypoplasia; ineffective thrombopoiesis caused by folic acid or vitamin B_{12} deficiency; pooling of platelets in an enlarged spleen; increased platelet destruction caused by drugs or immune disorders; disseminated intravascular coagulation; Bernard-Soulier syndrome; mechanical injury to platelets; or suppression of bone marrow function caused by chemotherapy or radiation therapy.

Potassium, serum

This quantitative analysis measures serum levels of potassium. Vital to homeostasis, potassium maintains cellular osmotic equilibrium. It also helps regulate muscle activity by maintaining electrical conduction within the cardiac and skeletal muscles. As well, potassium helps regulate enzyme activity and acid-base balance and influences kidney function.

Potassium levels are affected by variations in the secretion of adrenocortical hormones and by fluctuations in pH, serum glucose levels, and serum sodium levels. A reciprocal relationship appears to exist between potassium and sodium; a substantial intake of one element causes a corresponding decrease of the other.

Although the body readily conserves sodium, it has no efficient method of conserving potassium. The kidneys excrete daily nearly all the ingested potassium. Even in patients with potassium depletion, potassium excretion continues; therefore, potassium deficiency develops readily and commonly.

Purpose
■ To evaluate clinical signs of hyperkalemia or hypokalemia
■ To monitor renal function, acid-base balance, and glucose metabolism
■ To evaluate neuromuscular and endocrine disorders
■ To detect the origin of arrhythmias

Procedure–related nursing care
Explain the purpose of the test to the patient, and tell him it requires a blood sample. After applying a tourniquet, perform the venipuncture immediately, telling the patient *not* to make a fist.

(Repeated clenching of the fist may cause elevated potassium levels.) Collect the sample in a 10- to 15-ml red-top tube.

Reference values
Normally, serum potassium levels range from 3.8 to 5 mEq/L.

Abnormal results
Abnormally high serum potassium levels are common in patients with burns, crushing injuries, diabetic ketoacidosis, and myocardial infarction — conditions in which excessive cellular potassium enters the blood. Hyperkalemia may also indicate reduced sodium excretion, possibly because of renal failure (preventing normal sodium-potassium exchange) or Addison's disease (caused by the absence of aldosterone with consequent potassium buildup and sodium depletion).

Decreased potassium values commonly result from aldosteronism or Cushing's syndrome (marked by hypersecretion of adrenal steroid hormones), loss of body fluids (as in diuretic therapy), or excessive licorice ingestion (because of the aldosterone-like effect of glycyrrhizic acid).

Prostate-specific antigen

Prostate-specific antigen (PSA) appears in normal, benign hyperplastic, and malignant prostatic tissue as well as in metastatic prostatic carcinoma. Serum PSA levels are used to monitor the spread of recurrence of prostate cancer and to evaluate the patient's response to treatment. Measurement of serum PSA levels along with a digital rectal examination is now recommended as a screening test for prostate cancer in men older than age 50.

Purpose
■ To monitor the course of prostate cancer and aid evaluation of treatment
■ To screen for prostate cancer in conjunction with a digital rectal examination in men older than age 50.

Procedure-related nursing care
Explain the purpose of the test to the patient and tell him that this test requires a blood sample.

Perform a venipuncture, and collect the sample in a 7-ml red-top tube. Collect the sample either before a digital rectal examination or at least 48 hours after it to avoid falsely elevated PSA levels. Handle the sample gently to prevent hemolysis. Send the sample, on ice, to the laboratory immediately.

Reference values
Normal serum values for PSA shouldn't exceed 2 ng/ml in males age 40 and younger and 4 ng/ml in men ages 41 to 61. In men older age 61, values shouldn't exceed 7 ng/ml.

Abnormal findings
About 80% of patients with prostate cancer have pretreatment PSA values greater than 4 ng/ml. However, PSA results alone don't confirm a diagnosis of prostate cancer. About 20% of patients with benign prostatic hyperplasia also have levels greater than 4 ng/ml. Further assessment and testing, including tissue biopsy, are needed to confirm cancer.

Protein, urine

A quantitative test for proteinuria, a urine protein test aids in the diagnosis of renal disease. Normally, the glomerular capillary membrane allows only proteins of low molecular weight to enter the filtrate. The renal tubules then reabsorb most of these proteins, normally excreting a small amount that's undetectable by a screening test. However, with a damaged glomerular capillary membrane and impaired tubular reabsorption, detectable amounts of proteins will be excreted in the urine.

A qualitative screening test — a simple dipstick test performed on a random urine sample — is commonly done first. If the results are positive, the quantitative analysis of a 24-hour urine specimen by acid precipitation will follow. Electrophoresis can detect Bence Jones protein, hemoglobins, myoglobins, or albumin in the urine.

Purpose
■ To aid in the diagnosis of renal disease
■ To aid in the diagnosis of preeclampsia in a pregnant patient

Procedure-related nursing care
Collect a 24-hour urine specimen using a special specimen container obtained from the laboratory. Refrigerate the specimen or place it on ice during the collection period. After collecting the entire specimen, transport it to the laboratory immediately.

Reference values
Normally, up to 150 mg of protein is excreted in 24 hours.

Abnormal results
Heavy proteinuria (more than 4 g/ 24 hours) is commonly associated with nephrotic syndrome.

Moderate proteinuria (0.5 to 4 g/ 24 hours) occurs with several types of renal disease — acute or chronic glomerulonephritis, amyloidosis, toxic nephropathies — and with diseases in which renal failure commonly develops as a late complication of the disease, such as diabetes or heart failure.

Minimal proteinuria is most commonly associated with renal diseases in which glomerular involvement isn't a major factor such as chronic pyelo-nephritis.

When accompanied by an elevated white blood cell count, proteinuria indicates urinary tract infection; with hematuria, proteinuria indicates local or diffuse urinary tract disorders.

Not all forms of proteinuria have pathologic significance. Benign proteinuria can result from changes in body position. Functional proteinuria is associated with emotional or physiologic stress and is usually transient.

Protein electrophoresis, serum

This test measures serum levels of albumin and globulins, the major blood proteins, in an electric field by separating the proteins according to their size, shape, and electrical charge at a pH of 8.6. Because each protein fraction moves at a different rate, this movement separates the fractions into recognizable and measurable patterns.

Albumin, which accounts for more than 50% of total serum protein levels, maintains oncotic pressure (preventing capillary plasma leaks) and transports substances that are insoluble in water alone — such as bilirubin, fatty acids, hormones, and drugs.

Four types of globulins exist: $alpha_1$, $alpha_2$, beta, and gamma. The first three types act primarily as carrier proteins that transport lipids, hormones, and metals through the blood. The fourth type, gamma globulin, acts as an important component of the body's immune system.

Although electrophoresis is the most current method of measuring serum protein levels, determinations of total protein and the albumin-globulin (A-G) ratio (normally greater than one) are still commonly performed. No matter which test method is used, a single protein fraction is rarely significant by itself.

Purpose
■ To aid the diagnosis of hepatic disease, protein deficiency, blood dyscrasias, renal disorders, and GI and neoplastic diseases

Procedure-related nursing care
Explain the purpose of the test to the patient, and tell him that it requires a blood sample.

Perform a venipuncture, and collect the sample in a 7-ml red-top tube.

Reference values
Values normally fall in these ranges:
■ total serum protein levels, 6.6 to 7.9 g/dl (66 to 79 g/L)
■ albumin fraction, 3.3 to 4.5 g/dl (33 to 45 g/L)
■ $alpha_1$ globulin, 0.1 to 0.4 g/dl (1 to 4 g/L)
■ $alpha_2$ globulin, 0.5 to 1 g/dl (5 to 10 g/L)
■ beta globulin, 0.7 to 1.2 g/dl (7 to 12 g/L)
■ gamma globulin, 0.5 to 1.6 g/dl (5 to 16 g/L).

Abnormal results
An increase in total protein can indicate chronic inflammatory disease, dehydration, diabetic acidosis, fulminating or chronic infection, monocytic leukemia, or multiple myeloma. A decrease can signal benzene or carbon tetrachloride poisoning, blood dyscrasias, heart failure, essential hypertension, GI disease, hemorrhage, hepatic disease, or Hodgkin's disease. It can also result from hyperthyroidism, malabsorption, nephrosis, a severe burn, surgical or traumatic shock, toxemia of pregnancy, or uncontrolled diabetes mellitus.

An increase in albumin levels results from multiple myeloma. A decrease can stem from acute cholecystitis, collagen disease, essential hypertension, hepatic disease, Hodgkin's disease, hyperthyroidism, or hypogammaglobulinemia. Other possible causes include malnutrition, metastatic cancer, nephritis or nephrosis, peptic ulcer, plasma loss (from burns), rheumatoid arthritis, sarcoidosis, and systemic lupus erythematosus.

An alpha$_1$ globulin level increase can result from an acute infection, cancer, pregnancy, or tissue necrosis. A decrease indicates a genetic deficiency of alpha$_1$-antitrypsin.

An increase in alpha$_2$ globulin may indicate acute infection, an acute myocardial infarction, advanced cancer, nephrotic syndrome, rheumatic fever, rheumatoid arthritis, trauma, or a severe burn. A drop indicates hemolytic anemia or severe liver disease.

Elevated beta globulin levels can result from biliary cirrhosis, Cushing's disease, diabetes mellitus, hypothyroidism, malignant hypertension, or nephrotic syndrome. A decrease results from hypocholesterolemia.

A rise in gamma globulin levels can indicate chronic active liver disease, Hodgkin's disease, rheumatoid arthritis, or systemic lupus erythematosus. A decrease can result from lymphocytic leukemia, lymphosarcoma, or nephrotic syndrome.

The A-G ratio is usually evaluated in relation to the total protein level. A low total protein level with a reversed A-G ratio (decreased albumin and elevated globulins) suggests chronic liver disease. A normal total protein level with a reversed A-G ratio suggests myeloproliferative disease (leukemia or Hodgkin's disease) or certain chronic infectious diseases (tuberculosis or chronic hepatitis).

Prothrombin time

This test measures the time required for a fibrin clot to form in a citrated plasma sample after calcium ions and tissue thromboplastin (factor III) have been added. This prothrombin time (PT) is then compared with the fibrin clotting time in a control sample of plasma. The most accurate test results state both the patient's and the control sample's clotting times in seconds.

The test bypasses the extrinsic coagulation pathway and platelets, and instead it measures prothrombin activity and evaluates the extrinsic coagulation system — including factors V, VII, and X — as well as the levels of prothrombin and fibrinogen.

Purpose
■ To monitor a patient's response to oral anticoagulant therapy
■ To evaluate the extrinsic coagulation system
■ To aid the diagnosis of conditions associated with abnormal bleeding
■ To identify patients at risk for excessive bleeding during surgical or other invasive procedures
■ To differentiate deficiencies of specific clotting factors
■ To monitor the effects of certain diseases (hepatic disease or protein deficiency, for example) on hemostasis

Procedure-related nursing care
Explain the purpose of the test to the patient, and tell him it requires a blood sample. If the test is being done to monitor the effects of anticoagulants, explain that it will be done daily when therapy begins and will be repeated at longer intervals when medication levels stabilize.

Perform a venipuncture, avoiding excessive probing. Collect the sample in a 4.5-ml blue-top tube, ensuring that the tube is completely filled. Gently mix the sample and the anticoagulant, and send it to the laboratory promptly.

Reference values
PT values normally range from 11 to 13 seconds in both men and women.

However, values vary, depending on the source of tissue thromboplastin and the type of sensing devices used to measure clot formation.

Abnormal results

Prolonged PT may indicate deficiencies in fibrinogen, prothrombin, or factors V, VII, or X (specific assays can pinpoint such deficiencies); vitamin K deficiency; and hepatic disease. The prolonged time may also result from oral anticoagulant therapy. A prolonged PT that exceeds $2\frac{1}{2}$ times the control values is commonly associated with abnormal bleeding.

Red blood cell count

Part of a complete blood count, this test determines the number of red blood cells (RBCs) in a cubic millimeter (microliter) of whole blood. The RBC count (also called the erythrocyte count) can be used to calculate two RBC indices, mean corpuscular volume and mean corpuscular hemoglobin. These, in turn, reveal RBC size and hemoglobin concentration and weight.

Purpose
■ To supply figures for computing the RBC indices
■ To aid in diagnosis of anemia and polycythemia

Procedure-related nursing care
Explain the purpose of the test to the patient, and tell him you'll need a blood sample. Then draw a venous blood sample, using a 7-ml lavender-top tube. Fill the collection tube completely, and invert it gently several times to mix the sample and the anticoagulant. Handle the sample gently to prevent hemolysis.

Reference values
RBC values vary according to age, sex, the type of blood sample, and altitude. In men, normal RBC counts range from 4.5 to 6.2 million/µl (4.5 to 6.2 × 10^{12}/L) of venous blood; in women, from 4.2 to 5.4 million/µl (4.2 to 5.4 × 10^{12}/L). People living at high altitudes usually have higher values.

Abnormal results
An elevated RBC count may indicate primary or secondary polycythemia or dehydration. A depressed count may signify anemia, fluid overload, or recent hemorrhage. Further studies, such as stained RBC examination, hematocrit, total hemoglobin levels, RBC indices, and white blood cell counts, confirm a diagnosis.

Red blood cell indices

Based on the results of red blood cell (RBC) count, hematocrit, and total hemoglobin tests, RBC indices provide important information about the size of RBCs, and the hemoglobin concentration and weight of an average RBC.

The first index, the mean corpuscular volume (MCV) — a ratio of hematocrit, or packed cell volume, to RBC — gives average RBC size. The mean corpuscular hemoglobin (MCH), the ratio of hemoglobin to RBC, expresses the weight of hemoglobin in an average RBC. And the mean corpuscular hemoglobin concentration (MCHC), a ratio of hemoglobin weight to hematocrit, provides the concentration of hemoglobin in 100 ml of packed RBCs.

Purpose
■ To help diagnose and classify anemias

Procedure-related nursing care
Explain the purpose of the test to the patient, and tell him you'll need a blood

sample. Draw a venous blood sample, using a 7-ml lavender-top tube. Fill the collection tube completely, and invert it gently several times to mix the sample and the anticoagulant. Handle the sample gently to prevent hemolysis.

Check for factors that may alter test results. A high white blood cell count, for instance, will falsely elevate the RBC count when automated or semiautomated counters are used, invalidating all test results.

Reference values

Normal MCV ranges from 84 to 99 μm³/RBC; normal MCH, from 26 to 34 pg/RBC; and normal MCHC, from 30% to 36%.

Abnormal results

A high MCV suggests macrocytic anemias caused by folic acid or vitamin B_{12} deficiency, inherited disorders of deoxyribonucleic acid synthesis, or reticulocytosis. Decreased MCV and MCHC indicate microcytic hypochromic anemias caused by iron deficiency, pyridoxine-responsive anemia, or thalassemia.

Sodium, serum

This test measures the amount of sodium in the blood. Sodium affects body water distribution, maintains osmotic pressure of extracellular fluid, and helps promote neuromuscular function. It also helps maintain acid-base balance and influences chloride and potassium levels. Sodium is absorbed by the intestines and excreted primarily by the kidneys.

Extracellular sodium concentration helps the kidneys regulate body water. Decreased sodium levels promote water excretion, and increased levels promote retention. For this reason, serum sodium levels are evaluated in relation to the amount of water in the body.

Thus, a sodium deficit (hyponatremia) refers to a decreased level of sodium in relation to the body's water level.

The body normally regulates this sodium-water balance through aldosterone, which inhibits sodium excretion and promotes its resorption (with water) by the renal tubules. Decreased sodium levels stimulate aldosterone secretion; elevated levels depress it.

Purpose

■ To evaluate fluid-electrolyte and acid-base balance and related neuromuscular, renal, and adrenal functions
■ To evaluate the effects of drug therapy (such as diuretics) on serum sodium levels

Procedure-related nursing care

Explain the purpose of the test to the patient, and tell him it requires a blood sample. Then perform a venipuncture, collecting the sample in a 10- to 15-ml red-top tube. Handle the sample gently to prevent hemolysis.

Reference values

Serum sodium levels normally range from 135 to 145 mEq/L.

Abnormal results

Elevated serum sodium levels (hypernatremia) may result from inadequate water intake, water loss that exceeds sodium loss (as in diabetes insipidus, impaired renal function, and prolonged hyperventilation), and sodium retention (as in aldosteronism). Hypernatremia can also result from excessive sodium intake.

Hyponatremia may result from inadequate sodium intake or excessive sodium loss caused by profuse sweating, GI suctioning, diuretic therapy, diarrhea, vomiting, adrenal insufficiency, burns, or chronic renal insufficiency with acidosis.

Thyroid-stimulating hormone

Thyroid-stimulating hormone (TSH), or thyrotropin, promotes increases in the size, number, and activity of thyroid cells and stimulates the release of triiodothyronine and thyroxine. These hormones affect total body metabolism and are essential for normal growth and development.

This test measures serum TSH levels by radioimmunoassay. It can detect primary hypothyroidism and determine whether the hypothyroidism results from thyroid gland failure or from pituitary or hypothalamic dysfunction. Normal serum TSH levels rule out primary hypothyroidism. This test may not distinguish between low-normal and subnormal levels, especially in secondary hypothyroidism.

Purpose
■ To confirm or rule out primary hypothyroidism and distinguish it from secondary hypothyroidism
■ To monitor drug therapy in patients with primary hypothyroidism

Procedure-related nursing care
Explain the purpose of the test to the patient and tell him that the test requires a blood sample. Advise him that the laboratory requires up to 2 days to complete the analysis. As ordered, withhold steroids, thyroid hormones, aspirin, and other drugs that may influence test results. If these medications must be continued, note this on the laboratory request. Keep the patient relaxed and recumbent for 30 minutes before the test.

Perform a venipuncture between 6 a.m. and 8 a.m., and collect the sample in a 7-ml red-top or green-top tube.

Reference values
Normal TSH values range from 0.3 to 5 mIU/L.

Abnormal results
TSH levels may be slightly elevated in euthyroid patients with thyroid cancer. Extremely high levels suggest primary hypothyroidism or, possibly, endemic goiter.

Low or undetectable TSH levels may be normal but occasionally indicate secondary hypothyroidism (with inadequate secretion of TSH or thyrotropin-releasing hormone). Low TSH levels may also result from hyperthyroidism (Graves' disease) or thyroiditis; both are marked by hypersecretion of thyroid hormones, which suppresses TSH release.

Thyroxine

Thyroxine (T_4) is an amine secreted by the thyroid gland in response to thyroid-stimulating hormone (TSH) and, indirectly, thyrotropin-releasing hormone. A complex system of negative and positive feedback mechanisms normally regulates the rate of secretion.

Only a fraction of T_4 (about 0.05%) circulates freely in the blood; the rest binds strongly to plasma proteins, primarily thyroxine-binding globulin (TBG). This minute fraction is responsible for the clinical effects of thyroid hormone. TBG binds so tenaciously that T_4 survives in the plasma for a relatively long time, with a half-life of about 6 days. This immunoassay should be interpreted in conjunction with the TBG level or as part of a free thyroxine index.

Purpose
■ To evaluate thyroid function
■ To aid diagnosis of hyperthyroidism and hypothyroidism

■ To monitor response to antithyroid medication in patients with hyperthyroidism or to thyroid replacement therapy in patients with hypothyroidism

Procedure-related nursing care

Explain the purpose of the test to the patient, and tell him a blood sample is needed. As ordered, withhold any medications that may interfere with test results. If these medications must be continued, note this on the laboratory request. (If this test is being performed to monitor thyroid therapy, the patient continues to receive daily thyroid supplements.)

Perform a venipuncture and collect the sample in a 7-ml red-top tube. Handle the specimen carefully to avoid hemolysis.

Reference values

Normally, total T_4 levels range from 5 to 12.5 µg/dl.

Abnormal results

Abnormally elevated T_4 levels are consistent with primary and secondary hyperthyroidism, including excessive T_4 (levothyroxine) replacement therapy (factitious or iatrogenic hyperthyroidism). Subnormal levels suggest primary or secondary hypothyroidism or may be due to T_4 suppression by normal, elevated, or replacement levels of triiodothyronine (T_3). In doubtful cases of hypothyroidism, TSH levels may be indicated.

Normal T_4 levels don't guarantee euthyroidism; for example, normal readings occur in T_3 thyrotoxicosis. Overt signs of hyperthyroidism require further testing.

Thyroxine-binding globulin

This test measures the serum level of thyroxine-binding globulin (TBG), the predominant protein carrier for circulating thyroxine (T_4).

Any condition that affects TBG levels and subsequent binding capacity also affects the amount of free T_4 (FT_4) in circulation. An underlying TBG abnormality renders tests for total triiodothyronine (T_3) and T_4 inaccurate but doesn't affect the accuracy of tests for free T_3 (FT_3) and FT_4.

Purpose

■ To evaluate abnormal thyrometabolic states that don't correlate with thyroid hormone (T_3 or T_4) values (for example, a patient with overt signs of hypothyroidism and a low FT_4 level with a high total T_4 level due to a marked increase of TBG secondary to use of oral contraceptives)
■ To identify TBG abnormalities

Procedure-related nursing care

Explain the purpose of the test to the patient and tell him the test requires a blood sample. As ordered, withhold medications that may interfere with accurate testing, such as estrogens, anabolic steroids, phenytoin, salicylates, and thyroid preparations. If these medications must be continued, note this on the laboratory request. (They may be continued to determine if prescribed drugs are affecting TBG levels.)

Perform a venipuncture, collecting blood into a 7-ml red-top tube. Handle the sample gently because excessive agitation may cause hemolysis.

Reference values

Normal values vary by sex and age, as follows:

Males
■ ages 1 to 6 years: 17 to 26 µg/ml
■ ages 7 to 13 years: 15 to 24 µg/ml
■ ages 14 to 18 years: 13 to 22 µg/ml
■ ages 19 to 23 years: 11 to 20 µg/ml

■ age 24 years and older: 16 to 24 µg/ml

Females
■ ages 1 to 6 years: 17 to 26 µg/ml
■ ages 7 to 23 years: 15 to 26 µg/ml
■ age 24 years and older: 16 to 24 µg/ml

Abnormal results
Elevated TBG levels may indicate hypothyroidism, or congenital (genetic) excess, some forms of hepatic disease, or acute intermittent porphyria. TBG levels normally rise during pregnancy and are high in neonates. Suppressed levels may indicate hyperthyroidism or congenital deficiency and can occur in active acromegaly, nephrotic syndrome, and malnutrition associated with hypoproteinemia, acute illness, or surgical stress.

Patients with TBG abnormalities require additional testing, such as the serum FT_3 and serum T_4 tests, to evaluate thyroid function more precisely.

Triglycerides, serum

This test provides a quantitative analysis of triglycerides — the main storage form of lipids. Triglycerides consist of one molecule of glycerol bonded to three molecules of fatty acids. Thus, the degradation of triglycerides leads directly to the production of fatty acids. Together with carbohydrates, triglycerides furnish energy for metabolism.

Triglyceride testing shouldn't be performed while a patient is hospitalized for a myocardial infarction because this condition causes an increase in very-low-density lipoproteins and a decrease in low-density lipoproteins.

Purpose
■ To determine the risk of coronary artery disease (CAD)
■ To screen for hyperlipidemia

■ To identify disorders associated with altered triglyceride levels

Procedure-related nursing care
Explain the purpose of the test to the patient, and tell him it requires a blood sample. Instruct him to abstain from alcohol for 24 hours before the test and from food for 12 to 14 hours before the test. Also tell him not to take any medication, such as a corticosteroid, that could alter his test results.

Perform a venipuncture and collect the sample in a 7-ml lavender-top tube.

After the test, tell the patient he can resume his normal diet.

Reference values
Although triglyceride values are age- and sex-related, some controversy exists regarding the most appropriate normal ranges. Nonetheless, serum values of 40 to 160 mg/dl for men and 35 to 135 mg/dl for women are widely accepted.

Abnormal results
Increased or decreased serum triglyceride levels suggest a clinical abnormality that requires additional testing, such as cholesterol measurement, for a definitive diagnosis.

High levels of triglycerides and cholesterol reflect an increased risk of atherosclerosis or CAD.

Markedly increased levels without an identifiable cause reflect congenital hyperlipoproteinemia and require lipoprotein phenotyping to confirm the diagnosis.

A mild-to-moderate increase in serum triglyceride levels indicates biliary obstruction, diabetes mellitus, nephrotic syndrome, endocrinopathies, or excessive consumption of alcohol.

Decreased serum levels are rare, occurring mainly in patients with malnutrition or abetalipoproteinemia.

Triiodothyronine

This highly specific radioimmunoassay measures total (bound and free) serum content of triiodothyronine (T_3) to investigate clinical indications of thyroid dysfunction. Like thyroxine (T_4) secretion, T_3 secretion occurs in response to thyroid-stimulating hormone (TSH) and, secondarily, thyrotropin-releasing hormone.

Although T_3 is present in the bloodstream in minute quantities and is metabolically active for only a short time, its impact on body metabolism dominates that of T_4. Another significant difference between the two major thyroid hormones is that T_3 binds less firmly to thyroxine-binding globulin. Consequently, T_3 persists in the bloodstream for a short time; half disappears in about 1 day, whereas half of T_4 disappears in 6 days.

Purpose

- To aid diagnosis of T_3 toxicosis
- To aid diagnosis of hypothyroidism and hyperthyroidism
- To monitor clinical response to thyroid replacement therapy in patients with hypothyroidism

Procedure-related nursing care

Explain the purpose of the test to the patient, and tell him that the test requires a blood sample. As ordered, withhold medications that may influence thyroid function, such as steroids, propranolol, and cholestyramine. If such medications must be continued, record this information on the laboratory request.

Perform a venipuncture and collect the sample in a 7-ml red-top tube. If a patient must receive thyroid preparations such as T_3 (liothyronine), note the time of drug administration on the laboratory request. Otherwise, T_3 levels aren't reliable. Handle the sample gently to prevent hemolysis. Send the sample to the laboratory as soon as possible to avoid stasis and to allow early separation of serum from the clotted blood.

Reference values

Serum T_3 levels vary by age:
- 1 to 14 years: 125 to 250 ng/dl
- 15 to 23 years: 100 to 220 ng/dl
- 24 years and older: 80 to 200 ng/dl.

Abnormal results

Serum T_3 and serum T_4 levels usually rise and fall in tandem. However, in T_3 toxicosis, T_3 levels rise, and total and free T_4 levels remain normal. T_3 toxicosis occurs in patients with Graves' disease, toxic adenoma, or toxic nodular goiter. T_3 levels also surpass T_4 levels in patients receiving thyroid replacement therapy containing more T_3 than T_4. In iodine-deficient areas, the thyroid may produce larger amounts of the more cellularly active T_3 than of T_4 in an effort to maintain the euthyroid state.

Generally, T_3 levels appear to be a more accurate diagnostic indicator of hyperthyroidism. Although both T_3 and T_4 levels are increased in about 90% of patients with hyperthyroidism, there's a disproportionate increase in T_3. In some patients with hypothyroidism, T_3 levels may fall within the normal range and not be diagnostically significant.

A rise in serum T_3 levels normally occurs during pregnancy. Low T_3 levels may appear in euthyroid patients with systemic illness (especially hepatic or renal disease), during severe acute illness, and after trauma or major surgery; in such patients, TSH levels are within normal limits. Low serum T_3 levels are found in some euthyroid patients with malnutrition.

Triiodothyronine uptake

The triiodothyronine (T_3) uptake test indirectly measures free thyroxine (FT_4) levels by demonstrating the availability of serum protein-binding sites for thyroxine (T_4). The results of T_3 uptake are commonly combined with a T_4 radioimmunoassay or T_4(D) (competitive protein-binding test) to determine the FT_4 index, a mathematical calculation that's thought to reflect FT_4 by correcting for thyroxine-binding globulin (TBG) abnormalities.

The T_3 uptake test has become less popular recently because rapid tests for T_3, T_4, and thyroid-stimulating hormone are readily available.

Purpose
■ To aid diagnosis of hypothyroidism and hyperthyroidism when TBG is normal
■ To aid diagnosis of primary disorders of TBG levels

Procedure-related nursing care
Explain the purpose of the test to the patient, and tell him that a blood sample is needed. Tell him the laboratory requires several days to complete the analysis. Withhold any medications that could interfere with test results, such as estrogens, androgens, phenytoin, salicylates, and thyroid preparations. If they must be continued, note this on the laboratory request.

Perform a venipuncture and collect the sample in a 7-ml red-top tube. Handle the sample gently to prevent hemolysis.

Reference values
Normal T_3 uptake values are 25% to 35%.

Abnormal results
A high T_3 uptake percentage in the presence of elevated T_4 levels indicates hyperthyroidism (implying few TBG free binding sites and high FT_4 levels). A low uptake percentage, together with low T_4 levels, indicates hypothyroidism (implying more TBG free binding sites and low FT_4 levels). Thus, in patients with primary thyroid disease, T_4 and T_3 uptake vary in the same direction; availability of binding sites varies inversely.

Discordant variance in T_4 and T_3 uptake suggests abnormality of TBG. For example, a high T_3 uptake percentage and a low or normal FT_4 level suggest decreased TBG levels. Such decreased levels may result from protein loss (as in nephrotic syndrome), decreased production (due to androgen excess or genetic or idiopathic causes), or competition for T_4 binding sites by certain drugs (salicylates, phenylbutazone, and phenytoin). Conversely, a low T_3 uptake percentage and a high or normal FT_4 level suggest increased TBG levels. Such increased levels may be due to exogenous or endogenous estrogen (pregnancy) or result from idiopathic causes. Thus, in primary disorders of TBG levels, measured T_4 and free sites change in the same direction.

Troponin-I and troponin-T

Troponin is the contractile regulatory protein of striated muscle (slow-twitch and fast-twitch skeletal muscle, and cardiac muscle). Cardiac muscle produces specific forms of troponin, cardiac Troponin-I (cTnI) and Troponin-T (cTnT). These are released into the circulation after cellular necrosis.

Purpose
■ To rule out myocardial infarction (MI) on initial presentation, especially when presentation isn't immediately after onset of symptoms; highest sensitivity occurs after 10 hours

Procedure-related nursing care

Explain the purpose of the test to the patient, and tell him that the test may require multiple blood samples.

Perform a venipuncture and collect the specimen in a 7-ml red-top tube. Obtain each specimen on schedule, and note the date and collection time on each.

Reference values

Positive results vary with the laboratory, from any detectable enzyme to greater than 3 ng/ml, in part due to several different tests available. Some tests for cTnT levels greater than 0.5 ng/ml have high sensitivity in detecting an acute MI.

Abnormal results

The presence of cTnI indicates cellular necrosis.

The prolonged persistence of troponin gives it much greater sensitivity than creatine kinase MB (CK-MB) for diagnosis of an MI beyond the first 48 hours, and it replaces lactate dehydrogenase isoenzymes for the detection of infarction at these times. cTnI is more specific for an MI than CK-MB with a decreased sensitivity early in the course of infarction (less than 5 hours) but with near perfect sensitivity and specificity later (more than 10 hours). Troponin appears in serum about 4 hours after onset of chest pain, peaks at 8 to 12 hours, and drops after 5 to 7 days.

Uric acid, serum

This test measures serum levels of uric acid — the major end metabolite of purine. Large amounts of purine are present in nucleic acids and are derived from dietary and endogenous sources. Uric acid clears the body by glomerular filtration and tubular secretion.

Purpose

■ To confirm a diagnosis of gout
■ To help detect kidney dysfunction

Procedure-related nursing care

Explain the purpose of the test to the patient, instruct him to fast for 8 hours, and tell him it requires a blood sample. Then perform a venipuncture, collecting the sample in a 7-ml red-top tube. Handle the sample gently to prevent hemolysis.

Reference values

Serum uric acid levels normally range from 3.5 to 7.2 mg/dl in men and from 2.3 to 6.6 mg/dl in women.

Abnormal results

Increased serum uric acid levels usually indicate impaired renal function or gout. However, with gout, levels don't correlate with the severity of the disease. Levels also may rise in patients with heart failure, glycogen storage disease (type I, von Gierke's disease), acute infectious diseases (such as infectious mononucleosis), hemolytic or sickle cell anemia, hemoglobinopathies, polycythemia, leukemia, lymphoma, metastatic cancer, or psoriasis.

Depressed serum uric acid levels may indicate defective renal tubular reabsorption (as in Fanconi's syndrome and Wilson's disease) or acute hepatic atrophy.

Urinalysis, routine

Routine urinalysis is a common test that's used to screen for urinary and systemic disorders. Abnormal findings suggest disease and indicate the need for further urine or blood tests to identify the problem.

Laboratory methods used to detect or measure urine components include the evaluation of physical characteristics, such as color, odor, and opacity;

screening for pH, protein, sugars, and ketone bodies; refractometry for measuring specific gravity; and microscopic inspection of centrifuged sediment for cells, casts, organisms, and crystals.

Purpose
■ To screen for renal or urinary tract disease
■ To help detect metabolic or systemic disease

Procedure-related nursing care
Explain the purpose of the test to the patient, and tell him to avoid strenuous exercise before the test. Tell him to avoid excessive amounts of such foods as carrots, rhubarb, and beets, which may cause a change in urine color, and excessive amounts of such foods as meats and cranberry juice, which can lower pH.

Collect a random urine specimen of at least 10 ml. If possible, obtain a first-voided morning specimen. If the urine appears concentrated or diluted, assess the patient's fluid status — dehydration and a decreased or increased fluid intake can affect the urine.

Send the specimen to the laboratory immediately, or refrigerate it if analysis will be delayed longer than 1 hour.

Reference values
Normal urine is clear and straw-colored, with a slightly aromatic odor. It has a specific gravity of 1.005 to 1.035 and a pH of 6.0 to 7.0; it contains no protein, glucose, ketones, or other sugars.

On microscopic examination, normal urine contains 0 to 2 red blood cells (RBCs), 0 to 5 white blood cells (WBCs), and 0 to 5 epithelial cells per high-power field. It contains few bacteria or crystals and no yeast cells, parasites, or casts (except occasional hyaline casts).

Abnormal results
The following abnormal results generally suggest pathologic conditions.

Color
Changes in color can result from diet, drugs, and many metabolic, inflammatory, and infectious diseases.

Odor
In diabetes mellitus, starvation, and dehydration, a fruity odor accompanies formation of ketone bodies. In urinary tract infection (UTI), a fetid odor is common, especially if *Escherichia coli* is present. Maple syrup urine disease and phenylketonuria also cause distinctive odors.

Turbidity
Turbid urine may contain RBCs, WBCs, bacteria, fat, or chyle and may reflect renal infection.

Specific gravity
Low specific gravity (less than 1.005) is characteristic of diabetes insipidus, nephrogenic diabetes insipidus, acute tubular necrosis, and pyelonephritis. Fixed specific gravity, in which values remain 1.010 regardless of fluid intake, occurs in patients with chronic glomerulonephritis and severe renal damage. High specific gravity (greater than 1.020) occurs in patients with nephrotic syndrome, dehydration, acute glomerulonephritis, heart failure, liver failure, or shock.

pH
Alkaline urine pH may result from Fanconi's syndrome, UTI, or metabolic or respiratory alkalosis. Acid urine pH is associated with renal tuberculosis, pyrexia, phenylketonuria, alkaptonuria, and all forms of acidosis.

Protein

Proteinuria suggests renal disease, such as nephrosis, glomerulosclerosis, glomerulonephritis, nephrolithiasis, polycystic kidney disease, and renal failure. Proteinuria can also result from multiple myeloma or excessive exercise.

Sugars

Glycosuria usually indicates diabetes mellitus but may also result from pheochromocytoma, Cushing's syndrome, and increased intracranial pressure.

Ketones

Ketonuria occurs with diabetes mellitus when cellular energy needs exceed the available cellular glucose. If cells lack glucose, they metabolize fat, an alternate energy supply. Ketone bodies — the end products of incomplete fat metabolism — accumulate in plasma and are excreted in the urine. Ketonuria may also occur with starvation states and with conditions of acutely increased metabolic demand associated with decreased food intake, such as diarrhea or vomiting.

Cells

Hematuria indicates bleeding within the genitourinary tract and may result from infection, obstruction, inflammation, trauma, tumors, glomerulonephritis, renal hypertension, lupus nephritis, renal tuberculosis, renal vein thrombosis, hydronephrosis, pyelonephritis, scurvy, malaria, parasitic infection of the bladder, subacute bacterial endocarditis, polyarteritis nodosa, or hemorrhagic disorders. Numerous WBCs in urine usually suggest urinary tract inflammation, especially cystitis or pyelonephritis. WBCs and WBC casts in urine suggest renal infection. An excessive number of epithelial cells suggest renal tubular degeneration.

Casts

Plugs of gelled protein, known as casts, form in the distal renal tubules and collecting ducts by agglutination of protein cells or cellular debris. These casts are flushed loose by urine flow. An excessive number of casts indicates renal disease. Hyaline casts are associated with renal parenchymal disease, inflammation, and trauma to the glomerular capillary membrane; epithelial casts, with renal tubular damage, nephrosis, eclampsia, amyloidosis, and heavy metal poisoning; coarse and fine granular casts, with acute or chronic renal failure, pyelonephritis, and chronic lead intoxication; fatty and waxy casts, with nephrotic syndrome, chronic renal disease, and diabetes mellitus; RBC casts, with renal parenchymal disease (especially glomerulonephritis), renal infarction, subacute bacterial endocarditis, vascular disorders, sickle cell anemia, scurvy, blood dyscrasias, malignant hypertension, collagen disease, and acute inflammation; and WBC casts, with acute pyelonephritis and glomerulonephritis, nephrotic syndrome, pyogenic infection, and lupus nephritis.

Crystals

Some crystals normally appear in urine, but numerous calcium oxalate crystals suggest hypertyrosine. Cystine crystals (cystinuria) reflect an inborn metabolism error. Uric acid crystals suggest gout.

Other components

Yeast cells and parasites in urine sediment reflect genitourinary tract infection as well as contamination of external genitalia. Yeast cells, which may be mistaken for RBCs, can be identified by their ovoid shape, lack of color, variable size and, in many cases, signs of budding. The most common parasite in sediment is *Trichomonas vaginalis,* a flagellated protozoan that commonly causes vaginitis, urethritis, and prostatovesiculitis.

White blood cell count

Part of the complete blood count, the white blood cell (WBC) count reports the number of WBCs found in a cubic millimeter (microliter) of whole blood. On any given day, the WBC count can vary by as much as 2,000/µl. Such variations may result from strenuous exercise, stress, or digestion. The WBC count can rise or fall significantly with certain diseases, but the count is diagnostically useful only when interpreted in light of the WBC differential and the patient's current clinical status.

Purpose
■ To determine the presence of infection or inflammation
■ To determine the need for further tests, such as the WBC differential or bone marrow biopsy
■ To monitor a patient's response to chemotherapy or radiation therapy

Procedure-related nursing care
Explain the purpose of the test to the patient. Tell him to avoid strenuous exercise for 24 hours before the test and to avoid eating a heavy meal before the test. If he's receiving treatment for an infection, advise him that this test may be repeated to monitor his progress.

Perform a venipuncture, collecting the sample in a 7-ml lavender-top tube. Handle the sample gently to prevent hemolysis.

After the procedure, tell the patient he may resume normal activities.

Reference values
The WBC count normally ranges from 4,000 to 10,000/µl.

Abnormal results
An elevated WBC count (leukocytosis) usually signals infection, such as abscess, meningitis, or appendicitis. A high count may also result from leukemia, or from tissue necrosis caused by burns, myocardial infarction, or gangrene.

A low WBC count (leukopenia) indicates bone marrow depression that can result from viral infections or from toxic reactions after ingestion of mercury or other heavy metals, treatment with antineoplastics, or exposure to benzene or arsenicals. Leukopenia also characteristically accompanies influenza, typhoid fever, measles, infectious hepatitis, mononucleosis, and rubella.

White blood cell differential

Because the white blood cell (WBC) differential evaluates the distribution and morphology of WBCs, it provides more specific information about a patient's immune function than the WBC count. The differential count represents the relative number of each type of WBC in the blood. Multiplying the percentage value of each type by the total WBC count provides the absolute number of each type of WBC.

Purpose
■ To evaluate the body's capacity to resist and overcome infection
■ To detect and identify various types of leukemia
■ To determine the stage and severity of an infection
■ To detect allergic reactions
■ To assess the severity of allergic reactions (eosinophil count)
■ To detect parasitic infections

Procedure-related nursing care
Explain the purpose of the test to the patient, and tell him it requires a blood sample. Instruct him to avoid strenu-

ous exercise for 24 hours before the test. Then perform a venipuncture, collecting the sample in a 7-ml lavender-top tube.

Reference values

For adults, absolute values and percentages for each of the five WBC differentials are:
■ neutrophils — 1,800 to 7,500/µl; 30% to 70%
■ eosinophils — 40 to 500/µl; 1% to 5%
■ basophils — 0 to 200/µl; 0% to 1%
■ lymphocytes — 880 to 4,000/µl; 22% to 40%
■ monocytes — 120 to 1,000/µl; 3% to 10%

Abnormal results

Neutrophil levels are increased by:
■ infections — osteomyelitis, otitis media, salpingitis, septicemia, gonorrhea, endocarditis, smallpox, appendicitis, chickenpox, herpes, Rocky Mountain spotted fever
■ ischemic necrosis from myocardial infarction, burns, or cancer
■ metabolic disorders — diabetic acidosis, eclampsia, uremia, thyrotoxicosis
■ stress response from acute hemorrhage, surgery, excessive exercise, emotional distress, third trimester of pregnancy, or childbirth
■ inflammatory diseases — rheumatic fever, rheumatic arthritis, acute gout, vasculitis, myositis
■ neoplastic disease — acute myelogenous leukemia.
Neutrophil levels are decreased by:
■ bone marrow depression from radiation therapy or cytotoxic drugs
■ infections — typhoid fever, tularemia, brucellosis, hepatitis, influenza, measles, mumps, rubella, infectious mononucleosis

■ hypersplenism — hepatic disease and storage diseases
■ collagen vascular diseases — systemic lupus erythematosus, rheumatoid arthritis
■ deficiency of folic acid or vitamin B_{12}.
Eosinophil levels are increased by:
■ allergic disorders — asthma, hay fever, food or drug sensitivity, serum sickness, angioneurotic edema
■ parasitic infections — trichinosis, hookworm, roundworm, amebiasis
■ skin diseases — eczema, pemphigus, psoriasis, dermatitis, herpes
■ neoplastic diseases — chronic myelocytic leukemia, Hodgkin's disease, metastasis and necrosis of solid tumors
■ miscellaneous — collagen vascular disease, adrenocortical hypofunction, ulcerative colitis, polyarteritis nodosa, postsplenectomy, pernicious anemia, scarlet fever, excessive exercise.
Eosinophil levels are decreased by:
■ stress response from trauma, shock, burns, surgery, or mental distress
■ Cushing's syndrome.
Basophil levels are increased by chronic myelocytic leukemia, polycythemia vera, some chronic hemolytic anemias, Hodgkin's disease, systemic mastocytosis, myxedema, ulcerative colitis, chronic hypersensitivity states, nephrosis.
Basophil levels are decreased by miscellaneous hyperthyroidism, ovulation, pregnancy, stress.
Lymphocyte levels are increased by:
■ infections — pertussis, brucellosis, syphilis, tuberculosis, hepatitis, infectious mononucleosis, mumps, German measles, cytomegalovirus
■ miscellaneous — thyrotoxicosis, hypoadrenalism, ulcerative colitis, immune diseases, lymphocytic leukemia.
Lymphocyte levels are decreased by:
■ severe debilitating illness — heart failure, renal failure, advanced tuberculosis

■ miscellaneous — defective lymphatic circulation, high levels of adrenal corticosteroids, immunodeficiency due to immunosuppressant therapy.

Monocyte levels are increased by:
■ infections — subacute bacterial endocarditis, tuberculosis, hepatitis, malaria, Rocky Mountain spotted fever
■ collagen vascular diseases — systemic lupus erythematosus, rheumatoid arthritis, polyarteritis nodosa
■ neoplastic diseases — carcinomas, monocytic leukemia, lymphomas.

Monocyte levels are decreased by:
■ prednisone treatment
■ hairy cell leukemia.

5

Common disorders
Treating and preventing diseases

Acquired immunodeficiency syndrome

Acquired immunodeficiency syndrome (AIDS) is marked by progressive failure of the immune system and is characterized by gradual destruction of cell-mediated (T-cell) immunity, humoral immunity, and even autoimmunity. The resultant immunodeficiency makes the patient susceptible to opportunistic infections, unusual cancers, and other abnormalities that define AIDS. Depending on individual variations and the presence of cofactors that influence progression, the time elapsed from acute human immunodeficiency virus (HIV) infection to the appearance of symptoms (mild to severe) to the diagnosis of AIDS and, eventually, to death varies greatly.

Causes

HIV is transmitted by direct inoculation during intimate sexual contact, especially with the mucosal trauma of receptive rectal intercourse. It's also transmitted by transfusion of contaminated blood or blood products, sharing of contaminated needles, and transplacental or postpartum transmission from infected mother to fetus (by cervical or blood contact at delivery and in breast milk).

The virus gains access by binding to the $CD4^+$ molecule on the cell surface along with a coreceptor (thought to be the chemokine receptor CCR5). After invading a cell, HIV replicates, leading to cell death, or becomes latent. HIV infection leads to direct destruction of $CD4^+$ cells, other immune cells, and neuroglial cells, or indirectly, through the secondary effects of $CD4^+$ T-cell dysfunction and resultant immunosuppression. The average time between exposure to the virus and diagnosis of AIDS is 8 to 10 years.

Assessment findings

HIV infection manifests itself in many ways. After a high-risk exposure and inoculation, the infected person usually experiences a mononucleosis-like syndrome, which may be attributed to flu or other virus and then may remain asymptomatic for years. In this latent stage, the only sign of HIV infection is laboratory evidence of seroconversion.

Signs and symptoms include persistent generalized adenopathy, nonspecific signs and symptoms (weight loss, fatigue, night sweats, fevers), neurologic symptoms resulting from HIV encephalopathy, opportunistic infection, and cancer.

The clinical course varies slightly in children with AIDS. Their incubation time is shorter, with a mean of 17 months. Signs and symptoms resemble those in adults, except for findings related to sexually transmitted diseases. Children show most of the opportunistic infections observed in adults, with a higher risk of bacterial infections.

Diagnostic tests

The Centers for Disease Control and Prevention (CDC) defines AIDS as an illness characterized by one or more "indicator" diseases coexisting with laboratory evidence of HIV infection and other possible causes of immunosuppression. The CDC's current AIDS surveillance case definition requires laboratory confirmation of HIV infection in people who have a $CD4^+$ T-cell count of less than 200 cells/μl or who have an associated clinical condition or disease.

The recommended protocol requires that both people and blood products be initially screened with an enzyme-linked immunosorbent assay (ELISA). A positive ELISA should be repeated and then confirmed by an alternative method, usually the Western blot or an immunofluorescence assay. Because the body takes a variable amount of time to produce a detectable level of antibodies, a "window" varying from a few weeks to as long as 35 months can lapse. Antibody tests are also unreliable in neonates because transferred maternal antibodies persist for 6 to 10 months. To overcome these problems, direct testing is performed to detect HIV by antigen tests (p24 antigen), HIV cultures, nucleic acid probes of peripheral blood lymphocytes with determination of HIV-1 ribonucleic acid levels, and the polymerase chain reaction.

Treatment

No cure has yet been found for AIDS; however, primary therapy for HIV infection includes three types of antiretroviral agents:
■ protease inhibitors, such as ritonavir, indinavir, nelfinavir, and saquinavir
■ nucleoside reverse transcriptase inhibitors (nRTIs), such as zidovudine, didanosine, zalcitabine, lamivudine, and stavudine
■ nonnucleoside reverse transcriptase inhibitors, such as nevirapine and delavirdine.
These agents, used in various combinations, are designed to inhibit HIV viral replication. Other potential therapies include immunomodulatory agents designed to boost the weakened immune system and anti-infective and antineoplastic agents to combat opportunistic infections and associated cancers; some are used prophylactically to help patients resist opportunistic infections.

Treatment with zidovudine has proved effective in slowing the progression of HIV infection, decreasing opportunistic infections, and prolonging survival, but it commonly produces serious adverse and toxic reactions. The drug is usually combined with other agents (such as lamivudine) but has also been used as a single agent for pregnant HIV-positive women. Other nRTIs, such as didanosine and zalcitabine, may be used in combination regimens for patients who can't tolerate or who no longer respond to zidovudine.

Nursing interventions

■ Monitor the patient for fever, noting any pattern, and for signs of skin breakdown, cough, sore throat, and diarrhea. Assess the patient for swollen, tender lymph nodes, and check laboratory values regularly.
■ Record the patient's caloric intake.
■ Ensure adequate fluid intake during episodes of diarrhea.
■ Encourage the patient to maintain as much physical activity as he can tolerate. Make sure his schedule includes time for both exercise and rest.
■ Monitor opportunistic infections or signs of disease progression, and treat infections as ordered.

Patient teaching
■ Patients must understand that medication regimens must be followed closely and may be required for many years, if not throughout life.
■ Urge the patient to inform potential sexual partners and health care workers that he has HIV infection.
■ Teach the patient how to identify the signs of impending infection, and stress the importance of seeking immediate medical attention.

Alzheimer's disease

Alzheimer's disease is a progressive degenerative disorder of the cerebral cortex (especially the frontal lobe) that accounts for more than half of all cases of dementia. Because this is a primary progressive dementia, the prognosis for a patient with this disease is poor.

Causes

The cause of Alzheimer's disease is unknown, but several factors are closely connected to it. These include neurochemical factors, such as deficiencies of the neurotransmitters acetylcholine, somatostatin, substance P, and norepinephrine; environmental factors, such as aluminum and manganese; trauma; genetic factors; and viral factors such as slow-growing central nervous system viruses.

Assessment findings

The onset of this disorder is insidious, and the initial changes are almost imperceptible, but gradually progress to serious problems. The patient history is almost always obtained from a family member or caregiver.

Typically, the patient history shows initial onset of very small changes, such as forgetfulness and subtle memory loss without the loss of social skills and behavior patterns. It also reveals that over a period of time the patient began experiencing recent memory loss and had difficulty learning and remembering new information. The history may also reveal a general deterioration in personal hygiene and appearance and an inability to concentrate.

Depending on the severity of the disease, the patient history may reveal difficulty with abstract thinking and activities that require judgment; progressive difficulty in communicating; and a severe deterioration of memory, language, and motor function that can result in coordination loss and an inability to speak or write. The patient may also perform repetitive actions and ex-

perience restlessness; negative personality changes, such as irritability, depression, paranoia, hostility, and combativeness; nocturnal awakening; and disorientation.

The person giving the history may explain that the patient is suspicious and fearful of imaginary people and situations, misperceives his environment, misidentifies objects and people, and complains of stolen or misplaced objects.

He may also report that the patient seems overdependent on caregivers and has difficulty using correct words, often substituting meaningless words. He may report that conversations with the patient drift off into nonsensical phrases. The patient's emotions may be described as labile. Also, the patient may laugh or cry inappropriately and have mood swings, sudden angry outbursts, and sleep disturbances.

Neurologic examination confirms many of the problems revealed during the history. Also, it commonly reveals an impaired sense of smell (usually an early symptom), impaired stereognosis (inability to recognize and understand the form and nature of objects by touching them), gait disorders, tremors, and loss of recent memory. The patient's susceptibility to infection and accidents (due to the loss of the cough reflex) and to pulmonary disease (such as pneumonia) may result in death. The patient with Alzheimer's disease also has a positive snout reflex.

If the patient is in the final stages, he typically has urinary or fecal incontinence and may twitch and have seizures.

Diagnostic tests

Alzheimer's disease is diagnosed by exclusion. Various tests such as those described below are performed to rule out other disorders. The diagnosis can't be confirmed until death, when pathologic findings come to light at autopsy.

Position emission tomography measures the metabolic activity of the cerebral cortex and may help confirm early diagnosis.

Computed tomography scanning in some patients shows progressive brain atrophy in excess of that which occurs with normal aging. Magnetic resonance imaging may permit evaluation of the condition of the brain and rule out intracranial lesions as the source of dementia.

EEG allows evaluation of the brain's electrical activity and may show slowing of the brain waves in the late stages of the disease. This diagnostic test also helps identify tumors, abscesses, and other intracranial lesions that might cause the patient's symptoms.

Cerebrospinal fluid analysis may help determine if the patient's signs and symptoms stem from a chronic neurologic infection. Cerebral blood flow studies may detect abnormalities in blood flow to the brain.

Neuropsychology testing is a battery of tests designed to assess cognitive ability and reasoning. They can help differentiate Alzheimer's disease from other types of dementia.

Treatment

No cure or definitive treatment exists for Alzheimer's disease. Therapy consists of cerebral vasodilators, such as ergoloid mesylates, isoxsuprine, and cyclandelate to enhance the brain's circulation; hyperbaric oxygen to increase oxygenation to the brain; psychostimulators such as methylphenidate to enhance the patient's mood; and antidepressants if depression seems to exacerbate the patient's dementia.

Most other drug therapies being tried are experimental. These include choline salts, lecithin, physostigmine, enkephalins, and naloxone, which may slow the disease process. Drugs given to enhance cognition include donepezil hydrochloride (Aricept) and tacrine hydrochloride (Cognex).

Nursing interventions

■ Provide emotional support to the patient and family members. Encourage them to talk about their concerns.
■ Because the patient may misperceive his environment, use a soft tone and a slow, calm manner when speaking to him.
■ Allow the patient sufficient time to answer your questions.
■ If the patient has trouble swallowing, check with a pharmacist to see if tablets can be crushed or capsules can be opened and mixed with a semisoft food.
■ Protect the patient from injury by providing a safe, structured environment. Provide rest periods between activities because patients with Alzheimer's disease tire easily.
■ Encourage the patient to exercise, as ordered, to help maintain mobility.
■ Encourage patient independence, and allow ample time for the patient to perform tasks.
■ Encourage sufficient fluid intake and adequate nutrition. Give the patient semisolid foods if he has dysphagia. Insert and care for a nasogastric or gastrostomy tube, as ordered for feeding.
■ Assist the patient with hygiene and dressing as necessary.

Patient teaching
■ Teach the patient's family about the disease and its symptoms. Explain that the disease progresses at an unpredictable rate and that patients eventually suffer complete memory loss and total physical deterioration.

■ Review the diagnostic tests that are to be performed and the treatment the patient requires.

■ Advise family members to provide the patient with exercise. Suggest physical activities, such as walking or light housework, that occupy and satisfy the patient.

■ Stress the importance of diet. Instruct family members to limit the number of foods on the patient's plate so he doesn't have to make decisions. If the patient has coordination problems, tell family members to cut his food and to provide finger foods, such as fruit and sandwiches. Suggest using plates with rim guards, built-up utensils, and cups with lids and spouts.

■ Encourage family members to allow the patient as much independence as possible while ensuring his and others' safety. Tell them to create a routine for all of the patient's activities, which helps avoid confusion. If the patient becomes belligerent, advise family members to remain calm and try to distract him.

■ Refer family members to support groups such as the Alzheimer's Association. Set up an appointment with the social service department to help family members assess their needs.

Arterial occlusive disease

Arterial occlusive disease is an obstruction or narrowing of the lumen of the aorta and its major branches, which interrupts blood flow, usually to the legs and feet. Arterial occlusive disease may affect the carotid, vertebral, innominate, subclavian, mesenteric, and iliac, femoral, and popliteal arteries. The prognosis depends on the location of the occlusion, the development of collateral circulation to counteract reduced blood flow and, in acute disease, the time elapsed between the development of the occlusion and its removal.

Causes

Arterial occlusive disease is a common complication of atherosclerosis. Predisposing factors include smoking; aging; conditions such as hypertension, hyperlipidemia, and diabetes mellitus; and family history of vascular disorders, myocardial infarction, or cerebrovascular accident.

Occlusions may be acute or chronic and can cause severe ischemia, skin ulceration, and gangrene.

Assessment findings

Assessment findings vary, depending on the vessel involved. (See *Signs and symptoms of arterial occlusive disease*, page 196.) Acute arterial occlusion occurs suddenly, in many instances without warning. However, peripheral occlusion can generally be recognized by the five Ps:

■ *Pain*, the most common symptom, occurs suddenly and is localized to the affected arm or leg.

■ *Pallor* results from vasoconstriction distal to the occlusion.

■ *Pulselessness* occurs distal to the occlusion.

■ *Paralysis* and *paresthesia* occur in the affected arm or leg from disturbed nerve endings or skeletal muscles.

A sixth P, known as *poikilothermy*, refers to temperature changes that occur distal to the occlusion, making the skin feel cool.

Diagnostic tests

Arteriography demonstrates the type, location, and degree of obstruction and the establishment of collateral circulation. It's particularly useful for evaluating patients with chronic disease or for candidates for reconstructive surgery.

Ultrasonography and plethysmography are noninvasive tests that, in pa-

Signs and symptoms of arterial occlusive disease

A patient with arterial occlusive disease may have a variety of signs and symptoms, depending on which portion of the vasculature the disorder has affected.

Site of occlusion	Signs and symptoms
Internal and external carotid arteries	Transient ischemic attacks (TIAs) due to reduced cerebral circulation may produce unilateral sensory or motor dysfunction (transient monocular blindness, hemiparesis), aphasia or dysarthria, confusion, decreased mentation, and headache. These recurrent signs and symptoms usually last for 5 to 10 minutes but may persist for up to 24 hours and may indicate cerebrovascular accident. Also, absent or decreased pulsation with an auscultatory bruit over the affected vessels may occur.
Vertebral and basilar arteries	TIAs of brain stem and cerebellum, producing binocular visual disturbances, vertigo, dysarthria, and "drop attacks" (falling down without loss of consciousness) (less common than carotid TIA).
Innominate (brachiocephalic) artery	Signs and symptoms of vertebrobasilar occlusion, indications of ischemia (claudication) of right arm, possible bruit over right side of neck.
Subclavian artery	Subclavian steal syndrome characterized by backflow of blood from the brain through the vertebral artery on the same side as the occlusion, into the subclavian artery distal to the occlusion, clinical effects of vertebrobasilar occlusion and exercise-induced arm claudication, possible gangrene (usually limited to the digits).
Mesenteric artery	Bowel ischemia, infarct necrosis, and gangrene; sudden, acute abdominal pain; nausea and vomiting; diarrhea; leukocytosis; shock due to massive intraluminal and plasma loss.
Aortic bifurcation (saddle-block occlusion)	Sensory and motor deficits (muscle weakness, numbness, paresthesia, paralysis), signs and symptoms of ischemia (sudden pain; cold, pale legs with decreased or absent peripheral pulses) in both legs.
Iliac artery (Leriche's syndrome)	Intermittent claudication of lower back, buttocks, and thighs, that's relieved by rest; absent or reduced femoral or distal pulses; shiny, scaly skin, subcutaneous tissue loss, and no body hair on affected limb; nail deformities; increased capillary refill time; blanching of feet on elevation; possible bruit over femoral arteries; impotence in males.
Femoral and popliteal arteries (associated with aneurysm formation)	Intermittent claudication of the calves on exertion; ischemic pain in feet; pretrophic pain (indicates necrosis and ulceration); leg pallor and coolness; shiny, scaly skin, subcutaneous tissue loss, and no body hair on affected limb; nail deformities; increased capillary refill time; blanching of feet on elevation; gangrene; no palpable pulses distal to occlusion (auscultation over affected area may reveal a bruit).

tients with acute disease, show decreased blood flow distal to the occlusion. Doppler ultrasonography typically reveals a relatively low-pitched sound and a monophasic waveform. Segmental limb pressures and pulse volume measurements help evaluate the location and extent of the occlusion.

Ophthalmodynamometry helps determine the degree of obstruction in the internal carotid artery by comparing ophthalmic artery pressure with brachial artery pressure on the affected side. More than a 20% difference between pressures suggests arterial insufficiency. EEG and a computed tomography scan may be necessary to rule out brain lesions.

Treatment

For patients with mild chronic disease, treatment usually consists of supportive measures: smoking cessation, hypertension control, walking exercise, and foot and leg care. For patients with carotid artery occlusion, antiplatelet therapy may begin with dipyridamole and aspirin. For those patients with intermittent claudication caused by chronic arterial occlusive disease, pentoxifylline may improve blood flow through the capillaries. This drug is particularly useful for patients who aren't good candidates for surgery.

Thrombolytics — such as urokinase, streptokinase, and alteplase — can dissolve clots and relieve the obstruction caused by a thrombus. Acute arterial occlusive disease usually requires surgery, such as embolectomy, thromboendarterectomy, atherectomy, balloon angioplasty, laser angioplasty, placement of stents, or combined therapy of these treatments. Percutaneous transluminal coronary angioplasty (PTCA) or laser surgery may also be attempted, as may patch or bypass grafting. Depending on the condition of the sympathetic

nervous system, a lumbar sympathectomy may be an adjunct to reconstructive surgery. Amputation may be necessary if arterial reconstructive surgery fails or if gangrene, uncontrollable infection, or intractable pain develops.

Nursing interventions

For patients with chronic disease
■ Prevent trauma to the affected extremity. Use minimal pressure mattresses, heel protectors, a foot cradle, or a footboard to reduce pressure that could lead to skin breakdown.
■ Avoid using restrictive clothing such as antiembolism stockings.

For preoperative care during an acute episode
■ Assess the patient's circulatory status by checking for the most distal pulses and by inspecting his skin color and temperature.
■ Administer heparin or a thrombolytic by continuous I.V. drip as ordered. Use an infusion monitor or pump to ensure the proper flow rate.
■ Wrap the patient's affected foot in soft cotton batting, and reposition it frequently to prevent pressure on any one area. Strictly avoid elevating or applying heat to the affected leg.
■ Watch for signs of fluid and electrolyte imbalance, and monitor intake and output.
■ If the patient has carotid, innominate, vertebral, or subclavian artery occlusion, monitor him for symptoms of cerebrovascular accident, such as numbness in an arm or a leg and intermittent blindness.

For postoperative care
■ Monitor the patient's vital signs. Continuously assess his circulatory function by assessing skin color and temperature and by checking for distal

pulses. Watch closely for signs of hemorrhage and check dressings for excessive bleeding.

■ For patients with carotid, innominate, vertebral, or subclavian artery occlusion, assess the patient's neurologic status frequently for changes in level of consciousness, pupil size, and muscle strength.

■ For patients with mesenteric artery occlusion, connect a nasogastric tube to low intermittent suction. Monitor intake and output (low urine output may indicate damage to renal arteries during surgery). Check bowel sounds for the return of peristalsis. Increasing abdominal distention and tenderness may indicate extension of bowel ischemia with resulting gangrene, necessitating further excision, or it may indicate peritonitis.

■ For patients with saddle block occlusion, check distal pulses for adequate circulation. Watch for signs and symptoms of renal failure, mesenteric artery occlusion (severe abdominal pain), and cardiac arrhythmias, which may precipitate embolus formation.

■ For patients who have had a PTCA, perform sheath (catheter) care. The line must be kept open with a heparin infusion; monitor the insertion site for bleeding. Keep the catheterized leg immobile, and maintain strict bed rest. Monitor and record pulses in the catheterized leg.

■ For patients with iliac artery occlusion, monitor urine output for signs of renal failure from decreased perfusion to the kidneys as a result of surgery.

■ For patients with both femoral and popliteal artery occlusion, assist with early ambulation, and don't allow them to sit for an extended period.

Patient teaching
■ When preparing the patient for discharge, instruct him to watch for signs and symptoms of recurrence (such as pain, pallor, numbness, paralysis, or absence of pulse) that can result from graft occlusion or occlusion at another site. Caution against wearing constrictive clothing and crossing his legs. Tell him to avoid "bumping" injuries to affected limbs.

■ Warn the patient to avoid tobacco products and temperature extremes. If he must go outside in the cold, remind him to dress warmly and to keep his feet warm.

■ Instruct the patient to wash his feet daily and inspect them for signs of injury or infection. Remind him to report abnormalities to the doctor.

■ Advise the patient to wear sturdy, properly fitting shoes. Refer him to a podiatrist for any foot problems.

■ Teach the patient about preventive measures, such as smoking-cessation programs, regular exercise, weight control, reduction of dietary fat intake, and the avoidance of pressure and constriction to the extremities. These measures may reduce the risk of arterial occlusive disease, especially for patients with a history of cardiovascular disease.

Asthma

Asthma is a chronic reactive airway disorder that involves episodic, reversible airway obstruction resulting from bronchospasms, increased mucus secretions, and mucosal edema. Signs and symptoms range from mild wheezing and dyspnea to life-threatening respiratory failure. Signs and symptoms of bronchial airway obstruction may or may not persist between acute episodes.

Asthma may result from sensitivity to specific external allergens (extrinsic) or from internal, hypoallergenic factors (intrinsic). Allergens that cause extrinsic asthma (atopic asthma) include pollen, animal dander, house dust and mold, kapok and feather pillows, food additives containing sulfites, and other sensitizing substances. Extrinsic asthma begins in children and is commonly accompanied by other signs of atopy (type I, immunoglobulin E [IgE]–mediated allergy), such as eczema and allergic rhinitis.

In patients with intrinsic asthma (nonatopic asthma), no extrinsic substance can be identified. Most episodes are preceded by a severe respiratory tract infection (especially in adults). Irritants, emotional stress, fatigue, endocrine changes, temperature and humidity variations, and exposure to noxious fumes may aggravate intrinsic asthma attacks. In many asthmatics, especially children, intrinsic and extrinsic asthma coexist.

Causes

In patients with asthma, the tracheal and bronchial linings overreact to various stimuli, causing episodic smooth-muscle spasms that severely constrict the airways. Mucosal edema and thickened secretions further block the airways.

IgE antibodies, attached to histamine-containing mast cells and receptors on cell membranes, initiate intrinsic asthma attacks. When exposed to an antigen such as pollen, the IgE antibody combines with the antigen. On subsequent exposure to the antigen, mast cells degranulate and release mediators.

These mediators cause the bronchoconstriction and edema of an asthma attack. As a result, expiratory airflow decreases, trapping gas in the airways and causing alveolar hyperinflation. Atelectasis may develop in some lung regions. The increased airway resistance initiates labored breathing. Several factors may contribute to bronchoconstriction. These include hereditary predisposition; sensitivity to allergens

or irritants such as pollutants; viral infections; aspirin, beta-adrenergic blockers, nonsteroidal anti-inflammatory drugs, and other drugs; tartrazine (a yellow food dye); psychological stress; cold air; and exercise.

Assessment findings

An asthma attack may begin dramatically, with simultaneous onset of severe, multiple symptoms, or insidiously, with gradually increasing respiratory distress. Typically, the patient reports exposure to a particular allergen followed by sudden onset of dyspnea, wheezing, and tightness in the chest accompanied by a cough that produces thick, clear or yellow sputum.

The patient may complain of feeling suffocated. He may be visibly dyspneic and able to speak only a few words before pausing for breath. You may also observe accessory respiratory muscle use. He may sweat profusely, and you may note an increased anteroposterior thoracic diameter.

Percussion may produce hyperresonance. Palpation may reveal vocal fremitus. Auscultation may disclose tachycardia, tachypnea, mild systolic hypertension, harsh respirations with both inspiratory and expiratory wheezes, prolonged expiratory phase of respiration, and diminished breath sounds.

Cyanosis, confusion, and lethargy indicate the onset of life-threatening status asthmaticus and respiratory failure. (See *Determining asthma's severity*, page 200.)

Diagnostic tests

Pulmonary function studies reveal signs of airway obstructive disease (decreased flow rates and forced expiratory volume in 1 second [FEV_1]), low-normal or decreased vital capacity, and increased total lung and residual capac-

Determining asthma's severity

Signs and symptoms during acute phase	Diagnostic test results	Other assessment findings
MILD ASTHMA		
■ Brief wheezing, coughing, dyspnea with activity ■ Infrequent nocturnal coughing or wheezing ■ Adequate air exchange ■ Intermittent, brief (less than 1 hour) wheezing, coughing, or dyspnea once or twice a week ■ Asymptomatic between attacks	■ FEV_1 or peak flow 80% of normal values ■ pH normal or increased ■ PaO_2 normal or decreased ■ $PaCO_2$ normal or decreased ■ Chest X-ray normal	■ One attack per week (or none) ■ Positive response to bronchodilator therapy within 24 hours ■ No signs of asthma between episodes ■ No sleep interruption ■ No hyperventilation ■ Minimal evidence of airway obstruction ■ Minimal or no increase in lung volume
MODERATE ASTHMA		
■ Respiratory distress at rest ■ Hyperpnea ■ Marked coughing and wheezing ■ Air exchange normal or below normal ■ Exacerbations that may last several days	■ FEV_1 or peak flow 60% to 80% of normal values; may vary 20% to 30% with symptoms ■ pH generally elevated ■ PaO_2 increased ■ $PaCO_2$ generally decreased ■ Chest X-ray that shows hyperinflation	■ Symptoms occurring more than two times weekly ■ Coughing and wheezing between episodes ■ Diminished exercise tolerance ■ Possible sleep interruption ■ Increased lung volumes
SEVERE ASTHMA		
■ Marked respiratory distress ■ Marked wheezing or absent breath sounds ■ Paradoxical pulse greater than 10 mm Hg ■ Chest wall contractions ■ Continuous symptoms ■ Frequent exacerbations	■ FEV_1 or peak flow less than 60% of normal values; may normally vary 20% to 30% with routine medications and up to 50% with exacerbations ■ pH normal or reduced ■ PaO_2 decreased ■ $PaCO_2$ normal or increased ■ Chest X-ray that may show hyperinflation	■ Frequent severe attacks ■ Daily wheezing ■ Poor exercise tolerance ■ Frequent sleep interruption ■ Bronchodilator therapy that doesn't completely reverse airway obstruction ■ Markedly increased lung volume

ities. Despite abnormal findings during asthma attacks, pulmonary function may be normal between attacks.

Typically, the patient has decreased partial pressure of arterial oxygen and partial pressure of arterial carbon dioxide ($PaCO_2$). However, in patients with severe asthma, $PaCO_2$ may be normal or increased, indicating severe bronchial obstruction. In fact, FEV_1 is most likely less than 25% of the predicted value. Residual volume remains abnormal for up to 3 weeks after the attack.

Serum IgE levels may increase from an allergic reaction, and complete blood count with differential reveals increased eosinophil count. Skin testing may be used to identify specific allergens. Bronchial challenge testing is used to evaluate the clinical significance of allergens identified by skin testing.

Chest X-rays can be used to diagnose or monitor the progress of asthma. X-rays may show hyperinflation with areas of focal atelectasis.

Treatment

The best treatment for asthma is prevention, including identification and avoidance of precipitating factors, such as environmental allergens or irritants. The patient may also be desensitized to specific antigens.

Drug therapy, which usually includes a bronchodilator, is most effective when begun soon after the onset of signs and symptoms. Bronchodilators used include rapid-acting epinephrine, methylxanthines (theophylline and aminophylline), and beta$_2$-adrenergic antagonists (albuterol and terbutaline) to decrease bronchoconstriction. A corticosteroid (hydrocortisone sodium succinate, prednisone, methylprednisolone, or beclomethasone) may be used for its anti-inflammatory and immunosuppressant effects on the airways. Cromolyn and nedocromil help prevent the re-

lease of the chemical mediators (histamine and leukotrienes) that cause bronchoconstriction. An anticholinergic bronchodilator (such as ipratropium) may be used to block acetylcholine, another chemical mediator. Arterial blood gas (ABG) measurements help to determine the severity of an asthma attack and the patient's response to treatment. For the most part, medical treatment of asthma must be tailored to the patient. (See *Tailoring treatments to types of asthma,* page 202.)

Low-flow oxygen and fluid replacement may be required, as may an antibiotic if infection exists.

Status asthmaticus must be treated promptly to prevent progression to fatal respiratory failure. The patient with increasingly severe asthma who doesn't respond to drug therapy is usually admitted to the intensive care unit for treatment with a corticosteroid, epinephrine, a sympathomimetic aerosol spray, and I.V. aminophylline. He needs frequent ABG analysis and pulse oximetry to assess respiratory status. The patient may require endotracheal intubation and mechanical ventilation if his $PaCO_2$ increases.

Nursing interventions

During an acute attack

■ First assess the severity of asthma, administer the prescribed treatments, and assess the patient's response.

■ Place the patient in high Fowler's position. Encourage pursed-lip and diaphragmatic breathing. Help him to relax.

■ Monitor the patient's vital signs. Keep in mind that developing or increasing tachypnea may indicate worsening asthma and that tachycardia may indicate worsening asthma or toxic reaction to a drug. Blood pressure readings may reveal paradoxical pulse, indicating severe asthma. Hypertension

Tailoring treatments to types of asthma

For the most part, medical treatment of asthma attacks must be tailored to each patient. However, the following treatments are generally used.

Chronic mild asthma

A beta$_2$-adrenergic agonist by metered-dose inhaler is used (alone or with cromolyn) before exercise and exposure to an allergen or other stimuli to prevent symptoms. The beta$_2$-adrenergic agonist is used every 3 to 4 hours if symptoms occur.

Chronic moderate asthma

Initial treatment may include an inhaled beta-adrenergic bronchodilator, an inhaled corticosteroid, and cromolyn. An anticholinergic bronchodilator may also be added. If symptoms persist, the inhaled corticosteroid dose may be increased, and sustained-release theophylline or an oral beta$_2$-adrenergic agonist (or both) may be added. Short courses of oral corticosteroids may also be used.

Chronic severe asthma

Initially, around-the-clock oral bronchodilator therapy with a long-acting theophylline or a beta$_2$-adrenergic agonist may be required, supplemented with an inhaled corticosteroid with or without cromolyn. An oral corticosteroid such as prednisone may be added in acute exacerbations.

Acute asthma attack

Acute attacks that don't respond to maintenance treatment may require hospital care, a beta$_2$-adrenergic agonist by inhalation or subcutaneous injection (in three doses over 60 to 90 minutes) and, possibly, oxygen for hypoxemia. If the patient responds poorly, a systemic corticosteroid and, possibly, subcutaneous (S.C.) epinephrine may help. Beta$_2$-adrenergic agonist inhalation continues hourly. I.V. aminophylline may be added to the regimen, and I.V. fluid therapy is started. Patients who don't respond to this treatment, whose airways remain obstructed, and who have increasing respiratory difficulty are at risk for status asthmaticus and may require mechanical ventilation.

Status asthmaticus

Treatment consists of aggressive drug therapy: a beta$_2$-adrenergic agonist by nebulizer over 30 to 60 minutes, possibly supplemented with S.C. epinephrine, an I.V. corticosteroid, I.V. aminophylline, oxygen administration, I.V. fluid therapy, and intubation and mechanical ventilation for hypercapnia respiratory failure (partial pressure of arterial carbon dioxide of 40 mm Hg or more).

---

may indicate asthma-related hypoxemia.

■ Administer prescribed humidified oxygen, and monitor effects.

■ Anticipate intubation and mechanical ventilation if the patient fails to maintain adequate oxygenation.

■ Monitor serum theophylline levels, and observe the patient for signs and symptoms of toxic reaction (vomiting, diarrhea, headache) and subtherapeutic response (respiratory distress, increased wheezing).

■ Auscultate his lungs, noting adventitious or absent sounds. If his cough isn't productive and rhonchi are present, teach him effective coughing techniques. If the patient can tolerate postural drainage and chest percussion, perform these procedures to clear se-

Coping with asthma

Use these guidelines to help your patient cope with asthma at home.

■ Teach the parents and child about what triggers an attack. Evaluate their home to detect triggers, and help minimize them.
■ Assess the child's compliance with the medication regimen, and suggest ways to improve it.
■ Teach the parents and child how to use inhalers with spacer devices. First, show them how to set up the device, and stress the need for a tight seal around the mouthpiece. After demonstrating its use, watch the child use it. (He should press down to release medication into the chamber, inhale slowly, hold his breath for 5 seconds, exhale, and repeat the sequence again.) Explain the need to clean the mouthpiece with warm running water once a day and to dry it completely before placing it in its case.
■ Instruct the parents to replace the mouthpiece every 6 months and the reservoir bag every 2 to 3 weeks or as needed. If the bag develops a hole or tear, tell them to replace it immediately.
■ Suggest keeping a spare device available.
■ Discuss the signs of an impending attack, and identify measures to minimize it.
■ If the child must take a methylxanthine such as theophylline, advise the parents to call the doctor if adverse reactions occur and to return for follow-up laboratory tests.
■ If the child must take a corticosteroid, monitor for cushingoid effects. If such effects occur, tell the parents not to discontinue the drug abruptly but to gradually reduce the dosage.
■ Encourage the parents to let the child perform whatever activities he feels comfortable doing.
■ Recommend community resources, such as the American Lung Association or the Asthma and Allergy Foundation of America.

cretions. Suction an intubated patient as needed.
■ Treat dehydration with I.V. fluids until the patient can tolerate oral fluids, which helps loosen secretions.
■ If conservative treatment fails to improve the airway obstruction, anticipate bronchoscopy or bronchial lavage when the area of collapse is a lobe or larger.

During long-term care
■ Monitor the patient's respiratory status to detect baseline changes, assess response to treatment, and prevent or detect complications.
■ Auscultate the lungs frequently, noting the degree of wheezing and quality of air movement.

■ If the patient is taking a systemic corticosteroid, observe him for complications, such as elevated blood glucose levels, friable skin, and bruising.
■ If the patient is taking an inhaled corticosteroid, watch for signs of candidal infection in the mouth and pharynx. He may consider using an extender device and rinsing his mouth after administering the drug to prevent such infection.
■ For patients with moderate to severe chronic disease, regular use of an extender device may facilitate better delivery of inhaled medications.
■ Observe the patient's anxiety level. Keep in mind that measures to reduce hypoxemia and breathlessness should relieve anxiety.

■ Keep the room temperature comfortable, and use an air conditioner or a fan in hot, humid weather.

■ Control exercise-induced asthma by instructing the patient to use a bronchodilator or cromolyn 30 minutes before exercise. Also, instruct him to use pursed-lip breathing while exercising.

Patient teaching

■ Teach the patient and family members to avoid known allergens and irritants.

■ Describe prescribed drugs, including their names, dosages, actions, adverse effects, and special instructions.

■ Teach the patient how to use a metered-dose inhaler. He may need an extender device to optimize therapy.

■ If the patient has moderate to severe asthma, explain how to use a peak-flow meter to measure the degree of airway obstruction. Tell him to keep a record of peak-flow readings and to bring it to his medical appointments. Explain the importance of calling the doctor immediately if the peak flow drops suddenly. (A drop can signal severe respiratory problems.)

■ Tell the patient to notify the doctor if he develops a temperature higher than 100° F (37.8° C), chest pain, shortness of breath without coughing or exercising, or uncontrollable coughing. An uncontrollable asthma attack requires immediate attention.

■ Teach the patient diaphragmatic and pursed-lip breathing as well as effective coughing techniques.

■ Urge the patient to drink at least 3.2 qt (3 L) of fluids daily to help loosen secretions and maintain hydration. (See *Coping with asthma,* page 203.)

Breast cancer

Breast cancer is a leading killer of women ages 35 to 54. Early detection and treatment influences the prognosis considerably. The most reliable breast cancer detection method is regular breast self-examination, followed by immediate professional evaluation of any abnormality.

Causes

The causes of breast cancer remain elusive. Significant risk factors include having a family history of breast cancer (mother, sister, grandmother, aunt) and being a premenopausal woman older than age 45. Other risk factors may include a long menstrual cycle, early onset of menses, or late menopause; first pregnancy after age 31; a high-fat diet; endometrial or ovarian cancer; radiation exposure; estrogen therapy; antihypertensive therapy; alcohol and tobacco use; and preexisting fibrocystic disease. The recent discovery of the breast cancer gene BRCA 1 confirms the theory that the disease can be inherited from either the mother or the father.

About half of all breast cancers develop in the upper outer quadrant. Growth rates vary, and slow-growing breast cancer may take up to 8 years to become palpable at $3/8''$ (1 cm). It spreads by way of the lymphatic system and the bloodstream through the right side of the heart to the lungs and to the other breast, chest wall, liver, bone, and brain.

Assessment findings

The most reliable way to detect breast cancer is through monthly breast self-examination by the patient, followed by immediate evaluation of any abnormality. A patient will usually report that she detected a painless lump or mass in her breast or that she noticed a thickening of breast tissue. Otherwise, the disease typically appears on a mammogram before a lesion becomes palpable. The patient's history may indicate several risk factors for breast cancer.

Inspection may reveal clear, milky, or bloody nipple discharge, nipple retraction, scaly skin around the nipple, and skin changes, such as dimpling, peau d'orange, or inflammation. Arm edema, also identified on inspection, may indicate advanced nodal involvement. Palpation may identify a hard lump, mass, or thickening of breast tissue. Palpation of the cervical supraclavicular and axillary nodes may also disclose lumps or enlargement.

Diagnostic tests

Mammography, the essential test for breast cancer, can reveal a tumor that's too small to palpate. Fine-needle aspiration and excisional biopsy provide cells for histologic examination to confirm the diagnosis.

Ultrasonography can distinguish between a fluid-filled cyst and a solid mass. Chest X-rays can pinpoint metastases in the chest. Scans of the bone, brain, liver, and other organs can detect distant metastases.

Laboratory tests, such as alkaline phosphatase levels and liver function tests, can uncover distant metastases. Hormonal receptor assay can determine whether the tumor is estrogen- or progesterone-dependent. This test guides decisions to use therapy that blocks the action of the estrogen hormone that supports tumor growth.

Treatment

The choice of treatment usually depends on the stage and type of disease, woman's age and menopausal status, and disfiguring effects of surgery. Therapy may include any combination of surgery, radiation, chemotherapy, and hormone therapy.

Surgery includes lumpectomy (removal of tumor, surrounding tissue, and nearby lymph nodes only), partial mastectomy (in which one-quarter or more of the breast is removed), simple or total mastectomy (removal of breast only), modified radical mastectomy (removal of breast and axillary lymph nodes), and radical mastectomy (removal of breast, pectoralis major and minor, and axillary lymph nodes). Before or after tumor removal, primary radiation therapy may be effective for a patient who has a small tumor in early stages without distant metastases. Radiation therapy can also prevent or treat local recurrence. Preoperative breast irradiation also helps to sterilize the field, making the tumor more manageable surgically, especially in patients with inflammatory breast cancer.

Various cytotoxic drug combinations may be administered either as adjuvant therapy or as primary therapy, depending on the cancer's stage and hormonal receptor assay results. Chemotherapy commonly relies on a combination of drugs, such as cyclophosphamide, fluorouracil, methotrexate, doxorubicin, vincristine, paclitaxel, and prednisone. A typical regimen used in premenopausal and postmenopausal women includes cyclophosphamide, methotrexate, and fluorouracil.

Hormone therapy lowers levels of estrogen and other hormones suspected of nourishing breast cancer cells. For example, antiestrogen therapy (specifically tamoxifen, which is most effective against tumors identified as estrogen receptor-positive) is used in postmenopausal women. Breast cancer patients may also receive estrogen, progesterone, androgen, or antiandrogen aminoglutethimide therapy. The success of these therapies provides growing evidence that breast cancer is systemic, not local, and has led to a decline in ablation surgery.

Nursing interventions

General
■ Perform comfort measures, such as repositioning, to promote relaxation and relieve anxiety.
■ Watch for treatment complications, such as nausea, vomiting, anorexia, leukopenia, thrombocytopenia, GI ulceration, and bleeding. Provide comfort measures and prescribed treatments to relieve these complications.

After surgery
■ Inspect the dressing anteriorly and posteriorly and record the amount and color of drainage. Promptly report excessive bleeding. Inspect the incision, and encourage the patient to do the same.
■ Monitor vital signs. If a general anesthetic was given during surgery, monitor intake and output for at least 48 hours.
■ Prevent lymphedema of the arm, which may be an early complication of lymph node dissection.

Patient teaching
■ Clearly explain all procedures and treatments.
■ Besides the usual preoperative teaching, show the mastectomy patient how to ease postsurgical pain by lying on the affected side or by placing a hand or pillow on the incision. Point out where the incision will be. Inform the patient that after the operation she'll receive an analgesic to help with comfort.
■ Tell her that she may move about and get out of bed as soon as possible, usually as soon as the effects of the anesthetic subside or the first evening after surgery.
■ Explain that she may have an incisional drain or some type of suction to remove accumulated fluid, relieve ten-

sion on the suture line, and promote healing.
■ Urge the patient to avoid activities that could injure her arm and hand on the side of her surgery (including venipunctures, injections, blood pressure measurements or I.V. therapy).
■ To help prevent lymphedema, instruct the patient to exercise her hand and arm on the affected side regularly and to avoid activities that might allow infection of this hand or arm.
■ Inform the patient that she may experience "phantom breast syndrome," a tingling or pins-and-needles sensation in the area where the breast was removed.
■ Urge the patient to continue examining the other breast and to comply with recommended follow-up treatment.

Cerebrovascular accident

Also known as stroke, cerebrovascular accident (CVA) is a sudden impairment of cerebral circulation in one or more of the blood vessels supplying the brain. CVA interrupts or diminishes oxygen supply and commonly causes serious damage or necrosis in brain tissues. About half of those who survive CVA remain permanently disabled and experience a recurrence within weeks, months, or years.

CVAs are classified according to their course of progression. The least severe is the transient ischemic attack (TIA), which results from a temporary interruption of blood flow, usually in the carotid and vertebrobasilar arteries. (See *Transient ischemic attack: A warning sign of CVA.*) A progressive stroke, or stroke-in-evolution (thrombus-in-evolution), begins with a slight neurologic deficit and worsens in a day or two. In a completed stroke, neurologic deficits are at the maximum at the onset.

Transient ischemic attack: A warning sign of CVA

A transient ischemic attack (TIA) is a recurrent episode of neurologic deficit lasting less than 1 hour without permanent neurologic defects. It's usually considered a warning sign of an impending thrombotic cerebrovascular accident (CVA); TIAs are reported in 50% to 80% of patients with a cerebral infarction from such thrombosis. The age of onset varies. Incidence increases dramatically after age 50 and is highest among blacks and men.

In TIA, microemboli released from a thrombus may temporarily interrupt blood flow, especially in the small distal branches of the brain's arterial tree. Small spasms in those arterioles may impair blood flow and also precede TIA. Predisposing factors are the same as for thrombotic CVAs.

Signs and symptoms
The most distinctive characteristics of TIA are the transient duration of neurologic deficits and the complete return of normal function. The signs and symptoms of TIA correlate with the location of the affected artery. They include double vision, speech deficits (slurring or thickness), unilateral blindness, staggering or uncoordinated gait, unilateral weakness or numbness, falling because of weakness in the legs, and dizziness.

Treatment
During an active TIA, treatment aims to prevent a completed stroke and consists of aspirin, an antiplatelet drug, or an anticoagulant to minimize the risk of thrombosis. After or between attacks, preventive treatment includes carotid endarterectomy or cerebral microvascular bypass.

Causes

Major causes of CVA include cerebral thrombosis, embolism, and hemorrhage. Thrombosis is the most common cause of CVA in middle-aged and elderly people and results from obstruction of a blood vessel. Embolism (especially left middle cerebral artery) can occur rapidly at any age, especially among patients who have a history of heart disorders or cardiac arrhythmias or who have undergone open-heart surgery. Hemorrhage, the third most common cause of CVA, may also occur suddenly at any age and results from chronic hypertension or aneurysms, which cause sudden rupture of a cerebral artery.

Factors that increase the risk of CVA include a history of TIAs, heart disease, atherosclerosis, hypertension, arrhythmias, electrocardiogram changes, rheumatic heart disease, diabetes mellitus, gout, postural hypotension, cardiac enlargement, high serum triglyceride levels, lack of exercise, use of oral contraceptives, smoking, and a family history of cerebrovascular disease. Genetic risk factors include apolipoprotein E4, homocysteines, and factor V mutation.

Among the many possible complications of CVA are unstable blood pressure from loss of vasomotor control, fluid imbalances, malnutrition, infections (pneumonia), and visual or other sensory impairment. Altered level of consciousness (LOC), aspiration, contractures, and pulmonary emboli also may occur.

Assessment findings

Clinical features of CVA vary with the artery affected (and, consequently, the portion of the brain it supplies), the severity of the damage, and the extent of collateral circulation that develops to help the brain compensate for a decreased blood supply.

In assessment, if the CVA occurs in the left hemisphere, it produces signs and symptoms on the right side, and vice versa. A CVA that causes cranial nerve damage produces signs of cranial nerve dysfunction on the same side as the hemorrhage.

The patient's history may uncover one or more risk factors for CVA. It may also reveal sudden onset of hemiparesis or hemiplegia or a gradual onset of dizziness, mental disturbances, or seizures. The patient may also have lost consciousness or suddenly developed aphasia. Speaking with the patient during the history may reveal communication problems, such as dysarthria, dysphasia or aphasia, and apraxia.

Neurologic examination identifies most physical findings associated with CVA. These include unconsciousness or changes in LOC, such as a decreased attention span, difficulties with comprehension, forgetfulness, and a lack of motivation. Inspection may reveal related urinary incontinence.

Motor function tests and muscle strength tests commonly show a loss of voluntary muscle control and hemiparesis or hemiplegia on one side of the body. In the initial phase, flaccid paralysis with decreased deep tendon reflexes may occur. These reflexes return to normal after the initial phase, along with an increase in muscle tone and, in some cases, muscle spasticity on the affected side.

Vision testing commonly reveals hemianopias on the affected side of the body and, in patients with left-sided hemiplegia, problems with visuospatial relations. Sensory assessment may reveal sensory losses, ranging from slight impairment of touch to the inability to perceive the position and motion of body parts. The patient also may have difficulty interpreting visual, tactile, and auditory stimuli.

Diagnostic tests

Magnetic resonance imaging (MRI) and magnetic resonance angiography allow evaluation of the lesion's location and size without exposing the patient to radiation. MRI doesn't distinguish hemorrhage, tumor, and infarction as well as computed tomography (CT) scanning, but it provides superior images of the cerebellum and the brain stem.

Cerebral angiography details disruption or displacement of the cerebral circulation by occlusion or hemorrhages, especially the entire cerebral artery. Digital subtraction angiography is used to evaluate the patency of the cerebral vessels and identify their position in the head and neck. It's also used to detect and evaluate lesions and vascular abnormalities.

CT scanning detects structural abnormalities, edema, and lesions, such as nonhemorrhagic infarction and aneurysms. It differentiates CVA from such disorders as primary metastatic tumor and subdural, intracerebral, or epidural hematoma. Many patients with TIA have a normal CT scan.

Positron emission tomography provides data on cerebral metabolism and cerebral blood flow changes, especially in ischemic stroke. Single-photon emission tomography identifies cerebral blood flow and helps diagnose cerebral infarction. Transcranial Doppler studies evaluate the velocity of blood flow through major intracranial vessels, which can indicate the vessels' diameter. Carotid Doppler studies measure flow through the carotid arteries and can provide information on etiology of stroke. Cerebral blood flow studies measure blood flow to the brain and help detect abnormalities.

Ophthalmoscopy may show signs of hypertension and atherosclerotic changes in the retinal arteries. EEG may show reduced electrical activity in an area of cortical infarction. This test is especially useful when CT scan results are inconclusive. It can also differentiate seizure activity from CVA. Oculoplethysmography indirectly measures ophthalmic blood flow and carotid artery blood flow.

Treatment

Treatment should include careful blood pressure management. Labetalol is the vasopressor of choice to regulate blood pressure. Blood pressure that's too low increases the risk of ischemia; blood pressure that's too high increases the risk of hemorrhage. Tissue plasminogen activator may be used in emergency care of the patient within 3 hours of onset of the symptoms. Thrombolytic agents are a consideration when there's a sign of hemorrhage on CT, when there are no other contraindications, and when it's begun in a timely fashion.

Medical management of CVA commonly includes physical rehabilitation, dietary and drug regimens to help decrease risk factors, possibly surgery, and care measures to help the patient adapt to specific deficits, such as speech impairment and paralysis.

Depending on the cause and extent of the CVA, the patient may undergo a craniotomy to remove a hematoma, an endarterectomy to remove atherosclerotic plaques from the inner arterial wall, or an extracranial-intracranial bypass to circumvent an artery that's blocked by occlusion or stenosis. Ventricular shunts may be necessary to drain cerebrospinal fluid.

Medications useful for treating patients with CVA include anticonvulsants (phenytoin or phenobarbital) to treat or prevent seizures, stool softeners (to prevent increased intracranial pressure [ICP] by straining), anticoagulants to reduce the risk of thrombotic stroke, and analgesics (codeine) to relieve headache.

Nursing interventions

■ During the acute phase, provide continuing neurologic assessment, respiratory support, continuous monitoring of vital signs, careful positioning to prevent aspiration and contractures, management of GI problems, and careful monitoring of fluid, electrolyte, and nutritional intake.
■ Maintain a patent airway and oxygenation. If the patient is unconscious, he could aspirate saliva, so keep him in a lateral position to allow the secretions to drain naturally, or suction the secretions as needed. Insert an artificial airway, and start mechanical ventilation or supplemental oxygen, if necessary.
■ Check vital signs and neurologic status and record observations. Report significant changes to the doctor.
■ Watch for signs and symptoms of pulmonary emboli, such as chest pain, shortness of breath, dusky color, tachycardia, fever, changed sensorium, and increased partial pressure of arterial carbon dioxide (if the patient is unresponsive).
■ Maintain fluid and electrolyte balance. Administer oral or I.V. fluids as ordered; never give too much too fast because doing so can increase ICP.
■ Ensure adequate nutrition. Check for gag reflex before offering small oral feedings of semisolid foods. Place the food tray within the patient's visual field. If the patient has dysphagia or one-sided facial weakness, provide him with semisoft foods and tell him to chew on the unaffected side of his

mouth. If oral feedings aren't possible, insert a nasogastric tube for tube feedings as ordered.

■ If the patient vomits (usually during the first few days), keep him positioned on his side to prevent aspiration.

■ Provide careful mouth care.

■ Remove secretions from eyes with a cotton ball and normal saline solution. Instill eyedrops as ordered. Patch the patient's affected eye if he can't close his eyelid.

■ Position the patient and align his extremities correctly. Use high-topped sneakers as well as a convoluted foam, flotation, or pulsating mattress. To decrease the possibility of pneumonia, turn the patient at least every 2 hours. Elevate the affected hand to control dependent edema, and place it in a functional position.

■ Perform range-of-motion exercises for both the affected and unaffected sides. Teach and encourage the patient to use his unaffected side to exercise his affected side.

■ Establish and maintain communication with the patient.

■ Protect the patient from injury by padding bed side rails and keeping them up at all times.

■ If surgery is necessary, provide preoperative and postoperative care. Monitor vital signs, fluid and electrolyte balance, and intake and output. Care for the operative area, provide pain relief, and watch for complications from the surgery.

Patient teaching

■ Teach the patient and family members about the disorder. Explain the diagnostic tests, treatments, and rehabilitation the patient is to undergo.

■ If surgery is scheduled, provide preoperative teaching. Make sure the patient and family understand the surgery and its possible effects.

■ If necessary, teach the patient to wash, dress, and comb his hair. With the aid of a physical and an occupational therapist, obtain appliances, such as hand bars by the toilet and ramps, as needed.

■ To reinforce teaching, involve the patient's family in all aspects of rehabilitation. With their cooperation and support, devise a realistic discharge plan, and let them help decide when the patient can return home.

■ Teach the patient and, if needed, a family member about the schedule, dosage, actions, and adverse effects of prescribed drugs. Make sure the patient taking aspirin realizes that he can't substitute acetaminophen for aspirin.

■ Review ways to decrease risk of future CVA, such as smoking cessation, maintenance of ideal weight with prescribed diet, control of diabetes and hypertension, minimization of stress, and avoidance of prolonged bed rest.

■ Review signs of impending stroke, and advise patient to seek prompt treatment if signs occur.

Colorectal cancer

Colorectal cancer is the second most common visceral neoplasm in the United States and Europe. Malignant tumors of the colon or rectum are almost always adenocarcinomas. About half of these are sessile lesions of the rectosigmoid area; the rest are polypoid lesions. Colorectal cancer progresses slowly, remaining localized for a long time. It's potentially curable in 75% of patients if an early diagnosis allows resection before nodal involvement.

Causes

Although the exact cause of colorectal cancer is unknown, studies show a greater incidence in areas of higher economic development, suggesting that a diet that's high in animal fat, especially from beef, and low in fiber is somehow related to the cancer. Other factors that magnify the risk of developing colorectal cancer include diseases of the digestive tract, a history of ulcerative colitis, and familial polyposis.

Assessment findings

Signs and symptoms depend on the location of the tumor. If it develops on the right side of the colon, the patient probably won't have signs and symptoms in the early stages because the stool is still in liquid form in that part of the colon. He may have a history of black, tarry stools and report anemia, abdominal aching, pressure, and dull cramps. As the disease progresses, he may complain of weakness, diarrhea, constipation, anorexia, weight loss, and vomiting.

A tumor on the left side of the colon causes signs and symptoms of obstruction, even in the early disease stages, because stools are more completely formed when they reach this part of the colon. The patient may report rectal bleeding (commonly ascribed to hemorrhoids), intermittent abdominal fullness or cramping, and rectal pressure.

As the disease progresses, constipation, diarrhea, or ribbon- or pencil-shaped stools may develop. The patient may note that the passage of flatus or stool relieves his pain. He may also report obvious bleeding during defecation and dark or bright red blood in the feces and mucus in or on the stools.

A patient with a rectal tumor may report a change in bowel habits, typically beginning with an urgent need to defecate on arising (morning diarrhea) or constipation alternating with diarrhea. He also may notice blood or mucus in the stools and complain of a sense of incomplete evacuation. Late in the disease, he may complain of pain that begins as a feeling of rectal fullness and progresses to a dull, sometimes constant ache confined to the rectum or sacral region.

Inspection of the abdomen may reveal distention or visible masses. Abdominal veins may appear enlarged and visible from portal obstruction. The inguinal and supraclavicular nodes may also appear enlarged. You may note abnormal bowel sounds on abdominal auscultation. Palpation may reveal abdominal masses. Right-sided tumors usually feel bulky; tumors of the transverse portion are more easily detected.

Diagnostic tests

Several tests support a diagnosis of colorectal cancer:

■ Digital rectal examination can detect almost 15% of colorectal cancers. Specifically, it can detect suspicious rectal and perianal lesions. Fecal occult blood test can detect blood in stools, a warning sign of rectal cancer.

■ Proctoscopy or sigmoidoscopy permit visualization of the lower GI tract. Colonoscopy permits visual inspection and photography of the colon up to the ileocecal valve and provides access for polypectomies and biopsies of suspected lesions.

■ Barium enema studies, using a dual contrast of barium and air, help locate lesions that aren't detectable manually or visually. Barium examination shouldn't precede colonoscopy or excretory urography because barium sulfate interferes with these tests. A computed tomography scan allows better visualization if a barium enema yields inconclusive results or if metastasis to the pelvic lymph nodes is suspected.

■ Carcinoembryonic antigen, although not specific or sensitive enough for early diagnosis of colorectal cancer, permits patient monitoring before and after treatment to detect metastasis or recurrence.

Treatment

The most effective treatment for colorectal cancer is surgery to remove the malignant tumor and adjacent tissues, along with any lymph nodes that may contain cancer cells. After surgery, treatment continues with chemotherapy, radiation therapy, or both.

The type of surgery required depends on the location of the tumor. Tumors in the cecum and ascending colon may require right hemicolectomy (for advanced disease), or resection of the terminal segment of the ileum, cecum, ascending colon, and right half of the transverse colon with corresponding mesentery. Tumors of the proximal and middle transverse colon require right colectomy that includes the transverse colon and mesentery corresponding to midcolic vessels, or segmental resection of the transverse colon and associated midcolic vessels. Tumors of the sigmoid colon require surgery limited to that area and the mesentery. Tumors of the upper rectum usually require anterior or low-anterior resection. Tumors of the lower rectum may require an abdominoperineal resection and permanent sigmoid colostomy.

If metastasis has occurred, or if the patient has residual disease or a recurrent inoperable tumor, he needs chemotherapy. Drugs used in such treatment commonly include fluorouracil combined with levamisole or leucovorin. Researchers are evaluating the effectiveness of fluorouracil with recombinant interferon alfa-2a. Radiation therapy, used before or after surgery, induces tumor regression.

Nursing interventions

■ Before colorectal surgery, monitor the patient's diet modifications and administer laxatives, enemas, and antibiotics, as ordered.
■ After surgery, monitor the patient's vital signs, intake and output, and fluid and electrolyte balance. Also, monitor the patient for complications, including anastomotic leaks, hemorrhage, irregular bowel function, phantom rectum, ruptured pelvic peritoneum, stricture, urinary dysfunction, and wound infection.
■ Care for the patient's incision and, if appropriate, the stoma. To decrease discomfort, administer ordered analgesics as necessary, and perform comfort measures, such as repositioning.
■ Encourage the patient to look at the stoma and to participate in caring for it as soon as possible. Teach good hygiene and skin care. Allow him to shower or bathe as soon as the incision heals.
■ Consult with an enterostomal therapist, if available, for questions on setting up a postoperative regimen for the patient.
■ Watch for adverse reactions to radiation therapy (nausea, vomiting, hair loss, malaise) and provide comfort measures and reassurance.
■ During chemotherapy, watch for complications (such as infection) and expected adverse reactions. Prepare the patient for these problems.
■ Encourage the patient to identify actions and care measures that will promote his comfort and relaxation. Try to perform these measures, and encourage the patient and family members to do so as well. Whenever possible, include the patient and family members in care decisions.

Patient teaching

■ Throughout therapy, answer the patient's questions and tell him what to expect from surgery and other therapy.

■ If appropriate, explain that the stoma will be red, moist, and swollen; reassure the patient that postoperative swelling eventually subsides. Educate the patient regarding anatomy and the ostomy.

■ Preoperatively, teach the patient the coughing and deep-breathing exercises he should use postoperatively.

■ If appropriate, instruct the patient with a sigmoid colostomy to perform his own irrigation as soon as he's able after surgery.

■ Direct the patient to follow a high-fiber diet.

■ If flatus, diarrhea, or constipation occurs, tell the patient to eliminate suspected causative foods from his diet. Explain that he may reintroduce them later. Teach him which foods may alleviate constipation, and encourage him to increase his fluid and fiber intake.

■ If diarrhea is a problem, advise the patient to try eating applesauce, bananas, or rice. Caution him that he should only take a laxative or an antidiarrheal if one is prescribed.

■ When appropriate, explain that after several months, many patients with an ostomy establish control with irrigation and no longer need to wear a pouch. A stoma cap or gauze sponge placed over the stoma protects it and absorbs mucoid secretions. Explain that before achieving such control, the patient can resume physical activities — including sports — provided he isn't at risk for injuring the stoma or surrounding abdominal muscles.

■ If the patient wants to swim, he can place a pouch or stoma cap over the stoma. He should avoid heavy lifting, which can cause herniation or prolapse through weakened muscles in the abdominal wall. Suggest that he check with his doctor about starting a structured, progressive exercise program to strengthen his abdominal muscles.

■ Emphasize the need for keeping follow-up appointments.

■ If the patient is to undergo radiation therapy or chemotherapy, explain the treatment to him. Make sure he understands the common adverse reactions and the measures he can take to decrease their severity or prevent their occurrence.

■ Instruct the patient and family members about the American Cancer Society's guidelines for colorectal cancer screening: a digital rectal examination annually starting at age 40, periodic sigmoidoscopy and colonoscopy, and a stool test for occult blood annually starting at age 50.

■ For male patients, suggest sexual counseling; most are impotent for a time after colostomy.

Coronary artery disease

The foremost effect of coronary artery disease (CAD) is the loss of oxygen and nutrients to myocardial tissue because of diminished coronary blood flow. Fatty fibrous plaques or calcium-plaque deposits, or combinations of both, narrow the lumens of coronary arteries, reducing the volume of blood that can flow through them.

Causes

Atherosclerosis, the most common cause of CAD, has been linked to many risk factors. Some risk factors can't be controlled, such as age (usually occurs after age 40), sex (men are eight times more susceptible than premenopausal women), heredity, and race (white men are more susceptible than nonwhite men, and nonwhite women are more susceptible than white women).

The patient can modify other risk factors with good medical care and appropriate lifestyle changes. Controlling blood pressure, cholesterol levels, and weight as well as not smoking, performing regular exercise, reducing stress, and controlling other medical disorders (such as diabetes mellitus) can reduce the risk of atherosclerosis. Other modifiable risk factors include increased levels of serum fibrinogen and uric acid, elevated hematocrit, reduced vital capacity, high resting heart rate, thyrotoxicosis, and the use of oral contraceptives.

Uncommon causes of reduced coronary artery blood flow include dissecting aneurysms, infectious vasculitis, syphilis, and congenital defects in the coronary vascular system. Coronary artery spasms may also impede blood flow. (See *Understanding coronary artery spasm.*)

Assessment findings

The classic symptom of CAD disease is angina, the direct result of inadequate flow of oxygen to the myocardium. The patient usually describes angina as a burning, squeezing, or crushing tightness in the substernal or precordial chest that may radiate to the left arm, neck, jaw, or shoulder blade. Nausea, vomiting, fainting, sweating, and cool extremities may accompany the tightness. Angina can occur after physical exertion, emotional excitement, exposure to cold, or a large meal. It can also develop during sleep and awaken the patient.

The patient's history suggests a pattern to the type and onset of pain. If the pain is predictable and relieved by rest or nitrates, it's called stable angina. If it increases in frequency and duration and is more easily induced, it's referred to as unstable, or unpredictable, angina. Unstable angina generally indicates extensive or worsening disease and, un-

treated, may progress to myocardial infarction. An effort-induced pain that occurs with increasing frequency and with decreasing provocation is referred to as crescendo angina. If severe non-effort-produced pain occurs at rest without provocation, it's called variant, or Prinzmetal's, angina.

Inspection may reveal evidence of atherosclerotic disease, such as xanthelasma and xanthoma. Ophthalmoscopic inspection may show increased light reflexes and arteriovenous nicking, suggesting hypertension, an important risk factor for CAD. Palpation can uncover thickened or absent peripheral arteries, signs of cardiac enlargement, and abnormal contraction of the cardiac impulse, such as left ventricular akinesia or dyskinesia. Auscultation may detect bruits, a third or fourth heart sound, or a late systolic murmur (if mitral insufficiency is present).

Diagnostic tests

■ Electrocardiography (ECG) during angina shows ischemia in the form of T-wave inversion or ST-segment depression and, possibly, arrhythmias such as premature ventricular contractions. ECG results may be normal during pain-free periods. Arrhythmias may occur without infarction, secondary to ischemia. A Holter monitor may be used to obtain continuous graphic tracing of the ECG as the patient performs daily activities.
■ Treadmill or bicycle exercise test may provoke chest pain and ECG signs of myocardial ischemia in response to physical exertion. Monitoring of electrical rhythm may demonstrate T-wave inversion or ST-segment depression in the ischemic areas.
■ Coronary angiography reveals coronary artery stenosis or obstruction, collateral circulation, and the condition of the artery beyond the narrowing.

Understanding coronary artery spasm

In coronary artery spasm, a spontaneous, sustained contraction of one or more coronary arteries causes ischemia and dysfunction of the heart muscle. This disorder may also cause Prinzmetal's angina and even myocardial infarction (MI) in patients with nonoccluded coronary arteries.

Causes

The direct cause of coronary artery spasm is unknown, but possible contributing factors include:
- altered influx of calcium across the cell membrane
- intimal hemorrhage into the medial layer of the blood vessel
- hyperventilation
- elevated catecholamine levels
- fatty buildup in the lumen.

Signs and symptoms

The major symptom of coronary artery spasm is angina. Unlike classic angina, this pain commonly occurs spontaneously and may be unrelated to physical exertion or emotional stress; it may, however, follow cocaine use. It's usually more severe than classic angina, lasts longer, and may be cyclic — recurring every day at the same time. Ischemic episodes may cause arrhythmias, altered heart rate, lower blood pressure and, occasionally, fainting caused by decreased cardiac output. Spasm in the left coronary artery may result in mitral valve prolapse, producing a loud systolic murmur and, possibly, pulmonary edema, with dyspnea, crackles, and hemoptysis. MI and sudden death may occur.

Treatment

After diagnosis by coronary angiography and 12-lead electrocardiography, the patient may receive a calcium channel blocker (such as verapamil, nifedipine, or diltiazem) to decrease coronary artery spasm and vascular resistance and a nitrate (such as nitroglycerin or isosorbide dinitrate) to relieve chest pain. During cardiac catheterization, the patient with clean arteries may receive ergotamine to induce the spasm and aid in the diagnosis.

Nursing interventions

When caring for a patient with coronary artery spasm, explain all necessary procedures and teach him how to take his medications safely. For calcium channel blocker therapy, monitor the patient's blood pressure, pulse rate, and cardiac rhythm strips to detect arrhythmias.

For nifedipine and verapamil therapy, monitor digoxin levels, and check for signs of digoxin toxicity. Because nifedipine may cause peripheral and periorbital edema, watch for fluid retention.

Because coronary artery spasm is sometimes associated with atherosclerotic disease, advise the patient to stop smoking, avoid overeating, minimize alcohol intake, and maintain a balance between exercise and rest.

- Myocardial perfusion imaging with thallium-201 during treadmill exercise detects ischemic areas of the myocardium as "cold spots."
- In pharmacologic myocardial perfusion imaging, a patent coronary artery vasodilator, usually dipyridamole, is administered and the response is tested. This can be done in combination with stress testing. In normal arteries, coronary blood flow is increased to three or four times baseline. In arteries with stenosis, the decrease in blood flow is proportional to the percentage of occlusion.
- Multiple gated acquisition scanning examines cardiac-wall motion and injury to cardiac tissue.

Treatment

The goal of treatment is to reduce myocardial oxygen demand or increase the oxygen supply and reduce pain. Activity restrictions may be required to prevent onset of pain. Stress reduction techniques are also essential, especially if known stressors precipitate pain.

Drug therapy consists primarily of a nitrate, such as nitroglycerin; isosorbide dinitrate; a beta-adrenergic blocker; or a calcium channel blocker.

Obstructive lesions may necessitate atherectomy or coronary artery bypass graft (CABG) surgery, using vein grafts. Percutaneous transluminal coronary angioplasty (PTCA) may be performed during cardiac catheterization to compress fatty deposits and relieve occlusion. In patients with calcification, PTCA may reduce the obstruction by fracturing the plaque. PTCA is a viable alternative to grafting in elderly patients or in those who otherwise can't tolerate cardiac surgery. However, patients with a left main coronary artery occlusion, lesions in extremely tortuous vessels, or occlusions older than 3 months aren't candidates for PTCA.

PTCA may be done along with coronary stenting, or stents may be placed alone. Stents provide a framework to hold an artery open by securing flaps of tunica media against an artery wall. Intravascular coronary stenting is done to reduce the risk of restenosis. Prosthetic intravascular cylindrical stents made of stainless steel coil are positioned at the site of the occlusion. For the patient to be eligible for this procedure, he must be able to tolerate anticoagulant therapy, and the vessel to be stented must be at least $1/8''$ (3 mm) in diameter.

Laser angioplasty corrects occlusion by vaporizing fatty deposits with the excimer or hot-tip laser device. Percutaneous myocardial, or transmyocardial, revascularization, is an investigational procedure that uses a carbon dioxide laser to create transmural channels from the epicardial layer to the myocardium, extending into the left ventricle, in order to improve perfusion to the myocardium. The technique appears to be up to 90% effective in treating severe symptoms.

Other surgical treatments include rotational ablation and the angiojet system septa. Rotational ablation, or rotational atherectomy, removes atheromatous plaque with a high-speed, rotating bur covered with diamond crystals. An alternative to thrombolytic therapy, the angiojet system septa uses a jet stream of saline solution and a catheter to remove clots in symptomatic coronary arteries and CABGs. After the clot is removed, the patient can undergo angioplasty.

Nursing interventions

■ During anginal episodes, monitor the patient's blood pressure and heart rate. Take a 12-lead ECG during anginal episodes before administering nitroglycerin or other nitrates. Record the duration of pain, the amount of medication required to relieve it, and any accompanying symptoms.

■ During catheterization, monitor for dye reactions. Increase parenteral fluids as ordered, administer oxygen, place the patient in Trendelenburg's position, and administer I.V. atropine.

■ After catheterization, monitor the catheter site for bleeding and check for distal pulses. To counter the diuretic effect of the dye, increase the patient's fluid intake. Assess potassium levels, and replace potassium if necessary.

■ After PTCA and intravascular stenting, maintain heparinization, observe the patient for systemic bleeding and bleeding at the site, keeping the affected leg immobile. With percutaneous myocardial revascularization the patient must also remain immobile because the stents are left in until his clotting time is less than 180 seconds. Precordial blood must be taken every 8 hours for 24 hours for cardiac enzyme levels, and complete blood count and electrolyte levels must be monitored.

■ After rotational ablation, monitor the patient for chest pain, hypotension, coronary artery spasm, and bleeding from the catheter site.

■ After bypass surgery, monitor blood pressure, intake and output, breath sounds, chest tube drainage, and cardiac rhythm, watching for signs of ischemia and arrhythmias. Intra-aortic balloon pump insertion may be necessary until the patient's condition stabilizes.

Patient teaching

■ Before cardiac catheterization, explain the procedure, the reason it's necessary, and the risks. Make sure the patient realizes that he may need certain therapies, such as PTCA, surgery, atherectomy, or laser angioplasty.

■ If the patient is scheduled for surgery, explain the procedure and discuss postoperative care.

■ Help the patient determine which activities precipitate episodes of pain. Help him identify and select more effective coping mechanisms to deal with stress.

■ Encourage the patient to maintain the prescribed low-sodium diet and to start a low-calorie diet as well.

■ Explain that recurrent angina symptoms after PTCA or rotational ablation may signal reobstruction.

■ Encourage regular, moderate exercise. Refer the patient to a cardiac rehabilitation center or cardiovascular fitness program near his home or workplace.

■ Refer the patient to a program to stop smoking as appropriate.

Deep vein thrombophlebitis

Thrombophlebitis, which is an acute condition characterized by inflammation and thrombus formation, may occur in deep or superficial veins. It occurs at the valve cusps because venous stasis encourages accumulation and adherence of platelet and fibrin. It usually begins with localized inflammation alone (phlebitis), but such inflammation rapidly causes thrombi to form. Rarely, venous thrombosis develops without associated inflammation of the vein (phlebothrombosis).

Deep vein thrombophlebitis affects small veins, such as the lesser saphenous vein, or large veins, such as the venae cavae and the iliac, femoral, and popliteal veins. It's more serious than superficial vein thrombophlebitis because it affects the veins deep in the leg musculature that carry 90% of the venous outflow from the leg.

Causes

Deep vein thrombophlebitis may be idiopathic, but it usually results from endothelial damage, accelerated blood clotting, and reduced blood flow, such as in predisposing factors of prolonged bed rest, trauma, surgery, childbirth, and use of oral contraceptives such as estrogens. It's also more likely to occur with certain diseases, treatments, injuries, or other factors, such as hypercoagulable states, intimal damage, and neoplasms or venulitis (Behçet's disease, homocystinuria, or thromboangiitis obliterans).

Assessment findings

Clinical features vary with the site of inflammation and length of the affected vein. The patient may be asymptomatic, or he may complain of tenderness, aching, severe pain, fever, chills, and malaise. Inspection may reveal redness, swelling, and cyanosis of the affected leg or arm. Some patients may have a positive Homans' sign, but this is considered an unreliable sign. A positive cuff sign (elicited by inflating a blood pressure cuff until pain occurs) may be present in deep vein thrombophlebitis of either the arm or leg. When palpated, the affected leg or arm may feel warm.

Diagnostic tests

Doppler ultrasonography identifies reduced blood flow to a specific area and any obstruction to venous flow, particularly in iliofemoral deep vein thrombophlebitis. Plethysmography shows decreased circulation distal to the affected area and is more sensitive than ultrasonography in detecting deep vein thrombophlebitis. Phlebography usually confirms the diagnosis and shows filling defects and diverted blood flow. Other studies may be done to rule out comparable disorders.

Treatment

For deep vein thrombophlebitis, treatment includes bed rest, with elevation of the affected arm or leg; application of warm, moist compresses to the affected area; and an analgesic. After the acute episode subsides, the patient may begin to walk while wearing antiembolism stockings.

Treatment may include an anticoagulant (initially, heparin; later, warfarin) to prolong clotting time. After some types of surgery, especially major abdominal or pelvic operations, prophylactic doses of an anticoagulant may reduce the risk of deep vein thrombophlebitis.

For lysis of acute, extensive deep vein thrombophlebitis, treatment

should include streptokinase or urokinase — that is, if the risk of bleeding doesn't outweigh the potential benefits of thrombolytic treatment.

Rarely, deep vein thrombophlebitis may cause complete venous occlusion, which necessitates venous interruption through simple ligation to vein plication or clipping. Embolectomy may be done if clots are being shed to the pulmonary and systemic vasculature and other treatment is unsuccessful. Caval interruption with transvenous placement of an umbrella filter can trap emboli, preventing them from traveling to the pulmonary vasculature.

Nursing interventions

■ Enforce bed rest as ordered, and elevate the patient's affected arm or leg.
■ Apply warm compresses to increase circulation to the affected area and to relieve pain and inflammation.
■ Mark, measure, and record the circumference of the affected arm or leg daily, and compare this measurement with that of the other arm or leg.
■ Watch for signs and symptoms of bleeding, such as tarry stools, coffee-ground vomitus, and ecchymoses. Watch for oozing of blood at I.V. sites, and assess gums for excessive bleeding.
■ Watch for signs of pulmonary emboli (such as crackles, dyspnea, hemoptysis, sudden changes in mental status, restlessness, and hypotension).
■ To prevent thrombophlebitis in high-risk patients, perform range-of-motion exercises while the patient is on bed rest, use intermittent pneumatic calf massage during lengthy surgical or diagnostic procedures, apply antiembolism stockings postoperatively, and encourage early ambulation.

Patient teaching

■ Before discharge, emphasize the importance of follow-up blood studies to monitor anticoagulant therapy.

■ If the patient is being discharged on heparin therapy, teach him or his family how to give subcutaneous injections. If he requires further assistance, arrange for a home health care nurse.

■ Tell the patient to avoid prolonged sitting or standing to help prevent a recurrence, and teach him how to properly apply and use antiembolism stockings.

Diabetes mellitus

Diabetes mellitus is a chronic disease of absolute or relative insulin deficiency or resistance. It's characterized by disturbances in carbohydrate, protein, and fat metabolism. Insulin transports glucose into the cells for use as energy and storage as glycogen. It also stimulates protein synthesis and free fatty acid storage in adipose tissues. Insulin deficiency compromises the body tissues' access to essential nutrients for fuel and storage.

Diabetes mellitus occurs in two primary forms: type 1, characterized by absolute insufficiency, and the more prevalent type 2, characterized by insulin resistance with varying degrees of insulin secretory defects. Onset of type 1 usually occurs before age 30, although it may occur at any age; the patient usually is thin and requires exogenous insulin and dietary management to achieve control. Type 2 usually occurs in obese adults after age 40, although it's commonly seen in North American youths. It's typically treated with diet, exercise, and an antidiabetic; treatment may include insulin therapy.

Causes

The effects of diabetes mellitus result from insulin deficiency. Insulin transports glucose into the cell for use as energy and storage as glycogen. It also stimulates protein synthesis and free fatty acid storage. Insulin deficiency compromises the body tissues' access to essential nutrients for fuel and storage.

The cause of both type 1 and type 2 diabetes mellitus remains unknown. Genetic factors may play a part in the development of all types. Autoimmune disease and viral infections may be risk factors in type 1. Other risk factors include obesity, stress, pregnancy, and some medications that can antagonize the effects of insulin (thiazide diuretics, adrenal corticosteroids, and oral contraceptives).

Assessment findings

With type 1 diabetes, the patient's symptoms usually develop rapidly. With type 2 diabetes, the patient's symptoms are long-standing, and develop gradually. Insulin deficiency causes hyperglycemia, which pulls fluid from body tissues, causing osmotic diuresis, polyuria, dehydration, polydipsia, dry mucous membranes, and poor skin turgor. Patients with type 2 diabetes generally report a family history of diabetes mellitus, gestational diabetes or the delivery of a baby weighing more than 9 lb (4 kg), severe viral infection, other endocrine disease, recent stress or trauma, or use of drugs that increase blood glucose levels. In patients with ketoacidosis and hyperosmolar nonketotic state, dehydration can cause hypovolemia and shock.

Wasting of glucose in the urine usually produces weight loss and hunger in patients with uncontrolled type 1 diabetes mellitus, even if the patient eats voraciously. Patients may complain of weakness; vision changes; frequent skin and urinary tract infections; dry, itchy skin; sexual problems; and vaginal discomfort, all of which are signs and symptoms of hyperglycemia. The patient is more susceptible to infection because hyperglycemia impairs resistance.

Inspection may show retinopathy or cataract formation. Skin changes, especially on the legs and feet, may represent impaired peripheral circulation. Muscle wasting and loss of subcutaneous fat may be evident in patients with type 1 diabetes mellitus; type 2 is characterized by obesity, particularly in the abdominal area. Long-term effects produce signs of neuropathy, atherosclerosis, and peripheral and autonomic neuropathy. Peripheral neuropathy usually affects hands and feet and may produce numbness or pain. A patient with autonomic neuropathy may present with gastroparesis leading to delayed gastric emptying and a feeling of nausea or fullness after eating. Nocturnal diarrhea and impotence may also occur.

Palpation may reveal poor skin turgor and dry mucous membranes related to dehydration. Decreased peripheral pulses, cool skin temperature, and decreased reflexes may also be palpable. Auscultation may reveal orthostatic hypotension. Patients with ketoacidosis may have a characteristic "fruity" breath odor because of increased acetone production.

Patients with diabetes mellitus also have a higher risk of chronic illness, including cardiovascular disease, peripheral vascular disease, retinopathy, nephropathy, diabetic dermopathy, and peripheral and autonomic neuropathy. Infants of diabetic mothers have a two- to three-times-greater risk of congenital malformations and fetal distress. Patients with diabetes mellitus also have an increased incidence of cognitive depression.

Diagnostic tests

In nonpregnant adults, diabetes mellitus is diagnosed when they present with:
■ a fasting plasma glucose level greater than or equal to 126 mg/dl on at least two separate occasions
■ typical symptoms of uncontrolled diabetes and a random blood glucose level greater than or equal to 200 mg/dl
■ a blood glucose level greater than or equal to 200 mg/dl 2 hours after ingesting 75 g of oral dextrose.

Two of the above tests are required for diagnosis; they can be the same two tests or any combination and should be separated by more than 24 hours.

An ophthalmologic examination may show diabetic retinopathy. Other diagnostic and monitoring tests include urinalysis for acetone and blood testing for glycosylated hemoglobin, which reflects glucose control over the past 2 to 3 months.

Treatment

For patients with type 1 diabetes mellitus, treatment includes insulin replacement, diet, and exercise. Current forms of insulin-replacement include single-dose, mixed-dose, split-mixed dose, and multiple-dose regimens. The multiple-dose regimens may include use of an insulin pump. Pancreas transplantation is available and requires long-term immunosuppression.

Patients with type 2 diabetes mellitus may require an oral antidiabetic to stimulate endogenous insulin production, increase insulin sensitivity at the cellular level, suppress hepatic gluconeogenesis, and delay GI absorption of carbohydrates.

A patient with either type of diabetes requires a diet that's planned to meet nutritional needs, control blood glucose levels, and reach and maintain appropriate body weight. For the obese patient with type 2 diabetes mellitus, the calorie allotment may be high, depending on growth stage and activity level. For success, the diet must be followed consistently, with meals eaten at regular times.

Nursing interventions

■ Keep accurate records of vital signs, weight, fluid intake, urine output, and calorie intake. Monitor serum glucose and urine acetone levels.

■ Monitor the patient for acute complications of diabetic therapy, especially hypoglycemia (vagueness, slow cerebration, dizziness, weakness, pallor, tachycardia, diaphoresis, seizures, and coma); immediately give carbohydrates in the form of fruit juice, hard candy, honey or, if the patient is unconscious, glucagon or I.V. dextrose. Also, watch for signs and symptoms of hyperosmolar coma (polyuria, thirst, neurologic abnormalities, and stupor). This hyperglycemic crisis requires I.V. fluids and insulin replacement.

■ Monitor diabetic effects on the cardiovascular system — such as cerebrovascular, coronary artery, and peripheral vascular impairment — and on the peripheral and autonomic nervous systems.

■ Provide meticulous skin care, especially to the feet and legs. Treat all injuries, cuts, and blisters. Avoid constricting hose, slippers, or bed linens. Refer the patient to a podiatrist.

■ Observe the patient for signs of urinary tract and vaginal infections. Encourage adequate fluid intake.

■ Monitor the patient for signs and symptoms of diabetic neuropathy (numbness or pain in the hands and feet, footdrop, and neurogenic bladder).

■ Consult a dietitian to plan a diet with the recommended allowances of calories, protein, carbohydrates, and fats, based on the patient's particular requirements.

Patient teaching

■ Stress the importance of carefully adhering to the prescribed program for controlling his blood glucose levels. Tailor your teaching to the patient's needs, abilities, and developmental stage. Discuss diet, medications, exercise, monitoring techniques, and hygiene as well as how to prevent and recognize hypoglycemia and hyperglycemia.

■ To encourage compliance with lifestyle changes, emphasize how controlling blood glucose levels affects long-term health. Teach the patient how to care for his feet: Urge him to report any skin changes to the doctor. Advise him to wear comfortable, nonconstricting shoes and never to walk barefoot.

■ Urge regular annual ophthalmologic examinations for early detection of diabetic retinopathy.

■ Describe the signs and symptoms of diabetic neuropathy and emphasize the need for safety precautions because decreased sensation can mask injuries.

■ Teach the patient how to manage diabetes when he has a minor illness, such as a cold, flu, or upset stomach.

■ Teach the patient and family members how to monitor the patient's diet. Teach them how to read labels in the supermarket to identify fat, carbohydrate, protein, and sugar content.

■ Encourage the patient and family to contact the Juvenile Diabetes Foundation, the American Association of Diabetes Educators, and the American Diabetes Association to obtain additional information.

Emphysema

Emphysema is one of several diseases usually labeled collectively as chronic obstructive pulmonary disease. It's the most common cause of death from respiratory disease in the United States.

Causes

Emphysema may be caused by a genetic deficiency of $alpha_1$-antitrypsin or cigarette smoking. Recurrent inflammation causes abnormal, irreversible enlargement of the air spaces distal to the terminal bronchioles, leading to destruction of alveolar walls, which results in a breakdown of elasticity.

Complications may include peptic ulcer disease as well as recurrent respiratory tract infections, cor pulmonale, and respiratory failure. Alveolar blebs and bullae may rupture, leading to spontaneous pneumothorax or pneumomediastinum. (See *Understanding cor pulmonale*).

Assessment findings

The patient history may reveal that the patient is a long-time smoker. The patient may report shortness of breath and a chronic cough. The history may also reveal anorexia with resultant weight loss and a general feeling of malaise. Inspection may show a barrel-chested patient who breathes through pursed lips and uses accessory muscles. You may notice peripheral cyanosis, clubbed fingers and toes, and tachypnea.

Palpation may reveal decreased tactile fremitus and decreased chest expansion. Percussion may detect hyperresonance. On auscultation, you may hear decreased breath sounds, crackles and wheezing during inspiration, a prolonged expiratory phase with grunting respirations, and distant heart sounds.

Diagnostic tests

Chest X-rays in patients with advanced disease may show a flattened diaphragm, reduced vascular markings at the lung periphery, overaeration of the lungs, a vertical heart, enlarged anteroposterior chest diameter, and large retrosternal air space.

Pulmonary function tests typically indicate increased residual volume and total lung capacity, reduced diffusing capacity, and increased inspiratory flow. Arterial blood gas analysis usually shows reduced partial pressure of arterial oxygen and normal partial pressure of arterial carbon dioxide until late in the disease.

Electrocardiography may reveal tall, symmetrical P waves in leads II, III, and aV_F; vertical QRS complex; and signs of right ventricular hypertrophy late in the disease.

Treatment

Management usually includes a bronchodilator such as aminophylline to promote mucociliary clearance, an antibiotic to treat respiratory tract infection, and immunizations to prevent influenza and pneumococcal pneumonia. Other treatment measures include adequate hydration and (in selected patients) chest physiotherapy to mobilize secretions. Some patients may require oxygen therapy (at low settings) to correct hypoxia. They may also require transtracheal catheterization to receive oxygen at home. Counseling about avoiding smoking and air pollutants is necessary.

Nursing interventions

■ Encourage the patient to express his fears and concerns about his illness. Remain with him during periods of extreme stress and anxiety.

Understanding cor pulmonale

Cor pulmonale (right ventricular hypertrophy) is most common in patients who smoke and have chronic obstructive pulmonary disease (COPD). Because it usually occurs late in irreversible disorders of the lungs or associated structures, the prognosis is poor.

In cor pulmonale, pulmonary hypertension increases the heart's workload and the right ventricle hypertrophies to force blood through the lungs. As this compensatory mechanism fails, the right ventricle dilates. Due to hypoxia, the bone marrow produces more red blood cells and blood viscosity increases, aggravating pulmonary hypertension and causing heart failure.

Signs and symptoms

The underlying disorder may first cause a productive cough, exertional dyspnea, wheezing, fatigue, and weakness. Later, look for dyspnea at rest, tachypnea, orthopnea, edema, weakness, right upper quadrant discomfort, dependent edema and distended neck veins, altered consciousness, tachycardia, weak pulse, enlarged and tender liver, hepatojugular reflux, and a prominent parasternal or epigastric cardiac impulse. With COPD, note crackles, rhonchi, and diminished breath sounds.

The diagnosis is based on pulmonary artery catheterization that shows increased right-ventricular and pulmonary artery pressures, echocardiography or angiography showing ventricular enlargement, and evidence from chest X-rays, arterial blood gas analysis, electrocardiography, pulmonary function tests, hematocrit, and serum hepatic enzyme and bilirubin levels.

Treatment

Treatment may include bed rest, digoxin, an antibiotic, pulmonary artery vasodilators, an angiotensin-converting enzyme inhibitor, a calcium channel blocker, a prostaglandin, oxygen administration or mechanical ventilation, and dietary and diuretic measures. Phlebotomy, tracheotomy, anticoagulation therapy, and a corticosteroid may be used.

■ Include the patient and family members in care-related decisions. Refer the patient to appropriate support services as needed.

■ If ordered, perform chest physiotherapy, including postural drainage and chest percussion and vibration, several times daily.

■ Provide the patient with a high-calorie, protein-rich diet to promote health and healing. Give small, frequent meals to conserve energy and prevent fatigue.

■ Schedule respiratory treatments at least 1 hour before or after meals. Provide mouth care after bronchodilator therapy.

■ Make sure the patient receives plenty of fluids (at least 3.2 qt [3 L] a day) to loosen secretions.

■ Encourage daily activity, and provide diversionary activities as appropriate. To conserve energy and prevent fatigue, help the patient alternate periods of rest and activity.

■ Watch for complications, such as respiratory tract infections, cor pulmonale, spontaneous pneumothorax, respiratory failure, and peptic ulcer disease.

Patient teaching

■ For family members of patients with familial emphysema, recommend a blood test for AAT deficiency. If a deficiency is found, stress the importance of not smoking and, if possible, avoiding areas where smoking is permitted.

■ Advise the patient to avoid crowds and people with known infections and to obtain influenza and pneumococcus immunizations.

■ For the patient receiving home oxygen therapy, explain the rationales for oxygen therapy and proper use of equipment. If the patient requires a transtracheal catheter, teach him about catheter care, precautions, and follow-up.

■ Teach the patient and family members how to perform postural drainage and chest percussion. Instruct them to maintain each position for about 10 minutes and then perform percussion and cough. Also, teach the patient coughing and deep-breathing techniques to promote good ventilation and to mobilize secretions.

■ Review the patient's medications and explain the rationale, dosage, and adverse effects related to the prescribed drugs. Advise him to immediately report adverse reactions to the doctor. Show him how to use an inhaler correctly, if appropriate.

■ Encourage the patient to eat high-calorie, protein-rich foods. Urge him to drink plenty of fluids to prevent dehydration and to help loosen secretions.

■ If the patient smokes, encourage him to stop. Provide him with smoking-cessation resources or counseling, if necessary.

■ Urge the patient to avoid respiratory irritants, such as automobile exhaust fumes, aerosol sprays, and industrial pollutants.

■ Warn the patient that exposure to blasts of cold air may precipitate bronchospasm. Suggest that he avoid cold, windy weather or that he cover his mouth and nose with a scarf or mask if he must go outside.

■ Inform the patient about signs and symptoms that suggest ruptured alveolar blebs and bullae. Urge him to notify the

doctor if he feels sudden, sharp pleuritic pain that is exacerbated by chest movement, breathing, or coughing.

Gastroenteritis

Gastroenteritis (also called intestinal flu, traveler's diarrhea, viral enteritis, and food poisoning) is an inflammation of the stomach and small intestine that is self-limiting. The bowel reacts to any of the varied causes of gastroenteritis with hypermotility, producing severe diarrhea and secondary depletion of intracellular fluid.

Gastroenteritis occurs in people of all ages. It's a major cause of morbidity and mortality in underdeveloped nations. It can be life-threatening in elderly and debilitated patients.

Causes

Gastroenteritis has many possible causes, including bacteria, amoebae, parasites, and viruses. It's also caused by ingestion of toxins, such as poisonous plants and toadstools, drug reactions from antibiotics, and food allergens.

Assessment findings

Patient history commonly reveals the acute onset of diarrhea accompanied by abdominal pain and discomfort. The patient may complain of cramping, nausea, and vomiting. He may also report malaise, fatigue, anorexia, fever, abdominal distention, and rumbling in the lower abdomen. If diarrhea is severe, he may experience rectal burning, tenesmus, and bloody mucoid stools.

Investigate the patient's history to try to determine the cause of the signs and symptoms. Ask about ingestion of contaminated food or water. The cause may be apparent if the patient reports that others who ingested the same food or water have similar signs and symptoms. Also, ask about the health of other family members and about recent travels.

Inspection may reveal slight abdominal distention. On palpation, the patient's skin turgor may be poor, which is a sign of dehydration. Auscultation may disclose hyperactive bowel sounds and, if the patient is dehydrated, orthostatic hypotension or generalized hypotension. Temperature may be either normal or elevated.

Diagnostic tests

Laboratory studies are used to identify the causative bacteria, parasites, or amoebae. These studies include Gram stain, stool culture (by direct rectal swab), or blood culture.

Treatment

Medical management is usually supportive, consisting of bed rest, nutritional support, increased fluid intake and, occasionally, antidiarrheal therapy. If gastroenteritis is severe or affects a young child or an elderly or debilitated person, hospitalization may be required. Treatment may include I.V. fluid and electrolyte replacement and administration of an antidiarrheal, an antiemetic, and an antimicrobial.

An antidiarrheal, such as bismuth subsalicylate, may be used to treat diarrhea, or camphorated opium tincture (paregoric), diphenoxylate with atropine, and loperamide, may be ordered. An antiemetic (oral, I.V., or rectal suppository), such as prochlorperazine and trimethobenzamide, may be prescribed for severe vomiting, although they should be avoided in patients with viral or bacterial gastroenteritis. Specific antibiotic administration is restricted to patients who have bacterial gastroenteritis, as identified by diagnostic testing.

Nursing interventions

■ Plan your care to allow uninterrupted rest periods for the patient.
■ If the patient feels nauseous, advise him to avoid quick movements, which can increase the severity of nausea.
■ If the patient can tolerate oral fluid intake, replace lost fluids and electrolytes with broth, ginger ale, and lemonade, as tolerated. Warn him to avoid milk and milk products, which may provoke recurrence.
■ Monitor fluid status carefully. Take vital signs at least every 4 hours, weigh the patient daily, monitor for fluid and electrolyte balance, and record intake and output.
■ Watch for signs of dehydration, such as dry skin and mucous membranes, fever, and sunken eyes. If dehydration occurs, administer oral and I.V. fluids as ordered and replace potassium as needed.
■ To ease the anal irritation caused by diarrhea, clean the area carefully and apply a repellent cream such as petroleum jelly. Warm sitz baths and application of witch hazel compresses can also soothe irritation.
■ If food poisoning is probable, contact public health authorities so they can interview patients and food handlers and take samples of the suspected contaminated food.

Patient teaching
■ Teach the patient about gastroenteritis, describing its symptoms and varied causes. Explain diagnosis and treatments.
■ Instruct the patient to wait until his diarrhea subsides and then to start drinking unsweetened fruit juice, tea, bouillon, or other clear broths. He may also start eating bland, soft foods, such as cooked cereal, rice, and applesauce. Tell him to avoid foods that are spicy, greasy, or high in roughage, such as

whole-grain products and raw fruits or vegetables. Explain that eating these foods can cause diarrhea.

■ Carefully review the proper use of all prescribed medications with the patient, making sure that he fully understands the desired effects of the drugs and their possible adverse effects.

■ Teach preventive measures. If the patient expects to travel, advise him to pay close attention to what he eats and drinks, especially in developing nations. Review proper hygiene measures to prevent recurrence. Instruct the patient to thoroughly cook foods, especially pork; to refrigerate perishable foods, such as milk, mayonnaise, potato salad, and cream-filled pastry; to always wash his hands with warm water and soap before handling food, especially after using the bathroom; to clean utensils thoroughly; and to eliminate flies and roaches in the home.

Gastroesophageal reflux disease

Commonly known as heartburn, gastroesophageal reflux disease (GERD) is the backflow of gastric or duodenal contents, or both, into the esophagus and past the lower esophageal sphincter (LES), without associated belching or vomiting. Reflux may cause symptoms or pathologic changes. Persistent reflux can cause reflux esophagitis, an inflammation of the esophageal mucosa. The prognosis varies with the underlying cause.

Causes

Normally, gastric contents don't back up into the esophagus because the LES creates enough pressure around the lower end of the esophagus to close it. Reflux occurs when LES pressure is deficient or pressure in the stomach exceeds LES

pressure. When this happens, the LES relaxes, allowing gastric contents to regurgitate into the esophagus. Any of the following predisposing factors can lead to reflux: pyloric surgery, nasogastric intubation for more than 4 days, any agent that lowers LES pressure (food, alcohol, cigarettes, anticholinergics), other drugs (morphine, diazepam, calcium channel blockers, meperidine), hiatal hernia with incompetent sphincter, and any condition or position that increases intra-abdominal pressure.

Reflux esophagitis, the primary complication of GERD, can lead to other signs and symptoms, including esophageal stricture, esophageal ulcer, and replacement of the normal squamous epithelium with columnar epithelium (Barrett's epithelium). A patient with severe reflux esophagitis may also develop anemia from chronic low-grade bleeding of inflamed mucosa. Pulmonary complications may develop if the patient experiences reflux of gastric contents into the throat and subsequent aspiration. Reflux aspiration can lead to chronic pulmonary disease.

Assessment findings

The patient complains of heartburn that occurs 1 to 2 hours after eating. It typically worsens when exercising vigorously, bending, or lying down. Taking an antacid or sitting upright may provide relief. If asked, he may recall regurgitating, without associated nausea or belching. This symptom is commonly described as a feeling of warm fluid traveling up the throat, followed by a sour or bitter taste in the mouth if the fluid reaches the pharynx.

Heartburn is the most common feature of reflux, but the patient may report any of the following signs and symptoms:

■ odynophagia, possibly followed by a dull substernal ache. This symptom may indicate severe, long-term reflux dysphagia from esophageal spasm, stricture, or esophagitis.

■ bright red or dark brown blood in vomitus.

■ chronic pain that may mimic angina pectoris, radiating to the neck, jaw, and arm. (This pain may be associated with esophageal spasm and may result from reflux esophagitis.)

■ nocturnal hypersalivation, a rare symptom that the patient says awakens him with coughing, choking, and a mouth full of saliva.

In children, assessment findings may identify failure to thrive and forceful vomiting caused by esophageal irritation. Keep in mind that vomiting can lead to aspiration pneumonia.

Diagnostic tests

A careful history and physical examination are essential to the diagnosis. Several tests help to confirm it.

■ The esophageal acidity test, a standard test for acid reflux, is the most sensitive and accurate measure of gastroesophageal reflux. Gastroesophageal scintillation testing may also detect reflux.

■ Esophageal manometry is used to evaluate the resting pressure of the LES and determine sphincter competence.

■ An acid perfusion test confirms esophagitis.

■ Esophagoscopy and biopsy allow visualization and tissue sampling of the esophagus. These tests are used to evaluate the extent of the disease and confirm pathologic changes in the mucosa.

■ Barium swallow with fluoroscopy reveals normal findings except in patients with advanced disease. In children, barium esophagography under fluoroscopic control may show reflux.

Treatment

Effective management relieves symptoms by reducing reflux through gravity, strengthening the LES with drug therapy, neutralizing gastric contents, and reducing intra-abdominal pressure. Treatment should also include reviewing how the patient's lifestyle or dietary habits may affect his LES pressure and reflux symptoms.

In mild cases, diet therapy may reduce symptoms sufficiently so that no other treatment is required. Positional therapy, which relieves symptoms by reducing intra-abdominal pressure, is especially useful in infants and children with uncomplicated cases.

For intermittent reflux, an antacid given 1 hour before and 3 hours after meals and at bedtime may be effective. Drug therapy may also include a cholinergic drug, such as bethanechol, to increase LES pressure, and a histamine-2 receptor antagonist, such as famotidine and ranitidine, to reduce gastric acidity. A 4-week course of lansoprazole is useful in patients with acute GERD. Metoclopramide and sucralfate have also been used with beneficial results.

Surgery is usually reserved for patients with refractory symptoms or serious complications. Indications for surgery include pulmonary aspiration, hemorrhage, esophageal obstruction or perforation, intractable pain, incompetent LES, or associated hiatal hernia. Surgical procedures reduce reflux by creating an artificial closure at the gastroesophageal junction. Several surgical approaches involve wrapping the gastric fundus around the esophagus. Other surgical procedures include a vagotomy or pyloroplasty (which may be combined with an antireflux regimen) to modify gastric contents.

Nursing interventions

■ In consultation with a dietitian, develop a diet that takes the patient's food preferences into account but, at the same time, helps to minimize his reflux symptoms. If the patient is obese, place him on a weight reduction diet as ordered.

■ To reduce intra-abdominal pressure, have the patient sleep in a reverse Trendelenburg position (with the head of the bed elevated 6″ to 12″ [15 to 30.5 cm]). He should avoid lying down immediately after meals and eating late-night snacks.

■ After surgery, provide care as you would for any patient who has undergone a laparotomy. Pay particular attention to the patient's respiratory status because the surgical procedure is performed close to the diaphragm. Administer an analgesic, oxygen, and I.V. fluids, as prescribed. Monitor the patient's intake and output and check his vital signs. If surgery was performed using a thoracic approach, watch and record chest tube drainage. If needed, provide chest physiotherapy.

Patient teaching

■ Teach the patient about the causes of GERD, and review his antireflux regimen of medication, diet, and positional therapy.

■ Discuss recommended dietary changes. Advise the patient to sit upright after meals and snacks, and to eat small, frequent meals. Explain that he should eat meals at least 2 to 3 hours before lying down. Tell him to avoid highly seasoned food, acidic juices, alcoholic drinks, bedtime snacks, and foods high in fat because these reduce LES pressure.

■ Instruct the patient to avoid situations or activities that increase intra-abdominal pressure, such as bending, coughing, vigorous exercise, obesity, constipation, and wearing tight clothing. Caution him to avoid anything that reduces sphincter control, including cigarettes, alcohol, fatty foods, and certain drugs.

Heart failure

When the myocardium can't pump effectively enough to meet the body's metabolic needs, heart failure occurs. Pump failure usually occurs in a damaged left ventricle (called left-sided heart failure), but it may happen in the right ventricle (called right-sided heart failure) primarily, or secondary to left-sided heart failure. Usually, left-sided and right-sided heart failure develop simultaneously.

Heart failure is classified as high-output or low-output, acute or chronic, left-sided or right-sided, and forward or backward. (See *Classifying heart failure.*)

Causes

Heart failure commonly results from a primary abnormality of the heart muscle (such as an infarction) that impairs ventricular function to the point that the heart can no longer pump sufficient blood. Heart failure can also result from causes not related to myocardial function. These include:

■ mechanical disturbances in ventricular filling during diastole, which result from blood volume that's insufficient for the ventricle to pump. This occurs in mitral stenosis secondary to rheumatic heart disease or constrictive pericarditis and atrial fibrillation.

■ systolic hemodynamic disturbances — such as excessive cardiac workload caused by volume overload or pressure overload — that limit the heart's pumping ability. These disturbances can result from mitral or aortic insufficiency, which causes volume overload, and aortic stenosis or sys-

Classifying heart failure

Heart failure is usually classified by the site of heart failure (left ventricle, right ventricle, or both). Some practitioners may also classify heart failure by level of cardiac output, stage, and direction (high-output or low-output, acute or chronic, or systolic or diastolic). These classifications represent a guide to different clinical aspects of heart failure that may be helpful in practice and treatment.

Left-sided failure

Failure of the left ventricle to pump blood to the vital organs and periphery is usually caused by myocardial infarction (MI). Decreased left ventricular output causes fluid to accumulate in the lungs, which precipitates dyspnea, orthopnea, and paroxysmal nocturnal dyspnea.

Right-sided failure

Resulting from failure of the right ventricle to pump sufficient blood to the lungs, this type usually is caused by a disorder that increases pulmonary vascular resistance, such as pulmonary embolism, pulmonic stenosis, or pulmonary hypertension. Right-sided heart failure produces congestive hepatomegaly, ascites, and edema.

High-output failure

Failure with an elevated cardiac output occurs when tissue demands for oxygenated blood exceed the heart's ability to supply it. High-output failure occurs with arteriovenous fistula, hyperthyroidism, anemia, sickle cell anemia, beriberi, Paget's disease of the bone, and thyrotoxicosis.

Low-output failure

Failure with decreased cardiac output is caused by increased pumping ability of the myocardium. Low output failure occurs with coronary artery disease, hyper-

tension, primary myocardial disease, and valvular disease.

Acute failure

Acute heart failure occurs suddenly, such as with an MI or a ruptured cardiac valve. The sudden reduction in cardiac output results in systemic hypotension without peripheral edema. Acute heart failure may occur with a chronic condition, such as when a patient with chronic heart failure experiences acute heart failure with an MI. It may also occur with any condition that stresses a heart that's already diseased.

Chronic failure

Chronic failure occurs gradually and is sustained for long periods. The arterial blood pressure doesn't drop, but peripheral edema is present. Chronic failure may occur in cardiomyopathy or multivalvular disease, or in a healed, extensive MI.

Systolic failure

In systolic failure, the heart fails to expel enough blood into the arterial system. Sodium and water retention results from decreased renal perfusion and excessive proximal tubular sodium reabsorption or excessive distal tubular reabsorption, through activation of the renin-angiotensin-aldosterone system.

Diastolic failure

When diastolic failure occurs, one ventricle is unable to relax during filling and end-diastolic ventricular pressures rise. The pressures and volume in the atrium and venous system behind the failing ventricle also increase, and sodium and water retention occurs because of the elevated systemic venous and capillary pressures and the resulting transudation of fluid into the interstitial space.

temic hypertension, which results in increased resistance to ventricular emptying.

Also, certain conditions can predispose the patient to heart failure, particularly if he has some underlying heart disease. Such conditions include arrhythmias, pregnancy, thyrotoxicosis, pulmonary embolism, infections, anemia, increased physical activity, emotional stress, increased salt and water intake, and failure to comply with the prescribed treatment regimen for the underlying heart disease.

Assessment findings

The patient's history reveals a disorder or condition that can precipitate heart failure. The patient commonly complains of shortness of breath, which occurs in early stages during activity and, in late stages, also at rest. He may report that dyspnea worsens at night when he lies down. He may use two or three pillows to elevate his head to sleep or have to sleep sitting up in a chair. He may relate that his shortness of breath wakes him up shortly after he falls asleep, causing him to sit upright to catch his breath. He may remain dyspneic and cough and wheeze, even when he sits up. This is referred to as paroxysmal nocturnal dyspnea.

The patient may report that his shoes or rings have become too tight, a result of peripheral edema. He may also report increasing fatigue, weakness, insomnia, anorexia, nausea, and a sense of abdominal fullness (particularly if he has right-sided heart failure).

Inspection may reveal a dyspneic, anxious patient in respiratory distress. In mild cases, dyspnea may occur while the patient is lying down or active; in severe cases, it isn't related to position. The patient may have a cough that produces pink, frothy sputum. You may note cyanosis of the lips and nail beds, pale skin, diaphoresis, dependent peripheral and sacral edema, and jugular vein distention. Ascites may also be present, especially with right-sided heart failure. If the patient has chronic heart failure, he may appear cachectic.

When palpating the pulse, you may note that the skin feels cool and clammy. The pulse rate is rapid, and an alternating pulse may be present. Hepatomegaly and splenomegaly may also be present. Percussion reveals dullness over lung bases that are fluid filled.

Auscultation of the blood pressure may detect decreased pulse pressure, reflecting reduced stroke volume. Heart auscultation may disclose third and fourth heart sounds. Lung auscultation reveals moist, bibasilar crackles. If pulmonary edema is present, you hear crackles throughout the lung, accompanied by rhonchi and expiratory wheezing.

Diagnostic tests

Electrocardiography reflects heart strain or enlargement, or ischemia. It may also reveal atrial enlargement, tachycardia, and extrasystoles. Chest X-rays show increased pulmonary vascular markings, interstitial edema, or pleural effusion and cardiomegaly.

Pulmonary artery pressure monitoring typically demonstrates elevated pulmonary artery and pulmonary artery wedge pressures, left ventricular end-diastolic pressure in left-sided heart failure, and elevated right atrial or central venous pressure in right-sided heart failure.

Treatment

The aim of therapy is to improve pump function by reversing the compensatory

Managing pulmonary edema

Heart failure can cause fluid to accumulate in the extravascular spaces of the lungs. To intervene appropriately, you must accurately assess the severity of the patient's edema.

Initial stage

Signs and symptoms
- Persistent cough, which resembles throat-clearing when it begins
- Slight dyspnea and exercise intolerance
- Restlessness and anxiety
- Crackles at lung bases
- Diastolic gallop and a third heart sound (S_3)

Special considerations
- Check color and amount of expectoration.
- Start and maintain a keep-vein-open I.V. line.
- Position the patient for comfort, and elevate the head of the bed.
- Auscultate the chest for crackles and S_3.
- Administer medications as ordered; morphine is the drug of choice.
- Administer a diuretic and replace potassium, if necessary.
- Monitor arterial blood gas (ABG) and electrolyte levels.
- Calculate intake and output accurately.
- Monitor apical and radial pulses.
- Help the patient conserve strength.
- Provide emotional support.

Acute stage

Signs and symptoms
- Acute dyspnea
- Rapid, noisy respirations (audible wheeze, crackles) in all lung fields

- More intense cough with frothy blood-tinged sputum
- Cyanosis and cold, clammy skin
- Tachycardia and arrhythmias
- Hypotension
- Restlessness

Special considerations
- Administer supplemental oxygen as needed (preferably by high concentration mask or intermittent positive-pressure breathing apparatus).
- Aspirate the nasopharynx as needed.
- Give an inotropic drug such as digoxin as ordered.
- Give a nitrate, morphine, and a potent diuretic such as furosemide as ordered.
- Insert an indwelling urinary catheter.
- Monitor and record intake and output.
- Monitor ABG levels.
- Attach cardiac monitor leads; monitor heart rate and for arrhythmias. Keep resuscitation equipment available. Prepare for intubation and mechanical ventilation in case it's needed.
- Provide emotional support for the patient and family.

Advanced stage

Signs and symptoms
- Decreased level of consciousness
- Ventricular arrhythmias, bradycardia, and shock
- Diminished breath sounds

Special considerations
- Assist with intubation and mechanical ventilation.
- Resuscitate the patient, if necessary.

---

mechanisms producing the clinical effects. Heart failure can usually be controlled quickly with the proper treatment, including diuresis to reduce total blood volume and circulatory conges-

tion, prolonged bed rest, oxygen, and an inotropic drug such as digoxin to strengthen myocardial contractility. A sympathomimetic, such as dopamine or dobutamine, may be used for acute sit-

Dealing with heart failure

To help a patient with heart failure deal with the disorder at home, use the following interventions:
- Advise the patient to follow a low-sodium diet, if ordered. Identify low-sodium food substitutes and foods to avoid, and show how to read labels to assess sodium content. To evaluate compliance, analyze the patient's 24-hour dietary intake.
- Show the patient how to take a pulse by placing a finger on the radial artery and counting for 1 minute. Then have him demonstrate the procedure.
- Tell the patient to take digoxin at the same time each day, to check the pulse rate and rhythm before taking it, and to call the doctor if the rate is under 60 beats/minute or the rhythm is irregular.
- Teach the patient to report important signs and symptoms, such as dizziness, blurred vision, shortness of breath, persistent dry cough, palpitations, increased fatigue, paroxysmal nocturnal dyspnea, swollen ankles, and decreased urine output.
- Advise the patient to weigh himself at least three times per week and to report an increase of 3 to 5 lb (1.5 to 2.5 kg) in 1 week.
- Instruct the patient taking a potassium-depleting diuretic to eat high-potassium foods, such as bananas and orange juice.
- Instruct patient to avoid fatigue. Schedule activities to allow for rest periods.

uations. Inamrinone may be used to increase contractility and arterial vasodilation; a vasodilator, to increase cardiac output; or an angiotensin-converting enzyme inhibitor to decrease afterload. Also, antiembolism stockings may be used to prevent venostasis and thromboembolism formation.

Treatment of acute pulmonary edema requires morphine; nitroglycerin or nitroprusside to diminish blood return to the heart; dobutamine, dopamine, or inamrinone to increase myocardial contractility and cardiac output; a diuretic to reduce fluid volume; supplemental oxygen; and high Fowler's position. (See *Managing pulmonary edema,* page 231.)

After recovery, most patients must continue taking a cardiac glycoside, a diuretic, and a potassium supplement and must remain under medical supervision. If the patient with valve dysfunction has recurrent acute heart failure, surgical replacement may be necessary.

Nursing interventions

- Place the patient in Fowler's position and give him supplemental oxygen to help him breathe more easily. Organize all activity to provide maximum rest periods.
- Weigh the patient daily, and check for peripheral edema. Also, monitor I.V. intake and urine output.
- Assess vital signs and mental status. Auscultate for abnormal heart and breath sounds. Report any changes immediately.
- Frequently monitor blood urea nitrogen and serum creatinine, potassium, sodium, chloride, and magnesium levels.
- Provide continuous cardiac monitoring during acute and advanced stages to identify and treat arrhythmias promptly.

■ To prevent deep vein thrombosis due to vascular congestion, assist the patient with range-of-motion exercises. Enforce bed rest, and apply antiembolism stockings. Check for calf pain and tenderness.

Patient teaching
■ Advise the patient to avoid foods high in sodium, such as canned or commercially prepared foods and dairy products, to curb fluid overload.
■ Prepare the patient to manage the disorder at home. (See *Dealing with heart failure.*)

Hypertension

Hypertension is defined as an intermittent or sustained elevation of diastolic or systolic blood pressure. Serial blood pressure measurements greater than 140/90 mm Hg in patients younger than age 50 or greater than 150/95 mm Hg in those older than age 50 confirm hypertension.

Aside from characteristic high blood pressure, hypertension is classified according to its cause, severity, and type. The two major types are essential (also called primary or idiopathic) hypertension, the most common (90% to 95% of cases), and secondary hypertension, which results from renal disease or another identifiable cause. Malignant hypertension is a severe, fulminant form of hypertension that commonly arises from both types.

Essential hypertension usually begins insidiously as a benign disease, slowly progressing to an accelerated or malignant state. If untreated, even mild hypertension can cause significant complications and a high mortality. In many cases, treatment with stepped care offers patients an improved prognosis. (See *Stepped-care approach to antihypertensive therapy,* page 234.)

Causes

The cause of essential hypertension is unknown. Family history, race, stress, obesity, a diet high in sodium or saturated fat, use of tobacco or oral contraceptives, excess alcohol intake, sedentary lifestyle, and aging have all been studied to determine their role in the development of hypertension.

Secondary hypertension may result from renovascular disease; renal parenchymal disease; pheochromocytoma; primary hyperaldosteronism; Cushing's syndrome; diabetes mellitus; dysfunction of the thyroid, pituitary, or parathyroid gland; coarctation of the aorta; pregnancy; and neurologic disorders. Use of oral contraceptives may be the most common cause of secondary hypertension, probably because these drugs activate the renin-angiotensin-aldosterone system. Other medications contributing to secondary hypertension include glucocorticoids, mineralocorticoids, sympathomimetics, cyclosporine, cocaine, and epoetin alfa.

Hypertension is a major cause of cerebrovascular accident, cardiac disease, and renal failure. Complications occur late in the disease and can attack any organ system. Cardiac complications include coronary artery disease, angina, myocardial infarction, heart failure, arrhythmias, and sudden death. Neurologic complications include cerebral infarctions and hypertensive encephalopathy. Hypertensive retinopathy can cause blindness. Renovascular hypertension can lead to renal failure.

Assessment findings

In many cases, the hypertensive patient has no symptoms, and the disorder is revealed incidentally during evaluation for another disorder or during a routine

Stepped-care approach to antihypertensive therapy

The diagram below illustrates the four-step approach to antihypertensive therapy that the National Institutes of Health recommends. The progression of therapy is based on the patient's response, which is defined in two ways: the patient has achieved the target blood pressure that the doctor established, or the patient is making considerable progress toward this goal.

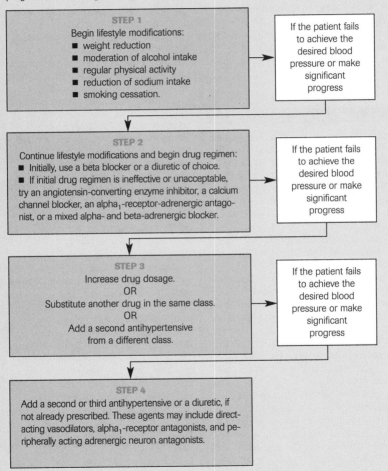

STEP 1
Begin lifestyle modifications:
- weight reduction
- moderation of alcohol intake
- regular physical activity
- reduction of sodium intake
- smoking cessation.

If the patient fails to achieve the desired blood pressure or make significant progress

STEP 2
Continue lifestyle modifications and begin drug regimen:
- Initially, use a beta blocker or a diuretic of choice.
- If initial drug regimen is ineffective or unacceptable, try an angiotensin-converting enzyme inhibitor, a calcium channel blocker, an alpha$_1$-receptor-adrenergic antagonist, or a mixed alpha- and beta-adrenergic blocker.

If the patient fails to achieve the desired blood pressure or make significant progress

STEP 3
Increase drug dosage.
OR
Substitute another drug in the same class.
OR
Add a second antihypertensive from a different class.

If the patient fails to achieve the desired blood pressure or make significant progress

STEP 4
Add a second or third antihypertensive or a diuretic, if not already prescribed. These agents may include direct-acting vasodilators, alpha$_1$-receptor antagonists, and peripherally acting adrenergic neuron antagonists.

Source: U.S. Department of Health and Human Services. National Institutes of Health. *Sixth Report of the Joint National Committee on Prevention, Detection, Evaluation, and Treatment of High Blood Pressure.* Washington, D.C. Government Printing Office, 1997.

blood pressure screening program. When symptoms do occur, they reflect the effect of hypertension on the organ systems.

The patient may report awakening with a headache in the occipital region, which subsides spontaneously after a few hours. This symptom usually is associated with severe hypertension. He may also complain of dizziness, palpitations, fatigue, and impotence.

With vascular involvement, the patient may complain of nosebleeds, bloody urine, weakness, and blurred vision. Complaints of chest pain and dyspnea may indicate cardiac involvement.

Inspection may reveal peripheral edema in late stages when heart failure is present. Ophthalmoscopic evaluation may reveal hemorrhages, exudates, and papilledema in late stages if hypertensive retinopathy is present. Palpation of the carotid artery may reveal stenosis or occlusion. Palpation of the abdomen may reveal a pulsating mass, suggesting an abdominal aneurysm. Enlarged kidneys may point to polycystic disease, a cause of secondary hypertension.

Systolic or diastolic pressure, or both may be elevated. An increase in diastolic blood pressure from a sitting to a standing position suggests essential hypertension, whereas a fall in blood pressure from the sitting to the standing position indicates secondary hypertension.

Auscultation may reveal an abdominal bruit to the right or left of the umbilicus midline or in the flanks if renal artery stenosis is present. Bruits may also be heard over the abdominal aorta and femoral arteries or the carotids.

Diagnostic tests

The following tests may be used to find predisposing factors and help identify the cause of hypertension.

■ Urinalysis may show protein, red blood cells, or white blood cells, suggesting renal disease; or glucose, suggesting diabetes mellitus.
■ Excretory urography may reveal renal atrophy, indicating chronic renal disease; one kidney that's more than $5/8''$ (1.5 cm) shorter than the other suggests unilateral renal disease.
■ Serum potassium levels less than 3.5 mEq/L may indicate adrenal dysfunction (primary hyperaldosteronism).
■ Blood urea nitrogen levels that are normal or elevated to more than 20 mg/dl and serum creatinine levels that are normal or elevated to more than 1.5 mg/dl suggest renal disease.

The following tests can help to detect cardiovascular damage and other complications.
■ Electrocardiography may show left ventricular hypertrophy or ischemia, and chest X-rays may show cardiomegaly.
■ Ophthalmoscopy reveals arteriovenous nicking and, in patients with hypertensive encephalopathy, edema.
■ An oral captopril challenge may be done to test for renovascular hypertension. This functional diagnostic test depends on the abrupt inhibition of circulatory angiotensin II by angiotensin-converting enzyme (ACE) inhibitors, removing the major support for perfusion through a stenotic kidney. The acutely ischemic kidney immediately releases more renin and undergoes a marked decrease in glomerular filtration rate and renal blood flow.
■ Renal arteriography may show renal artery stenosis.

Treatment

Although essential hypertension has no cure, drugs and modifications in diet and lifestyle can control it. Generally, nondrug treatment such as lifestyle modification is tried first, especially in early, mild cases. If this is ineffective, treatment progresses in a stepwise manner to include various types of antihypertensives. This stepped-care approach may need modification. For instance, most blacks respond poorly to beta-adrenergic blockers; however, for unclear reasons, they respond well to a combination of a diuretic and an ACE inhibitor. Many elderly patients can be treated with a diuretic alone.

Treatment for a patient with secondary hypertension includes correcting the underlying cause and controlling hypertensive effects.

Severely elevated blood pressure (hypertensive crisis) may be refractory to medications and may be fatal. Hypertensive emergencies require parenteral administration of a vasodilator or an adrenergic blocker or oral administration of a selected drug (such as nifedipine, captopril, clonidine, or labetalol), to rapidly reduce blood pressure.

Nursing interventions

■ If a patient is hospitalized with hypertension, find out if he was taking a prescribed antihypertensive.
■ When routine blood pressure screening reveals elevated pressure, make sure the sphygmomanometer cuff size is appropriate for the patient's upper arm circumference. Take the pressure in both arms in lying, sitting, and standing positions. Ask the patient if he smoked, drank a beverage containing caffeine, or was emotionally upset before the test. Advise him to return for blood pressure testing at frequent and regular intervals.
■ Carefully monitor the effects of treatments administered.

Patient teaching
■ Teach the patient to use a self-monitoring blood pressure cuff and to record the reading at least twice weekly in a journal so the doctor can review it at every office appointment. Tell the patient to take his blood pressure at the same hour each time with relatively the same type of activity preceding the measurement.
■ Tell the patient and family to keep a record of drugs used in the past, noting especially which ones are or aren't effective. Suggest recording this information on a card so the patient can show it to his doctor.
■ To encourage compliance with antihypertensive therapy, suggest establishing a daily routine for taking medication. Warn him that uncontrolled hypertension can cause a stroke or a heart attack. Tell him to report any adverse reactions to drugs. Advise him to avoid high-sodium antacids and over-the-counter cold and sinus medications containing harmful vasoconstrictors.
■ Help the patient examine and modify his lifestyle. Suggest stress-reduction groups, dietary changes, and an exercise program, particularly aerobic walking, to improve cardiac status and reduce obesity and serum cholesterol levels.
■ Encourage a change in dietary habits. Help the obese patient plan a diet to reduce weight. Tell him to avoid high-sodium foods (such as pickles, potato chips, canned soups, and cold cuts), table salt, and foods high in cholesterol and saturated fat.

Influenza

Also called the grippe or the flu, influenza is an acute, highly contagious respiratory tract infection. Although it affects patients of all ages, school-age children are affected the most. Those hit the hardest are young children, elderly patients, and those with chronic diseases. In these patients, influenza may even lead to death.

Causes

Influenza results from three types of virus. Type A, the most prevalent, strikes every year, with new serotypes causing epidemics every 3 years. Type B also strikes annually but only causes epidemics every 4 to 6 years. Type C is endemic and causes only sporadic cases. The infection can be transmitted if a respiratory droplet from an infected person is inhaled or if indirect contact is made; for example, if the patient drinks from a contaminated glass. The virus then invades the epithelium of the respiratory tract, causing inflammation and desquamation.

One remarkable feature of the influenza virus is its capacity for antigenic variation — that is, its ability to mutate into different strains so that no immunologic resistance is present in those at risk. Antigenic variation is characterized as antigenic drift (minor changes that occur yearly or every few years) and antigenic shift (major changes that lead to pandemics).

Assessment findings

The patient's history usually reveals recent exposure to a person with influenza. Most patients say that they didn't receive the influenza vaccine during the past season.

After an incubation period of 24 to 48 hours, flu signs and symptoms appear. The patient may report sudden onset of chills, fever ($101°$ to $104°$ F [$38.3°$ to $40°$ C]), headache, malaise, myalgia (particularly in the back and limbs), photophobia, a nonproductive cough, laryngitis, hoarseness, rhinitis, or rhinorrhea. Fever usually is higher in children, who may also show signs and symptoms of croup. These signs usually subside in 3 to 5 days, but cough and weakness may persist. Some patients (especially elderly people) may feel tired and listless for several weeks.

Initial inspection may reveal red, watery eyes; erythema of the nose and throat without exudate; and clear nasal discharge. As the disease progresses, respiratory findings become more apparent. The patient frequently coughs and looks tired. If pulmonary complications occur, tachypnea, cyanosis, and shortness of breath may be noted. With bacterial pneumonia, you'll see purulent or bloody sputum.

Palpation may reveal cervical adenopathy and tenderness, especially in children. Auscultation may disclose transient gurgles or crackles. With pneumonia, breath sounds may be diminished in areas of consolidation.

Diagnostic tests

At the beginning of an influenza epidemic, many patients are misdiagnosed with other respiratory tract disorders. Nose and throat cultures and increased serum antibody titers help confirm the diagnosis. When an epidemic is confirmed, diagnosis requires only observation of clinical signs and symptoms. Uncomplicated cases show decreased white blood cells with an increase in lymphocytes.

Treatment

The patient with uncomplicated influenza needs bed rest, adequate fluid intake, acetaminophen or aspirin to relieve fever and muscle pain (children should only receive acetaminophen), and guaifenesin or another expectorant to relieve nonproductive coughing. Prophylactic antibiotics aren't recommended because they have no effect on the influenza virus.

The antiviral amantadine effectively reduces the duration of the influenza A infection. Patients with influenza complicated by pneumonia need supportive care (fluid and electrolyte replacement, oxygen, and assisted ventilation) and treatment of bacterial superinfection with the appropriate antibiotic. No specific therapy exists for cardiac, central nervous system, or other complications.

Nursing interventions

■ Administer an analgesic, an antipyretic, and a decongestant, as ordered, and monitor the patient for effect.
■ Watch for signs and symptoms of developing pneumonia, such as crackles, increased fever, chest pain, dyspnea, and coughing accompanied by purulent or bloody sputum.
■ Provide cool, humidified air, but change the water daily to prevent *Pseudomonas* superinfection.
■ Encourage the patient to rest in bed and drink plenty of fluids. Administer I.V. fluids as ordered.
■ Administer oxygen therapy, if warranted.

Patient teaching
■ Influenza usually doesn't require hospitalization. Teach the home patient about supportive care measures and signs and symptoms of serious complications.
■ Advise the patient to use mouthwash or warm saline gargles to ease sore throat.
■ Teach the patient the importance of taking in plenty of fluids to prevent dehydration.
■ Suggest a warm bath or a heating pad to relieve myalgia.
■ Advise the patient to use a vaporizer to provide cool, moist air but to clean the reservoir and change the water every 8 hours.
■ Teach the patient the proper way to dispose of his tissues and wash his hands to prevent the virus from spreading.
■ Discuss influenza immunization. Suggest that high-risk patients and health care workers get an annual inoculation at the start of flu season (late autumn). Tell a patient receiving the vaccine about possible adverse effects (discomfort at the vaccination site, fever, malaise and, rarely, Guillain-Barré syndrome). Remember that the vaccine isn't recommended for pregnant women or anyone who is allergic to eggs, feathers, or chickens. (Amantadine is an effective alternative for these people.)

Lyme disease

Lyme disease affects multiple body systems. Persons of all ages and both sexes are affected, with onset during the summer months. It occurs in areas where the geographic ranges of certain ixodid ticks are located. It typically begins with the classic skin lesion called erythema chronicum migrans. Weeks or months later, cardiac, neurologic, or joint abnormalities develop, possibly followed by arthritis.

Causes

Lyme disease is caused by the spirochete *Borrelia burgdorferi.* Carried by the minute tick *Ixodes dammini* (or another tick in the Ixodidae family), the disease occurs when a tick injects spirochete-laden saliva into the bloodstream or deposits fecal matter on the skin. After incubating for 3 to 32 days, the spirochetes migrate outward on the skin, causing a rash and disseminating to other skin sites or organs by the bloodstream or lymph system. The spirochetes' life cycle isn't completely understood: They may survive for years in the joints, or they may die after triggering an inflammatory response in the host.

Myocarditis, pericarditis, arrhythmias, heart block, meningitis, encephalitis, cranial or peripheral neuropathies, and arthritis are among the known complications of Lyme disease.

Assessment findings

The patient's history may reveal recent exposure to ticks, especially if the patient lives, works, or plays in wooded areas where Lyme disease is endemic. He may report the onset of symptoms in warmer months. Typically reported symptoms include fatigue, malaise, and migratory myalgias, and arthralgias.

Nearly 10% of patients report cardiac symptoms, such as palpitations and mild dyspnea, especially in the early stage. Severe headache and stiff neck, which suggest meningeal irritation, may also occur in the early stage when the rash erupts. At a later stage, the patient may report neurologic symptoms, such as memory loss.

Especially in children, body temperature may increase to 104° F (40° C) in the early stage and be accompanied by chills. You may see erythema chronicum migrans, which begins as a red macule or papule at the tick bite site and may grow as large as 2″ (5.1 cm) in diameter. The patient may describe the lesion as hot and pruritic. Characteristic lesions (not seen in all patients) have bright red outer rims and white centers. They usually appear on the axillae, thighs, and groin. Within a few days, other lesions may erupt, as may a migratory, ringlike rash and conjunctivitis. In 3 to 4 weeks, the lesions fade to small red blotches, which persist for several more weeks.

Bell's palsy may be seen in the second stage and may occur alone. In the later stage, inspection may reveal signs and symptoms of intermittent arthritis:

joint swelling, redness, and limited movement. Typically, the disease affects one or only a few joints, especially large ones, such as the knee.

Palpation of the pulse may reveal tachycardia or irregular heartbeat. During the first or second stage, you may detect regional lymphadenopathy as well. The patient may complain of tenderness in the skin lesion site or the posterior cervical area. You'll note generalized lymphadenopathy less commonly.

If the patient has neurologic involvement, Kernig's and Brudzinski's signs usually aren't positive, and neck stiffness usually occurs only with extreme flexion.

Diagnostic tests

Blood tests, including antibody titers to identify *B. burgdorferi,* are the most practical diagnostic tests. The enzyme-linked immunosorbent assay may be ordered because it's more sensitive and more specific. However, serologic test results don't always confirm the diagnosis — especially if the disease is in the early stages, before the body produces antibodies — or seropositivity for *B. burgdorferi.* Also, the validity of test results depends on laboratory techniques and interpretation.

Mild anemia and elevated erythrocyte sedimentation rate, white blood cell count, serum immunoglobulin M levels, and aspartate aminotransferase levels support the diagnosis.

A lumbar puncture may be ordered if Lyme disease involves the central nervous system. Analysis of cerebrospinal fluid may detect antibodies to *B. burgdorferi.*

Treatment

A 10- to 20-day course of antibiotics is the treatment of choice. Adults typically receive doxycycline; amoxicillin, cefuroxime axetil, and erythromycin are alternatives. Children usually receive oral amoxicillin. Administered early in the disease, these medications can minimize later complications. In later stages, high-dose ceftriaxone, cefotaxime, or penicillin G sodium administered I.V. may produce good results.

Nursing interventions

■ Plan the patient's care to provide adequate rest.
■ Administer an analgesic and an antipyretic, as ordered, and monitor the effects.
■ If the patient has arthritis, help him with range-of-motion and strengthening exercises, but avoid overexerting him.
■ Protect the patient from sensory overload, and reorient him if needed. Also, encourage him to express his feelings and concerns about memory loss, if appropriate.

Patient teaching
■ Instruct the patient to take his antibiotic as prescribed.
■ Urge him to return for follow-up care and to report recurrent or new symptoms to the doctor.
■ Inform the patient, family members, and other caregivers about ways to prevent Lyme disease. Advise them to avoid tick-infested areas, if possible. If this isn't feasible, suggest covering the skin with clothing, using insect repellents, inspecting exposed skin for attached ticks at least every 4 hours, and removing ticks, if present, with tweezers or forceps and firm traction. A vaccine has been developed for persons at risk for Lyme disease. The patient can consult a doctor or local clinic for information.

Multiple sclerosis

Multiple sclerosis (MS) is a chronic disease caused by progressive demyelination of the white matter of the brain and spinal cord. These sporadic patches of demyelination in the central nervous system (CNS) cause widespread and varied neurologic dysfunction.

MS is a major cause of chronic disability in young adults ages 20 to 40. Exacerbations and remissions characterize it. MS may progress rapidly, causing death within months or disability by early adulthood. The prognosis varies; about 70% of patients lead active, productive lives with prolonged remissions.

Causes

The exact cause of MS is unknown but may be a slowly acting viral infection, an autoimmune response of the nervous system, or an allergic response. Other possible factors include trauma, anoxia, toxins, nutritional deficiencies, vascular lesions, and anorexia nervosa — all of which may help destroy axons and the myelin sheath. Emotional stress, overwork, fatigue, pregnancy, or acute respiratory tract infections may precede the onset of this illness. Genetic factors may also be involved.

Assessment findings

Clinical findings in patients with MS correspond to the extent and site of myelin destruction, extent of remyelination, and adequacy of subsequent restored synaptic transmission. Symptoms may be transient or may last for hours or weeks. They may vary from day to day, be unpredictable, and be difficult for the patient to describe. For most patients, visual problems and sensory impairment, such as burning, pins and needles, and tingling sensa-

Describing multiple sclerosis

Multiple sclerosis (MS) may be described in various terms:

■ Relapsing-remitting — clear relapses (or acute attacks or exacerbations) with full recovery and lasting disability. Between the attacks there's no worsening of the disease.

■ Primary progressive — to steady progression or worsening of the disease from the onset with minor recovery or plateaus. This form is uncommon and may involve different brain and spinal cord damage than other forms.

■ Secondary progressive — begins as a pattern of clear-cut relapses and recovery but becomes steadily progressive and worsens between acute attacks.

■ Progressive relapsing — steadily progressive from the onset but also has clear, acute attacks. This form is rare. In addition, differential diagnosis must rule out spinal cord compression, foramen magnum tumor (which may mimic the exacerbations and remission of MS), multiple small strokes, syphilis or another infection, thyroid disease, and chronic fatigue syndrome.

---

tions are the first indications that something is wrong.

The patient history commonly reveals initial visual problems and sensory impairment such as paresthesia. After the initial episode, findings may vary widely and include blurred vision or diplopia, urinary problems, emotional lability and, possibly, dysphagia.

As the patient speaks, you may notice poorly articulated speech. Neurologic examination and muscle function tests may reveal muscle weakness of the involved area and spasticity, hyperreflexia, intention tremor, gait ataxia, and paralysis, ranging from monoplegia to quadriplegia. Visual examination may reveal nystagmus, scotoma, optic neuritis, or ophthalmoplegia. (See *Describing multiple sclerosis*.)

The patient with MS may present with various signs and symptoms. Characteristic changes to look for in your assessment include:

■ ocular disturbances — optic neuritis, diplopia, ophthalmoplegia, blurred vision, and nystagmus

■ muscle dysfunction — weakness, paralysis ranging from monoplegia to quadriplegia, spasticity, hyperreflexia, intention tremor, and gait ataxia

■ urinary disturbances — incontinence, frequency, urgency, and frequent urinary tract infections

■ bowel disturbances — involuntary evacuation or constipation

■ fatigue — generally the most disabling symptom

■ neurologic problems — poorly articulated speech, scanning speech, or dysarthria disturbances.

Also, clinical effects may be so mild that the patient is unaware of them or so intense that they're disabling.

Diagnostic tests

This difficult diagnosis may require years of testing and observation. EEG results show abnormalities in one-third of patients. Cerebrospinal fluid (CSF) analysis reveals elevated immunoglobulin G (IgG) levels but normal total protein levels. Elevated IgG levels are significant only when serum gamma globulin levels are normal, and they reflect hyperactivity of the immune system due to chronic demyelination. The white blood cell count may be slightly increased.

Evoked potential studies demonstrate slowed conduction of nerve impulses in 80% of MS patients. Magnetic resonance imaging (MRI) is the most sensitive method of detecting MS lesions. More than 90% of patients with MS show multifocal white matter lesions when this test is performed. MRI is also used to evaluate disease progression. Computed tomography scanning may disclose lesions within the brain's white matter.

Electrophoresis can be used to detect oligoclonal bands of immunoglobulin in CSF. They're present in most patients and can be found even when the percentage of gamma globulin in CSF is normal. Other tests, such as neuropsychological tests, may help rule out other disorders.

Treatment

The goal of treatment is to treat acute exacerbations, the disease, and related signs and symptoms. Acute exacerbations are treated with I.V. methylprednisolone followed by oral prednisone. This is effective for speeding recovery from acute attacks. Other drugs, such as azathioprine (Imuran) or methotrexate and cytotoxin may be used.

Three drugs are used to treat the disease: interferon beta-1a (Avonex), interferon beta-1b (Betaseron), and glatiramer (Copaxone, copolymer-1), which may reduce the frequency and severity of relapses and slow CNS damage. Glatiramer is a combination of four amino acids; all the medications are immunomodulators, targeting the autoimmune response. They're all used for relapsing-remitting MS.

Associated signs and symptoms are treated with medications, supportive measures, and aggressive management to prevent deterioration. (See *Treating signs and symptoms of MS*.)

Nursing interventions

■ Assist with physical therapy. Increase the patient's comfort with massages and relaxing baths. Assist with active, resistive, and stretching exercises to maintain the patient's muscle tone and joint mobility, decrease spasticity, improve coordination, and boost morale. Provide rest periods between exercises because fatigue may contribute to exacerbations.
■ Administer medications as ordered, and watch for adverse reactions. For instance, dantrolene may cause muscle weakness and decreased muscle tone.
■ Promote emotional stability. Help the patient establish a daily routine to maintain optimal functioning. His tolerance level regulates his activity level. Encourage daily physical exercise and regular rest periods to prevent fatigue.
■ Keep the bedpan or urinal readily accessible because the need to void is immediate. Evaluate the need for bowel and bladder training, during hospitalization.
■ Reactions to glatiramer occur immediately after injection. The patient may experience transient flushing, chest pain, palpitations, and dyspnea that lasts only a few seconds. Usually no additional treatment is needed.
■ Patients receiving interferon beta-1a or interferon beta-1b require routine laboratory monitoring that includes blood urea nitrogen, creatinine and alanine aminotransferase levels, complete blood count with differential, and urinalysis.

Patient teaching
■ Review the disease process, emphasizing the need for optimizing the patient's potential and avoiding exacerbations if possible.

Treating signs and symptoms of MS

Signs and symptoms of multiple sclerosis (MS) include spasticity, fatigue, bladder and bowel problems. sensory symptoms, and cognitive and motor dysfunction. Each problem is treated with various medications and supportive measures.

■ Spasticity occurs as a result of opposing muscle groups relaxing and contracting at the same time. Stretching and range-of-motion exercises, coupled with correct positioning, are helpful in relaxing muscles and maintaining function. Drug therapy for spasticity includes baclofen (Lioresal) and tizanidine (Zanaflex). For severe spasticity, Botox injections, intrathecal injections, nerve blocks, and surgery may be necessary.

■ Fatigue is characterized by an overwhelming feeling of exhaustion that can occur at any time of the day without warning. The cause is unknown. Changes in environmental conditions, such as heat and humidity, can aggravate fatigue. Symmetrel, Cylert, and Ritalin are beneficial, as are certain antidepressants.

■ Bladder problems may arise from failure to store urine, failure to empty the bladder or, more commonly, a combination of both. Treatment ranges from simple strategies such as drinking cranberry juice to the placement of an indwelling urinary catheter and suprapubic tubes. Intermittent self-catheterization programs are beneficial. An anticholinergic may also be helpful.

■ Bowel problems, such as constipation and involuntary evacuation of stool, can be managed by increasing fiber. Bulking agents such as Metamucil assist in relief and prevention of bowel problems. Other bowel-training strategies, such as daily suppositories and rectal stimulation, may be necessary.

■ Sensory symptoms, such as pain, numbness, burning, and tingling sensations, can be well managed with low-dose tricyclic antidepressants, phenytoin, or carbamazepine.

■ Half of all patients with MS demonstrate cognitive dysfunction. Cognitive problems tend to be minor, with retrieval of information being the most common symptom. For more severe issues, a neuropsychological consultation could be beneficial.

■ Motor dysfunction, such as problems with balance, strength, and muscle coordination, may be present. Adaptive devices and physical therapy help to maintain mobility.

■ Other symptoms such as tremors may be treated with a beta-adrenergic blocker, a sedative, or a diuretic. Dysarthria requires speech therapy. Vertigo may be managed with an antihistamine, vision therapy, or exercises. Vision changes may require vision therapy or adaptive lenses.

■ Teach adverse effects of drug therapy and the medication regimen.
■ Emphasize the need to avoid stress, infections, and fatigue and to maintain independence by developing new ways of performing daily activities.
■ Tell the patient to avoid exposure to bacterial and viral infections.
■ Stress the importance of eating a nutritious, well-balanced diet that contains sufficient fiber to prevent constipation.
■ Encourage adequate fluid intake and regular urination.
■ Promote emotional stability. Help the patient establish a daily routine to maintain optimal functioning.
■ Inform the patient that exacerbations are unpredictable, necessitating physical and emotional adjustments in his lifestyle.

■ Refer the patient to the social service department when appropriate and to a local chapter of the National Multiple Sclerosis Society.

Myocardial infarction

Myocardial infarction (MI) results from reduced blood flow through one of the coronary arteries, which causes myocardial ischemia and necrosis. The infarction site depends on the vessels involved. For instance, occlusion of the circumflex coronary artery causes a lateral wall infarction; occlusion of the left anterior coronary artery causes an anterior-wall infarction. True posterior- and inferior-wall infarctions result from occlusion of the right coronary artery or one of its branches. Right ventricular infarctions can also result from right coronary artery occlusion, can accompany inferior infarctions, and may cause right-sided heart failure. In patients with a transmural (Q-wave) MI, tissue damage extends through all myocardial layers; in patients with a subendocardial (non-Q-wave) MI, usually only the innermost layer is damaged.

Causes

An MI results from occlusion of one of the coronary arteries. The occlusion can stem from atherosclerosis, thrombosis, platelet aggregation, or coronary artery stenosis or spasm. Predisposing factors include aging; diabetes mellitus; hypertension; obesity; smoking; elevated serum triglyceride, low-density lipoprotein, and cholesterol levels; decreased serum high-density lipoprotein levels; and excessive intake of saturated fats, carbohydrates, and salt. Additional factors include a positive family history of coronary artery disease (CAD), a sedentary lifestyle, and stress or a type A personality (aggressive, competitive attitude, addiction to work, chronic impatience). Also, the use of drugs, such as amphetamines or cocaine, can cause an MI.

Assessment findings

Typically, the patient reports persistent, crushing substernal pain that may radiate to the left arm, jaw, neck, and shoulder blades. He commonly describes the pain as heavy, squeezing, or crushing, and it may persist for 12 or more hours. In some patients — particularly elderly patients or those with diabetes — pain may not occur; in others, it may be mild and confused with indigestion.

Patients with CAD may report increasing anginal frequency, severity, or duration (especially when not precipitated by exertion, a heavy meal, or cold and wind). The patient may also report a feeling of impending doom, fatigue, nausea, vomiting, and shortness of breath. Sudden death, however, may be the first and only indication of an MI.

Inspection may reveal an extremely anxious and restless patient with dyspnea and diaphoresis. If right-sided heart failure is present, you may note jugular vein distention. Patients with an anterior-wall MI may exhibit sympathetic nervous system hyperactivity, such as tachycardia and hypertension, whereas patients with an inferior-wall MI may exhibit parasympathetic nervous system hyperactivity, such as bradycardia and hypotension.

In patients who develop ventricular dysfunction, auscultation may reveal a third and fourth heart sound, paradoxical splitting of the second heart sound, and decreased heart sounds. A systolic murmur of mitral insufficiency may be heard with papillary muscle dysfunction secondary to infarction. A pericardial friction rub may also be heard, especially in patients who have a transmural MI or have developed pericarditis. Fever is unusual at the onset of an MI, but a low-grade fever may develop during the next few days.

Diagnostic tests

In patients with an MI, diagnostic tests may provide the following results.
■ Serial 12-lead electrocardiography (ECG) readings may be normal or inconclusive during the first few hours after an MI. Characteristic abnormalities include serial ST-segment depression in a subendocardial MI and ST-segment elevation and Q waves in a transmural MI.
■ Serum creatine kinase (CK) level is elevated — specifically, the CK-MB isoenzyme level that signifies damage to cardiac muscle tissue.
■ Serum lactate dehydrogenase (LD) level is elevated. LD_1 is higher than LD_2.
■ Myoglobin is released with muscle damage and may be detected as soon as 2 hours after an MI.
■ Troponin I levels increase within 4 to 6 hours of myocardial injury and may remain elevated for 5 to 11 days.
■ Echocardiography shows ventricular-wall dyskinesia with a transmural MI and helps evaluate the ejection fraction.
■ Scans using I.V. technetium-99m pertechnetate can identify acutely damaged muscle by picking up accumulations of radioactive nucleotide, which appears as a "hot spot" on the film. Myocardial perfusion imaging with thallium-201 reveals a "cold spot" in most patients during the first few hours after a transmural MI.

Treatment

The goals of treatment are to relieve chest pain, to stabilize heart rhythm, and to reduce cardiac workload. Treatment includes revascularization to preserve myocardial tissue. Arrhythmias,

the most common problem during the first 48 hours after an MI, may require an antiarrhythmic, possibly a pacemaker and, rarely, cardioversion.

To preserve myocardial tissue, I.V. thrombolytic therapy should be started within 3 hours of the onset of symptoms (unless contraindicated). Thrombolytic therapy includes either streptokinase, alteplase, recombinant tissue plasminogen activator, reteplase, or urokinase. Percutaneous transluminal coronary angioplasty (PTCA) may be another option. If PTCA is performed soon after the onset of symptoms, the thrombolytic may be administered directly into the coronary artery.

Drug therapy usually includes aspirin (to inhibit platelet aggregation), lidocaine or comparable ventricular antiarrhythmic, atropine or a temporary pacemaker, and nitroglycerin. Other agents used include calcium channel blockers, diltiazem and verapamil, heparin I.V. (usually follows thrombolytic therapy), and morphine. The patient may also need a drug to increase contractility or blood pressure, an inotropic drug to treat reduced myocardial contractility, a beta-adrenergic blocker to help prevent reinfarction, and an angiotensin-converting inhibitor to improve survival rate in a low ejection fraction.

Other therapies include low-flow oxygen and bed rest with bedside commode. Pulmonary artery (PA) catheterization may be performed to detect left- or right-sided heart failure and to monitor response to treatment. Intra-aortic balloon pump may be used for patients with cardiogenic shock. Cardiac catheterization and coronary artery bypass grafting may also be performed.

Nursing interventions

■ Assess the patient's pain and give an analgesic if ordered. Record the severity, location, type, and duration of the pain. Don't give I.M. injections because absorption from the muscle is unpredictable, CK level may be falsely elevated, and I.V. administration gives more rapid relief of signs and symptoms.

■ Check the patient's blood pressure after giving nitroglycerin, especially the first dose.

■ Frequently monitor the ECG rhythm strips to detect rate changes and arrhythmias.

■ During episodes of chest pain, obtain ECG readings and blood pressure and PA catheter measurements (if applicable) to determine changes.

■ Watch for crackles, cough, tachypnea, and edema, which may indicate an impending left-sided heart failure. Carefully monitor daily weight, intake and output, respiratory rate, serum enzyme levels, ECG readings, and blood pressure. Auscultate for adventitious breath sounds.

■ Ask the dietary department to provide a clear liquid diet until the patient's nausea subsides. A low-cholesterol, low-sodium diet, without caffeine-containing beverages, may be ordered.

■ Provide a stool softener to prevent straining.

■ Assist with range-of-motion exercises. If the patient is immobilized by a severe MI, turn him often. Antiembolism stockings help prevent venostasis and thrombophlebitis.

■ If the patient has undergone PTCA, provide sheath care. Keep the sheath line open with a heparin drip, and observe for bleeding. Keep the leg with the sheath insertion site immobile, and maintain strict bed rest. Frequently check peripheral pulses in the affected leg. Provide analgesics for back pain, if needed.

■ After thrombolytic therapy, administer continuous heparin as ordered. Monitor the partial thromboplastin time every 6 hours, and monitor the patient for evidence of bleeding.

■ Monitor ECG rhythm strips for reperfusion arrhythmias and treat them according to facility protocol. If the artery reoccludes, the patient will experience the same symptoms as before. If this occurs, prepare the patient for return to the cardiac catheterization laboratory.

Patient teaching

■ To promote compliance with the prescribed medication regimen and other treatment measures, thoroughly explain dosages and therapy.

■ Review dietary restrictions with the patient. Ask the dietitian to speak to the patient and family members.

■ Encourage the patient to participate in a cardiac rehabilitation exercise program in a stepped-care program.

■ Counsel the patient to resume sexual activity progressively. He may need to take nitroglycerin before sexual intercourse to prevent chest pain from the increased activity.

■ Advise the patient to report typical or atypical chest pain. Post-MI syndrome may develop, producing chest pain that must be differentiated from a recurrent MI, pulmonary infarction, and heart failure.

■ Stress the need to stop smoking.

Osteoarthritis

Osteoarthritis is the most common form of arthritis. It causes deterioration of the joint cartilage and formation of reactive new bone at the margins and subchondral areas of the joints. This chronic degeneration results from a breakdown of chondrocytes, usually in the hips and knees. Depending on the site and severity of joint involvement, disability can range from minor limitation of the fingers to near immobility in people with hip or knee disease.

Progression rates vary; joints may remain stable for years in the early stage of deterioration.

Causes

Primary osteoarthritis may be related to aging, but researchers don't understand why. This form of the disease seems to lack any predisposing factors. In some patients, it may be hereditary. Secondary osteoarthritis usually follows an identifiable event — most commonly a traumatic injury or a congenital abnormality such as hip dysplasia. Endocrine disorders such as diabetes mellitus, metabolic disorders such as chondrocalcinosis, and other types of arthritis also can lead to secondary osteoarthritis.

Assessment findings

The patient usually complains of gradually increasing signs and symptoms. He may report a predisposing event such as a traumatic injury. The patient will typically have deep, aching joint pain, particularly after he exercises or bears weight on the affected joint. Rest may relieve the pain. Additional complaints include stiffness in the morning and after exercise, aching during changes in weather, a "grating" feeling when the joint moves, contractures, and limited movement. These symptoms tend to be worse in patients with poor posture, obesity, or occupational stress.

Inspection may reveal joint swelling, muscle atrophy, deformity of the involved areas, and gait abnormalities (when arthritis affects the hips or knees). Osteoarthritis of the interphalangeal joints produces hard nodes on the distal and proximal joints. Painless at first, these nodes eventually become red, swollen, and tender. The fingers may become numb and lose their dexterity. Palpation may reveal joint tenderness and warmth without redness, grating with movement, joint instability, muscle spasms, and limited movement.

Diagnostic tests

X-rays of the affected joint may help confirm the diagnosis, but findings may be normal in the early stages. Typical findings include a narrowing of the joint space or margin, cystlike bony deposits, sclerosis, joint deformity, bony growths, and joint fusion.

Synovial fluid analysis and radionuclide bone scan can be used to rule out inflammatory arthritis. Arthroscopy is used to identify soft-tissue swelling by showing internal joint structures. Magnetic resonance imaging produces clear cross-sectional images of the affected joint and adjacent bones. Results also show disease progression. Neuromuscular tests may disclose reduced muscle strength (reduced grip strength, for example).

Treatment

To relieve pain, improve mobility, and minimize disability, treatment includes medications, rest, physical therapy, assistive mobility devices and, possibly, surgery.

Medications include aspirin, other salicylates, nonsteroidal anti-inflammatory drugs, and intra-articular injections of corticosteroids, if needed.

Adequate rest is essential and should be balanced with activity. Physical therapy includes massage, moist heat, paraffin dips for the hands, supervised exercise to decrease muscle spasms and atrophy, and protective techniques for preventing undue joint stress. Some patients may reduce stress and increase stability by using crutches, braces, a cane, a walker, a cervical collar, or traction. Weight reduction may help an obese patient.

In some cases, a patient with severe disability or uncontrollable pain may undergo surgery. Techniques include arthroplasty (partial or total replacement of the deteriorated part of a joint with a prosthetic appliance), arthrodesis (surgical fusion of bones), osteoplasty (scraping and lavage of deteriorated bone from the joint) or osteotomy (excision or cutting of a wedge of bone to change alignment and relieve stress).

Nursing interventions

■ Provide emotional support and reassurance to help the patient cope with limited mobility. Include him and family members in all phases of his care.
■ Encourage the patient to perform as much self-care as his immobility and pain allow. Provide him with adequate time to perform activities at his own pace.
■ To help promote sleep, adjust pain medications to allow maximum rest. Provide the patient with normal sleep aids, such as a bath, back rub, or extra pillow.
■ For lumbosacral spinal joints, provide a firm mattress (or bed board); for cervical spinal joints, adjust the patient's cervical collar to prevent constriction and skin irritation; for the hip, use moist heat pads to relieve pain.
■ For the knee, assist with prescribed range-of-motion (ROM) exercises twice daily to maintain muscle tone. Help perform progressive resistance exercises to increase the patient's muscle strength.
■ Check crutches, cane, braces, or walker for proper fit.

Patient teaching
■ Instruct the patient to plan for adequate rest during the day, after exertion, and at night. Encourage him to take steps to conserve energy — for example, by pacing, simplifying work procedures, and protecting joints.
■ Advise against overexertion. Tell the patient that he should take care to stand and walk correctly, to minimize weight-bearing activities, and to be especially careful when stooping or picking up objects.
■ Tell the patient to wear well-fitting support shoes and to repair worn heels.
■ Recommend having safety devices installed in the home, such as grab bars in the bathroom.
■ Teach the patient to do ROM exercises, performing them as gently as possible.
■ Advise maintaining proper body weight to minimize strain on joints.
■ Teach the patient how to properly use crutches or other orthopedic devices. Stress the importance of proper fitting and regular professional readjustment of such devices. Warn that these aids can cause impaired sensation, which can result in tissue damage.
■ Recommend using cushions when sitting. Also, suggest using an elevated toilet seat. Both reduce stress when rising from a seated position.
■ As necessary, refer the patient to an occupational therapist or a home health nurse to help him cope with activities of daily living.

Otitis media

Otitis media, an inflammation of the middle ear associated with fluid accumulation, may be acute or chronic, suppurative or secretory. Acute otitis media is most common in infants and children because they have a shorter and more horizontal eustachian tube than adults, which predisposes them to middle ear infections.

With prompt treatment, the prognosis for acute otitis media is excellent. However, prolonged accumulation of fluid in the middle ear cavity can cause chronic serous otitis media, with possible perforation of the tympanic membrane. Chronic suppurative otitis media can lead to scarring, adhesions, and severe structural or functional ear damage. Chronic secretory otitis media, with its persistent inflammation and pressure, can cause conductive hearing loss.

Causes

Acute otitis media results from disruption of eustachian tube patency. Suppurative otitis media usually results from bacterial infection. In this disorder, respiratory tract infections, allergic reactions, and position changes, such as holding an infant in a supine position during feeding, allow reflux of nasopharyngeal flora through the eustachian tube and colonization in the middle ear. Chronic suppurative otitis media results from inadequate treatment of acute otitis episodes or from infection by resistant strains of bacteria.

Secretory otitis media stems from a viral infection, an allergy, or barotrauma (pressure injury from an inability to equalize pressures between the environment and the middle ear), such as that experienced during rapid aircraft descent or rapid underwater ascent in scuba diving (barotitis media). In this disorder, obstruction of the eustachian tube promotes transudation of sterile serous fluid from blood vessels in the middle ear membrane.

Chronic secretory otitis media is caused by adenoidal tissue overgrowth that obstructs the eustachian tube, edema resulting from allergic rhinitis, chronic sinus infection, or inadequate treatment of acute suppurative otitis media.

Spontaneous rupture of the tympanic membrane can cause persistent perforation that may develop into chronic otitis media. Other complications are mastoiditis, meningitis, cholesteatomas (cystlike masses in the middle ear), septicemia, abscesses, vertigo, lymphadenopathy, leukocytosis, and permanent hearing loss. Tympanosclerosis, which results from repeated ear infections, is a deposit of collagen and calcium in the middle ear that hardens around the ossicles, causing conduction hearing loss.

Assessment findings

The patient history may reveal an upper respiratory tract infection or history of allergies. The patient may complain of severe, deep, throbbing ear pain (from pressure behind the tympanic membrane) and dizziness, nausea, and vomiting. With acute secretory otitis media, the patient may describe a sensation of fullness in the ear and popping, crackling, or clicking sounds on swallowing or moving the jaw. The patient with an accumulation of fluid may describe hearing an echo when speaking and experiencing a vague feeling of top-heaviness. If the tympanic membrane has ruptured, the patient may state that the pain suddenly stopped. A history of recent air travel or scuba diving suggests barotitis media.

Inspection may reveal sneezing and coughing due to an upper respiratory tract infection. Vital sign assessment may reveal mild to very high fever. In chronic suppurative otitis media, inspection may reveal a painless, purulent discharge.

With acute suppurative otitis media, otoscopic examination may show obscured or distorted bony landmarks of the tympanic membrane. With acute secretory otitis media, otoscopy reveals tympanic membrane retraction, which causes the bony landmarks to appear more prominent. Otoscopy also reveals clear or amber fluid behind the tympanic membrane, possibly with a meniscus and bubbles. If hemorrhage into the middle ear has occurred, as in barotrauma, otoscopy exposes a blue-black tympanic membrane.

With chronic otitis media, otoscopic examination may show thickening and scarring of the tympanic membrane, decreased or absent tympanic membrane mobility, or cholesteatoma. If a tympanic perforation is present, a pulsating discharge may be visible.

With acute secretory otitis media, audiometric tests may reveal severe conductive hearing loss varying from 15 to 35 dB, depending on the thickness and amount of fluid in the middle ear cavity. With chronic suppurative otitis media, the associated conductive hearing loss varies with the size and type of tympanic membrane perforation and ossicular destruction.

Diagnostic tests

Otoscopic or neuroscopic examination is used to diagnose the disorder, remove debris, and perform minor surgery. Pneumatoscopy shows decreased tympanic membrane mobility. (This procedure is painful when the tympanic membrane is obviously bulging and erythematous.) Tympanometry is used to measure how well the tympanic membrane functions to detect hearing loss and evaluate the condition of the middle ear. Culture and sensitivity tests of exudate are used to identify the causative organism. Radiographic studies depict mastoid involvement. Audiometry is used to detect and measure the degree of hearing loss. Biopsy is used to rule out malignancy and identify tissues and a complete blood count is used to identify infection.

Treatment

For the patient with acute suppurative otitis media, antibiotic therapy includes ampicillin or amoxicillin and, also, amoxicillin clavulanate potassium (Augmentin) for infants, children, and adults. Therapy for patients allergic to penicillin derivatives may include a sulfonamide, erythromycin, a tetracycline, and other broad-spectrum antibiotics. Aspirin or acetaminophen is given to control pain and fever.

Severe, painful bulging of the tympanic membrane usually requires myringotomy. Codeine may be given to adults for severe pain, and sedatives may be given to small children.

A broad-spectrum antibiotic can help prevent acute suppurative otitis media in high-risk patients such as children with recurring episodes of otitis. In these patients, antibiotics must be used sparingly and with discretion, to prevent development of resistant bacteria.

For patients with acute secretory otitis media, performing Valsalva's maneuver several times a day to inflate the eustachian tube may be the only treatment required. If this isn't successful, nasopharyngeal decongestant therapy may be helpful; it should continue for at least 2 weeks and sometimes indefinitely, with periodic evaluation. If decongestant therapy fails, myringotomy and aspiration of middle ear fluid are necessary, followed by insertion of a polyethylene tube into the tympanic membrane to equalize pressure. This pressure-equalizing tube, called a tympanostomy tube, remains in place for 6 to 12 months, although it may fall out on its own. Concomitant treatment of the underlying cause (such as allergen elimination or adenoidectomy) also may be helpful.

Treatment for a patient with chronic otitis media may include an antibiotic for exacerbations of acute otitis media, elimination of eustachian tube obstruction, treatment of otitis externa (when present), myringoplasty (tympanic membrane graft), tympanoplasty to reconstruct middle ear structures when thickening and scarring are present, mastoidectomy, or cholesteatoma excision. A stapedectomy may be performed for a patient with otosclerosis.

Nursing interventions

■ If the patient has difficulty understanding procedures because of hearing loss, provide clear, concise explanations. Face him when speaking; enunciate clearly, slowly, and in a normal tone; and allow time for him to grasp what you've said. Provide a pencil and paper, and alert the staff to his communication problem.

■ After myringotomy, maintain the drainage flow. Don't place cotton or plugs deep in the ear canal; you may place sterile cotton loosely in the external ear to absorb drainage. To prevent infection, change the cotton when it gets damp, and wash your hands before and after ear care. As prescribed, give codeine and aspirin for pain and an antiemetic for nausea and vomiting.

■ After tympanoplasty, reinforce dressings and watch for excessive bleeding from the ear canal. Administer an analgesic if needed.

Patient teaching

■ Advise the patient with acute secretory otitis media, or his parents, to watch for and immediately report pain or fever, which indicates secondary infection.

■ Teach the patient and family members proper instillation of ointment, drops, and ear wash, as ordered.

■ Teach the patient and family members how to administer medications as ordered, and tell them about possible

adverse effects. Stress the importance of taking the antibiotic as prescribed to prevent secondary infection.

■ Tell the patient that some doctors require fitted earplugs for swimming after myringotomy and tympanostomy tube insertion. Advise the patient to notify the doctor if the tube falls out and if any ear pain, fever, or pus-filled ear discharge occurs.

■ Encourage a nutritious diet that includes the patient's favorite foods. To ensure adequate fluid intake, include electrolyte drinks. Ice pops, frozen fruit pops, and gelatin desserts are favorable alternatives.

■ Instruct the patient and parents to tell the doctor about any significant earache.

■ Reassure the patient that hearing loss caused by serious otitis media is temporary.

Parkinson's disease

Parkinson's disease characteristically produces progressive muscle rigidity, akinesia, and involuntary tremors. Deterioration commonly progresses, culminating in death, which usually results from aspiration pneumonia or some other infection. Parkinson's disease is also called parkinsonism, paralysis agitans, or shaking palsy.

Causes

The cause of Parkinson's disease is unknown in most cases. Studies of the extrapyramidal brain nuclei (corpus striatum, globus pallidus, and substantia nigra) have established that a dopamine deficiency prevents affected brain cells from performing their normal inhibitory function within the central nervous system. Some cases of Parkinson's disease are caused by exposure to toxins, such as manganese dust and carbon monoxide, that destroy cells in the substantia nigra.

Assessment findings

The patient history notes the cardinal signs of Parkinson's disease, which include muscle rigidity and akinesia, and an insidious tremor that begins in the fingers, commonly known as unilateral pill-rolling tremor. Although many patients can't pinpoint exactly when the tremors began, they typically increase with stress or anxiety and decrease with purposeful movement and sleep.

A patient with Parkinson's disease may also report dysphagia. He may complain that he becomes fatigued when he tries to perform activities of daily living (ADLs) and that he experiences muscle cramps of the legs, neck, and trunk. He may also mention oily skin, increased perspiration, insomnia, and mood changes. You may notice dysarthria and find that the patient speaks in a high-pitched monotone.

Inspection may reveal drooling, a masklike facial expression, and difficulty walking. The patient's gait generally will lack normal parallel motion and may be retropulsive or propulsive. Also, the patient may demonstrate a loss of posture control when he walks. Typically, the patient who loses posture control walks with the body bent forward. These signs result from akinesia.

Besides gait changes, musculoskeletal and neurologic assessment may point to muscle rigidity that results in resistance to passive muscle stretching. Such rigidity may be uniform (lead-pipe rigidity) or jerky (cogwheel rigidity). The patient may also pivot with difficulty and easily lose his balance.

As you assess this patient, keep in mind that Parkinson's disease itself doesn't impair the intellect but that a coexisting disorder such as arteriosclerosis may.

Diagnostic tests

Although urinalysis may reveal decreased dopamine levels, laboratory test results usually are of little value in identifying Parkinson's disease. Computed tomography scanning or magnetic resonance imaging may be performed to rule out other disorders such as intracranial tumors. A conclusive diagnosis is possible only after ruling out other causes of tremor, such as involutional depression, cerebral arteriosclerosis and, in patients younger than age 30, intracranial tremors, Wilson's disease, or toxic reactions to other substances such as the drug phenothiazine.

Treatment

No cure exists for Parkinson's disease, so the goal of treatment is to relieve the symptoms and keep the patient functional as long as possible. Treatment consists of drugs, physical therapy and, in severe disease unresponsive to drugs, stereotaxic neurosurgery.

Drug therapy usually includes levodopa, a dopamine replacement that's most effective for the first few years after it's initiated. When levodopa is ineffective or too toxic, alternative drug therapy includes an anticholinergic (such as trihexyphenidyl or benztropine) to control tremors and rigidity and antihistamines (such as diphenhydramine) to decrease tremors, with its central anticholinergic and sedative effects. Amantadine, an antiviral, is used early in treatment to reduce rigidity, tremors, and akinesia. Selegiline, an enzyme inhibitor, helps conserve dopamine and enhances the therapeutic effect of levodopa. A tricyclic antidepressant may be given to decrease the depression that commonly accompanies the disease.

When drug therapy fails, stereotaxic neurosurgery sometimes offers an effective alternative. In this procedure, electrical coagulation, freezing, radioactivity, or ultrasound destroys the ventrolateral nucleus of the thalamus to prevent involuntary movement. Such neurosurgery is most effective in comparatively young, otherwise healthy people with unilateral tremor or muscle rigidity. Like drug therapy, neurosurgery is a palliative measure that can only relieve symptoms.

Physical therapy complements drug treatment and neurosurgery to maintain the patient's normal muscle tone and function. Appropriate physical therapy includes active and passive range-of-motion exercises, routine daily activities, walking, and baths and massage to help relax muscles.

Nursing interventions

■ To promote independence, encourage the patient to participate in care decisions and to perform as much of his own care as possible.

■ Monitor drug treatment so dosage can be adjusted to minimize adverse reactions. Report adverse reactions.

■ If the patient has surgery, watch for signs of hemorrhage and increased intracranial pressure by frequently checking his level of consciousness and vital signs.

■ Encourage independence by helping the patient recognize the ADLs that he can perform. Provide assistive devices as appropriate.

■ To help the patient with severe tremors achieve partial control of his body, have him sit on a chair and use its arms to steady himself.

■ Remember that fatigue may cause the patient to depend more on others, so provide rest periods between activities.

■ Help the patient overcome problems related to eating and elimination. For example, if he has difficulty eating, offer supplementary feedings or small, frequent meals to increase caloric in-

take. Help establish a regular bowel elimination routine by encouraging him to drink at least 2.1 qt (2 L) of liquids daily and eat high-fiber foods. An elevated toilet seat assists the patient to stand, from the seated position.

■ Work with the physical therapist to develop a program of daily exercises to increase muscle strength, decrease muscle rigidity, prevent contractures, and improve coordination.

■ Provide frequent warm baths and massage to help relax muscles and relieve muscle cramps.

■ Protect the patient from injury by using the bed's side rails and assisting the patient as necessary when he walks and eats.

■ To decrease the possibility of aspiration, have the patient sit in an upright position when eating.

■ Provide the patient with a semisolid diet, which is easier to swallow than a diet consisting of solids and liquids.

Patient teaching

■ Teach the patient and family members about the disease, its progressive stages, and treatments that may help the patient. Explain the actions of prescribed medications and possible adverse effects.

■ Explain household safety measures, such as installing or using side rails in halls and stairs and removing throw rugs from frequently traveled floors to prevent patient injury.

■ To make dressing easier, teach the patient to wear clothing fitted with zippers or Velcro fasteners rather than buttons.

■ To improve communication, instruct the patient to make a conscious effort to speak, to speak slowly, to take a few deep breaths before he begins to speak, and to think about what he wants to say before he begins to speak.

■ If appropriate, advise the patient how to eat. Because these patients eat slowly, allow plenty of time for meals.
■ Refer the patient and family members to the National Parkinson Foundation, the American Parkinson Disease Association, or the United Parkinson Foundation for more information.

Peptic ulcers

Peptic ulcers, which are circumscribed lesions in the mucosal membrane, can develop in the lower esophagus, stomach, duodenum, or jejunum. Duodenal ulcers account for about 80% of peptic ulcers and affect the proximal part of the small intestine. These ulcers follow a chronic course characterized by remissions and exacerbations, and some cases necessitate surgery. Gastric ulcers affect the stomach mucosa.

Causes

Researchers have identified a bacterial infection with *Helicobacter pylori* (formerly known as *Campylobacter pylori*) as a leading cause of peptic ulcer disease. They also found that *H. pylori* releases a toxin that promotes mucosal inflammation and ulceration. In a peptic ulcer resulting from *H. pylori*, acid seems to be mainly a contributor to the consequences of the bacterial infection, with other risk factors including nonsteroidal anti-inflammatory drugs (NSAIDs), and pathologic hypersecretory states (such as Zollinger-Ellison syndrome).

Investigators think drug therapy — particularly with salicylates and other NSAIDs, reserpine, or caffeine — may erode the mucosal lining. Glucocorticoids also predispose the patient to ulcers. Because these drugs also decrease gastric pain, they can mask signs of ulcer development until hemorrhage or perforation occurs.

Certain illnesses — particularly pancreatitis, hepatic disease, Crohn's disease, preexisting gastritis, and Zollinger-Ellison syndrome — are believed to strongly influence ulcer development. Predisposing factors include genetic factors, exposure to irritants, cigarette smoking, trauma, psychogenic factors, and normal aging. Also, for unknown reasons, gastric ulcers commonly strike people who have type A blood; duodenal ulcers, people who have type O blood.

Assessment findings

Typically, the patient describes periods of exacerbation and remission of his symptoms. History may reveal possible causes or predisposing factors, such as smoking, use of aspirin or other medications, and associated disorders. The patient with a gastric ulcer may report a recent loss of weight or appetite, pain in the left epigastrium described as heartburn or indigestion, and feeling of fullness or distention. Commonly, the onset of pain signals the start of an attack. For a patient with a gastric ulcer, eating usually triggers or aggravates the pain of the ulcer; in a patient with a duodenal ulcer, food usually relieves the pain of the ulcer, so he may report a recent weight gain. Also, the patient with a duodenal ulcer reports waking up because of pain; the patient with a gastric ulcer doesn't.

The patient with a duodenal ulcer may have epigastric pain that he describes as sharp, gnawing, or burning, likening it to a sensation of hunger, abdominal pressure, or fullness. Typically, the pain occurs 90 minutes to 3 hours after eating.

If the patient is anemic from blood loss, you may notice pallor on inspection. Palpation in the midline and midway between the umbilicus and the xiphoid process may reveal epigastric tenderness. Auscultation may reveal hyperactive bowel sounds.

Diagnostic tests

A barium swallow or an upper GI and a small-bowel series may reveal the presence of the ulcer. An upper GI endoscopy or an esophagogastroduodenoscopy confirms the presence of an ulcer and permits cytologic studies and biopsy to rule out *H. pylori* or cancer. Laboratory analysis may disclose occult blood in stools.

Immunoglobulin A anti-*H. pylori* test on a venous blood sample can be used to accurately detect antibodies to *H. pylori*. Gastric secretory studies show hyperchlorhydria. Carbon 13 (^{13}C) urea breath test results reflect activity of *H. pylori*. (*H. pylori* contains the enzyme urease, which breaks down orally administered urea containing the radioisotope ^{13}C before it's absorbed systemically. Low levels of ^{13}C in exhaled breath point to *H. pylori* infection.)

Treatment

The goal of drug therapy is to eradicate *H. pylori*, reduce gastric secretions, protect the mucosa from further damage, and relieve pain. Medications may include bismuth and two other antimicrobials, usually tetracycline or amoxicillin and metronidazole. An antacid is used to reduce gastric acidity. A histamine-2 receptor antagonist, such as cimetidine or ranitidine, is used to reduce gastric secretion for up to 8 weeks, or a gastric acid pump inhibitor (lansoprazole) is used for 4 weeks. A coating agent, such as sucralfate, is used for a duodenal ulcer.

An antisecretory agent, such as misoprostol, is needed if the ulceration resulted from NSAID use, and the NSAID must be continued for another condition such as arthritis. A sedative

and tranquilizer, such as chlordiazepoxide and phenobarbital, are used for patients with a gastric ulcer. An anticholinergic such as propantheline is needed to inhibit the effect of the vagus nerve on the parietal cells and to reduce gastrin production and excessive gastric activity in patients with a duodenal ulcer. (These drugs are usually contraindicated in patients with a gastric ulcer.)

Standard therapy also includes physical rest and decreased activity, which help decrease the gastric secretions. Diet therapy may consist of six small meals daily (or small hourly meals) rather than three regular meals. Some doctors prescribe a milk and cream or bland diet, but the value of these measures is controversial.

If GI bleeding occurs, emergency treatment begins with passage of a nasogastric (NG) tube to allow iced saline lavage, possibly containing norepinephrine. Gastroscopy allows visualization of the bleeding site and coagulation by laser or cautery to control bleeding. This therapy allows surgery to be postponed until the patient's condition stabilizes.

Surgery is indicated for perforation, unresponsiveness to conservative treatment, suspected cancer, and other complications. The type of surgery chosen for peptic ulcers depends on the location and extent of the disorder. Major operations include bilateral vagotomy, pyloroplasty, and gastrectomy.

Nursing interventions

General
■ Provide six small meals or small hourly meals as ordered. Advise the patient to eat slowly, chew thoroughly, and have small snacks between meals.
■ Continuously monitor the patient for complications such as hemorrhage; perforation; obstruction; and penetra-

tion. If any of the above occurs, notify the doctor immediately.

After surgery

■ Keep the NG tube (inserted in the operating room) patent. If the tube isn't functioning, don't reposition it; you could damage the suture line or anastomosis. Instead, promptly notify the surgeon.

■ Monitor intake and output, including NG tube drainage. Also, check bowel sounds. Allow the patient nothing by mouth until peristalsis resumes and the NG tube is removed or clamped.

■ Replace fluids and electrolytes. Assess patient for signs of dehydration, sodium deficiency, and metabolic alkalosis, which can occur secondary to gastric suction.

■ Watch for complications, such as hemorrhage; shock; iron, folate, or vitamin B_{12} deficiency anemia; and dumping syndrome.

Patient teaching

■ Teach the patient about peptic ulcer disease, and help him to recognize its signs and symptoms. Review symptoms associated with complications, and urge him to notify the doctor if any of these occur. Emphasize the importance of complying with treatment, even after his symptoms are relieved.

■ Instruct the patient to take an antacid 1 hour after meals. If he follows a sodium-restricted diet, advise him to take only a low-sodium antacid. Caution him that antacids with magnesium may cause diarrhea; antacids with aluminum, constipation.

■ Check all medications the patient is using. Antacids inhibit the absorption of many other drugs, including digoxin. Work out a schedule for taking medications.

■ Warn against excessive intake of coffee and alcoholic beverages during exacerbations.

■ Encourage the patient to make appropriate lifestyle changes. Explain that emotional tension can precipitate an ulcer attack and prolong healing.

■ If the patient smokes, urge him to stop because smoking stimulates gastric acid secretion. Refer him to a smoking-cessation program.

■ Tell the patient to read labels of nonprescription medications and to avoid preparations that contain corticosteroids, aspirin, or other NSAIDs such as ibuprofen. Caution him to avoid systemic antacids such as sodium bicarbonate.

■ Tell the patient that, although cimetidine, famotidine, and other histamine-receptor antagonists are available over-the-counter, he shouldn't take them without consulting his doctor. These drugs may duplicate prescribed medications or suppress important symptoms.

■ To avoid dumping syndrome after gastric surgery, advise the patient to lie down after meals, to drink fluids between meals rather than with meals, to avoid eating large amounts of carbohydrates, and to eat four to six small high-protein, low-carbohydrate meals daily.

Pneumonia

Pneumonia is an acute infection of the lung parenchyma that often impairs gas exchange. Based on the microbiological cause, pneumonia can be classified as viral, bacterial, fungal, protozoal, mycobacterial, mycoplasmal, or rickettsial in origin. Based on the location, it can be classified as bronchopneumonia, lobular pneumonia, or lobar pneumonia. Bronchopneumonia involves distal airways and alveoli; lobular pneumonia, part of a lobe; and lobar pneumonia, an entire lobe.

The infection can also be classified as primary, secondary, or aspiration pneumonia. Primary pneumonia results directly from inhalation or aspiration of a pathogen, such as bacteria or a virus; it includes pneumococcal and viral pneumonia. Secondary pneumonia may follow initial lung damage from a noxious chemical or other insult (superinfection) or may result from hematogenous spread of bacteria from a distant area. Aspiration pneumonia results from inhalation of foreign matter, such as vomitus or food particles, into the bronchi. It's more likely to occur in elderly or debilitated patients, those receiving nasogastric (NG) tube feedings, and those with an impaired gag reflex, poor oral hygiene, or a decreased level of consciousness.

Causes

With bacterial pneumonia, which can occur in any part of the lungs, an infection initially triggers alveolar inflammation and edema. Capillaries become engorged with blood, causing stasis. As the alveolocapillary membrane breaks down, alveoli fill with blood and exudate, resulting in atelectasis. With severe bacterial infections, the lungs assume a heavy, liverlike appearance, as in adult respiratory distress syndrome (ARDS).

Viral infection, which typically causes diffuse pneumonia, first attacks bronchiolar epithelial cells, causing interstitial inflammation and desquamation. It then spreads to the alveoli, which fill with blood and fluid. With advanced infection, a hyaline membrane may form. As with bacterial infection, severe viral infection may clinically resemble ARDS.

With aspiration pneumonia, aspiration of gastric juices or hydrocarbons triggers similar inflammatory changes and also inactivates surfactant over a large area. Decreased surfactant leads to alveolar collapse. Acidic gastric juices

may directly damage the airways and alveoli. Particles with the aspirated gastric juices may obstruct the airways and reduce airflow, which, in turn, leads to secondary bacterial pneumonia.

Certain predisposing factors increase the risk of pneumonia. Bacterial and viral pneumonia may occur in patients with chronic illness and debilitation (such as patients with cancer, especially lung cancer; malnutrition; alcoholism; sickle cell disease; or chronic respiratory tract disease), atelectasis, common colds or other viral respiratory tract infections, influenza, tracheostomy, or aspiration. It may also occur in patients who have had abdominal or thoracic surgery, patients who smoke, patients who have been exposed to noxious gases, and patients who are undergoing immunosuppressive therapy.

Without proper treatment, pneumonia can lead to such life-threatening complications as septic shock, hypoxemia, and respiratory failure. The infection can also spread within the patient's lungs, causing empyema or lung abscess. It also may spread by way of the bloodstream or by cross-contamination to other parts of the body, causing bacteremia, endocarditis, pericarditis, or meningitis.

Assessment findings

A patient with bacterial pneumonia may report pleuritic chest pain, a cough, excessive sputum production, and chills. On assessment, you may note that the patient has a fever. During inspection, you may observe that the patient is shaking and coughs up sputum. Creamy yellow sputum suggests staphylococcal pneumonia; green sputum, *Pseudomonas* pneumonia; and sputum that looks like currant jelly, *Klebsiella* pneumonia. (Clear sputum means that the patient doesn't have an infection.)

With advanced cases of all types of pneumonia, you hear dullness when you percuss. Auscultation may disclose crackles, wheezing, or rhonchi over the affected lung area as well as decreased breath sounds and decreased vocal fremitus.

Diagnostic tests

Chest X-rays disclose infiltrates, confirming the diagnosis. Sputum specimen for Gram stain and culture and sensitivity tests show acute inflammatory cells. The white blood cell count indicates leukocytosis in patients with bacterial pneumonia and a normal or low count in patients with viral or mycoplasmal pneumonia. Blood cultures reflect bacteremia and help to determine the causative organism.

Arterial blood gas (ABG) levels vary depending on the severity of pneumonia and the underlying lung state. Bronchoscopy or transtracheal aspiration allows the collection of material for culture. Pleural fluid culture may also be obtained. Pulse oximetry may show a reduced level of arterial oxygen saturation.

Treatment

Antimicrobial therapy is based on the causative agent and should be reevaluated early in the course of treatment. Supportive measures include humidified oxygen therapy for hypoxia, a bronchodilator, an antitussive, mechanical ventilation for respiratory failure, a high-calorie diet and adequate fluid intake, bed rest, and an analgesic to relieve pleuritic chest pain. A patient with severe pneumonia on mechanical ventilation may need positive end-expiratory pressure to maintain adequate oxygenation.

Nursing interventions

■ Maintain a patent airway and adequate oxygenation. Measure the patient's ABG levels, especially if he's hypoxic, and monitor his response to oxygen therapy.
■ For patients with severe pneumonia who require endotracheal intubation or a tracheostomy with or without mechanical ventilation, provide thorough respiratory care, and suction often using sterile technique to remove secretions.
■ Administer I.V. fluids and electrolyte replacement, if needed, for fever and dehydration.
■ Provide a high-calorie, high-protein diet of soft foods to offset the calories the patient uses to fight the infection. If necessary, supplement oral feedings with NG feedings or parenteral nutrition.
■ To prevent aspiration during NG feedings, elevate the patient's head, check the tube position, and administer the feeding slowly. Don't give large volumes at one time because this can cause vomiting.
■ Monitor the patient's fluid intake and output.
■ Tell the patient to sneeze and cough into a disposable tissue, and tape a waxed bag to the side of the bed for used tissues.
■ Encourage him to identify actions and care measures that promote comfort and relaxation.

Patient teaching
■ Explain all procedures (especially intubation and suctioning) to the patient and family members.
■ Emphasize the importance of adequate rest to promote full recovery and prevent a relapse. Explain that the doctor will advise the patient when he can resume full activity and return to work.

■ Review the patient's medication regimen. Stress the need to take all medication, as prescribed, even if he feels better, to prevent a relapse.

■ Teach the patient how to clear lung secretions — for example, with deep-breathing and coughing exercises as well as home oxygen therapy. Explain deep breathing and pursed-lip breathing.

■ Urge the patient to drink 2.1 to 3.2 qt (2 to 3 L) of fluid a day to maintain adequate hydration and keep mucus secretions thin for easier removal.

■ Teach the patient and family members about chest physiotherapy. Explain that postural drainage, percussion, and vibration help to mobilize and remove mucus from the lungs.

■ Urge the patient to avoid irritants that stimulate secretions, such as cigarette smoke, dust, and significant environmental pollution. If necessary, refer him to community programs or agencies that can help him stop smoking.

Pulmonary embolism and infarction

Pulmonary embolism is an obstruction of the pulmonary arterial bed that occurs when a mass — such as a dislodged thrombus — lodges in a pulmonary artery branch, partially or completely obstructing it. This causes a ventilation-perfusion mismatch, resulting in hypoxemia, as well as intrapulmonary shunting.

Although pulmonary infarction that results from embolism may be so mild that it's asymptomatic, massive embolism (more than 50% obstruction of pulmonary arterial circulation) and infarction can cause rapid death.

Causes

In most patients, pulmonary embolism results from a dislodged thrombus (blood clot) that originates in the leg veins. More than half of such thrombi arise in the deep veins of the legs; usually multiple thrombi arise. Other, less common sources of thrombi include the pelvic, renal, and hepatic veins; the right side of the heart; and the upper extremities.

Rarely, pulmonary embolism results from other types of emboli, including bone, air, fat, amniotic fluid, tumor cells, or a foreign object, such as a needle, a catheter part, or talc (from drugs intended for oral administration that are injected I.V. by addicts).

The risk increases with long-term immobility, chronic pulmonary disease, heart failure or atrial fibrillation, thrombophlebitis, polycythemia vera, thrombocytosis, cardiac arrest, defibrillation, cardioversion, autoimmune hemolytic anemia, sickle cell disease, varicose veins, recent surgery, age older than 40, osteomyelitis, pregnancy, lower-extremity fractures or surgery, burns, obesity, vascular injury, cancer, and oral contraceptive use.

If the embolus totally obstructs the arterial blood supply, pulmonary infarction (lung tissue death) occurs, a complication that affects about 10% of pulmonary embolism patients. It's more likely to occur if the patient has chronic cardiac or pulmonary disease. Other complications include emboli extension, which blocks further vessels; hepatic congestion and necrosis; pulmonary abscess; shock and adult respiratory distress syndrome; massive atelectasis; venous overload; ventilation-perfusion mismatch; and death from massive embolism.

Assessment findings

The patient's history may reveal a predisposing condition. He may also complain of shortness of breath for no apparent reason, as well as pleuritic or anginal pain. The severity of these symptoms depends on the extent of damage. The signs and symptoms produced by small or fragmented emboli depend on their size, number, and location. If the embolus totally occludes the main pulmonary artery, the patient has severe signs and symptoms.

The patient may have tachycardia and low-grade fever. If circulatory collapse has occurred, he has a weak, rapid pulse rate and hypotension. On inspection, you may note a productive cough, possibly producing blood-tinged sputum. Less commonly, you may observe chest splinting, massive hemoptysis, leg edema and, with a large embolus, cyanosis, syncope, and distended neck veins. If you observe restlessness — a sign of hypoxia — the patient may have circulatory collapse.

Palpation may reveal a warm, tender area in the extremities, a possible area of thrombosis. On auscultation, you may hear transient pleural friction rub and crackles at the embolus site. You may also note third and fourth heart sounds, with increased intensity of the pulmonic component of the second heart sound.

A patient with pleural infarction may have a history of heart disease and left-sided heart failure. He may complain of sudden, sharp pleuritic chest pain accompanied by progressive dyspnea. On inspection, you may note that the patient has a fever and is coughing up blood-tinged sputum. Auscultation may reveal a pleural friction rub.

Diagnostic tests

Lung perfusion scan (lung scintiscan) reveals a pulmonary embolus, and ventilation scan (usually performed with a lung perfusion scan) confirms the diagnosis. Pulmonary angiography may show a pulmonary vessel filling defect or an abrupt vessel ending, both of which indicate pulmonary embolism.

Electrocardiography (ECG) helps to distinguish pulmonary embolism from myocardial infarction. If the patient has an extensive embolism, the ECG shows right axis deviation, right bundle-branch block, tall peaked P waves, ST-segment depression, T-wave inversion (a sign of right ventricular heart strain), and supraventricular tachyarrhythmias.

Chest X-ray helps to rule out other pulmonary diseases, although it's inconclusive in the 1 to 2 hours after embolism. It may also show areas of atelectasis, an elevated diaphragm, pleural effusion, a prominent pulmonary artery and, occasionally, the characteristic wedge-shaped infiltrate that suggests pulmonary infarction.

Arterial blood gas analysis sometimes reveals decreased levels of the partial pressures of arterial oxygen and carbon dioxide from tachypnea. Thoracentesis may rule out empyema, a sign of pneumonia, if the patient has pleural effusion.

Magnetic resonance imaging can identify blood flow changes that point to an embolus or identify the embolus itself.

Treatment

The goal of treatment is to maintain adequate cardiovascular and pulmonary function until the obstruction resolves and to prevent recurrence. (Most emboli resolve within 10 to 14 days.)

Treatment for an embolism caused by a thrombus generally consists of oxygen therapy as needed and anticoagulation with heparin to inhibit new thrombus formation. A patient undergoing heparin therapy needs daily or frequent coagulation studies (partial thromboplastin time [PTT]). The patient may also receive warfarin for 3 to 6 months, depending on his risk factors. The patient's prothrombin time should be monitored daily and then biweekly.

If the patient has a massive pulmonary embolism and shock, he may need fibrinolytic therapy with urokinase, streptokinase, or alteplase. Initially, these thrombolytics dissolve clots within 12 to 24 hours. Within 7 days, these drugs lyse clots to the same degree as heparin therapy alone.

If the embolus causes hypotension, the patient may need a vasopressor. A septic embolus requires an antibiotic, not an anticoagulant, and evaluation for the infection's source, which is most likely endocarditis.

If the patient can't take an anticoagulant or develops recurrent emboli during anticoagulant therapy, surgery is needed. Surgery consists of vena caval ligation, plication, or insertion of a device (umbrella filter) to filter blood returning to the heart and lungs. Angiographic demonstration of pulmonary embolism should take place before surgery. To prevent postoperative venous thromboembolism, the patient may require a vascular compression device applied to his legs. Or he can receive a combination of heparin and dihydroergotamine, which is more effective than heparin alone.

If the patient has a fat embolus, oxygen therapy is needed. He may also need mechanical ventilation, a corticosteroid and, if pulmonary edema arises, a diuretic.

Nursing interventions

■ As ordered, administer oxygen and monitor effects. If the patient's breathing is severely compromised, provide endotracheal intubation with assisted ventilation as ordered.
■ Administer heparin as ordered by I.V. push or continuous drip. Monitor coagulation studies frequently. Effective heparin therapy raises PTT to about 2 to 215 times normal.
■ During heparin therapy, watch closely for epistaxis, petechiae, and other signs of abnormal bleeding. Also check the patient's stools for occult blood. Don't administer I.M. injections.
■ After the patient's condition stabilizes, encourage him to move about, and assist with isometric and range-of-motion exercises. Check his temperature and the color of his feet to detect venous stasis. Never vigorously massage his legs; that could cause thrombi to dislodge.
■ Apply antiembolism stockings to promote venous return.
■ If the patient needs surgery, make sure he ambulates as soon as possible afterward to prevent venous stasis.
■ If the patient has pleuritic chest pain, administer the ordered analgesic.
■ If needed, provide incentive spirometry to help the patient with deep breathing.

Patient teaching
■ Teach the patient and family members the signs and symptoms of thrombophlebitis and pulmonary embolism.
■ Teach the patient on anticoagulant therapy the signs of bleeding to watch for — bloody stools, blood in urine, large bruises.
■ Tell the patient he can help prevent bleeding by shaving with an electric razor and by brushing his teeth with a soft toothbrush.

■ Tell him not to take other medications, especially aspirin, without asking the doctor.

■ Stress the importance of follow-up laboratory tests such as prothrombin time to monitor anticoagulant therapy.

■ Tell the patient that he must inform all his health care providers — including dentists — that he's taking an anticoagulant.

■ Instruct the patient taking warfarin not to significantly vary the amount of vitamin K he ingests daily. Doing so could interfere with anticoagulation stabilization.

■ To prevent pulmonary emboli in a high-risk patient, encourage him to walk and exercise his legs and to wear support or antiembolism stockings. Tell him not to cross or massage his legs.

Renal failure, acute

About 5% of all hospitalized patients develop acute renal failure, the sudden interruption of renal function resulting from obstruction, reduced circulation, or renal parenchymal disease. This condition is classified as prerenal, intrarenal, or postrenal and normally passes through three distinct phases: oliguric, diuretic, and recovery. It's usually reversible with medical treatment. If not treated, it may progress to end-stage renal disease, uremia, and death.

Causes

The three types of acute renal failure each have separate causes. Prerenal failure results from conditions that diminish blood flow to the kidneys. Between 40% and 80% of all cases of acute renal failure are caused by prerenal azotemia. Intrarenal failure (also called intrinsic or parenchymal renal failure) results from damage to the kidneys themselves, usually from acute tubular necrosis. Postrenal failure results from bilateral obstruction of urine outflow.

Ischemic acute tubular necrosis can lead to renal shutdown. Electrolyte imbalance, metabolic acidosis, and other severe effects follow as the patient becomes increasingly uremic and renal dysfunction disrupts other body systems. If left untreated, the patient dies. Even with treatment, an elderly patient is particularly susceptible to volume overload, precipitating acute pulmonary edema, hypertensive crisis, hyperkalemia, and infection.

Assessment findings

The patient's history may include a disorder that can cause renal failure, and he may have a recent history of fever, chills, central nervous system (CNS) problems such as headache, and GI problems, such as anorexia, nausea, vomiting, diarrhea, and constipation.

The patient may appear irritable, drowsy, and confused or demonstrate other alterations in his level of consciousness. In advanced stages, seizures and coma may occur. Depending on the stage of renal failure, his urine output may be oliguric (less than 400 ml/24 hours) or anuric (less than 100 ml/24 hours).

Inspection may uncover evidence of bleeding abnormalities, such as petechiae and ecchymoses. Hematemesis may occur. The skin may be dry and pruritic and, rarely, you may note uremic frost. Mucous membranes may be dry, and the patient's breath may have a uremic odor. If the patient has hyperkalemia, muscle weakness may occur.

Auscultation may reveal tachycardia and, possibly, an irregular rhythm. Bibasilar crackles may be heard if the patient has heart failure. Palpation and percussion may reveal abdominal pain if pancreatitis or peritonitis occurs and may reveal peripheral edema if the patient has heart failure.

Diagnostic tests

Blood test results indicating acute intrarenal failure include elevated blood urea nitrogen, serum creatinine, and potassium levels, and low blood pH, low bicarbonate and hemoglobin levels, and low hematocrit.

Urine specimens show casts, cellular debris, decreased specific gravity and, in patients with glomerular disease, proteinuria and urine osmolality close to serum osmolality. The urine sodium level is less than 20 mEq/L if oliguria results from decreased perfusion and more than 40 mEq/L if it results from an intrarenal problem. A creatinine clearance test measures the glomerular filtration rate and allows for an estimate of the number of remaining functioning nephrons.

Other studies used to determine the cause of renal failure include kidney ultrasonography, plain films of the abdomen, kidney-ureter-bladder radiography, excretory urography, renal scan, retrograde pyelography, computed tomography scans, and nephrotomography.

Treatment

Supportive measures include a diet high in calories and low in protein, sodium, and potassium, with supplemental vitamins and restricted fluids. Meticulous electrolyte monitoring is essential to detect hyperkalemia. If hyperkalemia occurs, acute therapy may include hypertonic glucose-and-insulin infusions and sodium bicarbonate — all administered I.V. — and sodium polystyrene sulfonate (Kayexalate) by mouth or enema to remove potassium from the body.

If measures fail to control uremic symptoms, the patient may require hemodialysis or peritoneal dialysis. Early initiation of diuretic therapy during the oliguric phase may benefit the patient.

Nursing interventions

■ Measure and record intake and output of all fluids, including wound drainage, nasogastric tube output, and diarrhea.
■ Weigh the patient daily. You may need to measure abdominal girth every day. Mark the skin with indelible ink so that measurements can be taken in the same place.
■ Evaluate all drugs the patient is taking to identify those that may affect or be affected by renal function.
■ Monitor vital signs. Watch for and report signs of pericarditis (pleuritic chest pain, tachycardia, and pericardial friction rub), inadequate renal perfusion (hypotension), and acidosis.
■ Maintain proper electrolyte balance. Strictly monitor potassium levels. Watch for signs and symptoms of hyperkalemia (malaise, anorexia, paresthesia, muscle weakness, and electrocardiogram changes), and report them immediately.
■ If the patient receives hypertonic glucose-and-insulin infusions, monitor potassium and glucose levels. If you give sodium polystyrene sulfonate rectally, make sure the patient doesn't retain it and become constipated. This can lead to bowel perforation.
■ Maintain nutritional status. Provide a diet high in calories and low in protein, sodium, and potassium, with vitamin supplements. Give the anorexic patient small, frequent meals.
■ Prevent complications of immobility by encouraging frequent coughing and deep breathing and by performing passive range-of-motion exercises. Help the patient walk as soon as possible. Add lubricating lotion to his bath water to combat skin dryness.

■ Provide mouth care frequently to lubricate dry mucous membranes. If stomatitis occurs, use an antibiotic solution, if ordered, and have the patient swish it around in the mouth before swallowing.

■ Monitor for GI bleeding by testing all stools for occult blood using the guaiac test. Administer medications carefully, especially antacids and stool softeners.

■ Use appropriate safety measures, such as bed rails and restraints, because the patient with CNS involvement may become dizzy or confused.

■ If the patient requires hemodialysis, check the blood access site (arteriovenous fistula or subclavian or femoral catheter) every 2 hours for patency and signs of clotting. Don't use the arm with the shunt or fistula for measuring blood pressure or drawing blood. Weigh the patient before beginning dialysis.

■ During hemodialysis, monitor vital signs, clotting times, blood flow, vascular access site function, and arterial and venous pressures. Watch for complications, such as septicemia, embolism, hepatitis, and rapid fluid and electrolyte losses.

■ After hemodialysis, monitor vital signs, check the vascular access site, weigh the patient, and watch for signs of fluid and electrolyte imbalances.

■ If the patient requires peritoneal dialysis, position him carefully, elevating the head of the bed to reduce pressure on the diaphragm and aid respiration. If pain occurs, reduce the amount of dialysate. Periodically monitor the diabetic patient's blood glucose levels, and administer insulin as ordered. Watch for complications, such as peritonitis, atelectasis, hypokalemia, pneumonia, and shock.

Patient teaching

■ Stress the importance of following the prescribed diet and fluid allowance.

■ Instruct the patient to weigh himself daily and report changes of 3 lb (1.4 kg) or more immediately.

■ Advise the patient to avoid overexertion. If he becomes dyspneic or short of breath during normal activity, tell him to report it to his doctor.

■ Teach the patient how to recognize edema, and tell him to report this finding to the doctor.

Renal failure, chronic

Chronic renal failure is usually the end result of a gradually progressive loss of renal function. It also occasionally results from a rapidly progressive disease of sudden onset that gradually destroys the nephrons and eventually causes irreversible renal damage. Few symptoms develop until after more than 75% of glomerular filtration is lost.

Chronic renal failure may progress through several stages. Reduced renal reserve occurs when the glomerular filtration rate (GFR) is 5% to 50% of normal; renal insufficiency, when the GFR is 20% to 35% of normal; renal failure, when the GFR is 20% to 25% of normal; and end-stage renal disease, when the GFR is less than 20% of normal. This syndrome is fatal without treatment, but maintenance dialysis or a kidney transplant can sustain life.

Causes

Chronic renal failure may result from chronic glomerular disease, chronic infections, congenital anomalies, vascular diseases, obstructive processes (such as calculi), collagen diseases (such as systemic lupus erythematosus), nephrotoxic agents, and endocrine diseases. If this condition continues unchecked, uremic toxins accumulate and produce potentially fatal physiologic changes in all major organ systems. Even if the patient can tolerate life-sustaining maintenance dialysis or a kidney transplant, he may still have anemia, peripheral neuropathy, cardiopulmonary and GI complications, sexual dysfunction, and skeletal defects.

Assessment findings

The patient's history may include a disease or condition that can cause renal failure, but he may not have symptoms for a long time. Symptoms usually occur by the time the GFR is 20% to 35% of normal; and almost all body systems are affected. Assessment findings reflect involvement of each system; many findings reflect involvement of more than one system.

■ *Renal*—With certain fluid and electrolyte imbalances, the kidneys can't retain salt, and hyponatremia occurs. The patient may complain of dry mouth, fatigue, and nausea. You may note hypotension, loss of skin turgor, and listlessness that may progress to somnolence and confusion. Later, as the number of functioning nephrons decreases, so does the kidneys' capacity to excrete sodium and potassium. Urine output decreases, and the urine is very dilute, with casts and crystals present. Accumulation of potassium causes muscle irritability and then muscle weakness, irregular pulses, and life-threatening cardiac arrhythmias as serum potassium levels increase. Sodium retention causes fluid overload, and edema is palpable. Metabolic acidosis also occurs.

■ *Cardiovascular*—When the cardiovascular system is involved, hypertension and life-threatening cardiac arrhythmias can occur. With pericardial involvement, you may auscultate a pericardial friction rub. Heart sounds may be distant if pericardial effusion is present. Bibasilar crackles may be aus-

cultated, and peripheral edema may be palpated if heart failure occurs.

■ *Respiratory*—Pulmonary changes include reduced pulmonary macrophage activity with increased susceptibility to infection. If pneumonia is present, breath sounds may be decreased over areas of consolidation. Bibasilar crackles indicate pulmonary edema. With pleural involvement, the patient may complain of pleuritic pain, and you may auscultate a pleural friction rub. Kussmaul's respirations occur with metabolic acidosis.

■ *GI*—With inflammation and ulceration of GI mucosa, inspection of the mouth may reveal gum ulceration and bleeding and, possibly, parotitis. The patient may complain of hiccups, a metallic taste in the mouth, anorexia, nausea, and vomiting caused by esophageal, stomach, or bowel involvement. You may note a uremic fetor (ammonia smell) to the breath. Abdominal palpation and percussion may elicit pain.

■ *Skin*—Inspection of the skin typically reveals a pallid, yellowish bronze color. The skin is dry and scaly with purpura, ecchymoses, petechiae, uremic frost (usually found in critically ill or terminal patients), and thin, brittle fingernails with characteristic lines. The hair is dry and brittle; it may change color and fall out easily. The patient usually complains of severe itching.

■ *Neurologic*—You may note that the patient has alterations in level of consciousness that may progress from mild behavior changes, shortened memory and attention span, apathy, drowsiness, and irritability to confusion, coma, and seizures. The patient may complain of muscle cramps, fasciculations, and twitching, which are caused by muscle irritability. He may also complain of restless leg syndrome. One of the first signs of peripheral neuropathy, restless leg syndrome causes pain, burning, and itching in the legs and feet that may be relieved by voluntarily shaking, moving, or rocking them. This condition eventually progresses to paresthesia, motor nerve dysfunction (usually bilateral footdrop) and, unless dialysis is initiated, flaccid paralysis.

■ *Endocrine* — Children with chronic renal failure exhibit growth retardation, even with elevated growth hormone levels. Adults may have a history of infertility, decreased libido, amenorrhea in women, and impotence in men.

■ *Hematologic* — Inspection may reveal purpura, GI bleeding and hemorrhage from body orifices, easy bruising, ecchymoses, and petechiae caused by thrombocytopenia and platelet defects.

■ *Musculoskeletal* — The patient may have a history of pathologic fractures and complain of bone and muscle pain caused by calcium-phosphorus imbalance and consequent parathyroid hormone imbalances. You may note gait abnormalities or, possibly, an inability to ambulate. Children may have impaired bone growth and bowed legs from rickets.

Diagnostic tests

Various laboratory findings aid in the diagnosis and monitoring of chronic renal failure. For example, blood studies show elevated blood urea nitrogen, serum creatinine, sodium, and potassium levels; decreased arterial pH and bicarbonate levels; low hemoglobin levels and hematocrit; decreased red blood cell (RBC) survival time; mild thrombocytopenia; platelet defects; and metabolic acidosis. They also show increased aldosterone secretion and increased blood glucose levels. Hypertriglyceridemia and decreased high-density lipoprotein levels are common.

Arterial blood gas analysis reveals metabolic acidosis. Urine specific gravity becomes fixed at 1.010; urinalysis may show proteinuria, glycosuria, RBCs, leukocytes, and casts and crystals, depending on the cause. X-ray studies, including kidney-ureter-bladder radiography, excretory urography, nephrotomography, renal scan, and renal arteriography show reduced kidney size. Renal biopsy allows histologic identification of the underlying pathology. EEG shows changes that indicate metabolic encephalopathy.

Treatment

The goal of conservative treatment is to correct specific symptoms. A low-protein diet reduces the production of end products of protein metabolism that the kidneys can't excrete. (A patient receiving continuous peritoneal dialysis should have a high-protein diet.) A high-calorie diet prevents ketoacidosis and the negative nitrogen balance that results in catabolism and tissue atrophy. The diet should restrict sodium, phosphorus, and potassium.

Maintaining fluid balance requires careful monitoring of vital signs, weight changes, and urine volume (if not anuric). Fluid retention can be reduced with a loop diuretic and with fluid restriction. Small doses of a cardiac glycoside may be used to mobilize the fluids causing the edema; an antihypertensive may be used to control blood pressure and associated edema.

An antiemetic taken before meals may relieve nausea and vomiting, and cimetidine or ranitidine may decrease gastric irritation. Methylcellulose or docusate can help prevent constipation. Anemia necessitates iron and folate supplements; severe anemia requires transfusions. Synthetic erythropoietin (epoetin alfa) stimulates production of RBCs.

Drug therapy commonly relieves associated symptoms. An antipruritic can relieve itching, and aluminum hydroxide gel can lower serum phosphate levels. The patient also may benefit from supplementary vitamins (particularly vitamins B and D) and essential amino acids. Severe hyperkalemia includes dialysis therapy and administration of 50% hypertonic glucose I.V., regular insulin, calcium gluconate I.V., sodium bicarbonate I.V., and cation exchange resins such as sodium polystyrene sulfonate. Cardiac tamponade resulting from pericardial effusion may require emergency pericardial tap or surgery. Calcium and phosphorus imbalances may be treated with phosphate binding agents, calcium supplements, and reduction of phosphorus in the diet. If hyperparathyroidism develops secondary to low serum calcium levels, a parathyroidectomy may be performed.

Intensive dialysis and thoracentesis can relieve pulmonary edema and pleural effusion. Hemodialysis or peritoneal dialysis (continuous ambulatory peritoneal dialysis and continuous cyclic peritoneal dialysis) can help control most signs and symptoms of end-stage renal disease. Altering the dialysate can correct fluid and electrolyte disturbances. However, maintenance dialysis itself may produce complications, including serum hepatitis (hepatitis B) from numerous blood transfusions, protein wasting, refractory ascites, and dialysis dementia.

Nursing interventions

■ Provide good skin care. Bathe the patient daily, using superfatted soaps, oatmeal baths, and skin lotion to ease pruritus. Pad the bed rails to guard against ecchymoses. Turn the patient often, and use a convoluted foam or low-pressure mattress to prevent skin breakdown.
■ Provide good oral hygiene. Hard candy and mouthwash minimize metallic taste in the mouth and alleviate thirst.
■ Offer small, palatable, nutritious meals and encourage intake of high-calorie foods.
■ As potassium levels increase, watch for muscle irritability, weak pulse rate, and electrocardiogram changes.
■ Carefully assess the patient's hydration status by intake and output (including drainage, emesis, diarrhea, and blood loss), daily weight, thirst, hypertension, and peripheral edema.
■ Monitor patient for bone or joint complications. Prevent pathologic fractures by turning the patient carefully and ensuring his safety. Perform passive range-of-motion exercises for the bedridden patient.
■ Encourage the patient to perform deep-breathing and coughing exercises to prevent pulmonary congestion. Watch for clinical signs of pulmonary edema.
■ Carefully monitor neurologic status, signs of bleeding, and complications (such as pericarditis and tamponade).
■ Schedule medication administration carefully. Give iron before meals, aluminum hydroxide gels after meals, and antiemetics (as necessary) a half hour before meals. Recommend antacid cookies as an alternative to aluminum hydroxide gels needed to bind GI phosphate. Don't give magnesium products because poor renal excretion can lead to toxic levels.
■ If the patient requires dialysis, check the vascular access site every 2 hours for patency and the arm used for adequate blood supply and intact nerve function (check temperature, pulse rate, capillary refill time, and sensation). Don't use the arm with the vascular access site to take blood pressure readings, draw blood, or give injections because these procedures may rupture the fistula or occlude blood flow.

■ Withhold the morning dose of antihypertensive on the day of dialysis, and instruct the patient to do the same.
■ After dialysis, check for disequilibrium syndrome, a result of sudden correction of blood chemistry abnormalities. Signs and symptoms range from a headache to seizures. Also, check for excessive bleeding from the dialysis site, and apply a pressure dressing or an absorbable gelatin sponge as indicated. Monitor blood pressure carefully after dialysis.

Patient teaching

■ Tell the patient to report leg cramps or excessive muscle twitching. Stress the importance of keeping follow-up appointments to have his electrolyte levels monitored.
■ Tell the patient to avoid high-sodium and high-potassium foods. Encourage adherence to fluid and protein restrictions. To prevent constipation, stress the need for exercise and sufficient dietary fiber.
■ If the patient requires dialysis, teach the patient and family members regarding the procedure.
■ Demonstrate how to care for the shunt, fistula, or other vascular access device and how to perform meticulous skin care. Discourage activity that might cause the patient to bump or irritate the access site.
■ Suggest that the patient wear a medical identification bracelet or carry pertinent information with him.

Rheumatoid arthritis

Rheumatoid arthritis is a chronic, systemic, symmetrical inflammatory disease. It primarily attacks peripheral joints and surrounding muscles, tendons, ligaments, and blood vessels. Spontaneous remissions and unpredictable exacerbations mark the course of this potentially crippling disease. A similar condition, psoriatic arthritis, has the same arthritic component along with psoriasis of the skin and nails.

Rheumatoid arthritis usually requires lifelong treatment and, sometimes, surgery. In most patients, the disease follows an intermittent course and allows normal activity. The prognosis worsens with the development of nodules, vasculitis, and high titers of rheumatoid factor (RF).

Causes

The cause of the chronic inflammation characteristic of rheumatoid arthritis isn't known, but infection (viral or bacterial), hormonal factors, and lifestyle may influence disease onset. Some patients develop an immunoglobulin (Ig) M antibody against their body's own IgG, which is called RF.

If joint inflammation isn't arrested, it progresses to destruction of the joint capsule and bone and eventual bone atrophy and misalignment, causing visible deformities. Muscle atrophy, imbalance and, possibly, partial dislocations or subluxations finally result with fibrous calcification, bony ankylosis, and immobility. Pain associated with movement may restrict active joint use and cause fibrous or bony ankylosis, soft-tissue contractures, and joint deformities. Vasculitis can lead to skin lesions, leg ulcers, and multisystem complications.

Assessment findings

The patient's history may reveal an insidious onset of nonspecific signs and symptoms, including fatigue, malaise, anorexia, persistent low-grade fever, weight loss, and vague articular symptoms. Later, more specific localized articular signs and symptoms develop, commonly in the fingers at the proximal interphalangeal, metacarpophalangeal, and metatarsophalangeal joints. These signs and symptoms usually occur bilaterally and symmetrically and can extend to the wrists, elbows, knees, and ankles. Articular signs and symptoms include painful, red, swollen arms and stiff joints.

The patient may report that affected joints stiffen after inactivity, especially on rising in the morning. He may complain that his joints are tender and painful, at first only when he moves them but eventually even at rest. Ultimately, joint function is diminished. He may experience paresthesia (in the fingers) and stiff, weak, or painful muscles. If the patient has peripheral neuropathy, numbness or tingling in the feet or weakness or loss of sensation in the fingers can occur. If pleuritis develops, he may complain of pain on inspiration. The patient with pulmonary nodules or fibrosis may complain of shortness of breath.

Inspection of the patient's joints may show deformities and contractures. Proximal interphalangeal joints may develop flexion deformities or become hyperextended. Metacarpophalangeal joints may swell dorsally, and volar subluxation and stretching of tendons may pull the fingers to the ulnar side (ulnar drift). The fingers may become spindle shaped and fixed in a swan-neck or boutonnière deformity. The hands appear foreshortened and the wrists appear boggy. Inspection of pressure areas may reveal rheumatoid nodules. If the patient has vasculitis, you may observe lesions, leg ulcers, and multisystem complications. If he has scleritis or episcleritis, you may observe redness of the eye.

Palpation may reveal joints that are warm to the touch. If the patient has pericarditis, auscultation may reveal pericardial friction rub (although pericarditis may produce no signs). If spinal cord compression occurs, your assessment may reveal signs of upper motor neuron disorder, such as a positive Babinski's sign and weakness. Other extra-articular findings include temporomandibular joint disease, infection, osteoporosis, myositis, cardiopulmonary lesions, lymphadenopathy, and peripheral neuritis.

Diagnostic tests

No test definitively diagnoses rheumatoid arthritis, but several are useful. In early stages, X-rays show bone demineralization and soft-tissue swelling. Later, they help determine the extent of cartilage and bone destruction, erosion, subluxations, and deformities. They also show the characteristic pattern of these abnormalities, particularly symmetrical involvement, although no particular pattern is conclusive for rheumatoid arthritis.

An RF test is positive in 75% to 80% of patients, as indicated by a titer of 1:160 or higher. Although the presence of RF doesn't confirm rheumatoid arthritis, it does help determine the prognosis; a patient with a high titer usually has more severe and progressive disease with extra-articular signs and symptoms.

Synovial fluid analysis shows increased volume and turbidity but decreased viscosity and complement (C3 and C4) levels. The white blood cell count often exceeds 10,000/µl. A serum protein electrophoresis test may show elevated serum globulin levels. The erythrocyte sedimentation rate (ESR) is elevated in 85% to 90% of patients. Because an elevated ESR typically parallels disease activity, this test may help monitor the patient's response to therapy (as may a C-reactive protein test).

Magnetic resonance imaging and computed tomography scans may provide information about the extent of damage.

Classifying rheumatoid arthritis

The American Rheumatism Association classifies rheumatoid arthritis according to certain basic criteria.

Guidelines

A patient who meets four of seven criteria is classified as having rheumatoid arthritis. He must experience the first four criteria for at least 6 weeks, and a doctor must observe the second through fifth criteria.

A patient with two or more other clinical diagnoses can also be diagnosed with rheumatoid arthritis.

Criteria

■ Morning stiffness in and around the joints that lasts for 1 hour before full improvement
■ Arthritis in three or more joint areas, with at least three joint areas (as observed by a doctor) exhibiting soft-tissue swelling or joint effusions, not just bony overgrowth (the 14 possible areas involved include the right and left proximal interphalangeal, metacarpophalangeal, wrist, elbow, knee, ankle, and metatarsophalangeal joints)
■ Arthritis of hand joints, including the wrist, the metacarpophalangeal joint, or the proximal interphalangeal joint
■ Arthritis that involves the same joint areas on both sides of the body
■ Subcutaneous rheumatoid nodules over bony prominences
■ Demonstration of abnormal amounts of serum rheumatoid factor by any method that produces a positive result in less than 5% of patients without rheumatoid arthritis
■ Radiographic changes, usually on posteroanterior hand and wrist radiographs; these changes must show erosions or unequivocal bony decalcification localized in or most noticeable adjacent to the involved joints.

The criteria for classifying rheumatoid arthritis developed by the American Rheumatism Association can also serve as guidelines for establishing a diagnosis. (See *Classifying rheumatoid arthritis*.)

Treatment

Treatment goals include reducing the patient's pain and inflammation, preserving functional capacity, resolving pathologic processes, and bringing about improvement.

Salicylates, particularly aspirin, are the mainstay of therapy because they decrease inflammation and relieve joint pain. The patient may also receive another nonsteroidal anti-inflammatory drug, an antimalarial, gold salts, penicillamine, and a corticosteroid, although corticosteroid therapy can cause osteoporosis. Other therapeutic drugs include immunosuppressants, which are used in the early stages of the disease.

Supportive measures include increased sleep (8 to 10 hours every night), frequent rest periods between daily activities, and splinting to rest inflamed joints (although, like corticosteroid therapy, immobilization can cause osteoporosis).

A physical therapy program that includes range-of-motion exercises and carefully individualized therapeutic exercises forestalls the loss of joint function; application of heat relaxes muscles and relieves pain. Moist heat (hot soaks, paraffin baths, whirlpools) usually works best for patients with chronic disease. Ice packs help during acute episodes.

Early intervention, under the guidance of an occupational therapist, with splinting and joint protection devices can delay the progression of joint deformities. A well-balanced diet and weight control along with the use of adaptive devices and ambulatory support (such as a cane, crutches, and a walker) are beneficial.

Useful surgical procedures include arthroplasty and insertion of a Silastic prosthesis between joints, arthrodesis (joint fusion), synovectomy, and osteotomy. Tendons that rupture spontaneously require surgical repair. Tendon transfers can prevent deformities or relieve contractures. The patient may need joint reconstruction or total joint arthroplasty in advanced disease.

Nursing interventions

General

■ Perform meticulous skin care. Check for rheumatoid nodules. Also, monitor for pressure ulcers and skin breakdown, especially if the patient is in traction or wearing splints.

■ Monitor the duration of morning stiffness. Duration, rather than intensity of the stiffness, more accurately reflects the severity of the disease.

■ Use occupational therapy and physical therapy to help the patient develop methods to make it easier for him to perform activities of daily living, such as dressing and feeding himself. Allow him enough time to calmly perform these tasks.

After total knee or hip arthroplasty

■ Monitor and record vital signs. Watch for complications, such as steroid crisis and shock in a patient receiving corticosteroids. Monitor the patient's distal leg pulses often, marking them with a waterproof marker to make them easier to find.

■ As soon as the patient awakens, have him perform active dorsiflexion. Supervise isometric exercises every 2 hours. After total hip arthroplasty, check traction for pressure areas, and keep the head of the bed raised between 30 and 45 degrees.

■ Change or reinforce dressings as needed using aseptic technique. Check wounds for hematoma, excessive drainage, color changes, and foul odor — all possible signs of hemorrhage or infection.

■ Monitor serum electrolyte and hemoglobin levels as well as hematocrit.

■ Have the patient turn, cough, and breathe deeply every 2 hours; then percuss his chest.

■ After total knee arthroplasty, keep the patient's leg extended and slightly elevated.

■ After total hip arthroplasty, keep the patient's hip in abduction to prevent dislocation. Watch for and immediately report any inability to rotate the hip or bear weight on it, increased pain, or a leg that appears shorter. All may indicate dislocation.

■ As soon as possible, help the patient get out of bed and sit in a chair, keeping his weight on the unaffected side. When he's ready to walk, consult with the physical therapist for walking instruction and aids.

Patient teaching

■ Explain the nature of rheumatoid arthritis. Make sure the patient and his family understand that rheumatoid arthritis is a chronic disease that may require major changes in lifestyle and that miracle cures don't work.

■ Encourage a balanced diet, stress the need for weight control because obesity further stresses the joints.

■ Discuss the patient's sexual concerns.

Living with rheumatoid arthritis

Follow these guidelines to help your patient learn to live with rheumatoid arthritis:

■ Teach the patient how to use correct posture when standing, sitting, and walking.

■ Recommend using chairs with high seats and armrests.

■ Recommend using a raised toilet seat.

■ Teach the patient proper body mechanics: avoiding flexion, keeping his hands close to the center of the body, and sliding rather than lifting objects.

■ Suggest that the patient take a hot shower or bath just before bed or in the morning to help relieve pain.

■ Refer the patient for physical and occupational therapy to help increase his mobility, strength, and ability to perform activities of daily living.

■ Reinforce instructions about the need for adaptive devices, such as dressing aids (long-handled shoehorn, reacher, elastic shoelaces, zipper pull, and buttonhook) and eating utensils.

■ Inspect the patient's home for possible safety hazards, and work with the patient and family to remove them. Encourage the use of grab bars and safety mats or strips in the tub or shower.

■ Advise the patient to save his strength by pacing his activities and dressing in a sitting position whenever possible.

■ Refer the patient to the Arthritis Foundation.

■ Review methods to assist the patient with day-to-day living. (See *Living with rheumatoid arthritis.*)

■ Teach postoperative exercises (such as isometrics), and supervise his practice. Also, teach the deep-breathing and coughing exercises he must perform after surgery.

■ Explain that total hip or knee arthroplasty requires frequent range-of-motion exercises of the leg after surgery; total knee arthroplasty also requires frequent leg-lift exercises.

■ Show the patient how to use a trapeze to move himself about in bed after surgery, and make sure he has a fracture bedpan handy.

■ After total knee arthroplasty, the patient's knee may be placed in a constant-passive-motion device to increase mobility and prevent emboli. After total hip arthroplasty, an abduction pillow is placed between the legs to help keep the hip prosthesis in place.

Seizure disorder

Seizure disorder, also known as epilepsy, is a condition of the brain characterized by a susceptibility to recurrent seizures. Seizures are paroxysmal events associated with abnormal electrical discharges of neurons in the brain. In most patients, this condition doesn't affect intelligence. About 80% of patients have good seizure control with strict adherence to prescribed treatment.

Causes

About half the cases of seizure disorders are idiopathic. No specific cause can be found, and the patient has no other neurologic abnormality. Nonidiopathic seizures may be caused by genetic abnormalities, perinatal injuries, metabolic abnormalities, brain tumors or other space-occupying lesions, infections (such as meningitis, encephalitis, or brain abscess), traumatic injury, ingestion of toxins (such as mercury, lead, or carbon monoxide), or cerebrovascular accident. Researchers also have detected hereditary EEG abnormalities in some families, and certain seizure disorders appear to have a familial incidence.

Assessment findings

Depending on the type and cause of the seizure, signs and symptoms vary. (See *Differentiating seizures,* pages 274 and 275.) Physical findings may be normal if the assessment is performed when the patient isn't having a seizure and the cause is idiopathic. If the seizure is associated with an underlying problem, the patient's history and physical examination should reveal signs and symptoms of that problem unless a brain tumor caused the seizure, in which case, no other symptoms may be apparent.

In many cases, the patient's history reveals that seizure occurrence is unpredictable and unrelated to activities. Occasionally, a patient may report precipitating factors or events. The patient may also report nonspecific changes, such as headache, mood changes, lethargy, and myoclonic jerking, occurring up to several hours before the onset of a seizure.

Patients who experience a generalized seizure may describe an aura (pungent smell, GI distress, a rising or sinking feeling in the stomach, a dreamy feeling, an unusual taste, or a visual disturbance such as a flashing light) that precedes seizure onset by a few seconds or minutes.

If you observe the patient during a seizure, note the type of seizure he's experiencing. Otherwise, details of what occurs during a seizure — obtained from a family member or friend, if necessary — may help to identify the seizure type.

Diagnostic tests

EEG can be used to identify paroxysmal abnormalities that may confirm the diagnosis of epilepsy by providing evidence of the continuing tendency to have seizures. A normal EEG doesn't rule out epilepsy because the paroxysmal abnormalities occur intermittently. The EEG also helps guide the prognosis and can help to classify the disorder.

Computed tomography scanning and magnetic resonance imaging provide density readings of the brain and may indicate abnormalities in internal structures. Other helpful tests include serum glucose and calcium studies, skull X-rays, lumbar puncture, brain scan, and cerebral angiography.

Treatment

Typically, treatment for seizures consists of drug therapy specific to the type of seizure. The most commonly prescribed drugs include phenytoin, carbamazepine, phenobarbital, and primidone administered individually for generalized tonic-clonic seizures and complex partial seizures. Valproic acid, clonazepam, and ethosuximide are commonly prescribed for absence seizures. Lamotrigine is also prescribed as adjunct therapy for partial seizures. Fosphenytoin is a new I.V. preparation that's effective in treatment.

If drug therapy fails, treatment may include surgical removal of a demonstrated focal lesion to attempt to end seizures. Surgery is also performed when epilepsy results from an underlying problem, such as intracranial tumors, a brain abscess or cyst, and vascular abnormalities.

Vagal nerve stimulation may be attempted. A pacemaker with a stimulator lead is placed on the vagus nerve. The nerve is stimulated for approximately 30 seconds every 5 minutes. This is useful

Differentiating seizures

The hallmark of epilepsy is recurring seizures, which can be classified as partial or generalized. Some patients may be affected by more than one type.

Partial seizures

Partial seizures arise from a localized area in the brain and cause specific symptoms. In some patients, partial seizure activity spreads to the entire brain, causing a generalized seizure. Partial seizures include simple partial (jacksonian motor-type and sensory-type), complex partial (psychomotor or temporal lobe), and secondarily generalized partial seizures.

Simple partial (jacksonian motor-type) seizure

This type of seizure begins as a localized motor seizure, which is characterized by a spread of abnormal activity to adjacent areas of the brain. Typically, the patient experiences stiffening or jerking in one extremity, accompanied by a tingling sensation in the same area. For example, the seizure may start in the thumb and spread to the entire hand and arm. The patient seldom loses consciousness, although the seizure may secondarily progress to a generalized tonic-clonic seizure.

Simple partial (sensory-type) seizure

Perception is distorted in this type of seizure. Signs and symptoms include hallucinations, flashing lights, tingling sensations, a foul odor, vertigo, and the feeling of having experienced something before.

Complex partial seizure

Signs and symptoms of complex partial seizure vary but usually include purposeless behavior. The patient may experience an aura and exhibit overt signs, including a glassy stare, picking at his clothes, aimless wandering, lip-smacking or chewing mo-

tions, and unintelligible speech. A seizure may last for a few seconds or as long as 20 minutes. Afterward, mental confusion may last for several minutes; as a result, an observer may mistakenly suspect psychosis or intoxication with alcohol or drugs. The patient has no memory of his actions during the seizure.

Secondarily generalized partial seizure

This type of seizure can be either simple or complex and can progress to generalized seizures. An aura may precede the progression. Loss of consciousness occurs immediately or within 1 to 2 minutes of the start of the progression.

Generalized seizures

As the term suggests, these seizures cause a generalized electrical abnormality in the brain. They include several distinct types.

Absence seizure

This type usually occurs in children but also may affect adults. It usually begins with a brief change in level of consciousness, indicated by blinking or rolling of the eyes, a blank stare, and slight mouth movements. The patient retains his posture and continues preseizure activity without difficulty. Typically, a seizure lasts from 1 to 10 seconds. The impairment is so brief that the patient is sometimes unaware of it. If not properly treated, these seizures can recur as often as 100 times a day. An absence seizure can progress to a generalized tonic-clonic seizure.

Myoclonic seizure

Myoclonic seizure — also called bilateral massive epileptic myoclonus — is marked by brief, involuntary muscular jerks of the body or extremities, which may occur in a

Differentiating seizures *(continued)*

rhythmic manner, and a brief loss of consciousness.

Generalized tonic–clonic seizure

Typically, this seizure begins with a loud cry, precipitated by air rushing from the lungs through the vocal cords. The patient falls to the ground, losing consciousness. The body stiffens (tonic phase) and then alternates between episodes of muscle spasm and relaxation (clonic phase). Tongue biting, incontinence, labored breathing, apnea, and subsequent cyanosis may also occur. The seizure stops in 2 to 5 minutes, when abnormal electrical conduction of the neurons is completed. The patient then regains consciousness but is somewhat confused and may have difficulty talking. If he can talk, he may complain of drowsiness, fatigue, headache, muscle soreness, and arm or leg weakness. He may fall into a deep sleep after the seizure.

Akinetic seizure

Akinetic seizure is characterized by a general loss of postural tone and a temporary loss of consciousness. This type of seizure occurs in young children. Sometimes it's called a drop attack because it causes the child to fall.

---

for those with refractory epilepsy because it decreases seizure frequency and intensity, diminishes the need for more medication, and increases the quality of life for some individuals.

Nursing interventions

■ If the patient is taking an anticonvulsant, constantly monitor him for signs and symptoms of toxic reaction, such as slurred speech, ataxia, lethargy, dizziness, drowsiness, nystagmus, irritability, nausea, and vomiting.
■ When administering phenytoin I.V., use a large vein, administer at a slow rate (not to exceed 50 mg/minute), and monitor the patient frequently.
■ If necessary, provide preoperative and postoperative care appropriate for the type of surgery the patient is to undergo.

Patient teaching

■ Answer any questions the patient and family members have about the condition. Help them to cope by dispelling myths. Provide assurance that most patients maintain a normal lifestyle.
■ Explain to the patient and family the need for compliance with the prescribed drug schedule. Reinforce dosage instructions, and find methods to help the patient remember to take medications. Caution the patient to monitor the amount of medication left so that he doesn't run out of it.
■ Explain the importance of having blood anticonvulsant levels checked at regular intervals, even if the seizures are under control.
■ If the patient is a candidate for surgery, provide appropriate preoperative teaching. Explain the care that the patient can expect postoperatively.
■ Know which social agencies in your community can help epileptic patients. Refer the patient to the Epilepsy Foundation of America for general information and to the state motor vehicle department for information about a driver's license.
■ Teach the patient's family how to care for the patient during a seizure.

Tuberculosis

Tuberculosis (TB) is an acute or chronic infection characterized by pulmonary infiltrates and by the formation of granulomas with caseation, fibrosis, and cavitation. Incidence is highest in people who live in crowded, poorly ventilated, unsanitary conditions, such as prisons, tenement houses, and homeless shelters. With proper treatment, the prognosis is usually excellent.

Causes

TB results from exposure to *Mycobacterium tuberculosis* and, sometimes, other strains of mycobacteria. Transmission occurs when an infected person coughs or sneezes, spreading infected droplets. TB can cause massive pulmonary tissue damage, with inflammation and tissue necrosis eventually leading to respiratory failure. Bronchopleural fistulas can develop from lung tissue damage, resulting in pneumothorax. The disease can also lead to hemorrhage, pleural effusion, and pneumonia. Small mycobacterial foci can infect other body organs, including the kidneys and the central nervous and skeletal systems. The patient may also develop complications such as liver involvement from drug therapy.

Assessment findings

The patient with a primary infection after an incubation period of 4 to 8 weeks is usually asymptomatic but may complain of weakness and fatigue, anorexia and weight loss, low-grade fever, and night sweats. The patient with reactivated TB may report chest pain and a cough that produces blood or mucopurulent or blood-tinged sputum. He may also have a low-grade fever.

When you percuss, you may note dullness over the affected area, a sign of consolidation or the presence of pleural fluid. On auscultation, you may hear crepitant crackles, bronchial breath sounds, wheezes, and whispered pectoriloquy.

Diagnostic tests

Several of the following tests may be necessary to distinguish TB from other diseases that may mimic it, such as lung carcinoma, lung abscess, pneumoconiosis, and bronchiectasis.

Chest X-rays show nodular lesions, patchy infiltrates (mainly in upper lobes), cavity formation, scar tissue, and calcium deposits. They may not help distinguish between active and inactive TB.

A tuberculin skin test reveals that the patient has been exposed to TB at some point, but it doesn't indicate active disease. In this test, intermediate-strength purified protein derivative or 5 tuberculin units (0.1 ml) are injected intradermally on the forearm and read in 48 to 72 hours. A positive reaction (greater than or equal to a 10-mm induration) develops within 2 to 10 weeks after exposure to the tubercle bacillus in both active and inactive TB.

Stains and cultures of sputum, cerebrospinal fluid, urine, drainage from abscess, or pleural fluid show heat-sensitive, nonmotile, aerobic, acid-fast bacilli.

Computed tomography scans or magnetic resonance imaging allow the evaluation of lung damage or confirm a difficult diagnosis. Bronchoscopy may be performed if the patient can't produce an adequate sputum specimen.

Treatment

Antituberculotic therapy — with daily oral doses of isoniazid, rifampin, and pyrazinamide (with ethambutol added in some cases) for at least 6 months —

usually cures TB. After 2 to 4 weeks, the disease is no longer infectious and the patient can resume normal activities, while continuing to take medication.

The patient with atypical mycobacterial disease or drug-resistant TB may require second-line drugs, such as capreomycin, streptomycin, paraaminosalicylic acid, pyrazinamide, and cycloserine.

Nursing interventions

■ Isolate the infectious patient in a quiet, properly ventilated room, as per guidelines from the Centers for Disease Control and Prevention, and maintain TB precautions.

■ Tell the patient to wear a mask when outside his room. Visitors and health care personnel should also take proper precautions while in the patient's room.

■ Provide the patient with well-balanced, high-calorie foods, preferably in small, frequent meals to conserve energy. (Small, frequent meals may also encourage the anorexic patient to eat more.) Record the patient's weight weekly.

■ Perform chest physiotherapy, including postural drainage and chest percussion, several times a day.

Patient teaching

■ Show the patient and family members how to perform postural drainage and chest percussion. Also, teach the patient coughing and deep-breathing techniques. Instruct him to maintain each position for 10 minutes and then to perform percussion and cough.

■ Emphasize the importance of regular follow-up examinations, and instruct the patient and family members concerning the signs and symptoms of recurring TB. Stress the importance of faithfully following long-term treatment.

■ Advise anyone exposed to an infected patient to receive tuberculin tests and, if a positive reaction occurs, chest X-rays and prophylactic isoniazid.

■ Warn the patient taking rifampin that the drug temporarily makes body secretions appear orange; reassure him that this effect is harmless. If the patient is a woman, warn her that oral contraceptives may be less effective while she's taking rifampin.

■ Instruct the patient to inform others of his disorder, such as dentists and other health care providers.

■ Stress the importance of hand washing and proper disposal of secretions.

■ Refer the patient to such support groups as the American Lung Association.

6

Surgical patient care
Reviewing the techniques

Preoperative care

Assessing the preoperative patient

A thorough preoperative assessment is the foundation of good surgical care, providing a baseline for comparison throughout a patient's treatment and recovery. This assessment also helps identify conditions that impair the patient's ability to tolerate the stress of surgery or to comply with postoperative routines.

Initial steps

Begin your preoperative assessment by focusing on problem areas suggested by the patient's history and on any body system directly affected by the surgical procedure:

■ Note your patient's general appearance. Does he look healthy and well nourished, or does he appear ill?
■ Record height, weight, and vital signs. Compare blood pressure bilaterally, using a cuff two-thirds the length of the patient's arm. Document the patient's position during this procedure.
■ Most patients are admitted the morning of surgery, so baseline vital signs are extremely important. Compare these values with any prehospital data, if available.
■ For inpatients, update vital sign measurements at least twice per day throughout the preoperative period. Use these measurements to establish a baseline.

Systematic examination

Examine your patient thoroughly from head to toe, using these procedures as a guide.

Head and neck

■ Check the patient's scalp for lesions or parasitic infection.
■ Check the jugular veins for distention.

■ Note the color of the sclerae; a yellowish color suggests jaundice.
■ Evert the lower eyelid and note the color of the conjunctiva; pale tissue suggests anemia.
■ Check the nose and throat for signs of respiratory tract infection.
■ Assess the mouth for sores, ulcerations, or bleeding of the tongue, gums, or cheeks. Check the lips for bluish or gray color, which may suggest cyanosis.
■ Check the neck for stiffness or cervical node enlargement.

Neurologic system

■ Assess the patient's level of consciousness. Note whether his pupils are uniform in size and shape.
■ Assess gross and fine motor movements.
■ Inform the doctor of any behavioral changes (for instance, from lethargy to agitation), which may indicate increased intracranial pressure.
■ Look for neurologic abnormalities such as slurred speech. If you know or suspect that your patient has a neurologic problem, conduct a complete neurologic examination.

Extremities and skin

■ Look for changes in skin color or temperature that suggest impaired circulation. Check for cyanotic nail beds and finger clubbing.
■ Note any skin lesions.
■ Assess skin turgor for signs of dehydration.
■ Check extremities for edema. Ask the patient if his feet, ankles, or fingers ever swell.
■ Note hair distribution on the patient's extremities. Uneven hair distribution suggests poor peripheral circulation.
■ Check all peripheral pulses (radial, pedal, femoral, and popliteal) bilaterally. Note any differences in quality, rate, or rhythm.

Respiratory system

■ Document the patient's respiratory rate and pattern. A patient with questionable pulmonary status may require an alternative to inhalation anesthesia such as a spinal block.

■ Assess breathing pattern. Check for asymmetrical chest expansion and accessory muscle use.

■ Auscultate the anterior and posterior chest for breath sounds. Listen for normal, abnormal, and adventitious sounds. Note dyspnea on exertion or resting.

■ Ask the patient whether he smokes. If he does, ask how many packs per day and whether he has recently tried to quit or cut down in anticipation of surgery. His doctor should have advised him to stop smoking 4 to 6 weeks before surgery.

Patient teaching tips While the immediate preoperative period isn't the time to have a lengthy discussion on smoking cessation, information can be placed with the patient's belongings and discussed postoperatively.

Cardiovascular system

■ Inspect the patient's chest for abnormal pulsations. Auscultate at the fifth intercostal space over the left midclavicular line. If you can't hear an apical pulse, ask the patient to turn onto his left side; the heart may shift closer to the chest wall. Note the rate and quality of the apical pulse.

■ Auscultate heart sounds. If you hear thrills, suspect mitral valve regurgitation or stenosis. Remember that murmurs you hear on the right side of the heart are more likely to change with respiration than those you hear on the left side.

■ Palpate the chest to find the point of maximal impulse.

GI system

■ Note the contour and symmetry of the abdomen; check for distention.

■ Note the position and color of the umbilicus; look for herniation.

■ Auscultate bowel sounds in each quadrant. Ask the patient if his bowel movements are regular. Note the date of his last bowel movement.

■ Percuss the abdomen for air and fluid.

■ Palpate the abdomen for softness, firmness, and bladder height. Note any tenderness.

■ Assess the six f's: fat, fluids, flatus, feces, fetus (if the patient is pregnant), and fibroid tissue (or any unusual mass).

Genitourinary system

■ Ask the patient if he ever experiences pain, burning, or bleeding during urination.

■ Also ask about urinary frequency and incontinence. Can he empty his bladder completely? Does he awaken at night to urinate?

■ If indicated, monitor urine output and try to correlate an excess or a deficit with blood urea nitrogen or creatinine levels. If urine output falls, first assess catheter patency and urinary drainage system patency, if applicable. Compare intake and output over the last several days as well as daily weights.

■ Note any discharge from the patient's genitalia.

■ If your patient is female, ask when her last menstrual period occurred and find out whether her cycle is regular. Also ask if she could be pregnant. If pregnancy is suspected, suggest that a pregnancy test be ordered.

Psychological status

■ Set aside time to allow the patient to discuss his feelings about the impending surgery. This step is important because depression and anxiety can significantly impact recovery. Offer the patient the option of seeing a member of the clergy.

■ Expect some anxiety. If the patient seems inappropriately relaxed or unconcerned, consider whether he's suppressing his fears. Such a patient may cope poorly with surgical stress, and it's important to encourage him to seek support from family or friends. If possible, allow family and friends to visit with the patient preoperatively. Also include them in your nursing plan of care.

Teaching the preoperative patient

Your teaching can help the patient cope with the physical and psychological stress of surgery. Because of the rising number of shorter hospital stays and same-day surgeries, preadmission and preoperative teaching have become more important than ever.

Explaining preoperative measures
Include in your teaching strategy an evaluation of the patient's understanding of his upcoming surgery so you can correct any misconceptions. Structure the teaching to accommodate a short time period, and use the following teaching tips as a guide:

■ Urge the patient to read the surgical consent form carefully and to ask questions of the surgeon before signing.

■ Explain that the results of chest X-rays, a complete blood count, urine studies, an electrocardiogram, and other preoperative tests will determine whether the patient is ready for surgery.

■ Discuss the rationale behind hair removal (if ordered) — that is, to prevent surgical wound infection by cleaning the skin of microorganisms found in body hair.

■ Stress the importance of withholding food and fluids for a specified time before surgery.

■ Inform the patient that after he has completed all preoperative routines, including dressing in a surgical cap and gown, he'll receive preanesthetic medication. Tell the patient that this medication will help him relax, although he probably won't fall asleep.

■ Tell the patient that he'll receive an I.V. line either before he goes to surgery or after he gets to the operating room.

■ Help the patient deal with fears about anesthesia. Assure him that the anesthesiologist will monitor his condition throughout surgery and provide the right amount of anesthetic. In most cases, an anesthesiologist will have met with the patient prior to hospitalization or on the morning of surgery.

■ Show the patient's family where they can wait during the operation. If they want to visit preoperatively, tell them to arrive 2 hours before surgery is scheduled.

🌀 *Age alert* When the patient is a child, you can help make the surgical experience less threatening by using therapeutic play. Follow these guidelines:

– Allow the parent or designee to remain with the child at all times (some hospitals allow the parent to accompany the child into the operating room).

– Allow the child to bring a familiar toy that can accompany him through the operating room and postanesthesia care unit.

– Allow the child to choose play articles.

– Provide materials specific to the child's experiences, such as a nasogastric tube, a syringe, or bandages.

– Allow play to be unstructured.

– Provide supervision to prevent accidental injury.

Previewing operating room procedures
Educate the patient on operating room procedures:

■ Warn the patient that he may have to wait a short time in the holding area, an area allocated to patients awaiting surgery, to allow the anesthetic to take effect. Explain that the doctors and nurses will wear surgical dress and will observe him closely.

■ Explain to the patient that he'll be repeatedly asked his name, the name of his surgeon, and the type of surgery he's having. Reassure him that this is a safety precaution used at most hospitals.

■ When discussing transfer procedures and techniques, describe sensations the patient will experience. Advise the patient that he'll be taken to the operating room on a stretcher and then transferred from the stretcher to the operating table. For his own safety, he'll be strapped securely to the table. The operating room nurses will check his vital signs frequently.

■ Educate the patient that the operating room may feel cool. Electrodes may be put on his chest to monitor his heart rate during surgery.

■ Explain to the patient that he'll have a blood pressure cuff placed on his arm and a clip on one of his fingers to monitor his blood pressure and oxygen levels.

■ Describe the drowsy, floating sensation he'll feel as the anesthetic takes effect. Tell him that it's important for him to relax at this time.

Getting ready for recovery

Prepare the patient for his stay in the postanesthesia care unit. Briefly describe the sensations the patient will experience when the anesthetic wears off. Tell him that the postanesthesia care unit nurse will call his name and then ask him to answer questions and follow simple commands such as wiggling his toes. He may feel pain at the surgical site, but medications can be given to minimize it.

■ Describe the oxygen delivery device, such as the nasal cannula, that he'll need after surgery.

■ Tell the patient that after he's recovered from the anesthesia, he'll return to his room. He'll be able to see his family, but he'll probably feel drowsy.

■ Make sure he's aware that you'll frequently be taking his blood pressure and pulse so that he won't be alarmed by these routine procedures.

■ Reduce the patient's anxiety about postoperative pain by informing him about the pain-control measures you'll be using. Explain that the doctor will order pain medication to be given according to the patient's needs.

Patient teaching tips Teach the patient how to use the 0-to-10 pain scale to rate his pain (with 0 equaling no pain and 10 describing unbearable pain). Also instruct the patient to describe pain in terms of its quality and location. Encourage him to let you know as soon as he feels pain, instead of waiting until it becomes intense.

■ Discuss the type of medication he'll receive, how it works, and the route of administration. Also describe other measures you'll take to relieve pain and promote patient comfort, such as positioning, diversionary activities, and splinting.

■ Teach the patient coughing exercises, unless he's scheduled for neurosurgery or eye surgery. If he's scheduled for chest or abdominal surgery, teach him how to splint his incision before he coughs. Instruct the patient to take a slow, deep breath, and then to breathe out through his mouth. Tell him to take a second breath in the same manner. Next, tell him to take a third deep breath and hold it. He should then cough two or three times to clear his breathing passages. Have him take three to five normal breaths,

Preoperative care 283

exhaling slowly and relaxing after each breath.

■ Also teach deep-breathing exercises. Instruct the patient to lie on his back in a comfortable position with one hand placed on his chest and the other over his upper abdomen. Instruct him to exhale normally, close his mouth, and inhale deeply through his nose. His chest shouldn't expand. Ask him to hold his breath and slowly count to five. Next, ask him to purse his lips and exhale completely through his mouth without letting his cheeks expand. Tell the patient to repeat the exercise 5 to 10 times.

■ Teach the patient the techniques of early mobility and ambulation.

■ Explain that postoperative exercises help to prevent complications, such as atelectasis, thrombophlebitis, constipation, and loss of muscle tone. Explain to the patient that he may have to wear leg wraps, called sequential compression devices, until he's ambulatory. These devices compress the calf muscles to simulate walking.

■ Demonstrate how to use an incentive spirometer, and have the patient do a return demonstration. Explain that this device will provide feedback when he's doing deep-breathing exercises. Explain how simple leg exercises, such as alternately contracting the calf muscles, will prevent venous pooling after surgery.

Identifying hazardous drugs

Some drugs may cause hazardous complications or interactions during or after surgery. Always review your patient's medication record carefully before he undergoes surgery. Use this chart to identify common drugs that can be hazardous to surgical patients.

Drug	Possible effects
ANTIANXIETY DRUGS	
diazepam Valium	■ Excessive sedation ■ Preoperative or postoperative nausea and vomiting ■ Local tissue irritation (with I.V. administration)
hydroxyzine hydrochloride Vistaril	■ Drowsiness and dry mouth
midazolam hydrochloride Versed	■ Respiratory depression (with high doses)
ANTIARRHYTHMICS	
All types	■ Laryngospasm ■ Intensified cardiac depression and reduced cardiac output
procainamide Pronestyl	■ Prolonged or enhanced effects of neuromuscular blockers ■ Hypotension

(continued)

Identifying hazardous drugs *(continued)*

Drug	Possible effects

propranolol
Inderal
- Prolonged or enhanced effects of neuromuscular blockers
- Depressed myocardial function
- Hypotension
- Laryngospasm

ANTIBIOTICS

All types
- Masked symptoms of infection

Aminoglycosides
amikacin, gentamicin,
kanamycin, neomycin,
netilmicin, streptomycin,
tobramycin
- Increased risk of neuromuscular blockade and respiratory paralysis

erythromycin
Erythrocin, E-Mycin
- Prolonged action of opiates

ANTICHOLINERGICS

atropine sulfate
- Excessive dryness of the mouth, tachycardia, flushing, and depressed sweating
- Increased intraocular pressure, blurred vision, and dilated pupils
- Urine retention
- Agitation and delirium (in elderly patients)

glycopyrrolate
Robinul
- Excessive dryness of the mouth, tachycardia, flushing, and depressed sweating
- Increased intraocular pressure, blurred vision, and dilated pupils
- Urine retention

scopolamine hydrobromide
Triptone, Isopto Hyoscine
- Excessive dryness of the mouth, tachycardia, and flushing
- Increased intraocular pressure, blurred vision, and dilated pupils
- Urine retention
- Excessive drowsiness
- Agitation and delirium (in elderly patients)

ANTICOAGULANTS

heparin
Liquaemin
warfarin
Coumadin
- Increased risk of hemorrhage

Identifying hazardous drugs *(continued)*

Drug	Possible effects
ANTICONVULSANTS	
magnesium sulfate	■ Increased risk of neuromuscular blockade
ANTIDIABETICS	
insulin	■ Increased insulin requirement during stress and healing ■ Diminished insulin requirement during fasting
ANTIHYPERTENSIVES	
All types	■ Worsened hypotension
CENTRAL NERVOUS SYSTEM DEPRESSANTS	
Alcohol, sedative hypnotics	■ If given with general anesthetics, increased risk of respiratory depression, apnea, or hypotension
CORTICOSTEROIDS	
betamethasone, cortisone, dexamethasone, hydrocortisone, methylprednisolone, paramethasone, prednisolone, prednisone, triamcinolone	■ Delayed wound healing ■ Risk of acute adrenal insufficiency ■ Increased risk of infection ■ Masked symptoms of infection ■ Increased risk of hemorrhage
DIURETICS	
furosemide Lasix **Potassium-wasting diuretics**	■ If given with certain anesthetics, increased risk of hypotension ■ Increased risk of complications associated with hypokalemia
HISTAMINE₂–RECEPTOR ANTAGONISTS	
cimetidine Tagamet **ranitidine** Zantac	■ Decreased clearance of diazepam, lidocaine, propranolol, and all other drugs

(continued)

Identifying hazardous drugs *(continued)*

Drug	Possible effects
MYOTICS	
demecarium, echothiophate, isoflurophate	■ If given with succinylcholine, increased risk of neuromuscular blockade, cardiovascular collapse, prolonged respiratory depression, or apnea (effects may occur up to a few months after the patient stops taking the drug)
NARCOTICS	
meperidine hydrochloride Demerol **morphine sulfate**	■ Depressed respiration, circulation, and gastric motility ■ Dizziness, tachycardia, and sweating ■ Hypotension, restlessness, and excitement ■ Preoperative or postoperative nausea and vomiting
OPIATES	
All types	■ If given with certain I.V. anesthetics (such as midazolam, propofol, thiopental, and droperidol), increased risk of respiratory depression, apnea, or hypotension
SEDATIVE-HYPNOTICS	
pentobarbital sodium Nembutal sodium	■ Confusion or excitement, especially in elderly patients or patients with severe pain
THYROID HORMONES	
All types	■ If given with ketamine, increased risk of hypertension and tachycardia
TRANQUILIZERS	
promethazine hydrochloride Phenergan	■ Postoperative hypotension

Reviewing care on the day of surgery

Early on the day of surgery, follow these procedures:
■ Verify that the patient has had nothing by mouth since midnight.
■ Verify that the patient took all prescribed medications as instructed.
■ Make sure diagnostic test results appear on the chart.
■ Ask the patient to remove jewelry, makeup, and nail polish; to shower with antimicrobial soap, if ordered; and to perform mouth care.
■ Instruct the patient to remove dentures or partial plates. Note on the chart whether he has dental crowns, caps, or braces. Also instruct him to remove contact lenses, glasses, prostheses, and hearing aids, if applicable. Hearing aid removal varies among health care facilities. Some may allow the patient to leave in the hearing aid if it helps him follow instructions. Document whether the patient is wearing a hearing aid into the operating room.
■ Tell the patient to void and to put on a surgical cap and gown.
■ Take and record vital signs.
■ Give preoperative medication, if ordered.

Preparing the bowel for surgery

The extent of bowel preparation depends on the type and site of surgery. For example, a patient scheduled for several days of postoperative bed rest who hasn't had a recent bowel movement may receive a mild laxative or enema. However, a patient scheduled for GI, pelvic, perianal, or rectal surgery will undergo more extensive intestinal preparation.

Preoperative enemas or an osmotic cathartic solution such as magnesium citrate may help empty the intestine, thereby minimizing injury to the colon and improving visualization of the operative site.

Expect to perform extensive intestinal preparation for patients undergoing elective colon surgery. During surgical opening of the colon, escaping bacteria may invade adjacent tissue, leading to infection. Perform a mechanical preparation and administer antimicrobials as ordered. Mechanical bowel preparation removes gross stool; oral antimicrobials suppress potent microflora without encouraging resistant strains.

If enemas are ordered to clear the bowel and the third enema still hasn't removed all the stool, notify the doctor. Repeated enemas may cause fluid and electrolyte imbalances.

Age alert Elderly patients who are allowed nothing by mouth and haven't received I.V. fluids are at high risk for fluid and electrolyte imbalances.

Preparing the skin for surgery

Before surgery, the patient's skin must be as free as possible from microorganisms to reduce the risk of infection at the incision site.

Hair removal should be done as close as possible to the time of surgery, such as while the patient is in the holding area, and should be performed with a clipper or shaver.

Reviewing common general anesthetics

Drug	Indications	Advantages
INHALATION AGENTS		
nitrous oxide	Maintains anesthesia; may provide an adjunct for inducing general anesthesia	■ Has little effect on heart rate, myocardial contractility, respiration, blood pressure, liver, kidneys, or metabolism in absence of hypoxia ■ Produces excellent analgesia ■ Allows for rapid induction and recovery ■ Doesn't increase capillary bleeding ■ Doesn't sensitize myocardium to epinephrine
halothane Fluothane	Maintains general anesthesia	■ Is easy to administer ■ Allows for rapid, smooth induction and recovery ■ Has a relatively pleasant odor and is nonirritating ■ Depresses salivary and bronchial secretions ■ Causes bronchodilation ■ Easily suppresses pharyngeal and laryngeal reflexes
enflurane Ethrane	Maintains anesthesia; occasionally is used to induce anesthesia	■ Allows for rapid induction and recovery ■ Is nonirritating and eliminates secretions ■ Causes bronchodilation ■ Provides good muscle relaxation ■ Allows cardiac rhythm to remain stable
isoflurane Forane	Maintains general anesthesia; occasionally is used to induce general anesthesia	■ Allows for rapid induction and recovery ■ Causes bronchodilation ■ Provides excellent muscle relaxation ■ Allows for extremely stable cardiac rhythm
methoxyflurane Penthrane	Maintains general anesthesia	■ Allows for rapid induction and recovery ■ Analgesic effects may extend into immediate postoperative period ■ Bronchiolar constriction or laryngeal spasm aren't usually provoked

Disadvantages	Nursing interventions
■ May cause hypoxia with excessive amounts ■ Doesn't relax muscles (procedures requiring muscular relaxation require addition of a neuromuscular blocker)	■ Monitor for signs of hypoxia.
■ May cause myocardial depression, leading to arrhythmias ■ Sensitizes heart to action of catecholamine ■ May cause circulatory or respiratory depression, depending on the dose ■ Has no analgesic property	■ Watch for arrhythmias, hypotension, respiratory depression. ■ Monitor for a fall in body temperature; the patient may shiver after prolonged use. Shivering increases oxygen consumption.
■ Causes myocardial depression ■ Lowers seizure threshold ■ Increases hypotension as depth of anesthesia increases ■ May cause shivering during recovery ■ May cause circulatory or respiratory depression, depending on the dose	■ Monitor for decreased heart and respiratory rates and hypotension. ■ Watch for shivering, which increases oxygen consumption.
■ May cause circulatory or respiratory depression, depending on the dose ■ Potentiates the action of nondepolarizing muscular relaxants ■ May cause the patient to shiver ■ Tends to lower blood pressure as depth of anesthesia increases; pulse remains somewhat elevated	■ Watch for respiratory depression and hypotension. ■ Watch for shivering, which increases oxygen consumption.
■ Doesn't provide skeletal muscle relaxation when used as a solo agent ■ May cause shivering during recovery	■ Watch for changes in the patient's vital signs. ■ Watch for shivering, which increases oxygen consumption.

(continued)

Reviewing common general anesthetics *(continued)*

Drug	Indications	Advantages
INHALATION AGENTS *(continued)*		
desflurane Suprane	Induces and maintains general anesthesia	■ Can use decreased doses for neuro-muscular blockers ■ Increased doses for maintenance anesthesia may produce dose-dependent hypotension
sevoflurane Ultane	Induces and maintains general anesthesia for adults and children	■ Nonpungent odor ■ No respiratory irritability ■ Suitable for use with mask induction
I.V. BARBITURATES		
thiopental sodium Pentothal	Is used primarily to induce general anesthesia	■ Promotes rapid, smooth, and pleasant induction and quick recovery ■ Infrequently causes complications ■ Doesn't sensitize autonomic tissues of heart to catecholamines
I.V. BENZODIAZEPINES		
diazepam Valium	Induces general anesthesia; provides amnesia during balanced anesthesia	■ Minimally affects the cardiovascular system ■ Acts as a potent anticonvulsant ■ Produces amnesia
midazolam hydrochloride Versed	Induces general anesthesia; provides amnesia during balanced anesthesia	■ Minimally affects the cardiovascular system ■ Acts as a potent anticonvulsant ■ Produces amnesia

Disadvantages	Nursing interventions
■ May increase heart rate ■ Respiratory irritant is more likely in adults during induction of anesthesia via mask ■ Not recommended for induction of general anesthesia in infants or children because of high incidence of laryngospasm or other respiratory adverse effects (after anesthesia is induced and tracheal intubation is achieved, it can be used for maintenance anesthesia) ■ Not indicated for patients with coronary artery disease or in those who will be adversely affected by increases in heart rate	■ Monitor the patient's vital signs, especially heart rate and blood pressure. ■ Watch for shivering, which increases oxygen consumption.
■ Dose-related cardiac depressant	■ Monitor the patient's vital signs. ■ Watch for shivering, which increases oxygen consumption.
■ Is associated with airway obstruction, respiratory depression, and laryngospasm, possibly leading to hypoxia ■ Doesn't provide muscle relaxation and produces little analgesia ■ May cause cardiovascular depression, especially in hypovolemic or debilitated patients	■ Watch for signs and symptoms of hypoxia, airway obstruction, and cardiovascular and respiratory depression.
■ May cause irritation when injected into a peripheral vein ■ Has a long elimination half-life	■ Monitor the patient's vital signs.
■ Can cause respiratory depression	■ Monitor the patient's vital signs, respiratory rate, and volume.

(continued)

Reviewing common general anesthetics *(continued)*

Drug	Indications	Advantages
I.V. NONBARBITURATES		
ketamine hydrochloride Ketalar	Produces a dissociative state of consciousness; induces anesthesia when a barbiturate is contraindicated; sole anesthetic for short diagnostic and surgical procedures not requiring skeletal muscle relaxation	■ Produces rapid anesthesia and profound analgesia ■ Doesn't irritate veins or tissues ■ Maintains a patent airway without endotracheal intubation because it suppresses laryngeal and pharyngeal reflexes
propofol Diprivan	Is used for induction and maintenance of anesthesia; is particularly useful for short procedures and outpatient surgery	■ Allows for quick, smooth induction ■ Permits rapid awakening and recovery ■ Causes less vomiting
I.V. TRANQUILIZERS		
droperidol Inapsine	Is used preoperatively and during induction and maintenance of anesthesia as an adjunct to general or regional anesthesia	■ Allows for rapid, smooth induction and recovery ■ Produces sleepiness and mental detachment for several hours
NARCOTICS		
fentanyl citrate Sublimaze	Is used preoperatively for minor and major surgery, urologic procedures, and gastroscopy; also used as an adjunct to regional anesthesia and for inducing and maintaining general anesthesia	■ Promotes rapid, smooth induction and recovery ■ Doesn't cause histamine release ■ Minimally affects cardiovascular system ■ Can be reversed by a narcotic antagonist (naloxone)
NEUROLEPTICS		
droperidol and fentanyl Innovar	Is used for short procedures during which the patient must remain conscious; also used as a premedication and as an adjunct for inducing and maintaining general anesthesia	■ Allows for rapid, smooth induction and recovery ■ Produces somnolence and psychological indifference to the environment without total unconsciousness ■ Eliminates voluntary movement ■ Makes it possible to use less analgesia postoperatively ■ Produces satisfactory amnesia

Disadvantages	Nursing interventions
■ May cause unpleasant dreams, hallucinations, and delirium during recovery ■ Increases heart rate, blood pressure, and intraocular pressure ■ Preserves muscle tone, leading to poor relaxation during surgery	■ Protect the patient from visual, tactile, and auditory stimuli during recovery. ■ Monitor the patient's vital signs.
■ Can cause hypotension ■ Can cause pain if injected into small veins ■ May cause clonic or myoclonic movements upon emergence ■ May interact with benzodiazepines, increasing propofol's effects ■ Doesn't cause profound analgesia	■ Monitor the patient for hypotension. ■ Prepare for rapid emergence.
■ May cause hypotension because it's a peripheral vasodilator	■ Monitor the patient for increased pulse rate and hypotension.
■ May cause respiratory depression, euphoria, bradycardia, bronchoconstriction, nausea, vomiting, and miosis ■ May cause skeletal-muscle and chest-wall rigidity	■ Observe the patient for respiratory depression. ■ Watch for nausea and vomiting. If vomiting occurs, position the patient to prevent aspiration. ■ Monitor blood pressure. ■ Decrease postoperative narcotics to one-third to one-fourth the usual dose.
■ May cause respiratory depression, extrapyramidal symptoms, apnea, laryngospasm, bronchospasm, bradycardia, and hallucinations	■ Closely monitor the patient's vital signs. ■ Decrease postoperative narcotics to one-third to one-fourth the usual dose for the first 8 hours.

Reviewing common neuromuscular blockers

Drug	Adverse effects	Special considerations
NONDEPOLARIZING NEUROMUSCULAR BLOCKERS		
atracurium besylate Tracrium	■ Slight hypotension in a few patients	■ Acts for 20 to 30 minutes ■ May cause slight histamine release ■ Doesn't accumulate with repeated doses ■ Is useful for patients with underlying hepatic, renal, and cardiac disease
gallamine triethiodide Flaxedil	■ Tachycardia and hypertension ■ Allergic reaction in patients sensitive to iodine	■ Acts for 15 to 35 minutes ■ May cause tachycardia after doses of 0.5 mg/kg; avoid using in cardiac disease ■ Doesn't cause bronchospasm ■ Accumulates; don't administer to patients with impaired renal function
metocurine iodide Metubine Iodide	■ Hypotension ■ Bronchospasm	■ Acts for 25 to 90 minutes; 60 minutes is average (depends on the dose and general anesthetic) ■ May cause histamine release
pancuronium bromide Pavulon	■ Tachycardia ■ Transient skin rashes and a burning sensation at the injection site	■ Acts for 35 to 45 minutes ■ Is five times more potent than curare ■ Doesn't cause ganglion blockage, so it doesn't usually lead to hypotension ■ Has a vagolytic action that increases heart rate
tubocurarine chloride Tubarine	■ Hypotension ■ Bronchospasm	■ Acts for 25 to 90 minutes with single large dose or multiple single doses; may last 24 hours in some patients ■ Causes histamine release; in higher doses, causes sympathetic ganglion blockade ■ May have prolonged action in elderly or debilitated patients and in those with renal or liver disease

Reviewing common neuromuscular blockers (continued)

Drug	Adverse effects	Special considerations
NONDEPOLARIZING NEUROMUSCULAR BLOCKERS (continued)		
vecuronium bromide Norcuron	■ Minimal and transient cardiovascular effects ■ Skeletal muscle weakness or paralysis; respiratory insufficiency; respiratory paralysis; prolonged, dose-related apnea	■ Acts for 25 to 40 minutes ■ Probably metabolized mostly in the liver ■ Has a short duration of action and causes fewer cardiovascular effects than other nondepolarizing neuromuscular blockers
DEPOLARIZING NEUROMUSCULAR BLOCKERS		
succinylcholine chloride (suxamethonium chloride) Anectine, Quelicin, Sucostrin	■ Respiratory depression ■ Bradycardia ■ Excessive salivation ■ Hypotension ■ Arrhythmias ■ Tachycardia ■ Hypertension ■ Increased intraocular and intragastric pressure ■ Fasciculations ■ Muscle pain ■ Malignant hyperthermia	■ Acts for 5 to 10 minutes ■ Is metabolized mostly in plasma by pseudocholinesterase; therefore, it's contraindicated in patients with a deficiency of plasma cholinesterase due to a genetic variant defect, liver disease, uremia, or malnutrition ■ Is used cautiously in patients with glaucoma or penetrating wounds of the eye; those undergoing eye surgery; or those with burns, severe trauma, spinal cord injuries, muscular dystrophy, or cardiovascular, hepatic, pulmonary, metabolic, or renal disorders; may cause sudden hyperkalemia and consequent cardiac arrest ■ Can cause pregnant patients who also receive magnesium sulfate to experience increased neuromuscular blockade because of decreased pseudocholinesterase levels

Postoperative care

Monitoring the postoperative patient

Monitoring the postoperative patient aims at minimizing complications through early detection and prompt treatment.

Equipment
Thermometer ◆ watch with second hand ◆ stethoscope ◆ sphygmomanometer or automated blood pressure machine ◆ postoperative flowchart or other documentation tool

Implementation
■ Obtain the patient's record from the postanesthesia care unit (PACU) nurse.

■ Transfer the patient from the PACU stretcher to the bed. Position him properly. Keep transfer movements smooth to minimize pain and complications.

■ If the patient has had orthopedic surgery, have a coworker move the affected extremity as you transfer the patient.

■ If the patient is in skeletal traction, have a coworker move the weights as you and another coworker transfer the patient.

■ Ensure the patient's comfort, and raise the side rails of the bed to ensure his safety.

■ Assess the patient's level of consciousness.

■ Monitor the patient's respiratory status by assessing his airway. Note breathing rate and depth; auscultate breath sounds. If ordered, administer oxygen and initiate oximetry.

■ Monitor the patient's postoperative pulse rate, which should be within 20% of the preoperative rate.

■ Compare postoperative blood pressure with preoperative blood pressure. It should be within 20% of the preoperative level unless the patient suffered a hypotensive episode during surgery.

■ Assess the patient's ability to wiggle his toes and the level of sensation if he has received spinal anesthesia.

■ Assess the patient's body temperature. If it's lower than 95.6° F (35.3° C), apply blankets and notify the doctor. Lowered body temperature produces shivering, which increases the body's consumption of oxygen and may strain the heart's normal function.

■ Assess the patient's infusion sites for redness, pain, swelling, and drainage.

■ Assess the surgical wound dressings. If they're soiled, assess the drainage and outline the soiled area. Note the date and time of assessment on the dressing. Check the soiled area often; if it enlarges, reinforce the dressing, and alert the doctor.

■ Note the presence and condition of any drains and tubes. Note the color, type, odor, and amount of drainage. Make sure all drains are properly connected and free from kinks and obstructions.

■ If the patient has had vascular or orthopedic surgery, assess the appropriate extremities. Notify the doctor of abnormalities.

■ As the patient recovers from anesthesia, monitor his respiratory and cardiovascular status closely. Watch for airway obstruction and hypoventilation caused by laryngospasm and for sedation, which can lead to hypoxemia.

■ Encourage coughing and deep-breathing exercises, unless the patient has had nasal, ophthalmic, or neurologic surgery.

■ Administer postoperative medications as ordered.

■ Remove all fluids from the patient's bedside until he's alert enough to eat and drink. Before giving liquids, assess his gag reflex.

Special considerations

■ If the patient has had epidural anesthesia or a postoperative continuous epidural narcotic, monitor his respiratory status closely. Respiratory rate and quality, along with oxygen saturation levels, should be assessed every hour for at least the first 24 hours.

Preventing postoperative complications

After surgery, take the following steps to avoid complications.

Turn and reposition the patient

Performed every 2 hours, turning and repositioning promotes circulation, thereby reducing the risk of skin breakdown — especially over bony prominences. When the patient is in a lateral recumbent position, tuck pillows under bony prominences to reduce friction and promote comfort. Each time you turn the patient, carefully inspect the skin to detect redness or other signs of breakdown.

Keep in mind that turning and repositioning may be contraindicated in some patients, such as those who have undergone neurologic or musculoskeletal surgery that demands postoperative immobilization.

Encourage coughing and deep breathing

Deep breathing promotes lung expansion, which helps clear anesthetics from the body. Coughing and deep breathing also lower the risk of pulmonary and fat emboli and of hypostatic pneumonia associated with secretion buildup in the airways.

Encourage the patient to deep-breathe at least every 2 hours and to cough. Show the patient how to splint his incision with his hands or a pillow to reduce pain. Also show him how to use an incentive spirometer. Because deep breathing doesn't increase intracranial pressure, it's safe to do after various neurosurgical procedures.

Monitor nutrition and fluids

Adequate nutrition and fluid intake are essential to ensure proper hydration, promote healing, and provide energy to match the increased basal metabolism associated with surgery. If the patient has a protein deficiency or compromised immune function preoperatively, expect to deliver supplemental protein by parenteral nutrition to promote healing. If he has renal failure, this treatment is contraindicated because his inability to break down protein could lead to dangerously high blood nitrogen levels.

Promote exercise and ambulation

Early postoperative exercise and ambulation can significantly reduce the risk of thromboembolism as well as improve ventilation.

Perform passive range-of-motion exercises to prevent joint contractures and muscle atrophy and promote circulation. These exercises can also help you assess the patient's strength and tolerance.

Before encouraging ambulation, ask the patient to dangle his legs over the side of the bed and perform deep-breathing exercises. How well a patient tolerates this step is commonly a key predictor of out-of-bed tolerance.

Begin ambulation by helping the patient walk a few feet from his bed to a sturdy chair. Then have him gradually progress each day from ambulating in his room to ambulating in the hallway, with or without assistance, as necessary. Document the frequency of ambulation and the patient's tolerance, including the use of an analgesic.

Managing postoperative complications

Despite your best efforts, complications can occur. By knowing how to recognize and manage them, you can limit their effects.

The following is a list of complications. Note that some complications are more likely to produce acute changes, whereas others produce symptoms slowly. Also, some complications are to be expected in the immediate postoperative period, and others are more prominent 2 or 3 days after surgery.

Abdominal distention, paralytic ileus, and constipation

Sluggish peristalsis and paralytic ileus usually last for 24 to 72 hours after surgery and cause abdominal distention. Paralytic ileus occurs whenever autonomic innervation of the GI tract becomes disrupted. Causes include intraoperative manipulation of intestinal organs, hypokalemia, wound infection, and use of codeine, morphine, or atropine. Postoperative constipation usually stems from colonic ileus caused by diminished GI motility and impaired perception of rectal fullness.

Assessment
■ To detect abdominal distention, monitor abdominal girth and ask the patient if he feels bloated.
■ To assess the patient for paralytic ileus, auscultate for bowel sounds in all four quadrants. Notify the doctor of decreased or absent bowel sounds.
■ Monitor flatus or stool passage and abdominal distention.
■ Ask about feelings of abdominal fullness or nausea.

Interventions
■ To treat abdominal distention, encourage ambulation and give nothing by mouth until bowel sounds return.
■ Insert a rectal or nasogastric tube as ordered. Keep the nasogastric tube patent and functioning properly.
■ To treat paralytic ileus, encourage ambulation and administer medications as ordered. If the ileus doesn't resolve within 24 to 48 hours, insert a nasogastric tube as ordered. Keep the nasogastric tube patent and functioning properly.
■ To treat constipation, encourage ambulation and administer a stool softener, laxative, or nonnarcotic analgesic as ordered.

Atelectasis and pneumonia
After surgery, atelectasis may result from hypoventilation and excessive retained secretions. This provides a medium for bacterial growth and sets the stage for stasis pneumonia.

Assessment
■ To detect atelectasis, auscultate for diminished or absent breath sounds over the affected area and note dullness on percussion.
■ Assess the patient for decreased chest expansion, mediastinal shift toward the side of collapse, fever, restlessness or confusion, worsening dyspnea, and elevated blood pressure, pulse rate, and respiratory rate.
■ To detect pneumonia, watch for sudden onset of shaking chills with high fever and headache.
■ Auscultate for diminished breath sounds or for telltale crackles over the affected lung area.
■ Assess the patient for dyspnea, tachypnea, sharp chest pain exacerbated by inspiration, productive cough with pinkish or rust-colored sputum, and cyanosis with hypoxemia that's confirmed by arterial blood gas measurement.
■ Chest X-rays show patchy infiltrates or consolidation areas.

Interventions
■ Encourage the patient to deep-breathe and cough every hour while he's awake. *Note:* Coughing is contraindicated in patients who have undergone neurosurgery or eye surgery.
■ Demonstrate how to use an incentive spirometer.
■ As ordered, perform chest physiotherapy, give an antibiotic, and administer humidified air or oxygen.
■ Reposition the patient every 2 hours. Elevate the head of the bed.

Hypovolemia
A total blood volume loss of 15% to 25% may result from blood loss and severe dehydration, third-space fluid sequestration (as in burns, peritonitis, intestinal obstruction, or acute pancre-

atitis), and fluid loss (as in excessive vomiting or diarrhea).

Assessment
■ Check for hypotension and a rapid, weak pulse.
■ Note cool, clammy and, perhaps, mottled skin.
■ Check for rapid, shallow respirations.
■ Assess the patient for oliguria or anuria and lethargy.

Interventions
■ To increase blood pressure, administer an I.V. crystalloid, such as normal saline solution or lactated Ringer's solution.
■ To restore urine output and fluid volume, give a colloid, such as plasma, albumin, or dextran.

Pericarditis
Pericarditis is an acute or chronic inflammation of the pericardium — the fibroserous sac that envelops, supports, and protects the heart. After surgery, pericarditis may result from bacterial, fungal, or viral infection or from postcardiac injury that leaves the pericardium intact but causes blood to leak into the pericardial cavity.

Assessment
■ To detect pericarditis, assess for sharp, sudden pain, starting over the sternum and radiating to the neck, shoulders, back, and arms.
■ Ask the patient to take a deep breath and then sit up and lean forward. Pericardial pain is commonly pleuritic, increasing with deep inspiration and decreasing when the patient sits up and leans forward. You also may hear a pericardial friction rub.

Interventions
■ Keep the patient on complete bed rest in an upright position.
■ Provide an analgesic and oxygen as ordered.
■ Assess pain in relation to respiration and body position to distinguish pericardial pain from myocardial ischemia pain.
■ Monitor the patient for signs of cardiac compression or cardiac tamponade. Signs include decreased blood pressure, increased central venous pressure, and paradoxic pulse. Because cardiac tamponade requires immediate treatment, keep a pericardiocentesis set at the patient's bedside whenever pericardial effusion is suspected.

Postoperative psychosis
Mental aberrations more likely stem from physiologic causes (cerebral anoxia, fluid and electrolyte imbalance, malnutrition, and such drugs as tranquilizers, sedatives, and narcotics). However, psychological causes (fear, pain, and disorientation) can also contribute.

Assessment
■ Assess the patient's mental status, and compare it with the preoperative baseline.

Interventions
■ Reorient the patient frequently to time, place, and person. Call him by his preferred name, and encourage him to move about.
■ Provide clean eyeglasses and a working hearing aid, if appropriate. Use sedatives and restraints only if necessary.

Septicemia and septic shock
Septicemia may stem from a break in asepsis during surgery or wound care or from peritonitis (as in ruptured ap-

pendix or ectopic pregnancy). The most common cause of postoperative septicemia is *Escherichia coli*. Septic shock occurs when bacteria release endotoxins into the bloodstream, decreasing vascular resistance and resulting in dramatic hypotension.

Assessment
■ To detect septicemia, check for fever, chills, rash, abdominal distention, prostration, pain, headache, nausea, and diarrhea.
■ Early indicators of septic shock include fever and chills; warm, dry, flushed skin; slightly altered mental status; increased pulse and respiratory rates; decreased or normal blood pressure; and reduced urine output.
■ Late indicators include pale, moist, cold skin and decreased mental status, pulse and respiratory rates, blood pressure, and urine output.

Interventions
■ To treat septicemia, obtain a urine specimen and blood and wound samples for culture and sensitivity tests.
■ Administer an antibiotic if ordered.
■ Monitor vital signs and level of consciousness.
■ To treat septic shock, administer an I.V. antibiotic if ordered.
■ Monitor serum peak and trough levels.
■ Give I.V. fluids and blood or blood products to restore circulating blood volume.

Thrombophlebitis and pulmonary embolism
Postoperative venous stasis associated with immobility may lead to thrombophlebitis — an inflammation of a vein, usually in the leg, accompanied by clot formation. If a clot breaks away, it may become lodged in the lung, causing a pulmonary embolism.

Assessment
■ To detect thrombophlebitis, ask high-risk patients about leg pain, functional impairment, and edema.
■ Inspect legs from feet to groin, and record calf circumference. Note any engorgement of the cavity behind the medial malleolus and increased temperature in the affected leg. Identify areas of cordlike venous segments.
■ To detect a pulmonary embolism, assess the patient for sudden anginal or pleuritic chest pain; dyspnea; rapid, shallow respirations; cyanosis; restlessness; and possibly a thready pulse.
■ Auscultate for fine-to-coarse crackles over the affected lung.

Interventions
■ To treat thrombophlebitis, elevate the affected leg and apply warm compresses.
■ Administer medications as ordered.
■ Monitor laboratory values, such as prothrombin and partial thromboplastin times, daily.
■ To treat a pulmonary embolism, administer oxygen and medications as ordered. Elevate the head of the bed.

Urine retention
The patient may not be able to void spontaneously within 12 hours after surgery. Urine retention is usually transient and reversible.

Assessment
■ Monitor intake and output.
■ Assess the patient for bladder distention above the level of the symphysis pubis, discomfort, and pain. Also note restlessness, anxiety, diaphoresis, and hypertension.

Interventions
■ To treat urine retention, help the patient ambulate as soon as possible after surgery, unless contraindicated.

■ Assist him to a normal voiding position and, if possible, leave him alone.
■ Turn the water on so the patient can hear it, and pour warm water over his perineum.

Wound infection

The most common wound complication, wound infection is also a major factor in wound dehiscence. Complete dehiscence leads to evisceration.

Assessment

■ To detect infection, assess surgical wounds for increased tenderness, deep pain, and edema, especially from the 3rd to 5th day after the operation.
■ Monitor the patient for increased pulse rate and temperature and an elevated white blood cell count.
■ Note a temperature pattern of spikes in the afternoon or evening, returning to normal by morning.

Interventions

■ As ordered, obtain a wound culture and sensitivity test, administer antibiotics, and irrigate the wound with an appropriate solution, if ordered.
■ Monitor wound drainage.

Caring for surgical wounds

Proper care of surgical wounds helps prevent infection, protects the skin from maceration and excoriation, allows removal and measurement of wound drainage, and promotes comfort. When a surgical incision is closed primarily, the incision is covered with a sterile dressing for 24 to 48 hours. After 48 hours, the incision can be covered by a dressing or left open to air.

Managing a draining wound involves two techniques: dressing and pouching. Dressing is indicated when drainage doesn't compromise skin integrity. Lightly seeping wounds with drains and wounds with minimal puru-

lent drainage can usually be managed with packing and gauze dressings. Surgical incisions left open at the skin level for a few days prior to closure by the doctor (delayed primary closure) are managed by packing with a sterile dressing. Incisions left open to heal by second intention are packed with sterile moist gauze and covered with a sterile dressing.

Wounds draining more than 100 ml in 24 hours and those with excoriating drainage require pouching.

Equipment and preparation

Waterproof trash bag or trash can ◆ clean gloves ◆ sterile gloves ◆ gown, if indicated ◆ sterile 4″ × 4″ gauze pads ◆ abdominal bandage dressing pads, if needed ◆ sterile cotton-tipped applicators ◆ topical medication or ointment, if ordered ◆ prescribed cleaning agent, if ordered ◆ sterile container ◆ adhesive or other tape ◆ soap and water ◆ optional: skin protectant, acetone-free adhesive remover or baby oil, sterile normal saline solution, a graduated container, and Montgomery straps or a T-binder

For a wound with a drain

Precut sterile 4″ × 4″ gauze pads ◆ adhesive tape

For pouching

Pouch with or without drainage port ◆ skin protectant ◆ sterile gauze pad

Determine the type of dressing needed. Assemble all equipment in the patient's room. Check the expiration date on each sterile package, and inspect for tears. Place the trash bag or trash can where you can avoid carrying articles across the sterile field or the wound when disposing of them.

Implementation

■ Check the doctor's order for wound care instructions. Some doctors prefer to not use any cleaning agents on surgical incisions unless the area has become soiled.

■ Note the location of drains to avoid dislodging them during the procedure.

■ Explain the procedure to the patient, and position him properly. Expose only the wound site.

■ Wash your hands. Put on a gown, if necessary, and clean gloves.

Removing the old dressing

■ Hold the skin and pull the tape or dressing toward the wound. This protects newly formed tissue. Use acetone-free adhesive remover or baby oil, if needed. Don't apply solvents to the incision.

■ Remove the soiled dressing. If needed, loosen gauze with sterile normal saline solution.

■ Check the dressing for the amount, type, color, and odor of drainage. Discard the dressing and gloves in the waterproof trash bag.

■ If ordered, obtain a wound culture.

Caring for the wound or incision

■ Establish a sterile field for equipment and supplies. Squeeze the needed amount of ordered ointment onto the sterile field. Pour into a sterile container. Put on sterile gloves.

■ If you aren't using prepackaged swabs, saturate sterile gauze pads with the prescribed cleaning agent. Avoid using cotton balls because these may shed particles in the wound.

■ Squeeze excess solution from the pad or swab. Wipe once from the top to the bottom of the incision; then discard the pad or swab. With a second pad, wipe from top to bottom in a vertical path next to the incision; then discard the pad.

■ Continue to work outward from the incision in lines running parallel to it. Always wipe from the clean area toward the less-clean area. Use each pad

or swab for only one stroke. Use sterile cotton-tipped applicators to clean tight-fitting wire sutures, deep wounds, or wounds with pockets.

■ If the patient has a surgical drain, clean the drain's surface last. Clean the surrounding skin by wiping in half or full circles from the drain site outward.

■ Clean to at least 1″ (2.5 cm) beyond the new dressing or 2″ (5.1 cm) beyond the incision.

■ Check for signs of infection, dehiscence, or evisceration. If you observe such signs or the patient reports pain, notify the doctor.

■ Wash the surrounding skin with soap and water, and pat dry. Apply prescribed topical medication and a skin protectant, if warranted.

■ Pack an open wound with sterile moist gauze using the wet-to-damp method. Avoid using cotton-lined gauze pads.

Apply a fresh gauze dressing

■ Place a sterile 4″ × 4″ gauze pad at the wound center, and move the pad outward to the edges of the wound site. Extend the gauze at least 1″ (2.5 cm) beyond the incision in each direction. Use enough sterile dressings to absorb all drainage until the next dressing change.

■ When the dressing is in place, remove and discard the gloves. Secure the dressing with strips of tape, a T-binder, or Montgomery straps.

■ For the recently postoperative patient or a patient with complications, check the dressing every 30 minutes or as ordered. If the wound is healing properly, check it at least every 8 hours.

Dressing a wound with a drain

■ Use a precut sterile 4″ × 4″ gauze pad.

■ Place the pad close to the skin around the drain so that the tubing fits into the slit. Press a second pad around the drain from the opposite direction to encircle the tubing.

■ Layer as many uncut sterile pads around the tubing as needed to absorb drainage. Secure the dressing with tape, a T-binder, or Montgomery straps.

Pouching a wound

■ To create a pouch, measure the wound and then cut an opening in the collection pouch's facing ⅛″ (0.3 cm) larger than the wound.

■ Make sure surrounding skin is clean and dry; then apply a skin protectant.

■ Make sure the drainage port at the bottom of the pouch is closed; then press the contoured pouch opening around the wound, beginning at its lower edge.

■ To empty the pouch, put on gloves, insert bottom half of the pouch into a graduated container, and open the drainage port. Note the color, consistency, odor, and amount of fluid.

■ Wipe the bottom of the pouch and the drainage port with a sterile gauze pad; reseal the port. Change the pouch if it leaks or comes loose.

Special considerations

■ Because many doctors prefer to change the first postoperative dressing, avoid changing it unless ordered. If you have no such order and drainage is seeping through the dressing, reinforce the dressing with fresh sterile gauze. To prevent bacterial growth, don't allow a reinforced dressing to remain in place longer than 24 hours. Immediately replace dressing that becomes wet from the outside.

■ Consider all dressings and drains infectious.

■ If the patient has two wounds in the same area, cover each separately with layers of sterile 4″ × 4″ gauze pads. Then cover both sites with an abdominal bandage dressing pad secured to the skin with tape.

Draining closed wounds

Inserted during surgery, a closed-wound drain promotes healing and prevents swelling by suctioning serosanguineous fluid at the wound site. By removing this fluid, the drain helps reduce the risk of infection and skin breakdown as well as the number of dressing changes.

A closed-wound drain consists of perforated tubing connected to a portable vacuum unit. The distal end of the tubing lies within the wound and usually leaves the body from a site other than the primary suture line, to preserve the integrity of the surgical wound. The tubing exit site is treated as an additional surgical wound; the drain is usually sutured to the skin. The drain may be left in place for longer than 1 week to accommodate heavy drainage.

Equipment

Graduated cylinder ◆ sterile laboratory container, if needed ◆ alcohol pad ◆ sterile gloves ◆ clean gloves ◆ sterile gauze pads ◆ antiseptic cleaning agent ◆ prepackaged povidone-iodine swabs ◆ waterproof trash bag or trash can

Implementation

■ Check the doctor's order and assess the patient's condition. Explain the procedure to the patient. Provide privacy. Wash your hands, and put on the clean gloves.

■ Unclip the vacuum unit. Using aseptic technique, remove the spout plug to release the vacuum.

■ Empty the unit's contents into a graduated cylinder. Note the amount and appearance of the drainage. If ordered, empty the drainage into a sterile laboratory container and send it to the laboratory for diagnostic testing.

■ Maintaining aseptic technique, clean the unit's spout and plug with an alcohol pad.

■ To reestablish the vacuum that creates the drain's suction power, fully compress the vacuum unit. Keep the unit compressed as you replace the spout plug.

■ Check the patency of the equipment. Make sure the tubing has no twists, kinks, or leaks because the drainage system must be airtight to work properly. Keep the vacuum unit compressed when you release manual pressure; rapid reinflation indicates an air leak. If this occurs, recompress the unit and secure the spout plug.

⟟ *Patient teaching tips* If it's anticipated that the patient will be discharged with the drain, teach the patient how to empty and reconstitute the drain at each session.

■ Secure the vacuum unit to the patient's bedding or, if he's ambulatory, to his gown. Fasten it below wound level to promote drainage. To prevent possible dislodgment, don't apply tension on drainage tubing. Remove and discard gloves, and wash your hands thoroughly.

■ Put on the sterile gloves. Check sutures for signs of pulling or tearing and for swelling or infection of the surrounding skin. Gently clean the sutures with sterile gauze pads soaked in an antiseptic cleaning agent or with a povidone-iodine swab.

■ Properly dispose of drainage, solutions, and waterproof trash bag, and clean or dispose of soiled equipment and supplies.

Special considerations

■ Empty the system and measure the contents once during each shift if drainage has accumulated; do so more often if drainage is excessive.

■ If the patient has more than one closed drain, number the drains so that you can record drainage from each site. *Note:* Be careful not to mistake chest tubes for closed-wound drains because

the vacuum of a chest tube should never be released.

Managing dehiscence and evisceration

Occasionally, the edges of a wound may fail to join, or they may separate after they seem to be healing normally. Called wound dehiscence, this abnormality may lead to a more serious complication: evisceration, in which a portion of the viscera protrudes through the incision. In turn, this can lead to peritonitis and septic shock.

Equipment

Two sterile towels ◆ 1 L of sterile normal saline solution ◆ sterile irrigation set, including a basin, a solution container, and a 50-ml catheter-tip syringe ◆ several large abdominal dressings ◆ sterile waterproof drape ◆ linen-saver pads ◆ sterile gloves

For patients who will return to the operating room
I.V. administration set and I.V. fluids ◆ nasogastric intubation equipment ◆ sedative as ordered ◆ suction apparatus

Implementation

■ Tell the patient to stay in bed. If possible, stay with him while someone else notifies the doctor and collects the equipment.

■ Place a linen-saver pad under the patient and create a sterile field. Place the basin, solution container, and 50-ml syringe on the sterile field.

■ Open the bottle of sterile normal saline solution and pour 400 ml into the solution container and 200 ml into the basin.

■ Place several large abdominal dressings on the sterile field. Wearing sterile gloves, place one or two dressings into the basin.

■ Place the moistened dressings over the exposed viscera. Cover with sterile towels and sterile waterproof drape.

■ Keep the dressings moist by gently moistening with the saline solution frequently. If the viscera appears dusky or black, notify the doctor immediately. Interrupted blood supply may cause a protruding organ to become ischemic and necrotic.

■ Keep the patient on strict bed rest in low Fowler's position (no more than a 20-degree angle elevation) with his knees flexed.

■ Monitor vital signs every 15 minutes to detect shock. Prepare to return to the operating room.

■ Prepare for nasogastric tube insertion and I.V. insertion, if ordered. Connect the nasogastric tube to the suction apparatus. Nasogastric intubation may make the patient gag, causing further evisceration. For this reason, the tube may be inserted in the operating room.

■ Administer preoperative sedative as ordered.

Special considerations

■ To help prevent dehiscence and evisceration, inspect the incision with each dressing change.

Patient teaching tips By the 5th to 9th postoperative day, teach the patient to feel for a healing ridge, which forms directly under the suture line. The lack of a healing ridge may indicate that the patient is at risk for dehiscence and evisceration.

■ Treat early signs of infection immediately. Make sure bandages aren't so tight that they limit the blood supply to the wound.

■ If the patient has weak abdominal walls, apply an abdominal binder. Encourage a high-risk patient to splint his abdomen with a pillow during straining, coughing, or sneezing.

■ If a postoperative patient detects a sudden gush of pinkish serous drainage on his wound dressing, inspect the incision for dehiscence. If the wound seems to be separating slowly and evisceration hasn't developed, place the patient in a supine position and call the doctor.

Planning for discharge

Begin planning for discharge during your first contact with the patient. The initial nursing history and preoperative assessment as well as subsequent assessments can provide useful information.

Recognizing potential problems early will help your discharge plan succeed. Assess the strengths and limitations of the patient and family. Consider physiologic factors (such as general physical and functional abilities, current medications, and general nutritional status), psychological factors (such as self-concept, motivation, and learning abilities), and social factors (such as duration of care needed, types of services available, and the family's involvement in the patient's care).

Medication

Explain the purpose of the drug therapy, the duration of the regimen, the proper dosages and routes, any special instructions, and potential adverse effects as well as when to notify the doctor. Try to establish a medication schedule that fits the patient's lifestyle.

Diet

Discuss dietary restrictions with the patient and, if appropriate, the person who will prepare his meals. Assess the patient's usual dietary intake. If appropriate, discuss how much the diet will cost and how restrictions may affect other family members. Refer the patient to a dietitian, if appropriate.

Activity

After surgery, many patients are advised not to lift heavy objects. Restrictions usually last 4 to 6 weeks after surgery. Discuss how limitations will affect the patient's daily routine. Let him know when he can return to work, drive, and resume sexual activity. If the patient seems unlikely to comply, discuss compromises.

Home care procedures

Use nontechnical language and include caregivers when teaching about home care. After the patient watches you demonstrate a procedure, have him repeat the demonstration.

Explain to the patient that he may not have to use the same equipment he used in the hospital; discuss what's available to him at home. If the patient needs to rent or purchase equipment, such as a hospital bed or walker, arrange for delivery prior to discharge.

Wound care

Teach the patient about changing his wound dressing. Tell him to keep the incision clean and dry, and teach proper hand-washing technique. Specify whether and when he should shower or bathe.

Potential complications

Teach the patient to recognize wound infection and other potential complications. Provide written instructions about reportable signs and symptoms, such as bleeding or discharge from the incision and acute pain. Advise the patient to call the doctor with any questions.

Return appointments

Stress the importance of scheduling and keeping checkup appointments, and make sure the patient has the doctor's office telephone number. If the patient has no transportation, refer him to an appropriate community resource.

Referrals

Reassess whether the patient needs referral to a home care agency or other community resource. Discuss with the family how they'll handle the patient's return home. In some facilities, the responsibility for making referrals falls to a home care coordinator or discharge planning nurse.

7

Common procedures
Performing them safely and accurately

Arterial pressure monitoring

Direct arterial pressure monitoring permits continuous measurement of systolic, diastolic, and mean pressures and allows arterial blood sampling. Because direct measurement reflects systemic vascular resistance as well as blood flow, it's generally more accurate than indirect methods (such as palpation and auscultation of Korotkoff, or audible pulse sounds), which are based on blood flow.

Direct monitoring is indicated when highly accurate or frequent blood pressure measurements are required — for example, in patients with low cardiac output and high systemic vascular resistance. It may be used for hospitalized patients who are obese or have severe edema, if these conditions make indirect measurement hard to perform. It may also be used for patients who are receiving titrated doses of vasoactive drugs or who need frequent blood sampling.

Indirect monitoring, which carries few associated risks, is commonly performed by applying pressure to an artery (such as by inflating a blood pressure cuff around the arm) to decrease blood flow. As pressure is released, flow resumes and can be palpated or auscultated. Korotkoff sounds presumably result from a combination of blood flow and arterial wall vibrations; with reduced flow, these vibrations may be less pronounced.

Equipment and preparation

Sheet protector ◆ gloves, gown, mask, protective eye wear

For arterial catheter insertion
Sterile gloves ◆ 16G to 20G catheter (type and length depend on the insertion site, patient's size, and other anticipated uses of the line) ◆ preassembled preparation kit (if available) ◆ sterile drapes ◆ sterile towels ◆ prepared pressure transducer system ◆ ordered local anesthetic ◆ sutures ◆ syringe and 21G to 25G 1″ needle ◆ tubing and medication labels ◆ site-care kit (containing sterile dressing, antimicrobial ointment, and hypoallergenic tape) ◆ arm board and soft wrist restraint (for a femoral site, an ankle restraint) ◆ optional: shaving kit (for femoral artery insertion)

For blood sample collection from an open system
Sterile 4″ × 4″ gauze pads ◆ 5- or 10-ml syringe for discard sample ◆ syringes of appropriate size and number for ordered laboratory tests ◆ laboratory requests and labels ◆ 16G or 18G needles (depending on facility policy) ◆ Vacutainers

For blood sample collection from a closed system
Syringes with attached cannula of appropriate size and number for ordered laboratory tests ◆ laboratory requests and labels ◆ alcohol swabs ◆ blood transfer unit ◆ Vacutainers

For arterial line tubing changes
Sheet protector ◆ preassembled arterial pressure tubing with flush device and disposable pressure transducer ◆ sterile gloves ◆ 500-ml bag of I.V. flush solution (such as dextrose 5% in water or normal saline solution) ◆ 500 or 1,000 units of heparin ◆ syringe and 21G to 25G 1″ needle ◆ I.V. pole ◆ alcohol swabs ◆ medication and tubing labels ◆ pressure bag ◆ site-care kit (containing a sterile dressing)

For arterial catheter removal
Sterile 4″ × 4″ gauze pad ◆ sheet protector ◆ sterile suture removal set ◆ dressing ◆ alcohol swabs ◆ hypoallergenic tape

For femoral line removal
Additional four sterile 4″ × 4″ gauze pads ◆ small sandbag (which you may wrap in a towel or place in a pillow-case) ◆ adhesive bandage

For a catheter-tip culture
Sterile 4″ × 4″ gauze pad ◆ sterile scissors ◆ sterile container ◆ specimen label
Before setting up and priming the monitoring system, wash your hands thoroughly. Maintain asepsis by wearing personal protective equipment throughout preparation.

When you've finished preparing the equipment, set the alarms on the bedside monitor according to facility policy.

Implementation

■ Explain the procedure to the patient and his family, including the purpose of arterial pressure monitoring and the anticipated duration of the catheter placement. Make sure the patient signs a consent form. If he's unable to sign, ask a responsible family member to give written consent.
■ Check the patient's history for an allergy or a hypersensitivity to iodine or the ordered local anesthetic.
■ Maintain asepsis by wearing personal protective equipment throughout all procedures described here.
■ Position the patient for easy access to the catheter insertion site. Place a sheet protector under the site.
■ If the catheter will be inserted into the radial artery, perform Allen's test to assess collateral circulation in the hand.

Inserting an arterial catheter
■ Using a preassembled preparation kit, the doctor prepares and anesthetizes the insertion site. He covers the surrounding area with either sterile drapes or sterile towels. The doctor then inserts the catheter into the artery using sterile gloves and other protective equipment, then the fluid-filled pressure tubing is attached.
■ While the doctor holds the catheter in place, activate the fast-flush release to flush blood from the catheter. After each fast-flush operation, observe the drip chamber to verify that the continuous flush rate is as desired. A waveform should appear on the bedside monitor.
■ The doctor may suture the catheter in place, or you may secure it with hypoallergenic tape. Apply antimicrobial ointment and cover the insertion site with a sterile dressing, as specified by facility policy.
■ Immobilize the insertion site. With a radial or brachial site, use an arm board and soft wrist restraint (if the patient's condition so requires). With a femoral site, assess the need for an ankle restraint; keep the patient on bed rest, with the head of the bed raised no more than 15 to 30 degrees, to prevent the catheter from kinking. Level the zeroing stopcock of the pressure transducer with the phlebostatic axis. Then zero the system to atmospheric pressure.
■ Activate monitor alarms as appropriate.

Obtaining a blood sample from an open system
■ Assemble the equipment, taking care not to contaminate the dead-end cap, stopcock, and syringes. Turn off or temporarily silence the monitor alarms, depending on facility policy. (Some facilities require that alarms be left on.)
■ Locate the stopcock nearest the patient. Open a sterile 4″ × 4″ gauze pad. Remove the dead-end cap from the stopcock, and place it on the gauze pad.
■ Insert the syringe for the discard sample into the stopcock. (This sample is discarded because it's diluted with flush solution.) Follow your facility's

policy on how much discard blood to collect. In most cases, you'll withdraw 5 to 10 ml through a 5- or 10-ml syringe.

■ Next, turn the stopcock off to the flush solution. Slowly retract the syringe to withdraw the discard sample. If you feel resistance, reposition the affected extremity, and check the insertion site for obvious problems (such as catheter kinking). After correcting the problem, withdraw the blood. Then turn the stopcock halfway back to the open position to close the system in all directions.

■ Remove the discard syringe, and dispose of the blood in the syringe, observing standard precautions.

■ Place the syringe for the laboratory sample in the stopcock, turn the stopcock off to the flush solution, and slowly withdraw the required amount of blood. For each additional sample required, repeat this procedure. If the doctor has ordered coagulation tests, obtain blood for this sample from the final syringe to prevent dilution from the flush device.

■ After you've obtained blood for the final sample, turn the stopcock off to the syringe and remove the syringe. Activate the fast-flush release to clear the tubing. Then turn off the stopcock to the patient, and repeat the fast flush to clear the stopcock port.

■ Turn the stopcock off to the stopcock port, and replace the dead-end cap. Reactivate the monitor alarms. Attach needles to the filled syringes, and transfer the blood samples to the appropriate Vacutainers, labeling them according to facility policy. Send all samples to the laboratory with the laboratory request.

■ Check the monitor for return of the arterial waveform and pressure reading. (See *Understanding the arterial waveform,* page 312.)

Obtaining a blood sample from a closed system

■ Assemble the equipment, maintaining aseptic technique. Locate the closed-system reservoir and blood sampling site. Turn off or temporarily silence monitor alarms, depending on facility policy. (Some facilities require that alarms be left on.)

■ Clean the sampling site with an alcohol swab.

■ Holding the reservoir upright, grasp the flexures and slowly fill the reservoir with blood over 3 to 5 seconds. (This blood is the discard blood.) If you feel resistance, reposition the affected extremity, and check the catheter site for obvious problems (such as kinking). Then withdraw the blood.

■ Turn off the one-way valve to the reservoir by turning the handle perpendicular to the tubing. Using a syringe with attached cannula, insert the cannula into the sampling site. (Make sure the plunger is depressed to the bottom of the syringe barrel.) Slowly fill the syringe. Then grasp the cannula near the sampling site, and remove the syringe and cannula as one unit. Repeat the procedure as needed to fill the required number of syringes. If the doctor has ordered coagulation tests, obtain blood for those tests from the final syringe to prevent dilution from the flush solution.

■ After filling the syringes, turn the one-way valve to its original position, parallel to the tubing. Now smoothly and evenly push down on the plunger until the flexures lock in place in the fully closed position and all fluid has been reinfused. The fluid should be reinfused over a 3- to 5-second period. Then activate the fast-flush release to clear blood from the tubing and reservoir.

■ Clean the sampling site with an alcohol swab. Reactivate the monitor alarms. Using the blood transfer unit,

Understanding the arterial waveform

Normal arterial blood pressure produces a characteristic waveform, representing ventricular systole and diastole. The waveform has five distinct components: the anacrotic limb, systolic peak, dicrotic limb, dicrotic notch, and end diastole.

The anacrotic limb marks the waveform's initial upstroke, which results as blood is rapidly ejected from the ventricle through the open aortic valve into the aorta. The rapid ejection causes a sharp rise in arterial pressure, which appears as the waveform's highest point. This is called the systolic peak.

As blood continues into the peripheral vessels, arterial pressure falls, and the waveform begins a downward trend. This part is called the dicrotic limb. Arterial pressure usually continues to fall until pressure in the ventricle is less than pressure in the aortic root. When this occurs, the aortic valve closes. This event appears as a small notch (the dicrotic notch) on the waveform's downside. When the aortic valve closes, diastole begins, progressing until the aortic root pressure gradually descends to its lowest point. On the waveform, this is known as end diastole.

Normal arterial waveform

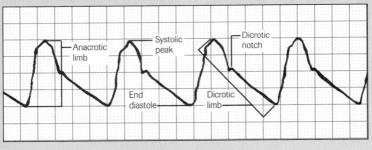

transfer blood samples to the appropriate Vacutainers, labeling them according to facility policy. Send all samples to the laboratory with the appropriate laboratory request forms.

Changing arterial line tubing

■ Wash your hands and follow standard precautions.
■ Check with facility policy to determine how much tubing length to change.
■ Check the pressure bag for air leaks after inflating it to 300 mm Hg. Then release the pressure.
■ Prepare the I.V. flush solution by adding the heparin to the flush solution as your facility policy states and

following doctors' orders. The heparin should be drawn up into the syringe with the needle attached and injected into the flush solutions after swabbing the port with alcohol, mixing thoroughly. Prime the pressure tubing and transducer system. Add medication and tubing labels. Apply 300 mm Hg of pressure to the system. Then hang the I.V. bag on a pole.
■ Place the sheet protector under the affected extremity. Remove the dressing from the catheter insertion site, taking care not to dislodge the catheter or cause vessel trauma. Turn off or temporarily silence monitor alarms, depending on facility policy. (Some facilities require that alarms be left on.)

■ Turn off the flow clamp of the tubing segment that you'll change. Disconnect the tubing from the catheter hub, taking care not to dislodge the catheter. Immediately insert the primed pressure tubing with transducer system into the catheter hub. Secure the tubing and then activate the fast-flush release to clear it.

■ Reactivate the monitor alarms. Apply an appropriate sterile dressing following your facility's protocol.

■ Level the zeroing stopcock of the transducer with the phlebostatic axis, and zero the system to atmospheric pressure.

Removing an arterial or a femoral line

■ Consult facility policy to determine whether you're permitted to perform this procedure.

■ Explain the procedure to the patient.

■ Assemble all equipment. Wash your hands. Observe standard precautions or this procedure, including wearing personal protective equipment.

■ Record the patient's systolic, diastolic, and mean blood pressures. If a manual, indirect blood pressure hasn't been assessed recently, obtain one now to establish a new baseline.

■ Turn off monitor alarms. Then turn off the flow clamp to the flush solution.

■ Carefully remove the dressing over the insertion site. Remove any sutures, using the sterile suture removal set, and then carefully check that all sutures have been removed.

■ Withdraw the catheter using a gentle, steady motion. Keep the catheter parallel to the artery during withdrawal to reduce the risk of traumatic injury.

■ Immediately after withdrawing the catheter, apply pressure to the site with a sterile 4″ × 4″ gauze pad. Maintain pressure for at least 10 minutes (longer if bleeding or oozing persists). Apply additional pressure if a femoral site was used or if the patient has coagulopathy or is receiving an anticoagulant.

■ Cover the site with an appropriate dressing, and secure it with hypoallergenic tape. If stipulated by facility policy, make a pressure dressing for a femoral site by folding in half four sterile 4″ × 4″ gauze pads, and apply the dressing. Cover the dressing tightly with an adhesive bandage; then cover the bandage with a small sandbag. Keep the patient on bed rest for 6 hours with the sandbag in place.

■ If the doctor has ordered a culture of the catheter tip (to diagnose a suspected infection), gently place the catheter tip on a sterile 4″ × 4″ gauze pad. When the bleeding is under control, hold the catheter over the sterile container. Using sterile scissors, cut the tip so it falls into the sterile container. Label the specimen, and send it to the laboratory.

■ Observe the site for bleeding. Assess circulation in the extremity distal to the site by evaluating color, pulses, and sensation. Repeat this assessment every 15 minutes for the first 4 hours, every 30 minutes for the next 2 hours, then hourly for the next 6 hours.

Special considerations

■ Observing the pressure waveform on the monitor can enhance assessment of arterial pressure. An abnormal waveform may reflect an arrhythmia (such as atrial fibrillation) or other cardiovascular problems, such as aortic stenosis, aortic insufficiency, alternating pulse, or paradoxical pulse. (See *Recognizing abnormal waveforms,* page 314.)

■ Following facility policy regarding frequency, change the pressure tubing (usually every 2 to 3 days), and change the dressing at the catheter site. Regularly assess the site for signs of infec-

Recognizing abnormal waveforms

Understanding a normal arterial waveform is relatively straightforward. An abnormal wave-form, however, is more difficult to decipher. Abnormal patterns and markings may provide important diagnostic clues to the patient's cardiovascular status, or they may simply signal trouble in the monitor. Use this chart to help you recognize and resolve waveform abnormalities.

Abnormality	Possible causes	Nursing interventions
Alternating high and low waves in a regular pattern	Ventricular bigeminy	■ Check the electrocardiogram to confirm ventricular bigeminy. The tracing should reflect premature ventricular contractions every second beat.
Flattened waveform	Overdamped wave-form or hypotensive patient	■ Check blood pressure with a sphygmomanometer. If the reading is high, suspect overdamping. Correct the problem by trying to aspirate the arterial line. If you succeed, flush the line. If the reading is very low or absent, suspect hypotension.
Slightly rounded waveform with consistent variations in systolic height	Patient on ventilator with positive end-expiratory pressure	■ Check systolic blood pressure regularly. The difference between the highest and lowest systolic pressure should be less than 10 mm Hg. If the difference exceeds that amount, suspect paradoxical pulse, possibly from cardiac tamponade.
Slow upstroke	Aortic stenosis	■ Check heart sounds for signs of aortic stenosis. Also, notify the doctor, who will document suspected aortic stenosis.
Diminished amplitude on inspiration	Paradoxical pulse, possibly from cardiac tamponade, constrictive pericarditis, or lung disease	■ Note systolic pressure during inspiration and expiration. If inspiratory pressure is at least 10 mm Hg less than expiratory pressure, call the doctor. ■ If you're also monitoring pulmonary artery pressure, watch for a diastolic plateau. This occurs when the mean central venous pressure (right atrial pressure), mean pulmonary artery pressure, and mean pulmonary artery wedge pressure (pulmonary artery obstructive pressure) are within 5 mm Hg of one another.

tion, such as redness and swelling. Notify the doctor immediately if you note any such signs.

■ Be aware that erroneous pressure readings may result from a catheter that is clotted or positional, loose connections, added stopcocks or extension tubing, inadvertent entry of air into the system, or improper calibration, leveling, or zeroing of the monitoring system. If the catheter lumen clots, the flush system may be improperly pressurized. Regularly assess the amount of flush solution in the I.V. bag, and maintain 300 mm Hg of pressure in the pressure bag.

■ Monitor for complications such as arterial bleeding, infection, air embolism, arterial spasm, and thrombosis.

Documentation

Document the date of the system setup so that all caregivers know when to change the components. Document systolic, diastolic, and mean pressure readings as well. Record circulation in the extremity distal to the site by assessing color, pulses, and sensation. Carefully document the amount of flush solution infused to avoid hypervolemia and volume overload and to ensure accurate assessment of the patient's fluid status.

Document the position of the patient when each blood pressure reading is obtained, to help determine trends.

Automated external defibrillation

Automated external defibrillators (AEDs) are commonly used today to meet the need for early defibrillation, which is considered the most effective treatment for ventricular fibrillation. Some facilities require an AED in every noncritical care unit. Their use is also

becoming common in such public places as shopping malls, sports stadiums, and airplanes. Instruction in using the AED is already required as part of Basic Life Support (BLS) and Advanced Cardiac Life Support (ACLS) training.

AEDs are used increasingly to provide early defibrillation — even when no health care provider is present. The AED interprets the victim's cardiac rhythm and gives the operator step-by-step directions on how to proceed if defibrillation is indicated. Most AEDs have a "quick look" feature that allows you to see the rhythm with the paddles before electrodes are connected.

The AED is equipped with a microcomputer that senses and analyzes a patient's heart rhythm at the push of a button. Then it audibly or visually prompts you to deliver a shock. AED models all have the same basic function but offer different operating options. For example, all AEDs communicate directions, either through messages on a display screen or by voice commands, or both. Some AEDs simultaneously display a patient's heart rhythm.

All devices record your interactions with the patient during defibrillation, either on a cassette tape or in a solid-state memory module. Some AEDs have an integral printer for immediate event documentation. Facility policy determines who is responsible for reviewing all AED interactions; the patient's doctor always has that option. Local and state regulations govern who is responsible for collecting AED case data for reporting purposes.

Equipment

AED ◆ two prepackaged electrodes ◆ electrode connector cables

Implementation

■ After discovering that your patient is unresponsive to your questions, pulseless, and apneic, follow BLS and ACLS protocols. Then ask a colleague to bring the AED into the patient's room and set it up before the code team arrives.

■ Open the foil packets containing the two electrode pads. Attach the white electrode cable connector to one pad and the red electrode cable connector to the other. The electrode pads aren't site specific.

■ Expose the patient's chest. Remove the plastic backing film from the electrode pads, and place the electrode pad attached to the white cable connector on the right upper portion of the patient's chest, just beneath his clavicle.

■ Place the pad attached to the red cable connector to the left of the heart's apex. To help remind yourself where to place the pads, think "white — right, red — ribs." (Placement for both electrode pads is the same for manual defibrillation or cardioversion.)

■ Firmly press the device's ON button, and wait while the machine performs a brief self-test. Most AEDs indicate their readiness by sounding a computerized voice that says "Stand clear" or by emitting a series of loud beeps. (If the AED isn't functioning properly, it conveys the message "Don't use the AED. Remove and continue cardiopulmonary resuscitation [CPR].") Remember to report any AED malfunctions according to facility procedure.

■ Now the machine is ready to analyze the patient's heart rhythm. Ask everyone to stand clear, and press the ANALYZE button when the machine prompts you to. Be careful not to touch or move the patient while the AED is in analysis mode. (If you get the message "Check electrodes," make sure the electrodes are correctly placed and the patient cable is securely attached; then press the ANALYZE button again.)

■ In 15 to 30 seconds, the AED will analyze the patient's rhythm. When the patient needs a shock, the AED will display a "Stand clear" message and emit a beep that changes into a steady tone as it's charging.

■ When an AED is fully charged and ready to deliver a shock, it prompts you to press the SHOCK button. (Some fully automatic AED models automatically deliver a shock within 15 seconds after analyzing the patient's rhythm. If a shock isn't needed, the AED displays a "No shock indicated" message and prompts you to "Check patient.")

■ Make sure that no one is touching the patient or his bed, and call out "Stand clear." Then press the SHOCK button on the AED. Most AEDs are ready to deliver a shock within 15 seconds.

■ After the first shock, the AED automatically reanalyzes the patient's heart rhythm. If no additional shock is needed, the machine prompts you to check the patient. However, if the patient is still in ventricular fibrillation, the AED automatically begins recharging at a higher joule level to prepare for a second shock. Repeat the steps you performed before shocking the patient. According to the AED algorithm, the patient can be shocked up to three times at increasing joule levels (200, 200 to 300, and 360 joules).

■ If the patient is still in ventricular fibrillation after three shocks, resume CPR for 1 minute. Then press the ANALYZE button on the AED to identify the heart rhythm. If the patient is still in ventricular fibrillation, continue the algorithm sequence until the code team leader arrives.

Special considerations

■ Defibrillators vary from one manufacturer to the next, so familiarize yourself with your facility's equipment.
■ Defibrillator operation should be checked at least every 8 hours and after each use.
■ Defibrillation can cause accidental electric shock to those providing care. Using an insufficient amount of conduction medium can lead to skin burns.

Documentation

After the code, remove and transcribe the AED's computer memory module or tape, or prompt the AED to print a rhythm strip with code data. Follow facility policy for analyzing and storing code data. Document the code on the appropriate form, including such information as the patient's name, age, medical history and reason for seeking care; the time you found the patient in arrest; the time CPR began; the time the AED was applied; the number of shocks the patient received; the time the pulse was regained; postarrest care given; and physical assessment findings.

Bladder irrigation, continuous

Continuous bladder irrigation can help prevent urinary tract obstruction by flushing out small blood clots that form after prostate or bladder surgery. It may also be used to treat an irritated, inflamed, or infected bladder lining.

This procedure requires placement of a triple-lumen catheter. One lumen controls balloon inflation, one allows irrigant inflow, and one allows irrigant outflow. The continuous flow of irrigating solution through the bladder also creates a mild tamponade that may help prevent venous hemorrhage. Although the patient typically receives the catheter while he's in the operating room after prostate or bladder surgery, he may have it inserted at his bedside if he isn't a surgical patient.

Equipment and preparation

One 4,000-ml container or two 2,000-ml containers of irrigating solution (usually normal saline solution) or the prescribed amount of medicated solution ◆ Y-type tubing made specifically for bladder irrigation ◆ alcohol or povidone-iodine pad ◆ I.V. pole or bedside pole attachment ◆ drainage bag and tubing

Normal saline solution is usually prescribed for bladder irrigation after prostate or bladder surgery. Large volumes of irrigating solution are usually required during the first 24 to 48 hours after surgery. This explains the use of Y-type tubing, which allows immediate irrigation with reserve solution.

Before starting continuous bladder irrigation, double-check the irrigating solution against the doctor's order. If the solution contains an antibiotic, check the patient's chart to make sure he isn't allergic to the drug. Unless specified otherwise, the patient should remain on bed rest throughout continuous bladder irrigation.

Implementation

■ Wash your hands. Assemble all equipment at the patient's bedside. Explain the procedure, and provide privacy.
■ Insert the spike of the Y-type tubing into the container of irrigating solution. (If you have a two-container system, insert one spike into each container.) (See *Setup for continuous bladder irrigation,* page 318.)

Setup for continuous bladder irrigation

During continuous bladder irrigation, a triple-lumen catheter allows irrigating solution to flow into the bladder through one lumen and flow out through another as shown in the inset. The third lumen is used to inflate the balloon that holds the catheter in place.

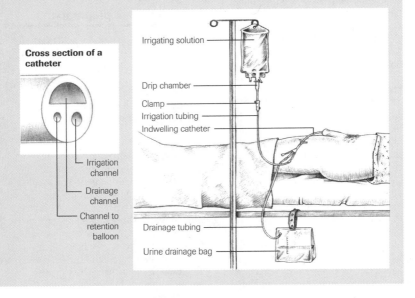

Cross section of a catheter

Irrigation channel

Drainage channel

Channel to retention balloon

Irrigating solution

Drip chamber

Clamp

Irrigation tubing

Indwelling catheter

Drainage tubing

Urine drainage bag

■ Squeeze the drip chamber on the spike of the tubing.

■ Open the flow clamp and flush the tubing to remove air, which could cause bladder distention. Then close the clamp.

■ To begin, hang the irrigating solution on the I.V. pole.

■ Clean the opening to the inflow lumen of the catheter with the alcohol or povidone-iodine pad.

■ Insert the distal end of the Y-type tubing securely into the inflow lumen (third port) of the catheter.

■ Make sure the catheter's outflow lumen is securely attached to the drainage bag tubing.

■ Open the flow clamp under the container of irrigating solution, and set the drip rate as ordered.

■ To prevent air from entering the system, don't let the primary container empty completely before replacing it.

■ If you have a two-container system, simultaneously close the flow clamp under the nearly empty container and open the flow clamp under the reserve container. This prevents reflux of irrigating solution from the reserve container into the nearly empty one. Hang a new reserve container on the I.V. pole and insert the tubing, maintaining asepsis.

■ Empty the drainage bag about every 4 hours or as often as needed. Use sterile technique to avoid the risk of contamination.

■ Monitor vital signs at least every 4 hours during irrigation; increase the frequency if the patient's condition becomes unstable.

Special considerations

■ Check the inflow and outflow lines periodically for kinks to make sure the solution is running freely. If the solution flows rapidly, check the lines frequently.

■ Measure the outflow volume accurately. It should, allowing for urine production, exceed inflow volume. If inflow volume exceeds outflow volume postoperatively, suspect bladder rupture at the suture lines or renal damage, and notify the doctor immediately.

■ Also, assess outflow for changes in appearance and for blood clots, especially if irrigation is being performed postoperatively to control bleeding. If drainage is bright red, irrigating solution is usually infused rapidly with the clamp wide open until drainage clears. Notify the doctor at once if you suspect hemorrhage. If drainage is clear, the solution is usually given at a rate of 40 to 60 gtt/minute. The doctor typically specifies the rate for antibiotic solutions.

■ Encourage oral fluid intake of 2 to 3 qt/day (2 to 3 L/day), unless contraindicated by another medical condition.

■ Watch for interruptions in the continuous irrigation system, which can predispose the patient to infection.

■ Check frequently for obstruction in the catheter's outflow lumen, which can lead to bladder distention.

Documentation

Each time you finish a container of solution, record the date, time, and

amount of fluid given on the intake and output record. Also, record the time and amount of fluid each time you empty the drainage bag. Note the appearance of the drainage and any complaints the patient has.

Cardiac monitoring

Because it allows continuous observation of the heart's electrical activity, cardiac monitoring is used for patients with conduction disturbances and for those at risk for life-threatening arrhythmias. Like other forms of electrocardiography (ECG), cardiac monitoring uses electrodes placed on the patient's chest to transmit electrical signals that are converted into a tracing of cardiac rhythm on an oscilloscope.

Two types of monitoring may be performed: hardwire and telemetry. With hardwire monitoring, the patient is connected to a monitor at his bedside, where the rhythm display appears, but it may also be transmitted to a console at a remote location. With telemetry monitoring, the patient is connected to a small transmitter that sends electrical signals to a monitor in another location. Battery-powered and portable, telemetry frees the patient from cumbersome wires and cables, so not only can he walk around, but he's also safely isolated from the electrical leakage and accidental shock occasionally associated with hardwire monitoring. Telemetry is especially useful for monitoring arrhythmias that occur during sleep, rest, exercise, or stressful situations. However, unlike hardwire monitoring, telemetry can monitor only cardiac rate and rhythm.

Regardless of the type, cardiac monitors can display the patient's heart rate and rhythm, produce a printed record of cardiac rhythm, and sound an alarm if the heart rate exceeds or falls below specified limits. Monitors also recognize and count abnormal heartbeats as well as changes. For example, a relatively new technique, ST-segment monitoring, helps detect myocardial ischemia, electrolyte imbalance, coronary artery spasm, and hypoxic events. The ST segment represents early ventricular repolarization, and any changes in this waveform component reflect alterations in myocardial oxygenation. Any monitoring lead that views an ischemic heart region will reveal ST-segment changes. The monitor's software establishes a template of the patient's normal QRST pattern from the selected leads; then the monitor displays ST-segment changes. Some monitors display such changes continuously, others only on command.

Equipment and preparation

For hardwire monitoring

Cardiac monitor ◆ leadwires ◆ patient cable ◆ disposable pregelled electrodes (number of electrodes varies from three to five, depending on patient's needs) ◆ alcohol pad ◆ 4″ × 4″ gauze pads ◆ optional: shaving supplies and washcloth

For telemetry monitoring

Transmitter ◆ pouch for transmitter ◆ telemetry battery pack, leadwires, and disposable pregelled electrodes

For hardwire monitoring, plug the cardiac monitor into an electrical outlet and turn it on to warm up the unit while you prepare the equipment and the patient. Insert the cable into the appropriate socket in the monitor. Connect the leadwires to the cable. In some systems, the leadwires are permanently secured to the cable. Each leadwire should indicate the location for attachment to the patient: right arm (RA), left arm (LA), right leg (RL), left leg (LL), and ground (C or V). This should appear on the leadwire — if it's permanently connected — or at the

connection of the leadwires and cable to the patient. Then connect an electrode to each of the leadwires, carefully checking that each leadwire is in its correct outlet.

For telemetry monitoring, insert a new battery into the transmitter. Make sure the poles on the battery match with the polar markings on the transmitter case. Press the button at the top of the unit to test the battery's charge; then test the unit to ensure that the battery is operational. If the leadwires aren't permanently affixed to the telemetry unit, attach them securely. If they must be attached individually, make sure you connect each one to the correct outlet.

Implementation

Hardwire monitoring

■ Explain the procedure to the patient, provide privacy, and ask him to expose his chest. Wash your hands.
■ Determine electrode positions on the patient's chest, based on which system and lead you're using. (See *Positioning monitoring leads.*)
■ If the leadwires and patient cable aren't permanently attached, verify that the electrode placement corresponds to the label on the patient cable.
■ If necessary, shave an area about 4″ (10 cm) in diameter around each electrode site. Clean the area with an alcohol pad, and dry it completely to remove skin secretions that may interfere with electrode function. Gently abrade the dried area by rubbing it briskly until it reddens to remove dead skin cells and to promote better electrical contact with living cells. (Some electrodes have a small, rough patch for abrading the skin; otherwise, use a dry washcloth or a dry gauze pad.)
■ Remove the backing from the disposable pregelled electrode. Check the gel for moistness. If the gel is dry, dis-

Positioning monitoring leads

This chart shows the correct electrode positions for the monitoring leads you'll use most often. For each lead, you'll see electrode placement for a five-leadwire system, a three-leadwire system, and a telemetry system.

In the two hardwire systems, the electrode positions for one lead may be identical to the electrode positions for another lead. In this case, you simply change the lead selector switch to the setting that corresponds to the lead you want. In some cases, you'll need to reposition the electrodes.

In the telemetry system, you can create the same lead with two electrodes that you do with three, simply by eliminating the ground electrode.

The illustrations below use these abbreviations: RA, right arm; LA, left arm; RL, right leg; LL, left leg; C, chest; and G, ground.

Five-leadwire system	**Three-leadwire system**	**Telemetry system**

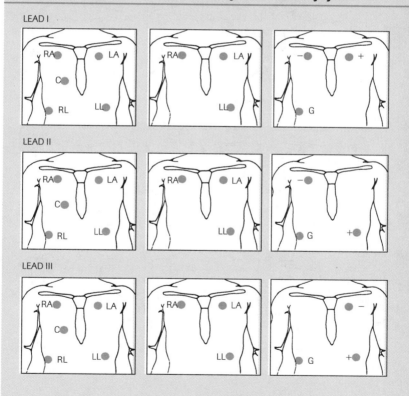

LEAD I

LEAD II

LEAD III

(continued)

Positioning monitoring leads *(continued)*

Five-leadwire system	Three-leadwire system	Telemetry system

LEAD MCL₁

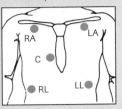 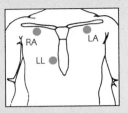 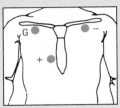

LEAD MCL₆

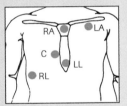 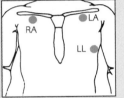 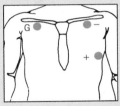

STERNAL LEAD

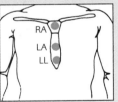 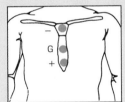

LEWIS LEAD

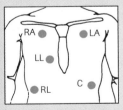 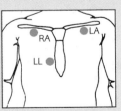 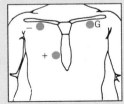

card it, and replace it with a fresh electrode.

■ Apply the electrode to the site and press firmly to ensure a tight seal. Repeat with the remaining electrodes.

■ When all electrodes are in place, check for a tracing on the cardiac monitor. Assess the quality of the ECG.

■ To verify that the monitor is detecting each beat, compare the digital heart rate display with your count of the patient's heart rate.

■ If necessary, use the gain control to adjust the size of the rhythm tracing, and use the position control to adjust the waveform position on the recording paper.

■ Set the upper and lower limits of the heart rate alarm, based on unit policy. Turn the alarm on.

Telemetry monitoring

■ Wash your hands. Explain the procedure to the patient and provide privacy.

■ Expose the patient's chest, and select the lead arrangement. Remove the backing from one of the disposable pregelled electrodes. Check the gel for moistness. If it's dry, discard the electrode, and obtain a new one.

■ Apply the electrode to the appropriate site by pressing one side of the electrode against the patient's skin, pulling gently, and then pressing the other side against the skin. Press your fingers in a circular motion around the electrode to fix the gel and stabilize the electrode. Repeat for each electrode.

■ Attach an electrode to the end of each leadwire.

■ Place the transmitter in the pouch. Tie the pouch strings around the patient's neck and waist, making sure that the pouch fits snugly without causing him discomfort. If no pouch is available, place the transmitter in the patient's bathrobe pocket.

■ Check the patient's waveform for clarity, position, and size. Adjust the gain and baseline as needed. (If necessary, ask the patient to remain resting or sitting in his room while you locate his telemetry monitor at the central station.)

■ To obtain a rhythm strip, press the RECORD key at the central station. Label the strip with the patient's name and room number, date, and time. Also, identify the rhythm. Place the rhythm strip in the appropriate location in the patient's chart.

Special considerations

■ Make sure that all electrical equipment and outlets are grounded to avoid electric shock and interference (artifacts). Also, ensure that the patient is clean and dry to prevent electric shock.

■ Avoid opening the electrode packages until just before using them, to prevent the gel from drying out.

■ Avoid placing the electrodes on bony prominences, hairy locations, areas where defibrillator pads will be placed, or areas where the chest will be compressed.

■ If the patient's skin is very oily, scaly, or diaphoretic, rub the electrode site with a dry 4″ × 4″ gauze pad before applying the electrode to help reduce interference in the tracing. Instruct the patient to breathe normally during the procedure. If his respirations distort the recording, ask him to hold his breath briefly to reduce baseline wander in the tracing.

■ Assess skin integrity, and reposition the electrodes every 24 hours or as necessary.

Patient teaching tips If the patient is being monitored by telemetry, show him how the transmitter works. If applicable, show him the button that can produce a recording of his ECG at the central station. Teach him how to push the button whenever he has symptoms. This causes the central console to print a rhythm strip. Tell the patient to remove the transmitter if he takes a shower or bath, but stress that he should let you know before he removes the unit.

Documentation

Record in your nurse's notes the date and time that monitoring begins and the monitoring lead used. Document a rhythm strip at least every 8 hours and with any changes in the patient's condition (or as stated by facility policy). Label the rhythm strip with the patient's name and room number, the date, and the time.

Cardiac output measurement

Cardiac output (CO) — the amount of blood ejected by the heart — helps evaluate cardiac function. The most widely used method of calculating this measurement is the bolus thermodilution technique. Performed at the patient's bedside, the thermodilution technique is the most practical method of evaluating the cardiac status of critically ill patients and those suspected of having cardiac disease. Other methods include the Fick method and the dye dilution test.

To measure CO, a quantity of solution colder than the patient's blood is injected into the right atrium via a port on a pulmonary artery (PA) catheter. This indicator solution mixes with the blood as it travels through the right ventricle into the pulmonary artery, and a thermistor on the catheter registers the change in the temperature of the flowing blood. A computer then plots the temperature change over time

as a curve and calculates flow based on the area under the curve.

Iced or room temperature injectant may be used. The choice should be based on facility policy as well as the patient's status. The accuracy of the bolus thermodilution technique depends on the computer being able to differentiate the temperature change that the injectant causes in the pulmonary artery as well as the temperature changes in that artery. Because it's colder than the room temperature injectant, iced injectant provides a stronger signal and thus is more easily detected.

Typically, however, room temperature injectant is more convenient and provides equally accurate measurements. Iced injectant may be more accurate for patients with high or low CO, hypothermic patients, or patients with volume restrictions and children, in whom smaller volumes of injectant (3 to 5 ml) must be used.

Equipment and preparation

For the thermodilution method
Thermodilution PA catheter in position ♦ CO computer and cable (or a module for the bedside cardiac monitor) ♦ closed or open injectant delivery system ♦ 10-ml syringe ♦ 500-ml bag of I.V. solution (dextrose 5% in water or normal saline solution) ♦ crushed ice and water and Styrofoam container (if iced injectant is used)

The newer bedside cardiac monitors measure CO continuously, either invasively or noninvasively. If your bedside monitor doesn't have this capability, you'll need a freestanding CO computer.

Wash your hands thoroughly, and assemble the equipment at the patient's bedside. Insert the closed injectant system tubing into the 500-ml bag of I.V. solution. Connect the 10-ml syringe to the system tubing, and prime the tubing with I.V. solution until all the air is out. Then clamp the tubing. The steps that follow differ, depending on the temperature of the injectant.

For room temperature injectant in a closed-delivery system

After clamping the tubing, connect the primed system to the stopcock of the proximal injectant lumen of the thermodilution PA catheter. Next, connect the temperature probe from the CO computer to the system's flow-through housing device. Connect the CO computer cable to the thermistor connector on the PA catheter, and verify the blood temperature reading. Finally, turn on the CO computer, and enter the correct computation constant, as provided by the catheter's manufacturer. The constant is determined by the volume and temperature of the injectant as well as the size and type of catheter.

🌀 *Age alert* For children, you'll need to adjust the computation constant to reflect a smaller volume and a smaller catheter size.

For iced injectant in a closed-delivery system

After clamping the tubing, place the coiled segment into the Styrofoam container, and add crushed ice and water to cover the entire coil. Let the solution cool for 15 to 20 minutes. The rest of the steps are the same as those for the room temperature injectant closed-delivery system.

Implementation

■ Make sure your patient is in a comfortable position. Tell him not to move during the procedure because movement can cause an error in measurement.

■ Explain to the patient that the procedure will help determine how well

his heart is pumping and that he'll feel no discomfort.

For room temperature injectant in a closed delivery system

■ Verify the presence of a PA waveform on the cardiac monitor.

■ Unclamp the I.V. tubing and withdraw exactly 10 ml of solution. Reclamp the tubing.

■ Turn the stopcock at the catheter injectant hub to open a fluid path between the injectant lumen of the thermodilution PA catheter and the syringe.

■ Press the START button on the CO computer or wait for an INJECT message to flash.

■ Inject the solution smoothly within 4 seconds, making sure it doesn't leak at the connectors.

■ If available, analyze the contour of the thermodilution washout curve on a strip chart recorder for a rapid upstroke and a gradual, smooth return to the baseline.

■ Repeat these steps until three values are within 10% to 15% of the median value. Compute the average, and record the patient's CO.

■ Return the stopcock to its original position, and make sure the injectant delivery system tubing is clamped.

■ Verify the presence of a PA waveform on the cardiac monitor.

■ Discontinue CO measurements when the patient's condition is hemodynamically stable and the patient is weaned from his vasoactive and inotropic medications. You can leave the PA catheter in place for pressure measurements.

■ Disconnect and discard the injectant delivery system and the I.V. bag. Cover any exposed stopcocks with air-occlusive caps.

■ Monitor the patient for signs and symptoms of inadequate perfusion, including restlessness, fatigue, changes in level of consciousness, decreased capillary refill time, diminished peripheral pulses, oliguria, and pale, cool skin.

For iced injectant in a closed-delivery system

■ Unclamp the I.V. tubing and withdraw 5 ml of solution into the syringe.

Age alert With children, withdraw 3 ml or less.

■ Inject the solution to flow past the temperature sensor while observing the injectant temperature that registers on the computer. Verify that the injectant temperature is between 43° and 54° F (6.1° and 12.2° C).

■ Verify the presence of a PA waveform on the cardiac monitor.

■ Withdraw exactly 10 ml of cooled solution before reclamping the tubing.

■ Turn the stopcock at the catheter injectant hub to open a fluid path between the injectant lumen of the PA catheter and syringe.

■ Press the START button on the CO computer, or wait for the INJECT message to flash.

■ Inject the solution smoothly within 4 seconds, making sure it doesn't leak at the connectors.

■ If available, analyze the contour of the thermodilution washout curve for a rapid upstroke and a gradual, smooth return to baseline.

■ Wait 1 minute between injections, and repeat the procedure until three values are within 10% to 15% of the median value. Compute the average, and record the patient's CO.

■ Return the stopcock to its original position, and make sure the injectant delivery system tubing is clamped.

■ Verify the presence of a PA waveform on the cardiac monitor.

Special considerations

■ The normal range for CO is 4 to 8 L/minute. The adequacy of a pa-

tient's CO is better assessed by calculating his cardiac index (CI), adjusted for his body size.

■ To calculate the patient's CI, divide his CO by his body surface area (BSA), a function of height and weight. For example, a CO of 4 L/minute might be adequate for a 5'5", 120-lb (1.65-m, 54.4-kg) patient (normally a BSA of 1.59 and a CI of 2.5) but would be inadequate for a 6'2", 230-lb (1.88-m, 104.3-kg) patient (normally a BSA of 2.26 and a CI of 1.8). The normal CI for adults ranges from 2.5 to 4.2 L/minute/m²; for pregnant women, 3.5 to 6.5 L/minute/m².

Age alert The normal CI for infants and children is 3.5 to 4 L/minute/m²; for elderly adults, 2 to 2.5 L/minute/m².

■ Add the fluid volume injected for CO determinations to the patient's total intake. Injectant delivery of 30 ml/hour will contribute 720 ml to the patient's 24-hour intake.

■ After CO measurement, make sure the clamp on the injectant bag is secured to prevent inadvertent delivery of the injectant to the patient.

Documentation

Document your patient's CO, CI, and other hemodynamic values and vital signs at the time of measurement. Note the patient's position during measurement and any other unusual occurrences, such as bradycardia or neurologic changes.

Central venous line insertion and removal

A central venous catheter (CVC) is a sterile catheter made of polyurethane, polyvinyl chloride, or silicone rubber (Silastic). It's inserted through a large vein such as the subclavian vein or, less commonly, the jugular vein.

By providing access to the central veins, central venous (CV) therapy offers several benefits. It allows monitoring of CV pressure, which indicates blood volume or pump efficiency and permits aspiration of blood samples for diagnostic tests. It also allows administration of I.V. fluids (in large amounts if necessary) when an emergency arises; when decreased peripheral circulation makes peripheral vein access difficult; when prolonged I.V. therapy reduces the number of accessible peripheral veins; when solutions must be diluted (for large fluid volumes or for irritating or hypertonic fluids, such as total parenteral nutrition solutions); and when a patient requires long-term venous access. Because multiple blood samples can be drawn through it without repeated venipuncture, the CV line decreases the patient's anxiety and preserves or restores peripheral veins.

As a variation of CV therapy, peripheral CV therapy involves insertion of a catheter into a peripheral vein instead of a central vein, but with the catheter tip still lying in the CV circulation. A peripherally inserted central catheter (PICC) usually enters at the basilic vein and terminates in the superior vena cava. PICCs may be inserted by a specially trained nurse. New catheters have longer needles and smaller lumens, facilitating this procedure. PICCs are commonly used in home I.V. therapy, but they may also be used if the patient has a chest injury; chest, neck, or shoulder burns; compromised respiratory function; or a surgical site that is close to a CV line placement site and if a doctor isn't available to insert a CV line.

CV therapy increases the risk of complications, such as pneumothorax, sepsis, thrombus formation, and vessel and adjacent organ perforation (all life-threatening conditions). Also, the CVC may decrease patient mobility, is difficult to insert, and costs more than a peripheral I.V. catheter.

Either at the end of therapy or at the onset of complications, a doctor or nurse removes the CVC, which is a sterile procedure. A specially trained nurse may remove a peripherally inserted central line. If the patient has an infection, the removal procedure includes collection of the catheter tip as a specimen for culture.

Equipment and preparation

For inserting a CVC
Shave preparation kit, if necessary ◆ sterile gloves and gowns ◆ blanket ◆ linen-saver pad ◆ sterile towel ◆ sterile drape ◆ masks ◆ alcohol pad ◆ 10% povidone-iodine pads and other approved antimicrobial solution, such as 70% isopropyl alcohol or tincture of iodine 2% ◆ normal saline solution ◆ antibiotic ointment, if necessary ◆ 3-ml syringe with 25G 10 needle ◆ 1% or 2% injectable lidocaine ◆ dextrose 5% in water (D_5W) ◆ syringes for blood sample collection ◆ suture material ◆ two 14G or 16G CVCs ◆ I.V. solution with administration set prepared for use ◆ infusion pump or controller as needed ◆ sterile 4″ × 4″ gauze pad ◆ 1″ adhesive tape ◆ sterile scissors ◆ heparin or normal saline flushes as needed ◆ portable X-ray machine ◆ optional: transparent semipermeable dressing, soap and water, nail clippers

For flushing a catheter
Normal saline solution or heparin flush solution ◆ alcohol pad ◆ 70% alcohol solution

For changing an injection cap
Alcohol or povidone-iodine pad ◆ injection cap ◆ padded clamp

For removing a CVC

Clean gloves and sterile gloves ◆ mask ◆ sterile suture removal set ◆ alcohol pad ◆ povidone-iodine solution ◆ sterile 4″ × 4″ and 2″ × 2″ gauze pads ◆ forceps ◆ tape ◆ sterile, plastic adhesive-backed dressing or transparent semipermeable dressing ◆ agar plate or culture tube, if necessary for culture ◆ povidone-iodine ointment

The type of catheter selected depends on the type of therapy to be used. Some facilities have prepared trays containing most of the equipment for catheter insertion. Before insertion of a CV catheter, confirm catheter type and size with the doctor; usually, a 14G or 16G catheter is selected. Set up the I.V. solution and prime the administration set using strict aseptic technique. Attach the line to the infusion pump or controller, if ordered. Recheck all connections to make sure they're tight. As ordered, notify the radiology department that a portable X-ray machine will be needed.

Implementation

■ Wash your hands thoroughly to prevent the spread of microorganisms.

Inserting a CVC

■ Reinforce the doctor's explanation of the procedure, and answer the patient's questions. Make sure that the patient has signed a consent form, if necessary, and check his history for hypersensitivity to iodine, latex, or the local anesthetic.

■ Place the patient in Trendelenburg's position to dilate the veins and reduce the risk of air embolism.

■ For subclavian insertion, place a rolled blanket lengthwise between the shoulders to increase venous distention. For jugular insertion, place a rolled blanket under the opposite shoulder to extend the neck, making anatomic landmarks more visible. Place a linen-saver pad under the patient to prevent soiling of the bed.

■ Turn the patient's head away from the site to prevent possible contamination from airborne pathogens and to make the site more accessible. Or, if dictated by facility policy, place a mask on the patient unless this increases his anxiety or is contraindicated because of his respiratory status.

■ Prepare the insertion site. Make sure the skin is free from hair because hair can harbor microorganisms. Infection-control practitioners recommend clipping the hair close to the skin rather than shaving. Shaving may cause skin irritation and create multiple small open wounds, increasing the risk of infection. (If the doctor orders that the area be shaved, try shaving it the evening before catheter insertion; this allows minor skin irritations to heal partially.) You may also need to wash the skin with soap and water first.

■ Establish a sterile field on a table, using a sterile towel or the wrapping from the instrument tray.

■ Put on a mask and sterile gloves and gown, and clean the area around the insertion site with alcohol pads and gauze pads soaked in 70% isopropyl alcohol followed by 10% povidone-iodine solution or other approved antimicrobial solution, working in a circular motion outward from the site. If the patient is sensitive to iodine, use a solution of 70% alcohol.

■ After the doctor puts on a mask, gown, and gloves and drapes the area to create a sterile field, open the packaging of the 3-ml syringe and 25G 10 needle and give the syringe to him using sterile technique.

■ Wipe the top of the lidocaine vial with an alcohol pad, and invert it. The doctor then fills the 3-ml syringe and injects the anesthetic into the site.

■ Open the CVC catheter, and give the catheter to the doctor using aseptic technique. The doctor then inserts the catheter.

■ During this time, prepare the I.V. administration set for immediate attachment to the catheter hub. Ask the patient to perform Valsalva's maneuver while the doctor attaches the I.V. line to the catheter hub. This increases intrathoracic pressure, reducing the possibility of an air embolus.

■ After the doctor attaches the I.V. line to the catheter hub, set the flow rate at a keep-vein-open rate to maintain venous access. (Alternatively, the catheter may be capped and flushed with heparin.) The doctor then sutures the catheter in place.

■ After an X-ray confirms correct catheter placement in the midsuperior vena cava, set the flow rate as ordered.

■ Use normal saline solution to remove dried blood that could harbor microorganisms. Secure the catheter with 1″ adhesive tape, and apply a sterile 4″ × 4″ gauze pad. You may also use a transparent semipermeable dressing either alone or placed over the gauze pad (as shown below).

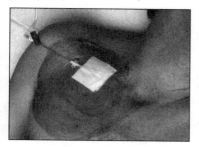

■ Expect some serosanguineous drainage during the first 24 hours. Label the dressing with the time and date of catheter insertion and catheter length and gauge, if not imprinted on the catheter as shown at top right.

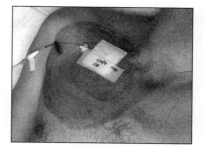

■ Place the patient in a comfortable position, and reassess his status.

Flushing a catheter

■ To maintain patency, flush the catheter routinely according to facility policy. If the system is being maintained as a heparin lock and the infusions are intermittent, the flushing procedure will vary according to policy, the medication administration schedule, and the type of catheter.

■ All lumens of a multilumen catheter must be flushed regularly. Most facilities use a heparin flush solution available in premixed 10-ml multidose vials. Recommended concentrations vary from 10 to 100 units of heparin per milliliter. Use normal saline solution instead of heparin to maintain patency in two-way valve devices, such as the Groshong type, because research suggests that heparin isn't always needed to keep the line open.

■ The recommended frequency for flushing CVCs varies from once every 12 hours to once weekly.

■ The recommended amount of flushing solution also varies. If the volume of the cannula and the add-on devices is known, most facilities recommend using twice this amount. If the volume is unknown, most facilities recommend 3 to 5 ml of solution to flush the catheter, although some facilities call for as much as 10 ml of solution. Different catheters require different amounts of solution.

■ To perform the flushing procedure, start by cleaning the cap with an alcohol pad (using 70% alcohol solution). Allow the cap to dry. If using the needleless system, follow the manufacturer's guidelines.

■ Access the cap and aspirate to confirm the patency of the CVC.

■ Inject the recommended type and amount of flush solution.

■ After flushing the catheter, maintain positive pressure by keeping your thumb on the plunger of the syringe while withdrawing the needle. This prevents blood backflow and clotting in the line. If flushing a valved catheter, close the clamp just before the last of the flush solution leaves the syringe.

Changing an injection cap

■ CVCs used for intermittent infusions have needle-free injection caps (short luer-lock devices similar to the heparin lock adapters used for peripheral I.V. therapy). These caps must be luer-lock types to prevent inadvertent disconnection and an air embolism. Unlike heparin lock adapters, these caps contain a minimal amount of empty space, so you don't have to preflush the cap before connecting it.

■ The frequency of cap changes varies according to what facility policy dictates and how often the cap is used. Use strict aseptic technique when changing the cap.

■ Clean the connection site with an alcohol pad or a povidone-iodine pad.

■ Instruct the patient to perform Valsalva's maneuver while you quickly disconnect the old cap and connect the new injection cap using aseptic technique. If he can't perform this maneuver, use a padded clamp to prevent air from entering the catheter.

Removing a CVC

■ If you'll be removing the CVC, first check the patient's record for the most recent placement (confirmed by an X-ray) to trace the catheter's path as it exits the body. Make sure that assistance is available if a complication (such as uncontrolled bleeding) occurs during catheter removal. (Some vessels, such as the subclavian vein, can be difficult to compress.) Before you remove the catheter, explain the procedure to the patient.

■ Place the patient in a supine position to prevent an embolism.

■ Wash your hands and put on clean gloves and a mask.

■ Turn off all infusions.

■ Remove and discard the old dressing, and change to sterile gloves.

■ Clean the site with an alcohol pad or a sterile 4″ × 4″ gauze pad soaked in povidone-iodine solution. Inspect the site for signs of drainage and inflammation.

■ Clip the sutures and, using forceps, remove the catheter in a slow, even motion. Have the patient perform Valsalva's maneuver as the catheter is withdrawn, to prevent an air embolism.

■ Apply pressure with a sterile gauze pad immediately after removing the catheter.

■ Apply povidone-iodine ointment to the insertion site to seal it. Cover the site with a sterile 2″ × 2″ gauze pad, and place a transparent semipermeable dressing over the gauze. Write the date and time of the removal and your initials on the dressing with indelible ink. Keep the site covered for 48 hours.

■ Inspect the catheter tip and measure the length of the catheter to ensure that the catheter has been completely removed. If you suspect that the catheter hasn't been completely removed, notify the doctor immediately, and monitor the patient closely for signs of distress. If you suspect an infection, swab the catheter on a fresh agar plate, and send the specimen to the laboratory for culture.

■ Dispose of the I.V. tubing and equipment properly.

Special considerations

■ While you're awaiting chest X-ray confirmation of proper catheter placement, infuse an I.V. solution such as D_5W or normal saline solution at a keep-vein-open rate, until correct placement is assured. Or use a heparin lock and flush the line. Infusing an isotonic solution avoids the risk of vessel-wall thrombosis.

■ Watch for signs of air embolism, including sudden onset of pallor, cyanosis, dyspnea, coughing, and tachycardia, progressing to syncope and shock. If any of these signs occur, place the patient on his left side in Trendelenburg's position, and notify the doctor.

■ After insertion, monitor the patient for signs and symptoms of pneumothorax, such as shortness of breath, uneven chest movement, tachycardia, and chest pain. Notify the doctor immediately if such signs appear.

■ If a gauze dressing is used, change it at least every 48 hours, or if a transparent semipermeable dressing is used, change it every 3 to 7 days, according to facility policy, or whenever it becomes moist or soiled. Change the tubing every 48 hours and the solution every 24 hours or according to facility policy while the CVC is in place. Dressing, tubing, and solution changes for a CVC should be performed using aseptic technique. (See *Key steps in changing a central venous dressing.*) Assess the site for signs and symptoms of infection, such as discharge, inflammation, and tenderness.

■ To prevent an air embolism, close the catheter clamp or have the patient perform Valsalva's maneuver each time the catheter hub is open to air. (A Groshong catheter doesn't require

Key steps in changing a central venous dressing

Expect to change your patient's central venous dressing every 3 to 7 days. Many facilities specify dressing changes whenever the dressing becomes soiled, moist, or loose. The following illustrations show the key steps you'll perform.

First, put on clean gloves, and remove the old dressing by pulling it toward the exit site of a long-term catheter or toward the insertion site of a short-term catheter. This technique helps you avoid pulling out the line. Remove and discard your gloves.

Next, put on sterile gloves, and clean the skin around the site three times, using a new alcohol pad each time. Start at the center and move outward, using a circular motion.

Allow the skin to dry, and repeat the same cleaning procedure using three swabs soaked in povidone-iodine solution (as shown below).

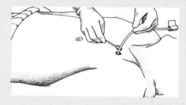

After the solution has dried, cover the site with a dressing, such as a gauze dressing or the transparent semipermeable dressing shown here. Write the time and date on the dressing.

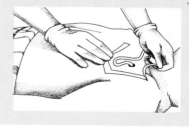

clamping because it has an internal valve.)

■ Long-term use of a CVC allows patients to receive caustic fluids and blood infusions at home. These catheters have a much longer life because they're less thrombogenic and less prone to infection than short-term devices.

Patient teaching tips
A candidate for home therapy must have a family member or friend who can safely and competently administer the I.V. fluids, a backup helper, a suitable home environment, a telephone, transportation, adequate reading skills, and the ability to prepare, handle, store, and dispose of the equipment. The care procedures used in the home are the same as those used in the facility, except that the home therapy patient uses clean instead of aseptic technique.

The overall goal of home therapy is patient safety, so your patient teaching must begin well before discharge. After discharge, a home therapy coordinator provides follow-up care until the patient or someone close to him can provide catheter care and infusion therapy independently. Many home therapy patients learn to care for the catheter themselves and infuse their own medications and solution.

■ Complications can occur at any time during infusion therapy. Traumatic complications such as pneumothorax typically occur on catheter insertion but may not be noticed until after the procedure is completed. Systemic complications such as sepsis typically occur later during infusion therapy. Other complications include phlebitis (especially in peripheral CV therapy), thrombus formation, and air embolism.

Documentation

Record the time and date of insertion, length and location of the catheter, solution infused, doctor's name, and patient's response to the procedure. Document the time of the X-ray, its results, and your notification of the doctor.

Also, record the time and date of removal and the type of antimicrobial ointment and dressing applied. Note the condition of the catheter insertion site and collection of a culture specimen.

Central venous pressure monitoring

In central venous pressure (CVP) monitoring, the doctor inserts a catheter through a vein and advances it until its tip lies in or near the right atrium. Because no major valves lie at the junction of the vena cava and right atrium, pressure at end diastole reflects back to the catheter. When connected to a manometer, the catheter measures CVP, an index of right ventricular function.

CVP monitoring helps you assess cardiac function, evaluate venous return to the heart, and indirectly gauge how well the heart is pumping. The central venous (CV) line also provides access to a large vessel for rapid, high-volume fluid administration and allows frequent blood withdrawal for laboratory samples.

CVP monitoring can be done intermittently or continuously. The catheter is inserted percutaneously or using a cutdown method. Typically, a single lumen CVP line is used for intermittent pressure readings. To measure the patient's volume status, a disposable plastic water manometer is attached between the I.V. line and the central catheter with a three- or four-way stopcock. CVP is recorded in centimeters of water (cm H_2O) or millimeters of mercury (mm Hg) and read from manometer markings.

Normal CVP ranges from 5 to 10 cm H_2O. Any condition that alters venous return, circulating blood volume, or cardiac performance can affect CVP. If circulating volume increases (such as with enhanced venous return to the heart), CVP rises. If circulating volume decreases (such as with reduced venous return), CVP drops.

Equipment

For intermittent CVP monitoring

Disposable CVP manometer set ◆ leveling device (such as a rod from a reusable CVP pole holder or a carpenter's level or rule) ◆ stopcock (to attach the CVP manometer to the catheter) ◆ I.V. pole ◆ I.V. solution

For continuous CVP monitoring

Pressure monitoring kit with disposable pressure transducer ◆ leveling device ◆ bedside pressure module ◆ continuous I.V. flush solution ◆ 1 unit/1 to 2 ml of heparin flush solution ◆ pressure bag

For removing a CV catheter

Gloves ◆ suture removal set ◆ sterile gauze pads ◆ povidone-iodine ointment ◆ dressing ◆ tape

Implementation

■ Gather the necessary equipment. Explain the procedure to the patient to reduce his anxiety.

■ Assist the doctor as he inserts the CV catheter. (The procedure is similar to that used for pulmonary artery pressure monitoring, except that the catheter is advanced only as far as the superior vena cava.)

Monitoring CVP intermittently with a water manometer

■ With the CV line in place, position the patient flat. Align the base of the disposable CVP manometer with the previously determined zero reference point by using a leveling device. Because CVP reflects right atrial pressure, you must align the right atrium (the zero reference point) with the zero mark on the manometer. To find the right atrium, locate the fourth intercostal space at the midaxillary line. Mark the appropriate place on the patient's chest so that all subsequent recordings will be made using the same location.

■ If the patient can't tolerate a flat position, place him in semi-Fowler's position. When the head of the bed is elevated, the phlebostatic axis remains constant but the midaxillary line changes. Use the same degree of elevation for all subsequent measurements.

■ Attach the manometer to an I.V. pole or place it next to the patient's chest. Make sure the zero reference point is level with the right atrium. (See *Measuring CVP with a water manometer*, page 334.)

■ Verify that the manometer is connected to the I.V. tubing. Typically, markings on the manometer range from −2 to 38 cm H_2O. However, manufacturer's markings may differ, so read the directions before setting up the manometer and obtaining readings.

■ Turn the stopcock off to the patient, and slowly fill the manometer with I.V. solution until the fluid level is 10 to 20 cm H_2O higher than the patient's expected CVP value. Don't overfill the tube because fluid that spills over the top can become a source of contamination.

■ Turn the stopcock off to the I.V. solution and open to the patient. The fluid level in the manometer will drop. When the fluid level comes to rest, it

Measuring CVP with a water manometer

To ensure accurate central venous pressure (CVP) readings, make sure the manometer base is aligned with the patient's right atrium (the zero reference point). The manometer set usually contains a leveling rod to allow you to determine this quickly.

After adjusting the manometer's position, examine the typical three-way stopcock. By turning it to any position shown at right, you can control the direction of fluid flow. Four-way stopcocks also are available.

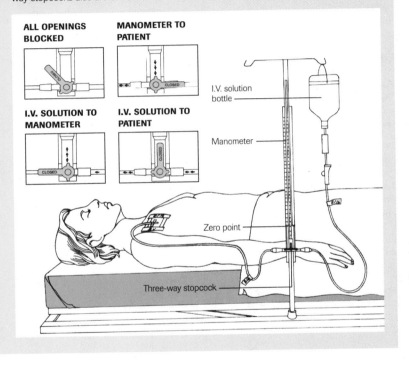

will fluctuate slightly with respirations. Expect it to drop during inspiration and to rise during expiration.

■ Record CVP at the end of inspiration, when intrathoracic pressure has a negligible effect. Depending on the type of water manometer used, note the value either at the bottom of the meniscus or at the midline of the small floating ball.

■ After you've obtained the CVP value, turn the stopcock to resume the I.V. infusion. Adjust the I.V. drip rate as required.

■ Place the patient in a comfortable position.

Monitoring CVP continuously with a water manometer

Follow the procedure as outlined for monitoring CVP intermittenly with a water manometer, except that the CVP system will be continuously hooked up for use.

■ Make sure the stopcock is turned so that the I.V. solution port, CVP column port, and patient port are open. Be aware that with this stopcock position, infusion of the I.V. solution increases CVP. Therefore, expect higher readings than those taken with the stopcock turned off to the I.V. solution. If the I.V. solution infuses at a constant rate, CVP will change as the patient's condition changes, although the initial reading will be higher. Assess the patient closely for changes.

Monitoring CVP continuously with a pressure monitoring system

■ Make sure the CV line or the proximal lumen of a pulmonary artery catheter is attached to the system. (If the patient has a CV line with multiple lumens, one lumen may be dedicated to continuous CVP monitoring and the other lumens used for fluid administration.)

■ Set up a pressure transducer system. Connect noncompliant pressure tubing from the CVP catheter hub to the transducer. Then connect the continuous I.V. flush solution to the pressure tubing.

■ To obtain values, position the patient flat. If he can't tolerate this position, use semi-Fowler's position. Locate the level of the right atrium by identifying the phlebostatic axis. Zero the transducer, leveling the transducer air-fluid interface stopcock with the right atrium. Read the CVP value from the digital display on the monitor, and note the waveform. Make sure the patient is still when the reading is taken to prevent artifact. (See *Identifying hemodynamic pressure monitoring problems,* pages 336 to 338.) Use this position for all subsequent readings.

Removing a CV catheter

■ You may assist the doctor in removing a CV catheter. (In some states, a nurse is permitted to remove the catheter when acting under a doctor's order or advanced collaborative standards of practice.)

■ If the head of the bed is elevated, minimize the risk of air embolism during catheter removal — for instance, by placing the patient in Trendelenburg's position if the line was inserted using a superior approach. If he can't tolerate this, position him flat.

■ Turn the patient's head to the side opposite the catheter insertion site. The doctor removes the dressing and exposes the insertion site. If sutures are in place, he removes them carefully.

■ Turn the I.V. solution off.

■ The doctor pulls the catheter out in a slow, smooth motion and then applies pressure to the insertion site.

■ Clean the insertion site, apply povidone-iodine ointment, and cover it with a sterile gauze pad dressing and tape as ordered.

■ Assess the patient for signs of respiratory distress, which may indicate an air embolism.

Special considerations

■ As ordered, arrange for daily chest X-rays to check catheter placement.

■ Care for the insertion site according to facility policy. Typically, you'll change the dressing every 24 to 48 hours.

■ Wash your hands before performing dressing changes, and use aseptic technique and sterile gloves when redressing the site. When removing the old dressing, observe the patient for signs of infection, such as redness, and note any patient complaints of tenderness. Apply ointment, and then cover the site with a sterile gauze dressing or a clear occlusive dressing.

(Text continues on page 338.)

Identifying hemodynamic pressure monitoring problems

Problem	Possible causes	Interventions
No waveform	■ Power supply turned off ■ Monitor screen pressure range set too low ■ Loose connection in line ■ Transducer not connected to amplifier ■ Stopcock off to patient ■ Catheter occluded or out of blood vessel	■ Check the power supply. ■ Raise the monitor screen pressure range, if necessary. ■ Rebalance and recalibrate the equipment. ■ Tighten loose connections. ■ Check and tighten the connection. ■ Position the stopcock correctly. ■ Use the fast-flush valve to flush the line, or try to aspirate blood from the catheter. If the line remains blocked, notify the doctor, and prepare to replace the line.
Drifting waveforms	■ Improper warm-up ■ Electrical cable kinked or compressed ■ Temperature change in room air or I.V. flush solution	■ Allow the monitor and transducer to warm up for 10 to 15 minutes. ■ Place the monitor's cable where it can't be stepped on or compressed. ■ Routinely zero and calibrate the equipment 30 minutes after setting it up. This allows I.V. fluid to warm to room temperature.
Line fails to flush	■ Stopcocks positioned incorrectly ■ Inadequate pressure from pressure bag ■ Kink in pressure tubing ■ Blood clot in catheter	■ Make sure stopcocks are positioned correctly. ■ Make sure the pressure bag gauge reads 300 mm Hg. ■ Check the pressure tubing for kinks. ■ Try to aspirate the clot with a syringe. If the line still won't flush, notify the doctor and prepare to replace the line, if necessary. *Important:* Never use a syringe to flush a hemodynamic line.
Artifact (waveform interference)	■ Patient movement ■ Electrical interference ■ Catheter fling (tip of pulmonary artery [PA] catheter moving rapidly in large blood vessel or heart chamber)	■ Wait until the patient is quiet before taking a reading. ■ Make sure electrical equipment is connected and grounded correctly. ■ Notify the doctor, who may try to reposition the catheter.

Identifying hemodynamic pressure monitoring problems *(continued)*

Problem	Possible causes	Interventions
Artifact (waveform interference) *(continued)*	■ Transducer balancing port positioned below the patient's right atrium ■ Flush solution flow rate is too fast ■ Air in system ■ Catheter fling (tip of PA catheter moving rapidly in large blood vessel or heart chamber)	■ Position the balancing port level with the patient's right atrium. ■ Check the flush solution flow rate. Maintain it at 3 to 4 ml/hour. ■ Remove air from the lines and the transducer. ■ Notify the doctor, who may try to reposition the catheter.
False-high readings	■ Transducer balancing port positioned above right atrium ■ Transducer imbalance ■ Loose connection	■ Position the balancing port level with the patient's right atrium. ■ Make sure the transducer's flow system isn't kinked or occluded, and rebalance and recalibrate the equipment. ■ Tighten loose connections. ■ Secure all connections.
False-low readings	■ Air bubbles ■ Blood clot in catheter ■ Blood flashback in line ■ Incorrect transducer position	■ Remove air from the lines and the transducer. ■ Check for and replace cracked equipment. ■ Refer to "Line fails to flush" (earlier in this chart). ■ Make sure stopcock positions are correct, tighten loose connections, replace cracked equipment, flush the line with the fast-flush valve, and replace the transducer dome if blood backs up into it. ■ Make sure the transducer is kept at the level of the right atrium at all times. Improper levels give false-high or false-low pressure readings.
Damped waveform	■ Arterial catheter out of blood vessel or pressed against vessel wall	■ Reposition the catheter if it's against the vessel wall. ■ Try to aspirate blood to confirm proper placement in the vessel. If you can't aspirate blood, notify the doctor and prepare to replace the line.

(continued)

Identifying hemodynamic pressure monitoring problems *(continued)*

Problem	Possible causes	Interventions
Damped waveform	■ Ruptured balloon	*Note:* Bloody drainage at the insertion site may indicate catheter displacement. Notify the doctor immediately.
Pulmonary artery wedge pressure tracing unobtainable	■ Incorrect amount of air in balloon	■ If you feel no resistance when injecting air, or if you see blood leaking from the balloon inflation lumen, stop injecting air and notify the doctor. If the catheter is left in, label the inflation lumen with a warning not to inflate.
	■ Catheter malpositioned	■ Deflate the balloon. Check the label on the catheter for correct volume. Reinflate slowly with the correct amount. To avoid rupturing the balloon, never use more than the stated volume. ■ Notify the doctor. Obtain a chest X-ray.

■ After the initial CVP reading, reevaluate readings frequently to establish a baseline for the patient. Authorities recommend obtaining readings at 15-, 30-, and 60-minute intervals to establish a baseline. If the patient's CVP fluctuates by more than 2 cm H_2O, suspect a change in his clinical status, and report this finding to the doctor.

■ Change the I.V. solution every 24 hours and the I.V. tubing every 48 hours, according to facility policy. Expect the doctor to change the catheter every 72 hours. Label the I.V. solution, tubing, and dressing with the date, time, and your initials.

■ Assess patient for complications of CVP monitoring, including pneumothorax (which typically occurs upon catheter insertion), sepsis, thrombus, vessel and adjacent organ puncture, and air embolism.

Documentation

Document all dressing, tubing, and solution changes. Document the patient's tolerance of the procedure, the date and time of catheter removal, and the type of dressing applied. Note the condition of the catheter insertion site and whether a culture specimen was collected. Note any complications and actions taken.

Chest physiotherapy

Chest physiotherapy (PT) includes postural drainage, chest percussion and vibration, and coughing and deep-breathing exercises. Together, these techniques mobilize and eliminate secretions, reexpand lung tissue, and promote efficient use of respiratory muscles. Of critical importance to the bedridden patient, chest PT helps prevent or treat atelectasis and may also help prevent pneumonia, two respiratory complications that can seriously impede recovery.

Postural drainage performed with percussion and vibration encourages peripheral pulmonary secretions to empty by gravity into the major bronchi or trachea and is accomplished by sequential repositioning of the patient. Usually, secretions drain best with the patient positioned so that the bronchi are perpendicular to the floor. Lower and middle lobe bronchi usually empty best with the patient in the head-down position; upper lobe bronchi, in the head-up position. Percussing the chest with cupped hands mechanically dislodges thick, tenacious secretions from the bronchial walls. Vibration can be used with percussion or as an alternative to it in a patient who is frail, in pain, or recovering from thoracic surgery or trauma.

Candidates for chest PT include patients who expectorate large amounts of sputum, such as those with bronchiectasis or cystic fibrosis. The procedure hasn't proved effective in treating patients with status asthmaticus, lobar pneumonia, or acute exacerbations of chronic bronchitis when the patient has scant secretions and is being mechanically ventilated. Chest PT has little value for treating patients with stable, chronic bronchitis.

Contraindications include active pulmonary bleeding with hemoptysis and the immediate posthemorrhage stage, fractured ribs or an unstable chest wall, lung contusions, pulmonary tuberculosis, untreated pneumothorax, acute asthma or bronchospasm, lung abscess or tumor, bony metastasis, head injury, and recent myocardial infarction.

Equipment and preparation

Stethoscope ◆ emesis basin ◆ facial tissues ◆ suction equipment as needed ◆ equipment for oral care ◆ trash bag

Gather the equipment at the patient's bedside. Set up suction equipment, if needed, and test its function.

Implementation

◼ Explain the procedure to the patient, provide privacy, and wash your hands.

◼ Auscultate the patient's lungs with a stethoscope to determine baseline respiratory status.

◼ Position the patient as ordered using pillows. For patients with generalized disease, drainage usually begins with the lower lobes, continues with the middle lobes, and ends with the upper lobes. For patients with localized disease, drainage begins with the affected lobes and then proceeds to the other lobes to avoid spreading the disease to uninvolved areas.

◼ Instruct the patient to remain in each position for 10 to 15 minutes. During this time, perform percussion and vibration as ordered. (See *Performing percussion and vibration,* page 340.)

◼ After postural drainage, percussion, or vibration, instruct the patient to cough to remove loosened secretions. First, tell him to inhale deeply through his nose and then exhale in three short huffs. Then instruct him to inhale deeply again and cough through a slightly open mouth. Three consecutive coughs are highly effective. An effective cough sounds deep, low, and hollow; an ineffective one, high-pitched. Have the patient perform exercises for about 1 minute and then have him rest for 2 minutes. Gradually progress to a 10-minute exercise period four times daily.

◼ Provide oral hygiene because secretions may have a foul taste or a stale odor. Dispose of secretions via suction equipment setup or in tissues and in trash bag. Provide an emesis basin if needed.

Performing percussion and vibration

To perform percussion, instruct the patient to breathe slowly and deeply, using the diaphragm, to promote relaxation. Hold your hands in a cupped shape, with fingers flexed and thumbs pressed tightly against your index fingers. Percuss each segment for 1 to 2 minutes by alternating your hands against the patient in a rhythmic manner. Listen for a hollow sound on percussion to verify correct performance of the technique.

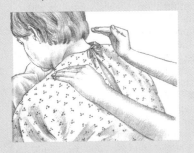

To perform vibration, ask the patient to inhale deeply and then exhale slowly through pursed lips. During exhalation, firmly press your fingers and the palms of your hands against the chest wall. Tense the muscles of your arms and shoulders in an isometric contraction to send fine vibrations through the chest wall. Vibrate during five exhalations over each chest segment.

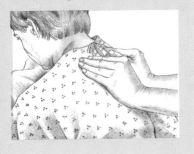

■ Auscultate the patient's lungs to evaluate the effectiveness of therapy.

Special considerations

■ For optimal effectiveness and safety, modify chest PT according to the patient's condition. For example, initiate or increase the flow of supplemental oxygen, if indicated. Also, suction the patient who has an ineffective cough reflex. If the patient tires quickly during therapy, shorten the sessions because fatigue leads to shallow respirations and increased hypoxia.

■ If the patient is receiving chest PT to prevent mucus dehydration and promote easier mobilization, make sure he takes in plenty of fluids. Avoid performing postural drainage immediately before or within $1\frac{1}{2}$ hours after meals to avoid nausea and aspiration of food or vomitus.

■ Because chest percussion can induce bronchospasm, any adjunct treatment (for example, intermittent positive-pressure breathing, aerosol, or nebulizer therapy) should precede chest PT.

■ Refrain from percussing over the spine, liver, kidneys, or spleen to avoid injury to the spine or internal organs. Also, avoid performing percussion on bare skin or the female patient's breasts. Percuss over soft clothing (but not over buttons, snaps, or zippers), or place a thin towel over the chest wall. Remember to remove jewelry that might scratch or bruise the patient.

Patient teaching tips
Explain coughing and deep-breathing exercises preoperatively so that the patient can practice them when he's pain-free and can concentrate better. Postoperatively, splint the patient's incision using your hands or, if possible, teach the patient to splint it himself to minimize pain during coughing.

■ Watch the patient for complications. During postural drainage in head-down positions, pressure on the diaphragm by abdominal contents can impair respiratory excursion and lead to hypoxia or postural hypotension. The head-down position also may lead to increased intracranial pressure, which precludes the use of chest PT in a patient with acute neurologic impairment. Vigorous percussion or vibration can cause rib fracture, especially if the patient has osteoporosis. In an emphysematous patient with blebs, coughing can lead to pneumothorax.

Documentation

Record the date and time of chest PT; positions for secretion drainage and length of time each is maintained; chest segments percussed or vibrated; color, amount, odor, and viscosity of secretions produced and the presence of any blood; any complications and nursing actions taken; and the patient's tolerance of treatment.

Colostomy and ileostomy care

A patient with an ascending or transverse colostomy or an ileostomy must wear an external pouch to collect emerging fecal matter, which is typically watery or pasty. In addition to collecting waste matter, the pouch helps to control odor and protect the stoma and peristomal skin. Most disposable pouching systems can be used for 2 to 7 days; some models last even longer.

All pouching systems need to be changed immediately if a leak develops, and every pouch must be emptied when it's one-third to one-half full. The patient with an ileostomy may need to empty his pouch four or five times daily.

Naturally, the best time to change the pouching system is when the bowel is least active, usually between 2 and 4 hours after meals. After a few months, most patients can predict the best changing time.

The selection of a pouching system should take into consideration which system provides the best adhesive seal and skin protection for the individual patient. The type of pouch selected also depends on the stoma's location and structure, availability of supplies, wear time, consistency of effluent, personal preference, and finances.

Equipment

Pouching system ◆ stoma measuring guide ◆ stoma paste (if drainage is watery to pasty or stoma secretes excess mucus) ◆ scissors ◆ water ◆ closure clamp ◆ toilet or bedpan ◆ gloves ◆ facial tissue ◆ optional: ostomy belt, paper tape, mild nonmoisturizing soap, skin shaving equipment ◆ prepared skin barrier ◆ gauze pad

Pouching systems may be drainable or closed-bottomed, disposable or reusable, adhesive-backed, and one- or two-piece. (See *Comparing ostomy pouching systems,* page 342.)

Implementation

■ Provide privacy and emotional support.

Fitting the pouch and skin barrier
■ For a pouch with an attached skin barrier, measure the stoma with the stoma measuring guide. Select the opening size that matches the stoma.
■ For an adhesive-backed pouch with a separate skin barrier, measure the stoma with the measuring guide and select the opening that matches the stoma. Trace the selected size opening onto the paper back of the skin barri-

Comparing ostomy pouching systems

Manufactured in many shapes and sizes, ostomy pouches are fashioned for comfort, safety, and easy application. For example, a disposable closed-end pouch may meet the needs of a patient who irrigates, who wants added security, or who wants to discard the pouch after each bowel movement. Another patient may prefer a reusable, drainable pouch. Some commonly available pouches are described below.

Disposable pouches

The patient who must empty his pouch often (because of diarrhea or a new colostomy or ileostomy) may prefer a one-piece, drainable, disposable pouch with a closure clamp attached to a skin barrier (below left).

These transparent or opaque, odor-proof, plastic pouches come with attached adhesive or karaya seals. Some pouches have microporous adhesive or belt tabs. The bottom opening allows for easy draining. This pouch may be used permanently or temporarily, until stoma size stabilizes.

Also disposable and made of transparent or opaque odor-proof plastic, a one-piece disposable closed-end pouch (below right) may come in a kit with adhesive seal, belt tabs, skin barrier, or carbon filter for gas release. A patient with a regular bowel elimination pattern may choose this style for added security and confidence.

A two-piece disposable drainable pouch with separate skin barrier (shown below) permits frequent changes and also minimizes skin breakdown. Also made of transparent or opaque odor-proof plastic, this style comes with belt tabs and usually snaps to the skin barrier with a flange mechanism.

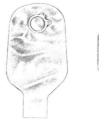

Reusable pouches

Typically manufactured from sturdy, opaque, hypoallergenic plastic, the reusable pouch comes with a separate custom-made faceplate and O-ring (as shown below). Some pouches have a pressure valve for releasing gas. The device has a 1- to 2-month life span, depending on how frequently the patient empties the pouch.

Reusable equipment may benefit a patient who needs a firm faceplate or who wishes to minimize cost. However, many reusable ostomy pouches aren't odor-proof.

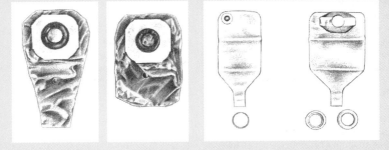

er's adhesive side. Cut out the opening. (If the pouch has precut openings, which can be handy for a round stoma, select an opening that is $1/8''$ [3 mm] larger than the stoma. If the pouch comes without an opening, cut the hole $1/8''$ wider than the measured tracing.) The cut-to-fit system works best for an irregularly shaped stoma.

■ For a two-piece pouching system with flanges, see *Applying a skin barrier and pouch,* page 344.

■ Avoid fitting the pouch too tightly because the stoma has no pain receptors. A constrictive opening could injure the stoma or skin tissue without the patient feeling the warning of discomfort. Also, avoid cutting the opening too big because this may expose the skin to fecal matter and moisture.

■ The patient with a descending or sigmoid colostomy who has formed stools and whose ostomy doesn't secrete much mucus may choose to wear only a pouch. In this case, make sure the pouch opening closely matches the stoma size.

■ Between 6 weeks and 1 year after surgery, the stoma will shrink to its permanent size. At that point, pattern-making preparations will be unnecessary unless the patient gains weight, has additional surgery, or injures the stoma.

Applying or changing the pouch

■ Collect all equipment.

■ Wash your hands and provide privacy.

■ Explain the procedure to the patient. As you perform each step, explain what you're doing and why because the patient will eventually perform the procedure himself.

■ Put on gloves.

■ Remove and discard the old pouch. Wipe the stoma and peristomal skin gently with a facial tissue.

■ Carefully wash the stoma with mild nonmoisturizing soap and water, and dry the peristomal skin by patting gently. Allow the skin to dry thoroughly. Inspect the peristomal skin and stoma. If necessary, shave surrounding hair (in a direction away from the stoma) to promote a better seal and avoid skin irritation from hair pulling against the adhesive.

■ If applying a separate skin barrier, peel off the paper backing of the prepared skin barrier, center the barrier over the stoma, and press gently to ensure adhesion.

■ You may want to outline the stoma on the back of the skin barrier (depending on the product) with a thin ring of stoma paste to provide extra skin protection. (Skip this step if the patient has a sigmoid or descending colostomy, formed stools, and little mucus.)

■ Remove the paper backing from the adhesive side of the pouching system and center the pouch opening over the stoma. Press gently to secure.

■ For a pouching system with flanges, align the lip of the pouch flange with the bottom edge of the skin barrier flange. Gently press around the circumference of the pouch flange, beginning at the bottom, until the pouch securely adheres to the barrier flange. (The pouch will click into its secured position.) Holding the barrier against the skin, gently pull on the pouch to confirm the seal between flanges.

■ Encourage the patient to stay quietly in position for about 5 minutes to improve adherence. The patient's body warmth also helps to improve adherence and to soften a rigid skin barrier.

■ Attach an ostomy belt to further secure the pouch, if desired. (Some pouches have belt loops, and others have plastic adapters for belts.)

Applying a skin barrier and pouch

Fitting a skin barrier and ostomy pouch properly can be done in a few steps. The commonly used, two-piece pouching system with flanges is shown below.

Measure the stoma using a measuring guide.

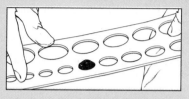

Trace the appropriate circle carefully on the back of the skin barrier.

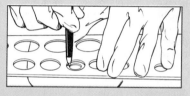

Cut the circular opening in the skin barrier. Bevel the edges to keep them from irritating the patient.

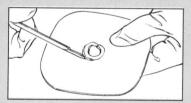

Remove the backing from the skin barrier and moisten it or apply barrier paste as needed along the edge of the circular opening.

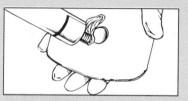

Center the skin barrier over the stoma, adhesive side down, and gently press it to the skin.

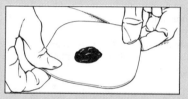

Gently press the pouch opening onto the ring until it snaps into place.

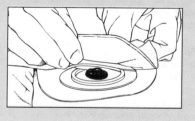

■ Leave a bit of air in the pouch to allow drainage to fall to the bottom.
■ Apply the closure clamp, if necessary.
■ If desired, apply paper tape in a picture-frame fashion to the pouch edges for additional security.

Emptying the pouch
■ Put on gloves.
■ Tilt the bottom of the pouch upward, and remove the closure clamp.
■ Turn up a cuff on the lower end of the pouch, and allow it to drain into the toilet or bedpan.

■ Wipe the bottom of the pouch with a gauze pad, and reapply the closure clamp.

■ If desired, the bottom portion of the pouch can be rinsed with cool tap water. Don't aim water up near the top of the pouch because this may loosen the seal on the skin.

■ A two-piece flanged system can also be emptied by unsnapping the pouch. Let the drainage flow into the toilet.

■ Release flatus through the gas release valve if the pouch has one. Otherwise, release flatus by tilting the pouch bottom upward, releasing the clamp, and expelling the flatus. To release flatus from a flanged system, loosen the seal between the flanges. (Some pouches have gas release valves.)

■ Never make a pinhole in a pouch to release gas. This destroys the odor-proof seal.

■ Remove gloves.

Special considerations

■ After performing and explaining the procedure to the patient, encourage the patient's increasing involvement in self-care.

■ Use adhesive solvents and removers only after patch-testing the patient's skin because some products may irritate the skin or produce hypersensitivity reactions. Consider using a liquid skin sealant, if available, to give skin tissue added protection from drainage and adhesive irritants.

■ Remove the pouching system if the patient reports burning or itching beneath it or purulent drainage around the stoma. Notify the doctor or therapist of any skin irritation, breakdown, rash, or unusual appearance of the stoma or peristomal area.

■ Use commercial pouch deodorants, if desired. However, most pouches are odor-free, and odor should only be evident when you empty the pouch or if it leaks. Before discharge, suggest that the patient avoid odor-causing foods, such as fish, eggs, onions, and garlic.

■ If the patient wears a reusable pouching system, suggest that he obtain two or more systems so that he can wear one while the other dries after cleaning with soap and water or a commercially prepared cleaning solution.

■ Failure to fit the pouch properly over the stoma or improper use of a belt can injure the stoma. Be alert for a possible allergic reaction to adhesives and other ostomy products.

Documentation

Record the date and time of the pouching system change; note the character of drainage, including color, amount, type, and consistency. Also, describe the appearance of the stoma and the peristomal skin. Document patient teaching. Describe the teaching content. Record the patient's response to self-care, and evaluate his learning progress.

Colostomy irrigation

Irrigation of a colostomy can serve two purposes: It allows a patient with a descending or sigmoid colostomy to regulate bowel function, and it cleans the large bowel before and after tests, surgery, or other procedures.

Colostomy irrigation may begin as soon as bowel function resumes after surgery. However, most clinicians recommend waiting until bowel movements are more predictable. Initially, the nurse or the patient irrigates the colostomy at the same time every day, recording the amount of output and any spillage between irrigations. Between 4 and 6 weeks may pass before colostomy irrigation establishes a predictable elimination pattern.

Equipment and preparation

Colostomy irrigation set (contains an irrigation drain or sleeve, an ostomy belt [if needed] to secure the drain or sleeve, water-soluble lubricant, drainage pouch clamp, and irrigation bag with clamp, tubing, and cone tip) ◆ 1 L of tap water irrigant warmed to about 100° F (37.8° C) ◆ warmed normal saline solution (for cleansing enemas) ◆ I.V. pole or wall hook ◆ washcloth and towel ◆ water ◆ ostomy pouching system ◆ linen-saver pad ◆ gloves ◆ optional: bedpan or chair, mild nonmoisturizing soap, rubber band or clip, and small dressing, bandage, or commercial stoma cap

Depending on the patient's condition, colostomy irrigation may be performed in bed using a bedpan or in the bathroom using the toilet or a chair. Set up the irrigation bag with tubing and cone tip. If irrigation will take place with the patient in bed, place the bedpan beside the bed, and elevate the head of the bed between 45 and 90 degrees, if allowed. If irrigation will take place in the bathroom, have the patient sit on the toilet or on a chair facing the toilet, whichever he finds more comfortable.

Fill the irrigation bag with warmed tap water (or normal saline solution, if the irrigation is to clean the bowel). Hang the bag on the I.V. pole or wall hook. The bottom of the bag should be at the patient's shoulder level to prevent the fluid from entering the bowel too quickly. Most irrigation sets also have a clamp that regulates the flow rate.

Prime the tubing with irrigant to prevent air from entering the colon and possibly causing cramps and gas pains.

Implementation

■ Explain every step of the procedure to the patient because he'll probably be irrigating the colostomy himself.
■ Provide privacy, and wash your hands.
■ If the patient is in bed, place a linen-saver pad under him to protect the sheets from getting soiled.
■ Put on gloves.
■ If the patient uses an ostomy pouch, remove it.
■ Place the irrigation sleeve over the stoma. If the sleeve doesn't have an adhesive backing, secure the sleeve with an ostomy belt. If the patient has a two-piece pouching system with flanges, snap off the pouch, and save it. Snap on the irrigation sleeve.
■ Place the open-ended bottom of the irrigation sleeve in the bedpan or toilet to promote drainage by gravity. If necessary, cut the sleeve so that it meets the water level inside the bedpan or toilet. Effluent may splash from a short sleeve or may not drain from a long sleeve.
■ Lubricate your gloved small finger with water-soluble lubricant and insert the finger into the stoma. If you're teaching the patient, have him do this to determine the bowel angle at which to insert the cone safely. Expect the stoma to tighten when the finger enters the bowel and then to relax in a few seconds.
■ Lubricate the cone with water-soluble lubricant to prevent it from irritating the mucosa.
■ Insert the cone into the top opening of the irrigation sleeve and then into the stoma. Angle the cone to match the bowel angle. Insert it gently but snugly; never force it in place.
■ Unclamp the irrigation tubing, and allow the water to flow slowly. If you don't have a clamp to control the irrigant's flow rate, pinch the tubing to

control the flow. The water should enter the colon over 10 to 15 minutes. (If the patient reports cramping, slow or stop the flow, keep the cone in place, and have the patient take a few deep breaths until the cramping stops.) Cramping during irrigation may result from a bowel that is ready to empty, water that is too cold, a rapid flow rate, or air in the tubing.

■ Have the patient remain stationary for 15 to 20 minutes so that the initial effluent can drain.

■ If the patient is ambulatory, he can stay in the bathroom until all effluent empties, or he can clamp the bottom of the drainage sleeve with a rubber band or clip and return to bed. Explain that ambulation and activity stimulate elimination. Suggest that the nonambulatory patient lean forward or massage his abdomen to stimulate elimination.

■ Wait about 45 minutes for the bowel to finish eliminating the irrigant and effluent. Then remove the irrigation sleeve.

■ If the irrigation was intended to clean the bowel, repeat the procedure with warmed normal saline solution until the return solution appears clear.

■ Using a washcloth, mild nonmoisturizing soap, and water, gently clean the area around the stoma. Rinse and dry the area thoroughly with a clean towel.

■ Inspect the skin and stoma for changes in appearance. Usually dark pink to red, stoma color may change with the patient's status. Notify the doctor of marked stoma color changes because a pale hue may result from anemia, and substantial darkening suggests a change in blood flow to the stoma.

■ Apply a clean pouch. If the patient has a regular bowel elimination pattern, he may prefer a small dressing, bandage, or commercial stoma cap.

■ Discard a disposable irrigation sleeve. Rinse a reusable irrigation sleeve, and hang it to dry along with the irrigation bag, tubing, and cone.

Special considerations

■ Irrigating a colostomy to establish a regular bowel elimination pattern doesn't work for all patients. If the bowel continues to move between irrigations, try decreasing the volume of irrigant. Increasing the irrigant won't help, because it serves only to stimulate peristalsis. Keep a record of results. Also consider irrigating every other day.

■ Irrigation may help to regulate bowel function in patients with a descending or sigmoid colostomy because this is the bowel's stool storage area. However, a patient with an ascending or transverse colostomy won't benefit from irrigation. Also, a patient with a descending or sigmoid colostomy who is missing part of the ascending or transverse colon may not be able to irrigate successfully, because his ostomy may function like an ascending or transverse colostomy.

■ If diarrhea develops, discontinue irrigations until stools form again. Keep in mind that irrigation alone won't achieve regularity for the patient. He must also observe a complementary diet and exercise regimen.

■ If the patient has a strictured stoma that prohibits cone insertion, remove the cone from the irrigation tubing, and replace it with a soft silicone catheter. Angle the catheter gently 2″ to 4″ (5 to 10 cm) into the bowel to instill the irrigant. Don't force the catheter into the stoma, and don't insert it farther than the recommended length, because you may perforate the bowel.

■ Observe the patient for complications. Bowel perforation may result if a catheter is incorrectly inserted into the stoma. Fluid and electrolyte imbalances may result from using too much irrigant.

Documentation

Record the date and time of irrigation and the type and amount of irrigant. Note the stoma's color and the character of drainage, including the drainage color, consistency, and amount. Record any patient teaching. Describe teaching content and patient response to self-care instruction. Evaluate the patient's learning progress.

Defibrillation

As the standard treatment for ventricular fibrillation, defibrillation involves using electrode paddles to direct an electric current through the patient's heart. The current causes the myocardium to depolarize, which in turn encourages the sinoatrial node to resume control of the heart's electrical activity. The electrode paddles delivering the current may be placed on the patient's chest or, during cardiac surgery, directly on the myocardium.

Because ventricular fibrillation leads to death if not corrected, the success of defibrillation depends on early recognition and quick treatment of this arrhythmia. In addition to treating ventricular fibrillation, defibrillation may be used to treat ventricular tachycardia that doesn't produce a pulse.

Patients with a history of ventricular fibrillation may be candidates for an implantable cardioverter-defibrillator, a sophisticated device that automatically discharges an electric current when it senses a ventricular tachyarrhythmia. (See *Understanding the ICD.*)

Equipment

Defibrillator ◆ external paddles ◆ conductive medium pads ◆ electrocardiogram (ECG) monitor with recorder ◆ supplemental oxygen therapy equipment ◆ emergency cardiac medications

Implementation

■ Assess the patient to determine if he lacks a pulse. Call for help, and perform cardiopulmonary resuscitation (CPR) until the defibrillator and other emergency equipment arrive.

■ If the defibrillator has "quick look" capability, place the external paddles on the patient's chest to quickly view his cardiac rhythm. Otherwise, connect the monitoring leads of the ECG monitor with recorder to the patient, and assess his cardiac rhythm.

■ Expose the patient's chest, and apply conductive medium pads at the paddle placement positions. For anterolateral placement, place one paddle to the right of the upper sternum, just below the right clavicle, and the other over the fifth or sixth intercostal space at the left anterior axillary line. For anteroposterior placement, place the anterior paddle directly over the heart at the precordium, to the left of the lower sternal border. Place the flat posterior paddle under the patient's body beneath the heart and immediately below the scapulae (but not under the vertebral column).

■ Turn on the defibrillator. If performing external defibrillation for an adult patient, set the energy level to 200 joules.

■ Charge the paddles by pressing the charge buttons, which are located either on the machine or on the paddles themselves.

■ Place the paddles over the conductive pads and press firmly against the

Understanding the ICD

The implantable cardioverter-defibrillator (ICD) has a programmable pulse generator and lead system that monitors the heart's activity, detects ventricular bradyarrhythmias and tachyarrhythmias, and responds with appropriate therapies. The range of therapies includes antitachycardia and bradycardia pacing, cardioversion, and defibrillation. Newer defibrillators also have the ability to pace both the atrium and the ventricle.

Implantation of an ICD is similar to that of a permanent pacemaker. The cardiologist positions the lead (or leads) transvenously in the endocardium of the right ventricle (and the right atrium, if both chambers require pacing). The lead connects to a generator box, which is implanted in the right or left upper chest near the clavicle.

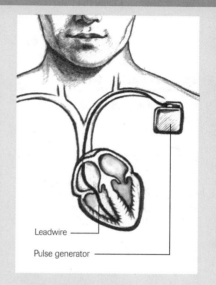

Leadwire

Pulse generator

---

patient's chest, using 25 lb (11.3 kg) of pressure.

■ Reassess the patient's cardiac rhythm.

■ If the patient remains in ventricular fibrillation or pulseless ventricular tachycardia, instruct all personnel to stand clear of the patient and the bed.

■ Discharge the current by pressing both paddle charge buttons simultaneously.

■ Leaving the paddles in position on the patient's chest, reassess the patient's cardiac rhythm, and have someone else assess the pulse.

■ If necessary, prepare to defibrillate a second time. Instruct a coworker to reset the energy level on the defibrillator to 200 to 300 joules. Announce that you're preparing to defibrillate, and follow the procedure described above.

■ Reassess the patient. If defibrillation is again necessary, instruct a coworker

to reset the energy level to 360 joules. Then follow the same procedure as before.

■ Perform the three countershocks in rapid succession, reassessing the patient's rhythm before each defibrillation.

■ If the patient still has no pulse after three initial defibrillations, resume CPR, give supplemental oxygen, and begin administering appropriate emergency cardiac medications such as epinephrine. Also, consider possible causes for failure of the patient's rhythm to convert, such as acidosis or hypoxia.

■ If defibrillation restores a normal rhythm, check the patient's central and peripheral pulses and obtain a blood pressure reading, heart rate, and respiratory rate. Assess the patient's level of consciousness, cardiac rhythm, breath sounds, skin color, and urine output. Obtain baseline arterial blood gas levels and a 12-lead ECG. Provide supplemental oxygen, ventilation, and medications as needed. Check the patient's chest for electrical burns and treat them as ordered with corticosteroid or lanolin-based creams. Also, prepare the defibrillator for immediate reuse.

Special considerations

■ Defibrillators vary from one manufacturer to the next, so familiarize yourself with your facility's equipment. Defibrillator operation should be checked at least every 8 hours and after each use.
■ Defibrillation can be affected by several factors, including paddle size and placement, condition of the patient's myocardium, duration of the arrhythmia, chest resistance, and the number of countershocks.
■ Defibrillation can cause accidental electric shock to those providing care. Use of an insufficient amount of conductive medium can lead to skin burns.

Documentation

Document the procedure, including the patient's ECG rhythms before and after defibrillation; the number of times defibrillation was performed; the voltage used during each attempt; whether a pulse returned; the dosage, route, and time of drug administration; whether CPR was used; the way the airway was maintained; and the patient's outcome.

Doppler use

More sensitive than palpation for determining pulse rate, the Doppler ultrasound blood flow detector is especially useful when a pulse is faint or weak. Unlike palpation, which detects arterial wall expansion and retraction, this instrument detects the motion of red blood cells (RBCs).

Equipment

Doppler ultrasound blood flow detector ◆ coupling or transmission gel ◆ soft cloth ◆ antiseptic solution or soapy water

Implementation

■ Apply a small amount of coupling or transmission gel (not water-soluble lubricant) to the ultrasound probe.
■ Position the probe on the skin directly over the selected artery.
■ When using a Doppler ultrasound blood flow detector model with a speaker, turn the instrument on, and moving counterclockwise, set the volume control to the lowest setting. If your model doesn't have a speaker, plug in the earphones, and slowly raise the volume. The Doppler ultrasound stethoscope is basically a stethoscope fitted with an audio unit, volume control, and transducer, which amplifies the movement of RBCs.
■ To obtain the best signals with either device, tilt the probe 45 degrees from the artery, and apply gel between the skin and the probe. Slowly move the probe in a circular motion to locate the center of the artery and the Doppler signal — a hissing noise at the heartbeat.
■ Avoid moving the probe rapidly because it distorts the signal.
■ Count the signals for 60 seconds to determine the pulse rate.
■ After you've measured the pulse rate, clean the probe with a soft cloth soaked in antiseptic solution or soapy water. Don't immerse the probe or bump it against a hard surface.

Documentation

Record the location and quality of the pulse, the pulse rate, and the time of measurement.

Feeding tube insertion and removal

Inserting a feeding tube nasally or orally into the stomach or duodenum provides nourishment to a patient who can't or won't eat. The feeding tube also permits administration of supplemental feedings to a patient who has very high nutritional requirements, such as an unconscious patient or one with extensive burns. Typically, a nurse inserts the feeding tube as ordered. The preferred feeding tube route is nasal, but the oral route may be used for patients with such conditions as a deviated septum or a head or nose injury.

The doctor may order duodenal feeding when the patient can't tolerate gastric feeding or when he expects gastric feeding to produce aspiration. Absence of bowel sounds or possible intestinal obstruction contraindicates using a feeding tube.

Feeding tubes differ somewhat from standard nasogastric tubes. Made of silicone, rubber, or polyurethane, feeding tubes have small diameters and great flexibility. This reduces oropharyngeal irritation, necrosis from pressure on the tracheoesophageal wall, distal esophageal irritation, and discomfort from swallowing. To facilitate passage, some feeding tubes are weighted with tungsten, and some need a guide wire to keep them from curling in the back of the throat.

These small-bore tubes usually have radiopaque markings and a water-activated coating, which provides a lubricated surface.

Equipment and preparation

For insertion
Feeding tube (#6 to #18 French, with or without a guide wire) ◆ linen-saver pad ◆ gloves ◆ hypoallergenic tape ◆ water-soluble lubricant ◆ skin preparation (such as tincture of benzoin) ◆ facial tissues ◆ penlight ◆ small cup of water with straw, or ice chips ◆ emesis basin ◆ 60-ml syringe ◆ stethoscope

For removal
Linen-saver pad ◆ tube clamp ◆ bulb syringe

Have the proper size tube available. Usually, the doctor orders the smallest-bore tube that will allow free passage of the liquid feeding formula. Read the instructions on the tubing package carefully because tube characteristics vary according to the manufacturer. (For example, some tubes have marks at the appropriate lengths for gastric, duodenal, and jejunal insertion.)

Examine the tube to make sure it's free from defects, such as cracks or rough or sharp edges. Next, run water through the tube. This checks for patency, activates the coating, and facilitates removal of the guide wire.

Implementation

■ Explain the procedure to the patient, and show him the feeding tube so that he knows what to expect and can cooperate more fully.
■ Provide privacy. Wash your hands and put on gloves.
■ Assist the patient into semi-Fowler's or high Fowler's position.
■ Place a linen-saver pad across the patient's chest to protect him from spills.
■ To determine the tube length needed to reach the stomach, first extend the distal end of the tube from the tip of the patient's nose to his earlobe. Coil this portion of the tube around your fingers so the end will remain curved until you insert it. Then extend the uncoiled portion from the earlobe to the xiphoid process. Use a small

piece of hypoallergenic tape to mark the total length of the two portions.

Inserting the tube nasally

■ Using the penlight, assess nasal patency. Inspect nasal passages for a deviated septum, polyps, or other obstructions. Occlude one nostril, then the other, to determine which has the better airflow. Assess the patient's history of nasal injury or surgery.

■ Lubricate the curved tip of the tube (and the feeding tube guide wire, if appropriate) with a small amount of water-soluble lubricant to ease insertion and prevent tissue injury.

■ Ask the patient to hold the emesis basin and facial tissues in case he needs them.

■ To advance the tube, insert the curved, lubricated tip into the more patent nostril and direct it along the nasal passage toward the ear on the same side. When it passes the nasopharyngeal junction, turn the tube 180 degrees to aim it downward into the esophagus. Tell the patient to lower his chin to his chest to close the trachea. Then give him a small cup of water with a straw or ice chips. Direct him to sip the water or suck on the ice and swallow frequently. This will ease the tube's passage. Advance the tube as he swallows.

Inserting the tube orally

■ Have the patient lower his chin to close his trachea, and ask him to open his mouth.

■ Place the tip of the tube at the back of the patient's tongue, give water, and instruct the patient to swallow. Remind him to avoid clamping his teeth down on the tube. Advance the tube as he swallows.

Positioning the tube

■ Keep passing the tube until the tape marking the appropriate length reaches the patient's nostril or lips.

■ To check tube placement, attach the syringe filled with 10 cc of air to the end of the tube. Gently inject the air into the tube as you auscultate the patient's abdomen with the stethoscope about 3″ (7.5 cm) below the sternum. Listen for a whooshing sound, which signals that the tube has reached its target in the stomach. If the tube remains coiled in the esophagus, you'll feel resistance when you inject the air, or the patient may belch.

■ If you hear the whooshing sound, gently try to aspirate gastric secretions. Successful aspiration confirms correct tube placement. If no gastric secretions return, the tube may be in the esophagus. You'll need to advance the tube or reinsert it before proceeding.

■ After confirming proper tube placement, remove the tape marking tube length.

■ Tape the tube to the patient's nose and remove the guide wire. *Note:* In some cases, an X-ray may be ordered to verify tube placement.

■ To advance the tube to the duodenum, especially a tungsten-weighted tube, position the patient on his right side. This lets gravity assist tube passage through the pylorus. Move the tube forward 2″ to 3″ (5 to 7.5 cm) hourly until X-ray studies confirm duodenal placement. (An X-ray must confirm placement before feeding begins because duodenal feeding can cause nausea and vomiting if accidentally delivered to the stomach.)

■ Apply a skin preparation to the patient's cheek before securing the tube with tape. This helps the tube adhere to the skin and also prevents irritation.

■ Tape the tube securely to the patient's cheek to avoid excessive pressure on his nostrils.

Removing the tube

■ Protect the patient's chest with a linen-saver pad.

■ Flush the tube with air with the bulb syringe, clamp or pinch it to prevent fluid aspiration during withdrawal, and withdraw it gently but quickly.

■ Promptly cover and discard the used tube.

Special considerations

■ Flush the feeding tube every 8 hours with up to 60 ml of normal saline solution or water to maintain patency. Retape the tube at least daily and as needed. Alternate taping the tube toward the inner and outer side of the nose to avoid constant pressure on the same nasal area. Inspect the skin for redness and breakdown.

■ Provide nasal hygiene daily using the cotton-tipped applicators and water-soluble lubricant to remove crusted secretions. Also, help the patient brush his teeth, gums, and tongue with mouthwash or a mild saltwater solution at least twice daily.

■ If the patient can't swallow the feeding tube, use a guide to aid insertion.

■ Precise feeding-tube placement is especially important because small-bore feeding tubes may slide into the trachea without causing immediate signs or symptoms of respiratory distress, such as coughing, choking, gasping, or cyanosis. However, the patient will usually cough if the tube enters the larynx. To be sure that the tube clears the larynx, ask the patient to speak. If he can't, the tube is in the larynx. Withdraw the tube at once and reinsert.

■ When aspirating gastric contents to check tube placement, pull gently on the syringe plunger to prevent trauma to the stomach lining or bowel. If you meet resistance during aspiration, stop the procedure because resistance may

result simply from the tube lying against the stomach wall. If the tube coils above the stomach, you won't be able to aspirate stomach contents. To rectify this, change the patient's position or withdraw the tube a few inches, readvance it, and try to aspirate again. If the tube was inserted with a guide wire, don't use the guide wire to reposition the tube. The doctor may do so, using fluoroscopic guidance.

Patient teaching tips If your patient will use a feeding tube at home, make appropriate home care nursing referrals and teach the patient and caregivers how to use and care for a feeding tube. Teach them how to obtain equipment, insert and remove the tube, prepare and store feeding formula, and solve problems with tube position and patency.

Teach your patient to watch for complications related to prolonged intubation such as skin erosion at the nostril, sinusitis, esophagitis, esophagotracheal fistula, gastric ulceration, and pulmonary and oral infection.

Documentation

For tube insertion, record the date, time, tube type and size, insertion site, area of placement, and confirmation of proper placement. Also record the name of the person performing the procedure. For tube removal, record the date and time and the patient's tolerance of the procedure.

Gastric lavage

After poisoning or drug overdose, especially in patients who have central nervous system depression or an inadequate gag reflex, gastric lavage flushes the stomach and removes ingested substances through a gastric lavage tube. The procedure is also used to empty the stomach in preparation for endoscopic examination. For patients with gastric or esophageal bleeding, lavage with tepid or iced water or normal saline solution may be used to stop bleeding. However, some controversy exists over the effectiveness of iced lavage for this purpose.

Gastric lavage can be continuous or intermittent. Typically, this procedure is done in the emergency department or intensive care unit by a doctor, gastroenterologist, or nurse; a wide-bore lavage tube is almost always inserted by a gastroenterologist.

Gastric lavage is contraindicated after ingestion of a corrosive substance (such as lye, a petroleum distillate, ammonia, an alkali, or a mineral acid) because the lavage tube may perforate the already compromised esophagus.

Correct lavage tube placement is essential for patient safety because accidental misplacement (in the lungs, for example) followed by lavage can be fatal. Other complications of gastric lavage include bradyarrhythmias and aspiration of gastric fluids.

Equipment and preparation

Lavage setup ◆ two graduated containers for drainage ◆ clamp or smooth hemostat ◆ 2 to 3 L of normal saline solution, tap water, or appropriate antidote as ordered ◆ basin of ice, if ordered ◆ Ewald tube or any large-lumen gastric or lavage tube, typically #36 to #40 French ◆ water-soluble lubricant or anesthetic ointment ◆ stethoscope ◆ 1/2" hypoallergenic tape ◆ 50 ml bulb or catheter-tip syringe ◆ gloves ◆ face shield ◆ linen-saver pad or towel ◆ tonsillar suction device ◆ labeled specimen container ◆ laboratory requests ◆ norepinephrine ◆ optional: patient restraints and charcoal

A prepackaged, syringe-type irrigation kit may be used for intermittent lavage. For poisoning or a drug overdose, however, the continuous lavage setup may be more appropriate to use because it's a faster and more effective means of diluting and removing the harmful substance.

Set up the lavage equipment. (See *Preparing for gastric lavage.*) If iced lavage is ordered, chill the desired irrigant (water or normal saline solution) in a basin of ice. Lubricate the end of the lavage tube with the water-soluble lubricant or anesthetic ointment.

Implementation

■ Explain the procedure to the patient, provide privacy, and wash your hands.
■ Put on gloves and a face shield.
■ Drape the towel or linen-saver pad over the patient's chest to protect him from spills.
■ The doctor inserts the lavage tube nasally and advances it slowly and gently because forceful insertion may injure tissues and cause epistaxis. He checks the tube's placement by injecting about 30 cc of air into the tube with the bulb syringe and then auscultating the patient's abdomen with a stethoscope. If the tube is in place, he'll hear the sound of air entering the stomach.
■ Because the patient may vomit when the lavage tube reaches the posterior pharynx during insertion, be prepared to suction the airway immediately with a tonsillar suction device.
■ When the lavage tube passes the posterior pharynx, help the patient into Trendelenburg's position and turn him toward his left side in a three-quarter prone posture. This position minimizes passage of gastric contents into the duodenum and may prevent the patient from aspirating vomitus.
■ After securing the lavage tube nasally or orally with hypoallergenic tape and making sure the irrigant inflow tube on the lavage setup is clamped, connect the unattached end

of this tube to the lavage tube. Allow the stomach contents to empty into a drainage graduated container before instilling any irrigant. This confirms proper tube placement and decreases the risk of overfilling the stomach with irrigant and inducing vomiting. If you're using a syringe irrigation kit, aspirate stomach contents with a 50-ml bulb or catheter-tip syringe before instilling the irrigant.

■ When you confirm proper tube placement, begin gastric lavage by instilling about 250 ml of irrigant to assess the patient's tolerance and prevent vomiting. If you're using a syringe, instill about 50 ml of solution at a time, until you've instilled between 250 and 500 ml.

■ Clamp the inflow tube with a smooth hemostat and unclamp the outflow tube to allow the irrigant to flow out. If you're using the syringe irrigation kit, aspirate the irrigant with the syringe, and empty it into a graduated container. Measure the outflow amount to make sure that it equals at least the amount of irrigant you instilled. This prevents accidental stomach distention and vomiting. If the drainage amount falls significantly short of the instilled amount, reposition the tube until sufficient solution flows out. Gently massage the abdomen over the stomach to promote outflow.

■ Repeat the inflow-outflow cycle until returned fluids appear clear. This signals that the stomach no longer holds harmful substances or that bleeding has stopped.

■ Assess the patient's vital signs, urine output, and level of consciousness (LOC) every 15 minutes. Notify the doctor of any changes.

■ If ordered, remove the lavage tube.

Special considerations

■ To control GI bleeding, the doctor may order continuous irrigation of the

Preparing for gastric lavage

Prepare the lavage setup as follows:
■ Connect one of the three pieces of large-lumen tubing to the irrigant container.
■ Insert the stem of the Y-connector in the other end of the tubing.
■ Connect the remaining two pieces of tubing to the free ends of the Y-connector.
■ Place the unattached end of one of the tubes into one of the drainage containers. (Later, you'll connect the other piece of tubing to the patient's gastric tube.)
■ Clamp the tube leading to the irrigant.
■ Suspend the entire setup from the I.V. pole, hanging the irrigant container at the highest level.

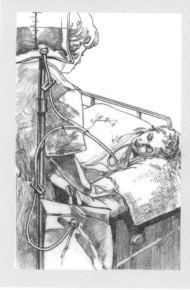

stomach with an irrigant and a vasoconstrictor, such as norepinephrine. After the stomach absorbs norepinephrine, the portal system delivers the drug directly to the liver, where it's metabolized. This prevents the drug from circulating systemically and initiating a hypertensive response. Or the doctor may direct you to clamp the outflow tube for a prescribed period after instilling the irrigant and the vasoconstrictor and before withdrawing it. This allows the mucosa time to absorb the drug.

■ Never leave a patient alone during gastric lavage. Observe him continuously for changes in LOC, and monitor vital signs frequently because the natural vagal response to intubation can depress the patient's heart rate.

■ If you need to restrain the patient, secure restraints on the same side of the bed or stretcher so you can free them quickly without moving to the other side of the bed. Don't restrain the patient in a "spread eagle" position; this position would keep him immobile and put him at risk for aspirating vomitus.

■ Remember also to keep tracheal suctioning equipment nearby and watch closely for airway obstruction caused by vomiting or excess oral secretions. Throughout gastric lavage, you may need to suction the oral cavity frequently to ensure an open airway and prevent aspiration. For the same reasons, and if he doesn't exhibit an adequate gag reflex, the patient may require an endotracheal tube before the procedure.

■ When aspirating the stomach for ingested poisons or drugs, save the contents in a labeled specimen container to send to the laboratory for analysis with the appropriate laboratory request. If ordered, after lavage to remove poisons or drugs, administer charcoal as directed through the nasogastric (NG) tube. The charcoal will absorb any remaining toxic substances. The tube may be clamped temporarily, allowed to drain via gravity, attached to intermittent suction, or removed.

■ When performing gastric lavage to stop bleeding, keep precise intake and output records to determine the amount of bleeding. When large volumes of fluid are instilled and withdrawn, serum electrolyte and arterial blood gas levels may be measured during or at the end of lavage.

■ Assess the patient for complications during gastric lavage. Vomiting and subsequent aspiration, the most common complications of gastric lavage, occur more commonly in a groggy patient. Bradyarrhythmias also may occur. After iced lavage especially, the patient's body temperature may drop, thereby triggering cardiac arrhythmias.

Documentation

Record the date and time of lavage, size and type of NG tube used, volume and type of irrigant, and amount of drained gastric contents. Document this information on the intake and output record sheet, and include your observations, including the color and consistency of drainage. Also, keep precise records of the patient's vital signs and LOC, any drugs instilled through the tube, the time the tube was removed, and the patient's response to the procedure.

Gastrostomy feeding button care

A gastrostomy feeding button serves as an alternative feeding device for an ambulatory patient who is receiving long-term enteral feedings. Approved by the Food and Drug Administration for 6-month implantation, feeding buttons can be used to replace gastrostomy tubes, if necessary.

The feeding button has a mushroom dome at one end and two wing tabs and a flexible safety plug at the other. When inserted into an established stoma, the button lies almost flush with the skin, with only the top of the safety plug visible.

The button can usually be inserted into a stoma in less than 15 minutes. In addition to its cosmetic appeal, the device is easily maintained, reduces skin irritation and breakdown, and is less likely to become dislodged or to migrate than an ordinary feeding tube. A one-way, antireflux valve mounted just inside the mushroom dome prevents accidental leakage of gastric contents. The device usually requires replacement after 3 to 4 months typically because the antireflux valve wears out.

Equipment

Gastrostomy feeding button of the correct size (all three sizes, if the correct one isn't known) ◆ gloves ◆ feeding accessories, including adapter, feeding catheter, food syringe or bag, and formula ◆ catheter clamp ◆ cleaning equipment, including water, cotton-tipped applicator, pipe cleaner, and mild soap or povidone-iodine solution ◆ optional: pump to provide continuous infusion over several hours

Implementation

■ Explain the insertion, reinsertion, and feeding procedure to the patient. Tell him the doctor will perform the initial insertion.
■ Wash your hands and put on gloves.
■ Attach the adapter and feeding catheter to the food syringe or bag. Clamp the catheter, and fill the syringe or bag and catheter with formula. Refill the syringe before it's empty. These steps prevent air from entering the stomach and distending the abdomen.
■ Open the safety plug, and attach the adapter and feeding catheter to the gastrostomy feeding button. Elevate the food syringe or bag above stomach level, and gravity-feed the formula for 15

to 30 minutes, varying the height as needed to alter the flow rate. Use a pump for continuous infusion or for feedings lasting several hours.
■ After the feeding, flush the button with 10 ml of water, and clean the inside of the feeding catheter with a cotton-tipped applicator and water to preserve patency and to dislodge formula or food particles. Then lower the food syringe or bag below stomach level to allow burping. Remove the adapter and feeding catheter. The antireflux valve should prevent gastric reflux. Then snap the safety plug into place to keep the lumen clean and prevent leakage if the antireflux valve fails. If the patient feels nauseated or vomits after the feeding, vent the button with the adapter and feeding catheter to help control the vomiting.
■ Wash the catheter and food syringe or bag in mild soap, and rinse thoroughly. Clean the catheter and adapter with a pipe cleaner. Rinse well before using for the next feeding. Soak the equipment once per week according to the manufacturer's recommendations.

Special considerations

■ If the button pops out during feeding, reinsert it (see *How to reinsert a gastrostomy feeding button,* page 358), estimate the amount of formula already delivered, and resume feeding.
■ Once daily, clean the peristomal skin with mild soap and water or povidone-iodine solution, and let the skin air-dry for 20 minutes to minimize skin irritation. Also clean the site whenever spillage from the feeding bag occurs.

Patient teaching tips Before discharge, make sure the patient can insert and care for the gastrostomy feeding button. If necessary, teach him or a family member how to reinsert the button by first practicing on a model. Offer written instructions, and answer his questions on obtaining replacement supplies.

How to reinsert a gastrostomy feeding button

If your patient's gastrostomy feeding button pops out (with coughing, for instance), you or he will need to reinsert the device. Here are some steps to follow.

Prepare the equipment

Collect the feeding button, an obturator, and water-soluble lubricant. If the button will be reinserted, wash it with soap and water, and rinse it thoroughly.

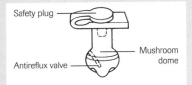

Safety plug

Antireflux valve

Mushroom dome

Insert the button

■ Check the depth of the patient's stoma to make sure you have a feeding button of the correct size. Then clean around the stoma.

■ Lubricate the obturator with a water-soluble lubricant, and distend the button several times to ensure the patency of the antireflux valve within the button.

■ Lubricate the mushroom dome and the stoma. Gently push the button through the stoma into the stomach.

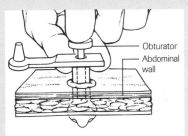

Obturator
Abdominal wall

■ Remove the obturator by gently rotating it as you withdraw it, to keep the antireflux valve from adhering to it. If the valve sticks, gently push the obturator back into the button until the valve closes.

■ After removing the obturator, make sure the valve is closed. Then close the flexible safety plug, which should be relatively flush with the skin surface.

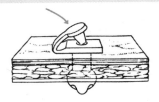

■ If you need to administer a feeding right away, open the safety plug and attach the feeding adapter and feeding tube. Deliver the feeding as ordered.

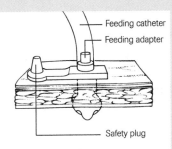

Feeding catheter
Feeding adapter

Safety plug

Documentation

Record feeding time and duration, amount and type of feeding formula used, and patient tolerance. Maintain intake and output records as necessary. Note the appearance of the stoma and surrounding skin.

Incentive spirometry

Incentive spirometry involves using a breathing device to help the patient achieve maximal ventilation. The device measures respiratory flow or respiratory volume and induces the patient to take a deep breath and hold it for several seconds. This deep breath increases lung volume, boosts alveolar inflation, and promotes venous return. This exercise also establishes alveolar hyperinflation for a longer time than is possible with a normal deep breath, thus preventing and reversing the alveolar collapse that causes atelectasis and pneumonitis.

Devices used for incentive spirometry provide a visual incentive to breathe deeply. Some are activated when the patient inhales a certain volume of air; the device then estimates the amount of air inhaled. Others contain plastic floats that rise according to the amount of air the patient pulls through the device when he inhales.

Patients at low risk for developing atelectasis may use a flow incentive spirometer. Patients at high risk may need a volume incentive spirometer, which measures lung inflation more precisely.

Incentive spirometry benefits the patient on prolonged bed rest, especially the postoperative patient who may regain his normal respiratory pattern slowly due to such predisposing factors as abdominal or thoracic surgery, advanced age, inactivity, obesity, smoking, and decreased ability to cough effectively and expel lung secretions.

Equipment and preparation

Flow or volume incentive spirometer as indicated, with sterile disposable tube and mouthpiece (The tube and mouthpiece are sterile on first use and clean on subsequent uses.) ◆ stethoscope ◆ warm water

Assemble the ordered equipment at the patient's bedside. Read the manufacturer's instructions for spirometer setup and operation. Remove the sterile disposable tube and mouthpiece from the package, and attach them to the device. Set the flow rate or volume goal as determined by the doctor or respiratory therapist and based on the patient's preoperative performance. Turn on the machine, if necessary.

Implementation

■ Assess the patient's condition.
■ Explain the procedure to the patient, making sure that he understands the importance of performing incentive spirometry regularly to maintain alveolar inflation. Wash your hands.
■ Help the patient into a comfortable sitting or semi-Fowler's position to promote optimal lung expansion. If you're using a flow incentive spirometer and the patient can't assume or maintain this position, he can perform the procedure in any position as long as the device remains upright. Tilting a flow incentive spirometer decreases the required patient effort and reduces the exercise's effectiveness.
■ Auscultate the patient's lungs with a stethoscope to provide a baseline for comparison with posttreatment auscultation.
■ Instruct the patient to insert the sterile mouthpiece and close his lips tightly around it because a weak seal may alter flow or volume readings.
■ Instruct the patient to exhale normally and then inhale as slowly and as

deeply as possible. If he has difficulty with this step, tell him to suck as he would through a straw but more slowly. Ask the patient to retain the entire volume of air he inhaled for 3 seconds or, if you're using a device with a light indicator, until the light turns off. This deep breath creates sustained transpulmonary pressure near the end of inspiration and is sometimes called a sustained maximal inspiration.

■ Tell the patient to remove the mouthpiece and exhale normally. Allow him to relax and take several normal breaths before attempting another breath with the spirometer. Repeat this sequence 5 to 10 times during every waking hour. Note tidal volumes.

■ Evaluate the patient's ability to cough effectively, and encourage him to cough after each effort because deep lung inflation may loosen secretions and facilitate their removal. Examine expectorated secretions.

■ Auscultate the patient's lungs, and compare findings with the first auscultation.

■ Instruct the patient to remove the mouthpiece. Wash the device in warm water, and shake it dry. Avoid immersing the spirometer itself because this enhances bacterial growth and impairs the internal filter's effectiveness in preventing inhalation of extraneous material.

■ Place the mouthpiece in a plastic storage bag between exercises, and label it and the spirometer, if applicable, with the patient's name so that another patient doesn't inadvertently use them.

Special considerations

■ If the patient is scheduled for surgery, assess beforehand his respiratory pattern and his ability to ensure development of appropriate postoperative goals. Teach him how to use the spirometer before surgery so that he can concentrate on your instructions and practice the exercise. A preoperative evaluation will also help in establishing postoperative therapeutic goals.

■ Avoid exercising at mealtime to prevent nausea. If the patient has difficulty breathing only through his mouth, provide a noseclip to fully measure each breath. Provide paper and pencil so the patient can note exercise times. Exercise frequency varies with condition and ability.

■ Immediately after surgery, monitor the exercise frequently to ensure compliance and assess achievement.

Documentation

Record any preoperative teaching that you provided. Document preoperative flow or volume levels, the date and time of the procedure, the type of spirometer, the flow or volume levels achieved, and the number of breaths taken. Also, note the patient's condition before and after the procedure, his tolerance of the procedure, and the results of both auscultations.

If you used a flow incentive spirometer, compute the volume by multiplying the setting by the duration that the patient kept the ball (or balls) suspended, as follows: If the patient suspended the ball for 3 seconds at a setting of 500 cc during each of 10 breaths, multiply 500 cc by 3 seconds and then record this total (1,500 cc) and the number of breaths, as follows: 1,500 cc × 10 breaths. If you used a volume incentive spirometer, take the volume reading directly from the spirometer. For example, record 1,000 cc × 5 breaths.

Latex allergy protocol

Latex, a natural product of the rubber tree, is commonly used in barrier protection products and medical equipment — and more and more nurses and patients are becoming hypersensitive to it. Those who are at increased risk for latex allergy include people who have had or will undergo multiple surgical procedures (especially those with a history of spina bifida), health care workers (especially those in the emergency department and operating room), workers who manufacture latex and latex-containing products, and people with a genetic predisposition to latex allergy.

People who are allergic to certain cross-reactive foods — including apricots, cherries, grapes, kiwis, passion fruit, bananas, avocados, chestnuts, tomatoes, and peaches — may also be allergic to latex. Exposure to latex elicits an allergic response similar to the ones these foods elicit.

For people with latex allergy, latex becomes a hazard when the protein in latex comes in direct contact with mucous membranes or is inhaled, which happens when powdered latex surgical gloves are used. People with asthma are at greater risk for developing worsening symptoms from airborne latex.

The diagnosis of latex allergy is based on the patient's history and physical examination. Laboratory testing should be performed to confirm or eliminate the diagnosis. Skin testing can be done, but the Alastat test, Hycor assay, and Pharmacia Cap test are the only blood tests that the Food and Drug Administration have approved. Some laboratories may also choose to perform an enzyme-linked immunosorbent assay.

Latex allergy can produce various signs and symptoms, including generalized itching (on the hands and arms, for example); itchy, watery, or burning eyes; sneezing and coughing (hay fever–type signs and symptoms); rash; hives; bronchial asthma, scratchy throat, or difficulty breathing; edema of the face, hands, or neck; and anaphylaxis.

To help identify people at risk for latex allergy, ask latex allergy–specific questions during the health history. (See *Latex allergy screening*, page 362.) If the patient's history reveals a latex sensitivity, the doctor assigns him to one of three categories based on the extent of his sensitization. Group 1 patients have a history of anaphylaxis or a systemic reaction when exposed to a natural latex product. Group 2 patients have a clear history of an allergic reaction of a nonsystemic type. Group 3 patients don't have a previous history of latex hypersensitivity but are designated as high risk because of an associated medical condition, occupation, or crossover allergy.

If you determine that your patient is sensitive to latex, make sure that he doesn't come in contact with it because such contact could result in a life-threatening hypersensitivity reaction. Creating a latex-free environment is the only way to safeguard your patient. Many facilities now designate latex-free equipment, which is usually kept on a cart that can be moved into the patient's room.

Equipment and preparation

Latex allergy patient identification wristband ◆ latex-free equipment, including room contents

After you've determined that the patient has a latex allergy or is sensitive to latex, arrange for him to be placed in a private room. If that isn't possible, make the room latex-free, even if the roommate hasn't been des-

Latex allergy screening

To determine if your patient has a latex sensitivity or allergy, ask the following screening questions:
■ What is your occupation?
■ Have you experienced an allergic reaction, local sensitivity, or itching after exposure to any latex products, such as balloons or condoms?
■ Do you have shortness of breath or wheezing after blowing up balloons or after a dental visit? Do you have itching in or around your mouth after eating a banana? If your patient answers "yes" to any of these questions, proceed with the following questions:
■ Do you have a history of allergies, dermatitis, or asthma? If so, what type of reaction do you have?

■ Do you have any congenital abnormalities? If yes, explain.
■ Do you have any food allergies? If so, what specific allergies do you have? Describe your reaction.
■ If you experience shortness of breath or wheezing when blowing up latex balloons, describe your reaction.
■ Have you had any previous surgical procedures? Did you experience associated complications? If so, describe them.
■ Have you had previous dental procedures? Did complications result? If so, describe them.
■ Are you exposed to latex in your occupation? Do you experience a reaction to latex products at work? If so, describe your reaction.

ignated as hypersensitive to latex, to prevent the spread of airborne particles from latex products used on the other patient.

Implementation

For all patients in groups 1 and 2
■ Assess for latex allergy all patients being admitted to the delivery room or short procedure unit or having a surgical procedure.
■ If the patient has a confirmed latex allergy, bring a cart with latex-free equipment into his room.
■ Document in the patient's chart (according to facility policy) that the patient has a latex allergy. If policy requires that the patient wear a latex allergy patient identification wristband, place it on the patient.
■ If the patient will be receiving anesthesia, make sure that LATEX ALLERGY is

clearly visible on the front of his chart. (See *Anesthesia induction and latex allergy.*) Notify the circulating nurse in the surgical unit, the postanesthesia care unit nurses, and any other team members that the patient has a latex allergy.
■ If the patient must be transported to another area of the facility, make sure that the latex-free cart accompanies him and that all health care workers who come in contact with him are wearing nonlatex gloves. The patient should wear a mask with cloth ties when leaving his room to protect him from inhaling airborne latex particles.
■ If the patient will have an I.V. line, make sure that only latex-free products are used to establish I.V. access. Post a LATEX ALLERGY sign on the I.V. tubing to prevent access of the line using latex products.

Anesthesia induction and latex allergy

Causes of intraoperative reaction	Signs and symptoms in a conscious patient	Signs and symptoms in an anesthetized patient
■ Latex contact with mucous membrane ■ Latex contact with intraperitoneal serosal lining ■ Inhalation of airborne latex particles during anesthesia ■ Injection of antibiotics and anesthetic agents through latex ports	■ Abnormal cramping ■ Anxiety ■ Bronchoconstriction ■ Diarrhea ■ Feeling of faintness ■ Generalized pruritus ■ Itchy eyes ■ Nausea ■ Shortness of breath ■ Swelling of soft tissue (hands, face, and tongue) ■ Vomiting	■ Bronchospasm ■ Cardiopulmonary arrest ■ Facial edema ■ Flushing ■ Hypotension ■ Laryngeal edema ■ Tachycardia ■ Urticaria ■ Wheezing

■ Flush I.V. tubing with 50 ml of I.V. solution because of latex ports in the I.V. tubing.

■ Place a warning label on I.V. bags that says DO NOT USE LATEX INJECTION PORTS.

■ Use a nonlatex tourniquet. If none are available, use a latex tourniquet over clothing.

■ Use latex-free oxygen administration equipment. Remove the elastic, and tie equipment on with gauze.

■ Wrap your stethoscope with a non-latex product to protect the patient from latex contact.

■ Wrap a transparent semipermeable dressing over the patient's finger before using pulse oximetry.

■ Use latex-free syringes when administering medication through a syringe.

■ If the patient has an allergic reaction to latex, act immediately. (See *Managing a latex allergy reaction,* page 364.)

Special considerations

■ Remember that signs and symptoms of latex allergy usually occur within 30 minutes after anesthesia is induced. However, the time of onset can range from 10 minutes to 5 hours.

■ Don't forget that, as a health care worker, you're in a position to develop a latex hypersensitivity. If you suspect that you're sensitive to latex, contact the employee health services department concerning facility protocol for latex-sensitive employees. Use latex-free products whenever possible to help reduce your exposure to latex.

■ Don't assume that if something doesn't look like rubber it isn't latex. Latex can be found in various equipment, including electrocardiograph leads, oral and nasal airway tubing, tourniquets, nerve stimulation pads, temperature strips, and blood pressure cuffs.

Managing a latex allergy reaction

If you determine that your patient is having an allergic reaction to a latex product, act immediately. Make sure that you perform emergency interventions using latex-free equipment. If the latex product that caused the reaction is known, remove it, and perform the following measures:
■ If the allergic reaction develops during medication administration or a procedure, stop it immediately.
■ Assess airway, breathing, and circulation.
■ Administer 100% oxygen with continuous pulse oximetry.
■ Start I.V. volume expanders with lactated Ringer's solution or normal saline solution.
■ Administer epinephrine according to the patient's symptoms as follows:
— cutaneous signs and symptoms of anaphylaxis (urticaria and angioedema): 0.3 to 0.5 ml of 1:1,000 aqueous epinephrine subcutaneously (S.C.); may be repeated every 15 to 20 minutes as needed, to a maximum of three doses
— pulmonary signs and symptoms of anaphylaxis (primarily laryngeal and pharyngeal edema) without airway obstruction or apnea: 0.3 to 0.5 ml of 1:1,000 aqueous epinephrine S.C.; may be repeated every 15 to 20 minutes as needed, to a maximum of three doses
— circulatory shock: 1 to 2 ml of aqueous epinephrine in 1:10,000 dilution (0.1 to 0.2 mg) I.V. over 2 to 3 minutes. In refrac-

tory cases, an epinephrine infusion via a 1:1,000,000 dilution can be administered using 1 ml of epinephrine 1:1,000 in 1,000 ml of dextrose 5% in water and adjusting the infusion rate from 6 to 30 ml/hour for a dosage range of 1 to 5 mcg/minute. This infusion rate should be titrated to the patient's blood pressure response or the development of arrhythmias.
■ Administer 20 mg of famotidine by I.V. push for 2 to 5 minutes, and then switch to oral administration as ordered.
■ If bronchospasm is evident, treat it with nebulized albuterol (0.25 to 0.5 ml diluted in 2.5 ml normal saline solution) as ordered.
■ Secondary treatment for latex allergy reaction is aimed at treating the swelling and tissue reaction to the latex as well as breaking the chain of events associated with the allergic reaction. It includes:
— 1 mg/kg of diphenhydramine I.V., to a maximum dose of 50 mg
— 2 mg/kg of methylprednisolone I.V., to a maximum dose of 125 mg
— 20 mg of famotidine every 12 hours by I.V. push over 2 to 5 minutes, to a maximum dose of 40 mg.
■ Document the event and the exact cause (if known). If latex particles have entered the I.V. line, insert a new I.V. line with a new catheter, new tubing, and new infusion attachments as soon as possible.

Adapted with permission of North Penn Hospital, Lansdale, Pa.

Lumbar puncture

Lumbar puncture involves the insertion of a sterile needle into the subarachnoid space of the spinal canal, usually between the third and fourth lumbar vertebrae. This procedure is used to detect increased intracranial pressure (ICP) or the presence of blood in cerebrospinal fluid (CSF), to obtain CSF specimens for laboratory analysis, and to inject dyes or gases for contrast in radiologic studies. It's also used to administer drugs or anesthetics and to relieve ICP by removing CSF.

Performed by a doctor with a nurse assisting, lumbar puncture requires sterile technique and careful patient positioning. This procedure is contraindicated in patients with lumbar deformity or infection at the puncture site. It should be performed cautiously in patients with increased ICP because the rapid reduction in pressure that follows withdrawal of CSF can cause tonsillar herniation and medullary compression.

Equipment and preparation

Overbed table ♦ two pairs of sterile gloves ♦ povidone-iodine solution ♦ sterile gauze pads ♦ alcohol pad ♦ sterile fenestrated drape ♦ 3-ml syringe for local anesthetic ♦ 25G ¾" sterile needle for injecting anesthetic ♦ local anesthetic (usually 1% lidocaine) ♦ 18G or 20G 3½" spinal needle with stylet (22G needle for children) ♦ three-way stopcock ♦ manometer ♦ small adhesive bandage ♦ three sterile collection tubes with stoppers ♦ laboratory requests ♦ labels ♦ light source such as a gooseneck lamp ♦ optional: patient-care reminder

Disposable lumbar puncture trays contain most of the needed sterile equipment.

Implementation

■ Explain the procedure to the patient to ease his anxiety and ensure his cooperation. Make sure he has signed a consent form.
■ Inform the patient that he may experience a headache after lumbar puncture, but reassure him that his cooperation during the procedure minimizes such an effect.
■ Immediately before the procedure, provide privacy, and instruct the patient to void.
■ Wash your hands thoroughly.

■ Open the disposable lumbar puncture tray on an overbed table, being careful not to contaminate the sterile field when you open the wrapper.
■ Provide an adequate light source at the puncture site, and adjust the height of the patient's bed to allow the doctor to perform the procedure comfortably.
■ Position the patient, and reemphasize the importance of remaining as still as possible to minimize discomfort and trauma. (See *Positioning for lumbar puncture*, page 366.)
■ The doctor cleans the puncture site with sterile gauze pads soaked in povidone-iodine solution, wiping in a circular motion away from the puncture site; he uses three different pads to prevent contamination of spinal tissues by the body's normal skin flora. Next, he drapes the area with the sterile fenestrated drape to provide a sterile field. (If the doctor uses povidone-iodine pads instead of sterile gauze pads, he may remove his sterile gloves and put on another pair to avoid introducing povidone-iodine into the subarachnoid space with the lumbar puncture needle.)
■ If no ampule of anesthetic is included on the equipment tray, clean the injection port of a multidose vial of anesthetic with an alcohol pad. Then invert the vial 45 degrees so that the doctor can insert a 25G needle and syringe and withdraw the anesthetic for injection.
■ Before the doctor injects the anesthetic, tell the patient he'll experience a transient burning sensation and local pain. Ask him to report any other persistent pain or sensations because they may indicate irritation or puncture of a nerve root, requiring repositioning of the needle.
■ When the doctor inserts the spinal needle with stylet into the subarachnoid space, instruct the patient to remain still and breathe normally. If necessary, hold the patient firmly in posi-

Positioning for lumbar puncture

To position a patient for a lumbar puncture have him lie on his side at the edge of the bed, with his chin tucked to his chest and his knees drawn up to his abdomen. Make sure the patient's spine is curved and his back is at the edge of the bed (as shown below). This position widens the spaces between the vertebrae, easing insertion of the needle.

To help the patient maintain this position, place one of your hands behind his neck and the other hand behind his knees, and pull gently. Hold the patient firmly in this position throughout the procedure to prevent accidental needle displacement.

Patient positioning

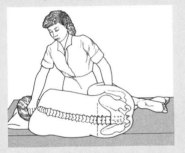

Typically, the doctor inserts the needle between the third and fourth lumbar vertebrae (as shown below).

Needle insertion

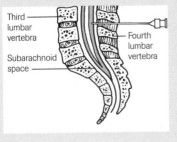

Third lumbar vertebra

Fourth lumbar vertebra

Subarachnoid space

tion to prevent sudden movement that may displace the needle.

■ If the lumbar puncture is being performed to administer contrast media for radiologic studies or spinal anesthetic, the doctor injects the dye or anesthetic at this time.

■ When the needle is in place, the doctor attaches a manometer with a three-way stopcock to the needle hub to read CSF pressure. If ordered, help the patient extend his legs to provide a more accurate pressure reading.

■ The doctor then detaches the manometer and allows CSF to drain from the needle hub into the collection tubes. When he has collected 2 to 3 ml in each tube, mark the tubes in sequence, insert stoppers to secure them, and label them.

■ If the doctor suspects an obstruction in the spinal subarachnoid space, he may check for Queckenstedt's sign. After he takes an initial CSF pressure reading, compress the patient's jugular vein for 10 seconds as ordered. This increases ICP and—if no subarachnoid block exists—causes CSF pressure to rise as well. The doctor then takes pressure readings every 10 seconds until the pressure stabilizes.

■ After the doctor collects the specimens and removes the spinal needle, clean the puncture site with povidone-iodine solution, and apply a small adhesive bandage.

■ Send the CSF specimens to the laboratory immediately, with the completed laboratory request.

Special considerations

■ During lumbar puncture, watch closely for signs of adverse reaction: elevated pulse rate, pallor, and clammy skin. Alert the doctor immediately to any significant changes.

■ The patient may be ordered to lie flat for 8 to 12 hours after the procedure. If necessary, place a patient-care reminder on his bed.

■ Collected CSF specimens must be sent to the laboratory immediately; they can't be refrigerated for later transport.

■ Assess the patient for complications after lumbar puncture. Headache is the most common adverse effect of lumbar puncture. Others include a reaction to the anesthetic, meningitis, epidural and subdural abscess, bleeding into the spinal canal, CSF leakage through the dural defect remaining after needle withdrawal, local pain caused by nerve root irritation, edema and hematoma at the puncture site, transient difficulty voiding, and fever. The most serious complications of lumbar puncture, although rare, are tonsillar herniation and medullary compression.

Documentation

Record the initiation and completion times of the procedure, the patient's response, administration of drugs, number of specimen tubes collected, time of transport to the laboratory, and color, consistency, and any other characteristics of the collected specimens.

Manual ventilation

Manual ventilation involves using a handheld resuscitation bag, which is an inflatable device that can be attached to a face mask or directly to an endotracheal (ET) or tracheostomy tube to allow manual delivery of oxygen or room air to the lungs of a patient who can't breathe by himself. Usually used in an emergency, manual ventilation also can be performed while the patient is disconnected temporarily from a mechanical ventilator, such as during a tubing change, during transport, or before suctioning. In such instances, use of the handheld resuscitation bag maintains ventilation. Oxygen administration with a resuscitation bag can help improve a compromised cardiorespiratory system.

Equipment and preparation

Handheld resuscitation bag ◆ mask ◆ oxygen source (wall unit or tank) ◆ oxygen tubing ◆ nipple adapter attached to oxygen flowmeter ◆ optional: oxygen accumulator and positive end–expiratory pressure (PEEP) valve ◆ optional: oropharyngeal airway or nasopharyngeal airway

Unless the patient is intubated or has a tracheostomy, select a mask that fits snugly over the mouth and nose. Attach the mask to the resuscitation bag. If oxygen is readily available, connect the handheld resuscitation bag to the oxygen. Attach one end of the oxygen tubing to the bottom of the bag and the other end to the nipple adapter on the flowmeter of the oxygen source.

Turn on the oxygen, and adjust the flow rate according to the patient's condition. For example, if the patient has a low partial pressure of arterial oxygen, he'll need a higher fraction of inspired oxygen (FIO_2). To increase the concentration of inspired oxygen, you can add an oxygen accumulator (also called an oxygen reservoir). This device, which attaches to an adapter on the bottom of the bag, permits an FIO_2 of up to 100%. Then, if time allows, set up suction equipment.

Implementation

■ Before using the handheld resuscitation bag, remove any objects from the patient's upper airway. (This alone may restore spontaneous respirations in some instances.) Also, suction the patient to remove any secretions that may obstruct the airway, impeding resuscitation efforts. If necessary, insert an oropharyngeal or nasopharyngeal airway to maintain airway patency. If

How to apply a handheld resuscitation bag and mask

Place the mask over the patient's face so that the apex of the triangle covers the bridge of his nose and the base lies between his lower lip and chin.

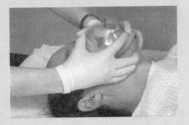

Make sure that the patient's mouth remains open underneath the mask. Attach the bag to the mask and to the tubing leading to the oxygen source.

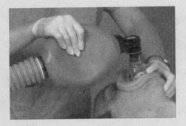

Or, if the patient has a tracheostomy tube or an endotracheal tube in place, remove the mask from the bag and attach the handheld resuscitation bag directly to the tube.

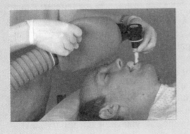

the patient has a tracheostomy or ET tube in place, suction the tube.

■ If appropriate, remove the bed's headboard and stand at the head of the bed to help keep the patient's neck extended and to free space at the side of the bed for other activities such as cardiopulmonary resuscitation.

■ Tilt the patient's head backward, if not contraindicated, and pull his jaw forward to move the tongue away from the base of the pharynx and prevent obstruction of the airway. (See *How to apply a handheld resuscitation bag and mask.*)

■ Keeping your nondominant hand on the patient's mask, exert downward pressure to seal the mask against his face. For an adult patient, use your dominant hand to compress the bag every 5 seconds to deliver about 1 L (1,000 cc) of air.

Age alert For infants and children, use a pediatric handheld resuscitation bag. For a child, deliver 15 breaths/minute, or one compression of the bag every 4 seconds; for an infant, 20 breaths/minute, or one compression every 3 seconds. Infants and children should receive 250 to 500 cc of air with each bag compression.

■ Deliver breaths with the patient's own inspiratory effort, if any is present. Don't attempt to deliver a breath as the patient exhales.

■ Observe the patient's chest to ensure that it rises and falls with each compression. If ventilation fails to occur, check the fit of the mask and the patency of the patient's airway; if necessary, reposition his head and ensure patency with an oral airway.

Special considerations

■ Add PEEP to manual ventilation by attaching a PEEP valve to the resuscitation bag. This may improve oxygenation if the patient hasn't responded to

increased fraction of inspired oxygen levels. Always use a PEEP valve to manually ventilate a patient who has been receiving PEEP on the ventilator.
■ If the patient has a cervical injury, avoid neck hyperextension; instead, use the jaw-thrust technique to open the airway. If you need both hands to keep the patient's mask in place and maintain hyperextension, use the lower part of your arm to compress the bag against your side.
■ Observe the patient for vomiting through the clear part of the mask. If vomiting occurs, stop the procedure immediately, lift the mask, wipe and suction the vomitus, and resume resuscitation.
■ Underventilation commonly occurs because the handheld resuscitation bag is difficult to keep positioned tightly on the patient's face while ensuring an open airway. What's more, the volume of air delivered to the patient varies with the type of bag used and the hand size of the person compressing the bag. An adult with a small or medium-sized hand may not consistently deliver 1 L (1,000 cc) of air. For these reasons, have someone assist with the procedure, if possible.
■ Aspiration of vomitus can result in pneumonia, and gastric distention may result from air forced into the patient's stomach.

Documentation

In an emergency, record the date and time of the procedure, manual ventilation efforts, any complications and the nursing action taken, and the patient's response to treatment, according to facility protocol for respiratory arrest.

In a nonemergency situation, record the date and time of the procedure, reason and length of time the patient was disconnected from mechanical ventilation and received manual ventilation, any complications and the nursing action taken, and the patient's tolerance of the procedure.

Mechanical ventilation

Mechanical ventilation involves using a mechanical ventilator that moves air in and out of a patient's lungs. Although the equipment serves to ventilate a patient, it doesn't ensure adequate gas exchange. Mechanical ventilators may use either positive or negative pressure to ventilate patients.

Positive-pressure ventilators exert a positive pressure on the airway, which causes inspiration while increasing tidal volume (V_T). The inspiratory cycles of these ventilators may vary in volume, pressure, or time. For example, a volume-cycle ventilator — the type most commonly used — delivers a preset volume of air each time, regardless of lung resistance. A pressure-cycle ventilator generates flow until the machine reaches a preset pressure, regardless of the volume delivered or the time required to achieve the pressure. A time-cycle ventilator generates flow for a preset amount of time. A high-frequency ventilator uses high respiratory rates and low V_T to maintain alveolar ventilation.

Negative-pressure ventilators act by creating negative pressure, which pulls the thorax outward and allows air to flow into the lungs. Examples of such ventilators are the iron lung, the cuirass (chest shell), and the body wrap. Negative-pressure ventilators are used mainly to treat neuromuscular disorders, such as Guillain-Barré syndrome, myasthenia gravis, and poliomyelitis.

Other indications for ventilator use include central nervous system disorders, such as cerebral hemorrhage and spinal cord transsection, adult respiratory distress syndrome, pulmonary edema, chronic obstructive pulmonary disease, flail chest, and acute hypoventilation.

Equipment and preparation

Oxygen source ◆ air source that can supply 50 psi ◆ mechanical ventilator ◆ humidifier ◆ ventilator circuit tubing, connectors, and adapters ◆ condensation collection trap ◆ spirometer, respirometer, or electronic device to measure flow and volume ◆ in-line thermometer ◆ probe for gas sampling and measuring airway pressure ◆ gloves ◆ handheld resuscitation bag with reservoir ◆ suction equipment ◆ sterile distilled water ◆ equipment for arterial blood gas (ABG) analysis ◆ soft restraints, if indicated ◆ optional: oximeter

In most facilities, respiratory therapists assume responsibility for setting up the ventilator. If necessary, check the manufacturer's instructions for setting it up. In most cases, you'll need to add sterile distilled water to the humidifier and connect the ventilator to the appropriate gas source.

Implementation

■ Verify the doctor's order for ventilator support. If the patient isn't already intubated, prepare him for intubation.
■ When possible, explain the procedure to the patient and his family to help reduce anxiety and fear. Assure the patient and his family that staff members are nearby to provide care.
■ Perform a complete physical assessment, and draw blood for ABG analysis to establish a baseline.
■ Suction the patient, if necessary.
■ Plug the mechanical ventilator into the electrical outlet, connect it to the oxygen source, and turn it on. Adjust the settings on the ventilator as ordered. Make sure that the ventilator's alarms are set as ordered and that the

humidifier is filled with sterile distilled water.
■ Put on gloves if you haven't already. Connect the endotracheal tube to the ventilator. Observe for chest expansion, and auscultate for bilateral breath sounds to verify that the patient is being ventilated.
■ Monitor the patient's ABG values after the initial ventilator setup (usually 20 to 30 minutes), after any changes in ventilator settings, and as the patient's clinical condition indicates to determine whether the patient is being adequately ventilated and to prevent oxygen toxicity. Be prepared to adjust ventilator settings based on the ABG analysis.
■ Check the ventilator circuit tubing frequently for condensation, which can cause airflow resistance and infection if the patient aspirates it. As needed, drain the condensate into a collection trap or briefly disconnect the patient from the ventilator (ventilating him with a handheld resuscitation bag if necessary), and empty the water into a receptacle. Don't drain the condensate into the humidifier because the condensate may be contaminated with the patient's secretions.
■ Check the in-line thermometer to make sure that the temperature of the air delivered to the patient is close to body temperature. Flow volume and airway pressure need to be monitored according to facility policy.
■ When monitoring the patient's vital signs, count spontaneous breaths as well as ventilator-delivered breaths.
■ Change, clean, or dispose of the ventilator tubing and equipment according to facility policy, to reduce the risk of bacterial contamination. Typically, ventilator tubing should be changed every 48 to 72 hours and sometimes more often.
■ When ordered, begin to wean the patient from the ventilator.

Special considerations

■ Provide the patient with emotional support during all phases of mechanical ventilation to reduce his anxiety and promote successful treatment. Even if the patient is unresponsive, continue to explain all procedures and treatments to him.

■ Make sure that the ventilator alarms are on at all times. These alarms alert nursing staff to potentially hazardous conditions and changes in patient status. If an alarm sounds and the problem can't be identified easily, disconnect the patient from the ventilator, and use a handheld resuscitation bag to ventilate him.

■ Unless contraindicated, turn the patient from side to side every 1 to 2 hours to facilitate lung expansion and removal of secretions. Perform active or passive range-of-motion exercises for all extremities to reduce the hazards of immobility. If the patient's condition permits, position him upright at regular intervals to increase lung expansion. When moving the patient or the ventilator tubing, make sure condensation in the tubing doesn't flow into the lungs, because aspiration of this contaminated moisture can cause infection. Provide care for the patient's artificial airway as needed.

■ Assess the patient's peripheral circulation, and monitor his urine output for signs of decreased cardiac output (CO). Watch for signs and symptoms of fluid volume excess or dehydration.

■ Place the call light within the patient's reach, and establish a method of communication, such as a communication board, because intubation and mechanical ventilation impair the patient's ability to speak. An artificial airway may help the patient to speak by allowing air to pass through his vocal cords.

■ Administer a sedative or neuromuscular blocker as ordered to relax the patient or to eliminate spontaneous breathing efforts that can interfere with the ventilator's action. Remember that the patient receiving a neuromuscular blocker requires close observation because of his inability to breathe or communicate.

■ If the patient is receiving a neuromuscular blocker, make sure that he also receives a sedative. Neuromuscular blockers cause paralysis without altering the patient's level of consciousness (LOC). Reassure the patient and his family that the paralysis is temporary. Also, make sure that emergency equipment is readily available in case the ventilator malfunctions or the patient is accidentally extubated. Continue to explain all procedures to the patient, and take additional steps to ensure his safety, such as raising the side rails of his bed while turning him and covering and lubricating his eyes.

■ Ensure that the patient gets adequate rest and sleep because fatigue can delay weaning from the ventilator. Provide subdued lighting, safely muffle equipment noises, and restrict staff access to the area to promote quiet during rest periods.

■ When weaning the patient, watch him for signs of hypoxia. Schedule weaning to fit comfortably and realistically with the patient's daily regimen. Avoid scheduling sessions after meals, baths, or lengthy therapeutic or diagnostic procedures. Have the patient help you set up the schedule to give him some sense of control over the procedure. As the patient's tolerance for weaning increases, help him sit up out of bed to improve his breathing and sense of well-being. Suggest diversionary activities to take his mind off breathing.

Patient teaching tips If the patient will be discharged on a ventilator, evaluate the family's or the caregiver's ability and motivation to provide such care. Well before discharge, develop a teaching plan that will address the patient's needs. For example, teaching should include information about ventilator care and settings, artificial airway care, suctioning, respiratory therapy, communication, nutrition, therapeutic exercise, the signs and symptoms of infection, and ways to troubleshoot minor equipment malfunctions.

■ Also, evaluate the patient's need for adaptive equipment, such as a hospital bed, wheelchair or walker with a ventilator tray, patient lift, and bedside commode. Determine whether the patient needs to travel; if so, select appropriate portable and backup equipment.

■ Before discharge, have the patient's caregiver demonstrate his ability to use the equipment. At discharge, contact a durable medical equipment vendor and a home health nurse to follow up with the patient. Also, refer the patient to community resources, if available.

■ Assess the patient for complications. Mechanical ventilation can cause tension pneumothorax, decreased CO, oxygen toxicity, fluid volume excess caused by humidification, infection, and such GI complications as distention or bleeding from stress ulcers.

Documentation

Document the date and time mechanical ventilation is initiated. Name the type of ventilator used for the patient, and note its settings. Describe the patient's subjective and objective responses to mechanical ventilation, including vital signs, breath sounds, use of accessory muscles, intake and output, and weight. List any complications and nursing actions taken. Record all pertinent laboratory data, including ABG analysis results and oxygen saturation levels.

During weaning, record the date and time of each session, the weaning method, and baseline and subsequent vital signs, oxygen saturation levels, and ABG values. Again describe the patient's subjective and objective responses, including LOC, respiratory effort, arrhythmias, skin color, and need for suctioning.

List all complications and nursing actions taken. If the patient was receiving pressure support ventilation or using a T-piece or tracheostomy collar, note the duration of spontaneous breathing and the patient's ability to maintain the weaning schedule. If using intermittent mandatory ventilation, with or without pressure support ventilation, record the control breath rate, the time of each breath reduction, and the rate of spontaneous respirations.

Nasogastric tube insertion and removal

Usually inserted to decompress the stomach, a nasogastric (NG) tube can prevent vomiting after major surgery. An NG tube is typically in place for 48 to 72 hours after surgery, by which time peristalsis usually resumes. It may remain in place for shorter or longer periods, however, depending on its use.

The NG tube has other diagnostic and therapeutic applications, especially in assessing and treating upper GI bleeding, collecting gastric contents for analysis, performing gastric lavage, aspirating gastric secretions, and administering medications and nutrients.

Inserting an NG tube requires close observation of the patient and verification of proper placement. Removing

Types of NG tubes

The doctor will choose the type and diameter of the nasogastric (NG) tube that best suits the patient's needs, including lavage, aspiration, enteral therapy, or stomach decompression. Choices may include the Levin tube and the Salem sump tube.

Levin tube

The Levin tube is a rubber or plastic tube that has a single lumen, a length of 42″ to 50″ (106.5 to 127 cm), and holes at the tip and along the side.

Salem sump tube

The Salem sump tube is a double-lumen tube, which is made of clear plastic and has a blue sump port (pigtail) that allows atmospheric air to enter the patient's stomach. Thus, the tube floats freely and doesn't adhere to or damage gastric mucosa. The larger port of this 48″ (121.9-cm) tube serves as the main suction conduit. The tube has openings at 45, 55, 65, and 75 cm as well as a radiopaque line to verify placement.

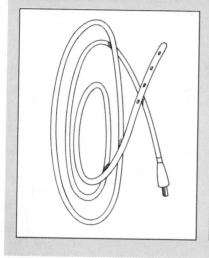

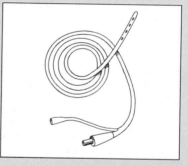

the tube requires careful handling to prevent injury or aspiration. The tube must be inserted with extra care in pregnant patients and in those with an increased risk of complications. For example, the doctor will order an NG tube for a patient with aortic aneurysm, myocardial infarction, gastric hemorrhage, or esophageal varices only if he believes that the benefits outweigh the risks of intubation.

Most NG tubes have a radiopaque marker or strip at the distal end so that the tube's position can be verified by X-ray. If X-ray fails to confirm placement, the doctor may order fluoroscopy.

The most common NG tubes are the Levin tube, which has one lumen, and the Salem sump tube, which has two lumens, one for suction and drainage and a smaller one for ventilation. Air flows through the vent lumen continuously. This protects the delicate gastric mucosa by preventing a vacuum from forming should the tube adhere to the stomach lining. The Moss tube, which has a triple lumen, is usually inserted during surgery. (See *Types of NG tubes*.)

Equipment and preparation

For inserting an NG tube

NG tube (usually #12, #14, #16, or #18 French for a normal adult) ◆ towel or linen-saver pad ◆ facial tissues ◆ emesis basin ◆ penlight ◆ 1″ or 2″ hypoallergenic tape ◆ gloves ◆ water-soluble lubricant ◆ cup or glass of water with straw (if appropriate) ◆ stethoscope ◆ tongue blade ◆ catheter-tip or bulb syringe or irrigation set ◆ safety pin ◆ ordered suction equipment ◆ optional: ice, alcohol pad, warm water, and rubber band

For removing an NG tube

Gloves ◆ catheter-tip syringe ◆ normal saline solution ◆ towel or linen-saver pad ◆ adhesive remover ◆ optional: clamp

Inspect the NG tube for defects, such as rough edges or partially closed lumens. Then check the tube's patency by flushing it with water. To ease insertion, increase a stiff tube's flexibility by coiling it around your gloved fingers for a few seconds or by dipping it into warm water. Stiffen a limp rubber tube by briefly chilling it in ice.

Implementation

■ Whether you're inserting or removing an NG tube, provide privacy, wash your hands, and put on gloves before inserting the tube. Check the doctor's order to determine the type of tube that should be inserted.

Inserting an NG tube

■ Explain the procedure to the patient to ease anxiety and promote cooperation. Inform her that she may experience some nasal discomfort, that she may gag, and that her eyes may water. Emphasize that swallowing will ease the tube's advancement.

■ Agree on a signal that the patient can use if she wants you to stop briefly during the procedure.

■ Gather and prepare all necessary equipment.

■ Help the patient into high Fowler's position, unless contraindicated.

■ Stand at the patient's right side if you're right-handed or at her left side if you're left-handed, to ease insertion.

■ Drape the towel or linen-saver pad over the patient's chest to protect her gown and bed linens from spills.

■ Have the patient gently blow her nose to clear her nostrils.

■ Place the facial tissues and emesis basin well within the patient's reach.

■ Help the patient face forward with her neck in a neutral position.

■ To determine how long the NG tube must be to reach the stomach, hold the end of the tube at the tip of the patient's nose. Extend the tube to the patient's earlobe and then down to the xiphoid process.

■ Mark this distance on the tubing with the tape. (Average measurements for an adult range from 22″ to 26″ [56 to 66 cm].) It may be necessary to add 2″ (5 cm) to this measurement for tall individuals, to ensure entry into the stomach.

■ To determine which nostril will allow easier access, use a penlight and inspect for a deviated septum or other abnormalities. Ask the patient if she ever had nasal surgery or a nasal injury. Assess airflow in both nostrils by occluding one nostril at a time while the patient breathes through her nose. Choose the nostril with the better airflow.

■ Lubricate the first 3″ (7.6 cm) of the tube with a water-soluble lubricant to minimize injury to the nasal passages. Using a water-soluble lubricant prevents lipoid pneumonia, which may result from aspiration of an oil-based lubricant or from accidental slippage of the tube into the trachea.

■ Instruct the patient to hold her head straight and upright.

■ Grasp the tube with the end pointing downward, curve it, if necessary, and carefully insert it into the more patent nostril(as shown below).

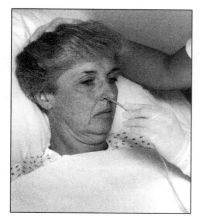

■ Aim the tube downward and toward the ear closer to the chosen nostril. Advance it slowly to avoid pressure on the turbinates and resultant pain and bleeding.

■ When the tube reaches the nasopharynx, you'll feel resistance. Instruct the patient to lower her head slightly to close the trachea and open the esophagus. Then rotate the tube 180 degrees toward the opposite nostril to redirect it so that the tube won't enter the patient's mouth.

■ Unless contraindicated, offer the patient a cup or glass of water with a straw. Direct her to sip and swallow as you slowly advance the tube (as shown below). This helps the tube pass to the esophagus. (If you aren't using water, ask the patient to swallow.)

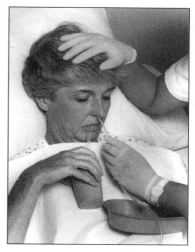

Ensuring proper tube placement

■ Use a tongue blade and penlight to examine the patient's mouth and throat for signs of a coiled section of tubing (especially in an unconscious patient). Coiling indicates an obstruction.

■ Keep an emesis basin and facial tissues readily available for the patient.

■ As you carefully advance the tube and the patient swallows, watch for signs of respiratory distress, which may indicate that the tube is in the bronchus and must be removed immediately.

■ Stop advancing the tube when the tape mark reaches the patient's nostril.

■ Attach a catheter-tip or bulb syringe to the tube, and try to aspirate stomach contents. If you don't obtain stomach contents, position the patient on her left side to move the contents into the stomach's greater curvature, and aspirate again.

Note: When confirming tube placement, never place the tube's end in a container of water. If the tube is mispositioned in the trachea, the patient may aspirate water. Furthermore, water without bubbles doesn't confirm proper placement. Instead, the tube may be coiled in the trachea or the esophagus.

■ If you still can't aspirate stomach contents, advance the tube 1″ to 2″ (2.5 to 5 cm). Then inject 10 cc of air into the tube. At the same time, auscultate for air sounds with your stethoscope placed over the epigastric region. You should hear a whooshing sound if the tube is patent and properly positioned in the stomach.

■ If these tests don't confirm proper tube placement, you'll need X-ray verification.

■ Secure the NG tube to the patient's nose with hypoallergenic tape (or other designated tube holder). If the patient's skin is oily, wipe the bridge of the nose with an alcohol pad, and allow to dry. You'll need about 4″ (10.2 cm) of 1″ tape. Split one end of the tape up the center about 1½″ (3.8 cm). Make tabs on the split ends (by folding sticky sides together). Stick the uncut tape end on the patient's nose so that the split in the tape starts about ½″ (1.3 cm) to 1½″ from the tip of her nose. Crisscross the tabbed ends around the tube (as shown at top right).

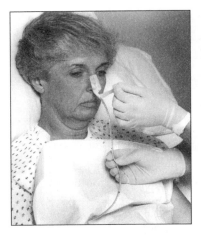

Then apply another piece of tape over the bridge of the nose to secure the tube.

■ Alternatively, stabilize the tube with a prepackaged product that secures and cushions it at the nose.

■ To reduce discomfort from the weight of the tube, tie a slipknot around the tube with a rubber band, and then secure the rubber band to the patient's gown with a safety pin, or wrap another piece of tape around the end of the tube and leave a tab. Then fasten the tape tab to the patient's gown.

■ Attach the tube to suction equipment, if ordered, and set the designated suction pressure.

■ Provide frequent nose and mouth care while the tube is in place.

Removing an NG tube

■ Explain the procedure to the patient, informing her that it may cause some nasal discomfort and sneezing or gagging.

■ Assess bowel function by auscultating for peristalsis or flatus.

■ Help the patient into semi-Fowler's position. Then drape a towel or linen-saver pad across her chest to protect her gown and bed linens from spills.

■ Using a catheter-tip syringe, flush the tube with 10 ml of normal saline solution to ensure that the tube doesn't contain stomach contents that could irritate tissues during tube removal.

■ Untape the tube from the patient's nose, and then unpin it from her gown.

■ Clamp the tube by folding it in your hand.

■ Ask the patient to hold her breath to close the epiglottis. Then withdraw the tube gently and steadily. (When the distal end of the tube reaches the nasopharynx, you can pull it quickly.)

■ When possible, immediately cover and remove the tube because its sight and odor may nauseate the patient.

■ Assist the patient with thorough mouth care, and clean the tape residue from her nose with adhesive remover.

■ For the next 48 hours, monitor the patient for signs and symptoms of GI dysfunction, including nausea, vomiting, abdominal distention, and food intolerance. GI dysfunction may necessitate reinsertion of the tube.

Special considerations

■ A helpful device for calculating the correct tube length is Ross-Hanson tape. Place the narrow end of this measuring tape at the tip of the patient's nose. Extend the tape to the patient's earlobe and down to the tip of the xiphoid process. Mark this distance on the edge of the tape labeled NOSE TO EAR TO XIPHOID. The corresponding measurement on the opposite edge of the tape is the proper insertion length.

■ If the patient has a deviated septum or other nasal condition that prevents nasal insertion, pass the tube orally after removing any dentures, if necessary.

Sliding the tube over the tongue, proceed as you would for nasal insertion.

■ When using the oral route, remember to coil the end of the tube around your hand. This helps curve and direct the tube downward at the pharynx.

■ If your patient is unconscious, tilt her chin toward her chest to close the trachea. Then advance the tube between respirations to ensure that it doesn't enter the trachea.

■ While advancing the tube in an unconscious patient (or in a patient who can't swallow), stroke the patient's neck to encourage the swallowing reflex and facilitate passage down the esophagus.

■ While advancing the tube, watch for signs that it has entered the trachea, such as choking or breathing difficulties in a conscious patient and cyanosis in an unconscious patient or a patient without a cough reflex. If these signs occur, remove the tube immediately. Allow the patient time to rest; then try to reinsert the tube.

■ After tube placement, vomiting suggests tubal obstruction or incorrect position. Assess the patient immediately to determine the cause.

■ An NG tube may be inserted or removed at home. Indications for insertion include gastric decompression and short-term feeding. A home care nurse or the patient may insert the tube, deliver the feeding, and remove the tube.

■ Assess the patient for potential complications of prolonged intubation, such as skin erosion at the nostril, sinusitis, esophagitis, esophagotracheal fistula, gastric ulceration, and pulmonary and oral infection. Additional complications that may result from suction include electrolyte imbalances and dehydration.

Documentation

Record the type and size of the NG tube and the date, time, and route of insertion. Also, note the type and amount of suction, if used, and describe the drainage, including the amount, color, character, consistency, and odor. Note the patient's tolerance of the procedure.

When you remove the tube, record the date and time. Describe the color, consistency, and amount of gastric drainage. Again, note the patient's tolerance of the procedure.

Peripheral I.V. line insertion

Peripheral I.V. line insertion involves selection of a venipuncture device and an insertion site, application of a tourniquet, preparation of the site, and venipuncture. Selection of a venipuncture device and site depends on the type of solution to be used; frequency and duration of infusion; patency and location of accessible veins; the patient's age, size, and condition; and, when possible, the patient's preference.

If possible, choose a vein in the nondominant arm or hand. Preferred venipuncture sites are the cephalic and basilic veins in the lower arm and the veins in the dorsum of the hand; least favorable are the leg and foot veins because of the increased risk of thrombophlebitis. Antecubital veins can be used if no other venous access is available as well as to accommodate a large-bore needle and to administer drugs that require large-volume dilution.

A peripheral line allows administration of fluids, medication, blood, and blood components and maintains I.V. access to the patient. Insertion is contraindicated in a sclerotic vein, an edematous or impaired arm or hand, or a postmastectomy arm and in patients with a mastectomy, burns, or an arteriovenous fistula. Subsequent venipunctures should be performed proximal to a previously used or injured vein.

Equipment and preparation

Alcohol pads or other approved antimicrobial solution, such as tincture of iodine 2% or 10% povidone-iodine ◆ gloves ◆ tourniquet (rubber tubing or a blood pressure cuff) ◆ I.V. access devices ◆ I.V. solution with attached and primed administration set ◆ I.V. pole ◆ sharps container ◆ sterile 2″ × 2″ gauze pads or a transparent semipermeable dressing ◆ 1″ hypoallergenic tape ◆ optional: arm board, roller gauze, and warm packs ◆ adhesive bandage

Commercial venipuncture kits come with or without an I.V. access device. In many facilities, venipuncture equipment is kept on a tray or cart, allowing a choice of correct access devices and easy replacement of contaminated items.

Check the information on the label of the I.V. solution container, including the patient's name and room number, type of solution, time and date of its preparation, preparer's name, and ordered infusion rate. Compare the doctor's orders with the solution label to verify that the solution is correct. Then select the smallest-gauge device that is appropriate for the infusion (unless subsequent therapy will require a larger one). Smaller gauges cause less trauma to veins, allow greater blood flow around their tips, and reduce the risk of clotting. The device may be an over-the-needle cannula or through-the-needle cannula.

If you're using a winged infusion set, connect the adapter to the administration set, and unclamp the line until fluid flows from the open end of the needle cover. Then close the clamp and place the needle on a sterile surface, such as the inside of its packaging. If you're using a catheter device, open its package to allow easy access.

Implementation

■ Place the I.V. pole in the proper slot in the patient's bed frame. If you're using a portable I.V. pole, position it close to the patient.

■ Hang the I.V. solution with attached primed administration set on the I.V. pole.

■ Verify the patient's identity by comparing the information on the solution container with the patient's wristband.

■ Wash your hands thoroughly. Then explain the procedure to the patient to ensure his cooperation and reduce anxiety. Anxiety can cause a vasomotor response resulting in venous constriction.

Selecting the site

■ Select the puncture site. If long-term therapy is anticipated, start with a vein at the most distal site so that you can move proximally as needed for subsequent I.V. insertion sites. For infusion of an irritating medication, choose a large vein distal to any nearby joint. Make sure the intended vein can accommodate the I.V. access device.

■ Place the patient in a comfortable, reclining position, leaving the arm in a dependent position to increase capillary fill of the lower arms and hands. If the patient's skin is cold, warm it by rubbing and stroking the arm, or cover the entire arm with warm packs for 5 to 10 minutes.

Applying the tourniquet

■ Apply a tourniquet about 6″ (15 cm) above the intended puncture site to dilate the vein. Check for a radial pulse. If it isn't present, release the tourniquet, and reapply it with less tension to prevent arterial occlusion.

■ Lightly palpate the vein with the index and middle fingers of your nondominant hand. Stretch the skin to anchor the vein. If the vein feels hard or ropelike, select another.

■ If the vein is easily palpable but not sufficiently dilated, one or more of the following techniques may help raise the vein. Place the extremity in a dependent position for several seconds, and gently tap your finger over the vein or rub or stroke the skin upward toward the tourniquet. If you have selected a vein in the arm or hand, tell the patient to open and close his fist several times.

■ Leave the tourniquet in place for no longer than 3 minutes. If you can't find a suitable vein and prepare the site in that time, release the tourniquet for a few minutes. Then reapply it and continue the procedure.

Preparing the site

■ Put on gloves. Clip the hair around the insertion site if needed. Clean the site with alcohol pads or another approved antimicrobial solution, according to your facility's policy. Don't apply alcohol after applying 10% povidone-iodine because the alcohol negates the beneficial effect of the povidone-iodine. Work in a circular motion outward from the site to a diameter of 2″ to 4″ (5 to 10 cm) to remove flora that would otherwise be introduced into the vascular system with the venipuncture. Allow the antimicrobial solution to dry.

■ If ordered, administer a local anesthetic. Make sure the patient isn't sensitive to lidocaine.

■ Lightly press the vein with the thumb of your nondominant hand about 1½″ (3.8 cm) from the intended insertion site. The vein should feel round, firm, fully engorged, and resilient.

■ Grasp the access cannula. If you're using a winged infusion set, hold the short edges of the wings (with the needle's bevel facing upward) between the thumb and forefinger of your dominant hand. Then squeeze the wings together. If you're using an over-the-needle cannula, grasp the plastic hub with your dominant hand, remove the cover, and examine the cannula tip. If the edge isn't smooth, discard and replace the device. If you're using a through-the-needle cannula, grasp the needle hub with one hand, and unsnap the needle cover. Then rotate the access device until the bevel faces upward.

■ Using the thumb of your nondominant hand, stretch the skin taut below the puncture site to stabilize the vein (as shown below).

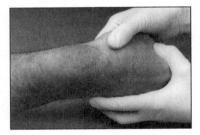

■ Tell the patient that you're about to insert the device.

■ Hold the needle bevel up, and enter the skin directly over the vein at a 15- to 25-degree angle (as shown below).

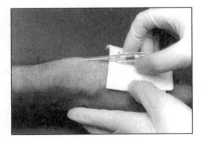

■ Aggressively push the needle directly through the skin and into the vein in one motion. Check the flashback chamber behind the hub for blood return, signifying that the vein has been properly accessed. (You may not see a blood return in a small vein.)

■ Then level the insertion device slightly by lifting the tip of the device up to prevent puncturing the back wall of the vein with the access device.

■ If you're using a winged infusion set, advance the needle fully, if possible, and hold it in place. Release the tourniquet, open the administration set clamp slightly, and check for free flow or infiltration.

■ If you're using an over-the-needle cannula, advance the device to at least half its length to ensure that the cannula itself — not just the introducer needle — has entered the vein. Then remove the tourniquet.

■ Grasp the cannula hub to hold it in the vein, and withdraw the needle. As you withdraw it, press lightly on the catheter tip to prevent bleeding.

■ Advance the cannula up to the hub or until you meet resistance.

■ To advance the cannula while infusing I.V. solution, release the tourniquet and remove the inner needle. Using aseptic technique, attach the I.V. tubing and begin the infusion. While stabilizing the vein with one hand, use the other to advance the catheter into the vein. When the catheter is advanced, decrease the I.V. flow rate. This method reduces the risk of puncturing the vein's opposite wall because the catheter is advanced without the steel needle and because the rapid flow dilates the vein.

■ To advance the cannula before starting the infusion, first release the tourniquet. While stabilizing the vein with one hand, use the other to advance the catheter up to the hub (as shown at top right). Next, remove the inner needle and, using aseptic technique, quickly attach the I.V. tubing. This method typically results in less blood being spilled.

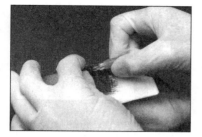

■ If you're using a through-the-needle cannula, remove the tourniquet, hold the needle in place with one hand and, with your opposite hand, grasp the cannula through the protective sleeve. Then slowly thread the cannula through the needle until the hub is within the needle collar. Never pull back on the cannula without pulling back on the needle, to avoid severing and releasing the cannula into the circulation, causing an embolus. If you feel resistance from the valve, withdraw the cannula and needle slightly and reinsert them, rotating the cannula as you pass the valve. Then withdraw the metal needle, split the needle along the perforated edge (according to the manufacturer's instructions), and carefully remove it from around the cannula. Dispose of the needle pieces appropriately. Remove the stylet and protective sleeve, and attach the administration set to the cannula hub. Open the administration set clamp slightly, and check for free flow or infiltration.

Dressing the site

■ After the venous access device has been inserted, clean the skin completely. If necessary, dispose of the stylet in a sharps container. Then regulate the flow rate.

■ You may use a transparent semipermeable dressing to secure the device.

■ If you don't use a transparent dressing, cover the site with a sterile gauze pad or small adhesive bandage.

■ Loop the I.V. tubing on the patient's limb, and secure the tubing with hypoallergenic tape. The loop allows some slack to prevent dislodgment of the cannula from tension on the line. (See *Methods of taping a venous access site*, page 382.)

■ Label the last piece of tape with the type, gauge of needle, and length of cannula; date and time of insertion; and your initials. Adjust the flow rate as ordered.

■ If the puncture site is near a movable joint, place an arm board under the joint, and secure it with roller gauze or tape to provide stability because excessive movement can dislodge the venous access device and increase the risk of thrombophlebitis and infection.

Removing a peripheral I.V. line

■ A peripheral I.V. line is removed on completion of therapy, for cannula site changes, and for suspected infection or infiltration; the procedure usually requires gloves, a sterile gauze pad, and an adhesive bandage.

■ To remove the I.V. line, first clamp the I.V. tubing to stop the flow of solution. Then gently remove the transparent dressing and all tape from the skin.

■ Using aseptic technique, open the gauze pad and adhesive bandage and place them within reach. Put on gloves. Hold the sterile gauze pad over the puncture site with one hand, and use your other hand to withdraw the cannula slowly and smoothly, keeping it parallel to the skin. (Inspect the cannula tip; if it isn't smooth, assess the patient immediately, and notify the doctor.)

■ Using the gauze pad, apply firm pressure over the puncture site for 1 to 2 minutes after removal or until bleeding has stopped.

■ Clean the site and apply the adhesive bandage or, if blood oozes, apply a pressure bandage.

Methods of taping a venous access site

When using tape to secure the venous access device to the insertion site, use one of the basic methods described below. Only sterile tape should be used under a transparent semipermeable dressing.

Chevron method

- Cut a long strip of ½" tape, and place it sticky side up under the cannula and parallel to the short strip of tape.
- Cross the ends of the tape over the cannula so that the tape sticks to the patient's skin (as shown).
- Apply a piece of 1" tape across the two wings of the chevron.
- Loop the tubing, and secure it with another piece of 1" tape. When the dressing is secured, apply a label. On the label, write the date and time of insertion, type and gauge of the needle, and your initials.

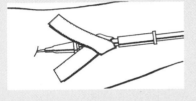

H method

- Cut three strips of 1" tape.
- Place one strip of tape over each wing, keeping the tape parallel to the cannula (as shown).
- Now place the other strip of tape perpendicular to the first two. Put it either directly on top of the wings or just below the wings, directly on top of the tubing.
- Make sure the cannula is secure; then apply a dressing and a label. On the label, write the date and time of insertion, type and gauge of needle or cannula, and your initials.

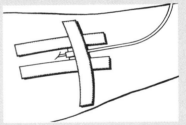

U method

- Cut a 2" (5-cm) strip of ½" tape. With the sticky side up, place it under the hub of the cannula.
- Bring each side of the tape up, folding it over the wings of the cannula in a U shape (as shown). Press it down parallel to the hub.
- Apply tape to stabilize the catheter.
- When a dressing is secured, apply a label. On the label, write the date and time of insertion, type and gauge of the needle or cannula, and your initials.

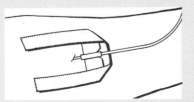

X method

- Place a transparent semipermeable dressing over the insertion site.
- Cut two 2" strips of ½" tape.
- Place one strip diagonal over the hub of the cannula.
- Now place the second strip diagonal to the hub in the opposite direction forming an X with the other piece (as shown).

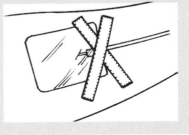

■ If drainage appears at the puncture site, send the tip of the device and a sample of the drainage to the laboratory to be cultured, according to facility policy. (A draining site may or may not be infected.) Then clean the area, apply a sterile dressing, and notify the doctor.

■ Instruct the patient to restrict activity for about 10 minutes and to leave the dressing in place for at least 1 hour. If the patient experiences lingering tenderness at the site, apply warm packs, and notify the doctor.

Special considerations

Age alert Apply the tourniquet carefully to avoid pinching the skin. If necessary, apply it over the patient's gown. Make sure skin preparation materials are at room temperature to avoid vasoconstriction from lower temperatures.

■ If the patient is allergic to compounds that contain iodine, clean the skin with alcohol.

■ If you fail to see blood flashback after the needle enters the vein, pull back slightly and rotate the device. If you still fail to see flashback, remove the cannula, and try again or proceed according to your facility's policy.

■ Change a gauze or transparent dressing whenever you change the administration set (every 48 to 72 hours or according to facility policy).

■ Rotate the I.V. site, usually every 48 to 72 hours or according to facility policy.

Patient teaching tips Most patients who receive I.V. therapy at home have a central venous line. But if you're caring for a patient going home with a peripheral line, you should teach him how to care for the I.V. site and identify certain complications. If the patient must observe movement restrictions, make sure he understands them.

■ Teach the patient how to examine the site, and instruct him to notify the doctor or home care nurse if redness, swelling, or discomfort develops; if the dressing becomes moist; or if blood appears in the tubing.

■ Also, tell the patient to report any problems with the I.V. line, for instance, if the solution stops infusing or if an alarm goes off on an infusion pump. Explain that the I.V. site will be changed at established intervals by a home care nurse.

■ If the patient is using an intermittent infusion device, teach him how and when to flush it. Finally, teach the patient to document daily whether the I.V. site is free from pain, swelling, and redness.

■ Teach the patient about possible complications related to peripheral lines. Complications can result from the needle or catheter (infection, phlebitis, and embolism) or from the solution (circulatory overload, infiltration, sepsis, and allergic reaction). (See *Risks of peripheral I.V. therapy,* pages 384 to 391.)

Documentation

In your notes or on the appropriate I.V. sheets, record the date and time of the venipuncture; type and gauge of the needle and length of the cannula; anatomic location of the insertion site; and reason the site was changed.

Also, document the number of attempts at venipuncture, type and flow rate of the I.V. solution, name and amount of medication in the solution (if any), any adverse reactions and actions taken to correct them, patient teaching and evidence of patient understanding, and your initials.

(Text continues on page 392.)

Risks of peripheral I.V. therapy

Complications	Signs and symptoms
LOCAL COMPLICATIONS	
Phlebitis	■ Tenderness proximal to venous access device ■ Redness at tip of cannula and along vein ■ Puffy area over vein ■ Vein hard on palpation ■ Elevated temperature
Infiltration	■ Swelling at and above I.V. site (may extend along entire limb) ■ Discomfort, burning, or pain at site (may be painless) ■ Tight feeling at site ■ Decreased skin temperature around site ■ Blanching at site ■ Continuing fluid infusion even when vein is occluded (although rate may decrease) ■ Absent backflow of blood ■ Loose tape
Cannula dislodgment	■ Cannula partly backed out of vein ■ Solution infiltrating
Occlusion	■ No increase in flow rate when I.V. container is raised ■ Blood backflow in line ■ Discomfort at insertion site

Possible causes	Nursing interventions
■ Poor blood flow around venous access device ■ Friction from cannula movement in vein ■ Venous access device left in vein too long ■ Clotting at cannula tip (thrombophlebitis) ■ Drug or solution with high or low pH or high osmolarity	■ Remove venous access device. ■ Apply warm soaks. ■ Notify doctor if patient has a fever. ■ Document patient's condition and your interventions. **Prevention** ■ Restart infusion using larger vein for irritating solution, or restart with smaller-gauge device to ensure adequate blood flow. ■ Use filter to reduce risk of phlebitis. ■ Tape device securely to prevent motion.
■ Venous access device dislodged from vein, or perforated vein	■ Stop infusion. If extravasation is likely, infiltrate the site with an antidote. ■ Apply warm soaks to aid absorption. Elevate limb. ■ Check for pulse and capillary refill periodically to assess circulation. ■ Restart infusion above infiltration site or in another limb. ■ Document patient's condition and your interventions. **Prevention** ■ Check I.V. site frequently. ■ Don't obscure area above site with tape. ■ Teach patient to observe I.V. site, and report pain or swelling.
■ Loosened tape, or tubing snagged in bed linens, resulting in partial retraction of cannula; pulled out by confused patient	■ If no infiltration occurs, retape without pushing cannula back into vein. If pulled out, apply pressure to I.V. site with sterile dressing. **Prevention** ■ Tape venipuncture device securely on insertion.
■ I.V. flow interrupted ■ Heparin lock not flushed ■ Blood backflow in line when patient walks ■ Line clamped too long	■ Use mild flush injection. Don't force it. If unsuccessful, remove I.V. line and insert a new one. **Prevention** ■ Maintain I.V. flow rate. ■ Flush promptly after intermittent piggyback administration. ■ Have patient walk with his arm bent at the elbow to reduce risk of blood backflow.

(continued)

Risks of peripheral I.V. therapy *(continued)*

Complications	Signs and symptoms
LOCAL COMPLICATIONS *(continued)*	
Vein irritation or pain at I.V. site	■ Pain during infusion ■ Possible blanching if vasospasm occurs ■ Red skin over vein during infusion ■ Rapidly developing signs of phlebitis
Hematoma	■ Tenderness at venipuncture site ■ Bruised area around site ■ Inability to advance or flush I.V. line
Severed cannula	■ Leakage from cannula shaft
Venous spasm	■ Pain along vein ■ Flow rate sluggish when clamp completely open ■ Blanched skin over vein
Vasovagal reaction	■ Sudden collapse of vein during venipuncture ■ Sudden pallor, sweating, faintness, dizziness, and nausea ■ Decreased blood pressure

Possible causes	Nursing interventions
■ Solution with high or low pH or high osmolarity, such as 40 mEq/L of potassium chloride, phenytoin, and some antibiotics (erythromycin, nafcillin, and vancomycin)	■ Decrease flow rate. ■ Try using an electronic flow device to achieve a steady flow. **Prevention** ■ Dilute solutions before administration. For example, give antibiotics in 250-ml solution rather than 100-ml solution. If drug has low pH, ask pharmacist if drug can be buffered with sodium bicarbonate. (Check facility policy.) ■ If long-term therapy of irritating drug is planned, ask doctor to use central I.V. line.
■ Vein punctured through opposite wall at time of insertion ■ Leakage of blood from needle displacement ■ Inadequate pressure applied when cannula is discontinued	■ Remove venous access device. ■ Apply pressure and warm soaks to affected area. ■ Recheck for bleeding. ■ Document patient's condition and your interventions. **Prevention** ■ Choose a vein that can accommodate the size of venous access device. ■ Release tourniquet as soon as insertion is successful.
■ Cannula inadvertently cut by scissors ■ Reinsertion of needle into cannula	■ If broken part is visible, attempt to retrieve it. If unsuccessful, notify the doctor. ■ If portion of cannula enters bloodstream, place tourniquet above I.V. site to prevent progression of broken part. ■ Notify doctor and radiology department. ■ Document patient's condition and your interventions. **Prevention** ■ Don't use scissors around I.V. site. ■ Never reinsert needle into cannula. ■ Remove unsuccessfully inserted cannula and needle together.
■ Severe vein irritation from irritating drugs or fluids ■ Administration of cold fluids or blood ■ Very rapid flow rate (with fluids at room temperature)	■ Apply warm soaks over vein and surrounding area. ■ Decrease flow rate. **Prevention** ■ Use a blood warmer for blood or packed red blood cells.
■ Vasospasm from anxiety or pain	■ Lower head of bed. ■ Have patient take deep breaths. ■ Check vital signs. **Prevention** ■ Prepare patient for therapy to relieve his anxiety. ■ Use local anesthetic to prevent pain.

(continued)

Risks of peripheral I.V. therapy *(continued)*

Complications	Signs and symptoms
LOCAL COMPLICATIONS *(continued)*	
Thrombosis	■ Painful, reddened, and swollen vein ■ Sluggish or stopped I.V. flow
Thrombophlebitis	■ Severe discomfort ■ Reddened, swollen, and hardened vein
Nerve, tendon, or ligament damage	■ Extreme pain (similar to electrical shock when nerve is punctured) ■ Numbness and muscle contraction ■ Delayed effects, including paralysis, numbness, and deformity
SYSTEMIC COMPLICATIONS	
Systemic infection (septicemia or bacteremia)	■ Fever, chills, and malaise for no apparent reason ■ Contaminated I.V. site, usually with no visible signs of infection at site

Possible causes	Nursing interventions
■ Injury to endothelial cells of vein wall, allowing platelets to adhere and thrombi to form	■ Remove venous access device; restart infusion in opposite limb, if possible. ■ Apply warm soaks. ■ Watch for I.V. therapy–related infection; thrombi provide an excellent environment for bacterial growth. **Prevention** ■ Use proper venipuncture techniques to reduce injury to vein.
■ Thrombosis and inflammation	■ Follow the procedure for thrombosis. **Prevention** ■ Check site frequently. Remove venous access device at first sign of redness and tenderness.
■ Improper venipuncture technique, resulting in injury to surrounding nerves, tendons, or ligaments ■ Tight taping or improper splinting with arm board	■ Stop procedure. **Prevention** ■ Don't repeatedly penetrate tissues with venous access device. ■ Don't apply excessive pressure when taping; don't encircle limb with tape. ■ Pad arm boards, and secure arm boards with tape, if possible.
■ Failure to maintain aseptic technique during insertion or site care ■ Severe phlebitis, which can set up ideal conditions for organism growth ■ Poor taping that permits venous access device to move, which can introduce organisms into bloodstream ■ Prolonged indwelling time of device ■ Weak immune system	■ Notify the doctor. ■ Administer medications as prescribed. ■ Culture the site and device. ■ Monitor vital signs. **Prevention** ■ Use aseptic technique when handling solutions and tubing, inserting venous access device, and discontinuing infusion. ■ Secure all connections. ■ Change I.V. solutions, tubing, and venous access device at recommended times. ■ Use I.V. filters.

(continued)

Risks of peripheral I.V. therapy *(continued)*

Complications	Signs and symptoms

SYSTEMIC COMPLICATIONS *(continued)*

Complications	Signs and symptoms
Allergic reaction	■ Itching ■ Watery eyes and nose ■ Bronchospasm ■ Wheezing ■ Urticarial rash ■ Edema at I.V. site ■ Anaphylactic reaction (flushing, chills, anxiety, itching, palpitations, paresthesia, wheezing, seizures, cardiac arrest) up to 1 hour after exposure
Circulatory overload	■ Discomfort ■ Neck vein engorgement ■ Respiratory distress ■ Increased blood pressure ■ Crackles ■ Increased difference between fluid intake and output
Air embolism	■ Respiratory distress ■ Unequal breath sounds ■ Weak pulse ■ Increased central venous pressure ■ Decreased blood pressure ■ Loss of consciousness

Possible causes	Nursing interventions
■ Allergens such as medications	■ If reaction occurs, stop infusion immediately. ■ Maintain a patent airway. ■ Notify the doctor. ■ Administer an antihistaminic steroid, an anti-inflammatory, and an antipyretic as prescribed. ■ Give 0.2 to 0.5 ml of 1:1,000 aqueous epinephrine S.C. as prescribed. Repeat at 3-minute intervals and as needed and prescribed. **Prevention** ■ Obtain patient's allergy history. Be aware of cross-allergies. ■ Assist with test dosing and document any new allergies. ■ Monitor patient carefully during first 15 minutes of administration of a new drug.
■ Roller clamp loosened to allow run-on infusion ■ Flow rate too rapid ■ Miscalculation of fluid requirements	■ Raise head of bed. ■ Administer oxygen as needed. ■ Notify the doctor. ■ Administer medications (probably furosemide) as prescribed. **Prevention** ■ Use pump, controller, or rate minder for elderly or compromised patients. ■ Recheck calculations of fluid requirements. ■ Monitor infusion frequently.
■ Solution container empty ■ Solution container emptying, and added container pushing air down the line (if line not purged first)	■ Discontinue infusion. ■ Place patient on his left side in Trendelenburg's position to allow air to enter right atrium and disperse by way of pulmonary artery. ■ Administer oxygen. ■ Notify the doctor. ■ Document patient's condition and your interventions. **Prevention** ■ Purge tubing of air completely before starting infusion. ■ Use air-detection device on pump or air-eliminating filter proximal to I.V. site. ■ Secure connections.

Peripheral I.V. line maintenance

Routine maintenance of I.V. sites and systems includes regular assessment and rotation of the site and periodic changes of the dressing, tubing, and solution. These measures help prevent complications, such as thrombophlebitis and infection. They should be performed according to facility policy.

Typically, I.V. dressings are changed every 48 hours or whenever the dressing becomes wet, soiled, or nonocclusive. I.V. tubing is changed every 48 to 72 hours or according to policy, and I.V. solution is changed every 24 hours or as needed. The site should be assessed every 2 hours if a transparent semipermeable dressing is used or with every dressing change otherwise and should be rotated every 48 to 72 hours. Sometimes limited venous access prevents frequent site changes; if so, assess the site frequently.

Equipment and preparation

For dressing changes
Sterile gloves ◆ povidone-iodine or alcohol pad ◆ povidone-iodine or other antimicrobial ointment, according to facility policy ◆ adhesive bandage, sterile 2″ × 2″ gauze pad, or transparent semipermeable dressing ◆ 1″ adhesive tape

For solution changes
Solution container as ordered (bag or bottle) ◆ alcohol pad

For tubing changes
I.V. administration set ◆ sterile gloves ◆ sterile 2″ × 2″ gauze pad ◆ adhesive tape for labeling ◆ hypoallergenic tape ◆ optional: hemostats

For I.V. site changes
Commercial kits containing the equipment for dressing changes are available.

If your facility keeps I.V. equipment and dressings in a tray or cart, have it nearby, if possible, because you may have to select a new venipuncture site, depending on the current site's condition. If you're changing the solution and the tubing, attach and prime the I.V. administration set before entering the patient's room.

Implementation

■ Wash your hands thoroughly to prevent the spread of microorganisms. Remember to wear sterile gloves whenever working near the venipuncture site.
■ Explain the procedure to the patient to allay his fears and ensure cooperation.

Changing the dressing
■ Remove the old dressing, open all supply packages, and put on sterile gloves.
■ Hold the cannula in place with your nondominant hand to prevent accidental movement or dislodgment, which could puncture the vein and cause infiltration.
■ Assess the venipuncture site for signs and symptoms of infection (redness and pain at the puncture site), infiltration (coolness, blanching, and edema at the site), and thrombophlebitis (redness, firmness, pain along the path of the vein, and edema). If such signs and symptoms are present, cover the area with a sterile 2″ × 2″ gauze pad and remove the catheter or needle. Apply pressure to the area until the bleeding stops, and apply an adhesive bandage. Then start the I.V. in another appropriate site, preferably on the opposite extremity. Don't use the same I.V. tubing and solution — change the solution and tubing.

If the venipuncture site is intact, stabilize the cannula and carefully clean around the puncture site with a povidone-iodine or an alcohol pad. Work in a circular motion outward from the site to avoid introducing bacteria into the clean area. Allow the area to dry completely.

Apply povidone-iodine or other antimicrobial ointment if facility policy dictates, and cover the site with transparent semipermeable dressing. The transparent dressing allows visibility of the insertion site and maintains sterility. It's placed over the insertion site to halfway up the cannula.

Changing the solution

Wash your hands.

Inspect the new solution container for cracks, leaks, and other damage. Check the solution for discoloration, turbidity, and particulates. Note the date and time the solution was mixed and its expiration date.

Clamp the tubing when inverting it to prevent air from entering the tubing. Keep the drip chamber half full.

If you're replacing a bag, remove the seal or tab from the new bag and remove the old bag from the pole. Remove the spike, insert it into the new bag, and adjust the flow rate.

If you're replacing a bottle, remove the cap and seal from the new bottle and wipe the rubber port with an alcohol pad. Clamp the line, remove the spike from the old bottle, and insert the spike into the new bottle. Then hang the new bottle, and adjust the flow rate.

Changing the tubing

Reduce the I.V. flow rate, remove the old spike from the container, and hang it on the I.V. pole. Place the cover of the new spike loosely over the old one.

Keeping the old spike in an upright position above the patient's heart level, insert the new spike into the I.V. container.

Prime the system. Hang the new I.V. container and primed set on the pole, and grasp the new adapter in one hand. Then stop the flow rate in the old tubing.

Put on sterile gloves.

Place a sterile gauze pad under the needle or cannula hub to create a sterile field. Press one of your fingers over the cannula to prevent bleeding.

Gently disconnect the old tubing (as shown below), being careful not to dislodge or move the I.V. device. (If you have trouble disconnecting the old tubing, use a hemostat to hold the hub securely while twisting the tubing to remove it. Or use one hemostat on the venipuncture device and another on the hard plastic end of the tubing. Then pull the hemostats in opposite directions. Don't clamp the hemostats shut; this could crack the tubing adapter or the venipuncture device.)

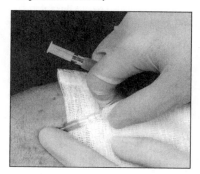

Remove the protective cap from the new tubing, and connect the new adapter to the cannula. Hold the hub securely to prevent dislodging the needle or cannula tip.

Observe for blood backflow into the new tubing to verify that the needle or cannula is still in place. (You may not be able to do this with small-gauge cannulas.)

■ Adjust the clamp to maintain the appropriate flow rate.

■ Retape the cannula hub and I.V. tubing, and recheck the I.V. flow rate because taping may alter it.

■ Label the new tubing and container with the date and time. Label the solution container with a time strip.

Special considerations

Check the prescribed I.V. flow rate before each solution change to prevent errors. If you crack the adapter or hub (or if you accidentally dislodge the cannula from the vein), remove the cannula. Apply pressure and an adhesive bandage to stop any bleeding. Perform a venipuncture at another site, and restart the I.V.

Documentation

Record the time, date, and rate and type of solution (and any additives) in the I.V. flowchart. Also record this information, dressing or tubing changes, and appearance of the site in your notes.

Peritoneal dialysis, continuous ambulatory

Continuous ambulatory peritoneal dialysis (CAPD) requires insertion of a permanent peritoneal catheter (such as a Tenckhoff catheter) to constantly circulate dialysate in the peritoneal cavity. Inserted under local anesthetic, the catheter is sutured in place and its distal portion tunneled subcutaneously (S.C.) to the skin surface. There it serves as a port for the dialysate, which flows in and out of the peritoneal cavity by gravity.

CAPD is usually used for patients with end-stage renal disease. CAPD can be a welcome alternative to hemodialysis because it gives the patient more independence and requires less travel for treatments. It also provides more stable fluid and electrolyte levels than conventional hemodialysis.

Patients or family members can usually learn to perform CAPD after only 2 weeks of training. Furthermore, because the patient can resume normal daily activities between solution changes, CAPD helps promote independence and a return to a near-normal lifestyle. It also costs less than hemodialysis.

Conditions that may prohibit CAPD include recent abdominal surgery, abdominal adhesions, an infected abdominal wall, diaphragmatic tears, ileus, and respiratory insufficiency.

Equipment

To infuse dialysate
Prescribed amount of dialysate (usually in 2-L bags) ◆ basin of hot water or commercial warmer ◆ three surgical masks ◆ 42″ (106.7-cm) connective tubing with drain clamp ◆ six to eight packages of sterile 4″ × 4″ gauze pads ◆ medication, if ordered ◆ povidone-iodine pads ◆ hypoallergenic tape ◆ plastic snap-top container ◆ povidone-iodine solution ◆ sterile basin ◆ container of alcohol ◆ sterile gloves ◆ belt or small fabric pouch ◆ two sterile waterproof paper drapes (one fenestrated) ◆ optional: syringes and labeled specimen container

To temporarily discontinue dialysis
Three sterile waterproof paper drapes (two fenestrated) ◆ 4″ × 4″ gauze pads (for cleaning and dressing the catheter) ◆ two surgical masks ◆ sterile basin ◆ hypoallergenic tape ◆ povidone-iodine solution ◆ sterile gloves ◆ sterile rubber catheter cap

All equipment for infusing the dialysate and discontinuing the procedure must be sterile. Commercially prepared sterile CAPD kits are available. Check the concentration of the dialysate against the doctor's order. Also check the expiration date and appearance of the solution — it should be clear, not cloudy. Warm the solution to body temperature with a heating pad or a commercial warmer if one is available. Don't warm the solution in a microwave oven because the temperature is unpredictable.

To minimize the risk of contaminating the bag's port, leave the dialysate container's wrapper in place. This also keeps the bag dry, which makes examining it for leakage easier after you remove the wrapper.

Wash your hands, and put on a surgical mask. Remove the dialysate container from the warming setup, and remove its protective wrapper. Squeeze the bag firmly to check for leaks.

If ordered, use a syringe to add any prescribed medication to the dialysate, using sterile technique to avoid contamination. (The ideal approach is to add medication under a laminar flow hood.) Disinfect multiple-dose vials in a 5-minute povidone-iodine soak. Insert the connective tubing into the dialysate container. Open the drain clamp to prime the tube. Then close the clamp.

Place a povidone-iodine pad on the dialysate container's port. Cover the port with a dry gauze pad, and secure the pad with hypoallergenic tape. Remove and discard the surgical mask. Tear the tape so it will be ready to secure the new dressing. Commercial devices with povidone-iodine pads are available for covering the dialysate container and tubing connection.

Implementation

■ Weigh the patient to establish a baseline level. Weigh him at the same time every day to help monitor fluid balance.

Infusing dialysate

■ Assemble all equipment at the patient's bedside, and explain the procedure to him. Prepare the sterile field by placing a sterile waterproof paper drape on a dry surface near the patient. Take care to maintain the drape's sterility.

■ Fill the plastic snap-top container with povidone-iodine solution, and place it on the sterile field. Place the basin of hot water on the sterile field. Then place four pairs of sterile gauze pads in the sterile basin, and saturate them with the povidone-iodine solution. Drop the remaining gauze pads on the sterile field. Loosen the cap on the alcohol container, and place it next to the sterile field.

■ Put on a surgical mask, and provide one for the patient.

■ Carefully remove the dressing covering the peritoneal catheter, and discard it. Avoid touching the catheter or skin. Check skin integrity at the catheter site, and look for signs of infection such as purulent drainage. If drainage is present, obtain a specimen, put it in a labeled specimen container, and notify the doctor.

■ Put on the sterile gloves, and palpate the insertion site and S.C. tunnel route for tenderness or pain. If these symptoms occur, notify the doctor.

■ If the patient experiences drainage, tenderness, or pain, don't proceed with the infusion without specific orders.

■ Wrap one gauze pad saturated with povidone-iodine solution around the distal end of the catheter, and leave it in place for 5 minutes. Clean the catheter and insertion site with the rest of the gauze pads, moving in concentric circles away from the insertion site. Use straight strokes to clean the catheter, beginning at the insertion site and moving outward. Use a clean area of the pad for each stroke. Loosen the catheter cap one notch, and clean the exposed area. Place each used pad at the base of the catheter to help support it. After using the third pair of pads, place the sterile waterproof, fenestrated paper drape around the base of the catheter. Continue cleaning the catheter for another minute with one of the remaining pads soaked with povidone-iodine.

■ Remove the povidone-iodine pad on the catheter cap, remove the cap, and use the remaining povidone-iodine pad to clean the end of the catheter hub. Attach the connective tubing from the dialysate container to the catheter. Make sure you secure the luer-lock connector tightly.

■ Open the drain clamp on the dialysate container to allow solution to enter the peritoneal cavity by gravity over a period of 5 to 10 minutes. Leave a small amount of fluid in the bag to make folding it easier. Close the drain clamp.

■ Fold the bag and secure it with a belt, or tuck it in the patient's clothing or in a small fabric pouch.

■ After the prescribed dwell time (usually 4 to 6 hours), unfold the bag, open the clamp, and allow peritoneal fluid to drain back into the bag by gravity.

■ When drainage is complete, attach a new bag of dialysate, and repeat the infusion.

■ Discard used supplies appropriately.

Discontinuing dialysis temporarily

■ Wash your hands, put on a surgical mask, and provide one for the patient. Explain the procedure to him.

■ Using sterile gloves, remove and discard the dressing over the peritoneal catheter.

■ Set up a sterile field next to the patient by covering a clean, dry surface with a sterile waterproof paper drape. Take care to maintain the drape's sterility. Place all equipment on the sterile field, and place the 4″ × 4″ gauze pads in the sterile basin. Saturate them with the povidone-iodine solution. Open the 4″ × 4″ gauze pads to be used as the dressing, and drop them onto the sterile field. Tear pieces of hypoallergenic tape as needed.

■ Tape the dialysate tubing to the side rail of the bed to keep the catheter and tubing off the patient's abdomen.

■ Change to another pair of sterile gloves. Then place one of the fenestrated drapes around the base of the catheter.

■ Use a pair of povidone-iodine pads to clean about 6″ (15 cm) of the dialysis tubing. Clean for 1 minute, moving in one direction only, away from the catheter. Then clean the catheter, moving from the insertion site to the junction of the catheter and dialysis tubing. Place used pads at the base of the catheter to prop it up. Use two more pairs of pads to clean the junction for a total of 3 minutes.

■ Place the second fenestrated drape over the first at the base of the catheter. With the fourth pair of pads, clean the junction of the catheter and 6″ of the dialysate tubing for another minute.

■ Disconnect the dialysate tubing from the catheter. Pick up the sterile rubber catheter cap, and fasten it to the catheter, making sure it fits securely over both notches of the hard plastic catheter tip.

■ Clean the insertion site and a 2″ (5 cm) radius around it with povidone-iodine pads, working from the insertion site outward. Let the skin air-dry before applying the dressing.

■ Properly dispose of used supplies.

Continuous-cycle peritoneal dialysis

Continuous ambulatory peritoneal dialysis is an easy method for the patient who uses an automated continuous cycler system. When set up, this system runs the dialysis treatment automatically until all the dialysate is infused. The system remains closed throughout the treatment, which cuts the risk of contamination. Continuous-cycle peritoneal dialysis (CCPD) can be performed while the patient is awake or asleep. The system's alarms warn about general system, dialysate, and patient problems.

The cycler can be set to an intermittent or continuous dialysate schedule at home or in a health care facility. The patient typically initiates CCPD at bedtime and undergoes three to seven exchanges, depending on individual prescriptions. Upon awakening, the patient infuses the prescribed dialysis volume, disconnects himself from the unit, and carries the dialysate in his peritoneal cavity during the day.

The continuous cycler follows the same aseptic care and maintenance procedures as the manual method.

Special considerations

■ If inflow and outflow are slow or absent, check the tubing for kinks. You can also try raising the solution or repositioning the patient to increase the inflow rate. Repositioning the patient or applying manual pressure to the lateral aspects of the patient's abdomen may also help increase drainage.

■ Make sure that the patient keeps an accurate record of fluid intake and output. Excessive fluid loss may result from a concentrated (4.25%) dialysate solution, improper or inaccurate monitoring of inflow and outflow, or inadequate oral fluid intake. Excessive fluid retention may result from improper or inaccurate monitoring of inflow and outflow, or excessive salt or oral fluid intake.

Patient teaching tips Teach the patient and family how to use sterile technique throughout the procedure, especially for cleaning the insertion site and changing the dressing, to prevent complications such as peritonitis. Also teach them the signs and symptoms of peritonitis — cloudy fluid, fever, abdominal pain, and tenderness — and stress the importance of notifying the doctor immediately if such signs and symptoms arise. Encourage them to call the doctor immediately if redness and drainage occur; these are also signs of infection. Peritonitis is the most common complication of CAPD. Although treatable, it can permanently scar the peritoneal membrane, decreasing its permeability and reducing the efficiency of dialysis. Untreated peritonitis can cause septicemia and death.

Inform the patient about the advantages of an automated continuous cycler system for home use. (See *Continuous-cycle peritoneal dialysis.*) Instruct the patient to record his weight and blood pressure daily and to check regularly for swelling of the extremities.

Documentation

Record the type and amount of fluid instilled and returned for each exchange, the time and duration of the exchange, and any medications added to the dialysate. Note the color and clarity of the returned exchange fluid, and check it for mucus, pus, and blood. Also note any discrepancy in the balance of fluid intake and output as well as any signs of fluid imbalance, such as weight changes, decreased breath sounds, peripheral edema, ascites, and changes in skin turgor. Record the patient's weight, blood pressure, and pulse rate after his last fluid exchange for the day.

Pressure ulcer care

As their name implies, pressure ulcers result when pressure — applied with great force for a short period or with less force over a longer period — impairs circulation, depriving tissues of oxygen and other life-sustaining nutrients. This process damages skin and underlying structures. Untreated, the ischemic lesions that result can lead to serious infection.

Most pressure ulcers develop over bony prominences, where friction and shearing force combine with pressure to break down skin and underlying tissues. Common sites include the sacrum, coccyx, ischial tuberosities, and greater trochanters. Other common sites include the skin over the vertebrae, scapulae, elbows, knees, and heels in bedridden and relatively immobile patients.

Successful pressure ulcer treatment involves relieving pressure, restoring circulation and, if possible, resolving or managing related disorders. Typically, the effectiveness and duration of treatment depend on the pressure ulcer's characteristics. (See *Assessing pressure ulcers.*)

Ideally, prevention is the key to avoiding extensive therapy. Preventive measures include ensuring adequate nourishment and mobility to relieve pressure and promote circulation.

When a pressure ulcer develops despite preventive efforts, treatment includes methods to decrease pressure, such as frequent repositioning to shorten pressure duration and the use of special equipment to reduce pressure intensity. Treatment also may involve special

pressure-reducing devices, such as beds, mattresses, mattress overlays, and chair cushions. Other therapeutic measures include risk factor reduction and the use of topical treatments, wound cleaning, debridement, and moist dressings to support wound healing.

Nurses usually perform or coordinate treatments according to facility policy. The procedures detailed below address cleaning and dressing the pressure ulcer. Always follow the standard precautions guidelines of the Centers for Disease Control and Prevention.

Equipment and preparation

Hypoallergenic tape or elastic netting ◆ piston-type irrigating system ◆ two pairs of gloves ◆ normal saline solution as ordered ◆ sterile 4″ × 4″ gauze pads ◆ selected topical dressing (moist saline gauze, hydrocolloid, transparent, alginate, foam, or hydrogel) ◆ linen-saver pads ◆ impervious plastic trash bag ◆ disposable wound-measuring device ◆ sterile cotton swabs ◆ optional: 21G needle and syringe, alcohol pad, sterile 4″ × 4″ gauze pads, pressure-reducing device, turning sheet

Assemble equipment at the patient's bedside. Cut tape into strips for securing dressings. Loosen lids on cleaning solutions and medications for easy removal. Make sure impervious plastic trash bag is within reach.

Implementation

■ Before any dressing change, wash your hands and review the principles of standard precautions.

Cleaning the pressure ulcer
■ Provide privacy, and explain the procedure to the patient to allay his fears and promote cooperation.
■ Position the patient in a way that maximizes his comfort while allowing easy access to the pressure ulcer site.

Assessing pressure ulcers

To select the most effective treatment for a pressure ulcer, you first need to assess its characteristics. The pressure ulcer staging system described here, used by the National Pressure Ulcer Advisory Panel and the Agency for Health Care and Quality Research, reflects the anatomic depth of exposed tissue. Keep in mind that if the wound contains necrotic tissue, you won't be able to determine the stage until you can see the wound base.

Stage 1
The heralding lesion of a pressure ulcer is persistent redness in lightly pigmented skin and persistent red, blue, or purple hues on darker skin. Other indicators include changes in temperature, consistency, or sensation.

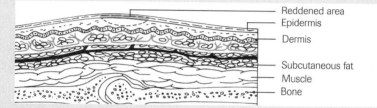

- Reddened area
- Epidermis
- Dermis
- Subcutaneous fat
- Muscle
- Bone

Stage 2
This stage is marked by partial-thickness skin loss involving the epidermis, the dermis, or both. The ulcer is superficial and appears as an abrasion, a blister, or a shallow crater.

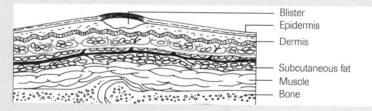

- Blister
- Epidermis
- Dermis
- Subcutaneous fat
- Muscle
- Bone

Stage 3
The ulcer constitutes a full-thickness wound penetrating the subcutaneous tissue, which may extend to – but not through – underlying fascia. The ulcer resembles a deep crater and may or may not undermine adjacent tissue.

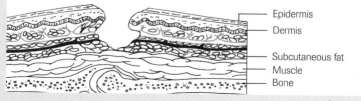

- Epidermis
- Dermis
- Subcutaneous fat
- Muscle
- Bone

(continued)

Assessing pressure ulcers *(continued)*

Stage 4

The ulcer extends through the skin, accompanied by extensive destruction, tissue necrosis, or damage to muscle, bone, or supporting structures (such as tendons and joint capsules).

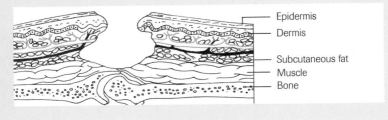

Epidermis
Dermis
Subcutaneous fat
Muscle
Bone

■ Cover bed linens with a linen-saver pad to prevent soiling.

■ Open the normal saline solution container and the piston syringe. Carefully pour normal saline solution into an irrigation container to avoid splashing. (The container may be clean or sterile, depending on facility policy.) Put the piston syringe into the opening provided in the irrigation container.

■ Open the packages of supplies.

■ Put on gloves to remove the old dressing and expose the pressure ulcer. Discard the soiled dressing in the impervious plastic trash bag to avoid contaminating the sterile field and spreading infection.

■ Inspect the wound. Note the color, amount, and odor of drainage and necrotic debris. Measure the wound perimeter with the disposable wound-measuring device (a square, transparent card with concentric circles arranged in bull's-eye fashion and bordered with a straightedge ruler).

■ Using the piston syringe, apply full force to irrigate the pressure ulcer to remove necrotic debris and help decrease bacteria in the wound.

■ Remove and discard your soiled gloves, and put on a fresh pair.

■ Insert a gloved finger or sterile cotton swab into the wound to assess wound tunneling or undermining. Tunneling usually signals wound extension along fascial planes. Gauge tunnel depth by determining how far you can insert your finger or the cotton swab.

■ Next, reassess the condition of the skin and the ulcer. Note the character of the clean wound bed and the surrounding skin.

■ If you observe adherent necrotic material, notify a wound care specialist or a doctor to ensure appropriate debridement.

■ Prepare to apply the selected topical dressing. Directions for typical moist saline gauze, hydrocolloid, transparent, alginate, foam, and hydrogel dressings follow. For other dressings or topical agents, follow facility protocol or manufacturer's instructions.

Choosing a pressure ulcer dressing

The patient's needs and the ulcer's characteristics determine which type of dressing to use on a pressure ulcer.

Gauze dressings

Made of absorptive cotton or synthetic fabric, gauze dressings are permeable to water, water vapor, and oxygen and may be impregnated with petroleum jelly or other agent. When uncertain about which dressing to use, you may apply a gauze dressing moistened in a normal saline solution until a wound specialist recommends definitive treatment.

Hydrocolloid dressings

Hydrocolloid dressings are adhesive, moldable wafers that are made of a carbohydrate-based material and usually have waterproof backings. They're impermeable to oxygen, water, and water vapor, and most have some absorptive properties.

Transparent film dressings

Clear, adherent, and nonabsorptive, transparent film dressings are polymer-based dressings that are permeable to oxygen and water vapor but not to water. Their transparency allows visual inspection. Because they can't absorb drainage, these dressings are used on partial-thickness wounds with minimal exudate.

Alginate dressings

Made from seaweed, alginate dressings are nonwoven, absorptive dressings, available as soft white sterile pads or ropes. They absorb excessive exudate and may be used on infected wounds. As these dressings absorb exudate, they turn into a gel that keeps the wound bed moist and promotes healing. When exudate is no longer excessive, switch to another type of dressing.

Foam dressings

Foam dressings are spongelike polymer dressings that may be impregnated or coated with other materials. Somewhat absorptive, they may or may not be adherent. These dressings promote moist wound healing and are useful when a nonadherent surface is desired.

Hydrogel dressings

Water-based and nonadherent, hydrogel dressings are polymer-based dressings that have some absorptive properties. They're available as a gel in a tube, as flexible sheets, and as saturated gauze packing strips. They may have a cooling effect, which eases pain.

Applying a moist saline gauze dressing

■ Irrigate the pressure ulcer with normal saline solution. Blot the surrounding skin dry.
■ Moisten the gauze dressing with normal saline solution.
■ Gently place the dressing over the surface of the ulcer. To separate surfaces within the wound, gently place a dressing between opposing wound surfaces. To avoid damage to tissues, don't pack the gauze tightly.

■ Change the dressing often enough to keep the wound moist. (See *Choosing a pressure ulcer dressing*.)

Applying a hydrocolloid dressing

■ Irrigate the pressure ulcer with normal saline solution. Blot the surrounding skin dry.
■ Choose a clean, dry, presized dressing, or cut one to overlap the pressure ulcer by about 1″ (2.5 cm). Remove the dressing from its package, pull the release paper from the adherent side of

the dressing, and apply the dressing to the wound. To minimize irritation, carefully smooth out wrinkles as you apply the dressing.

■ If the dressing's edges need to be secured with hypoallergenic tape, apply a skin sealant to the intact skin around the ulcer. After the area dries, tape the dressing to the skin. The sealant protects the skin and promotes tape adherence. Avoid using tension or pressure when applying the tape.

■ Remove your gloves, and discard them in the impervious plastic trash bag. Dispose of refuse according to facility policy, and wash your hands.

■ Change a hydrocolloid dressing every 2 to 7 days as necessary — for example, if the patient complains of pain, the dressing no longer adheres, or leakage occurs.

Applying a transparent dressing

■ Irrigate the pressure ulcer with normal saline solution. Blot the surrounding skin dry.

■ Clean and dry the wound as described above.

■ Select a dressing to overlap the ulcer by 2″ (5.1 cm).

■ Gently lay the dressing over the ulcer. To prevent shearing force, don't stretch the dressing. Press firmly on the edges of the dressing to promote adherence. Although this type of dressing is self-adhesive, you may have to tape the edges to prevent them from curling.

■ If necessary, aspirate accumulated fluid with a 21G needle and syringe. After aspirating the pocket of fluid, clean the aspiration site with an alcohol pad, and cover it with another strip of transparent dressing.

■ Change the dressing every 3 to 7 days, depending on the amount of drainage.

Applying an alginate dressing

■ Irrigate the pressure ulcer with normal saline solution. Blot the surrounding skin dry with a sterile 4″ × 4″ gauze pad.

■ Apply the alginate dressing to the ulcer surface. Cover the area with a secondary dressing (such as gauze pads) as ordered. Secure the dressing with hypoallergenic tape or elastic netting.

■ If the wound is draining heavily, change the dressing once or twice daily for the first 3 to 5 days. As drainage decreases, change the dressing less frequently — every 2 to 4 days or as ordered. When the drainage stops or the wound bed looks dry, stop using alginate dressing.

Applying a foam dressing

■ Irrigate the pressure ulcer with normal saline solution. Blot the surrounding skin dry.

■ Gently lay the foam dressing over the ulcer.

■ Use hypoallergenic tape, elastic netting, or gauze to hold the dressing in place.

■ Change the dressing when the foam no longer absorbs the exudate.

Applying a hydrogel dressing

■ Irrigate the pressure ulcer with normal saline solution. Blot the surrounding skin dry.

■ Apply gel to the wound bed.

■ Cover the area with a secondary dressing.

■ Change the dressing daily or as needed to keep the wound bed moist.

■ If the dressing you select comes in sheet form, cut the dressing to match the wound base; otherwise, the intact surrounding skin can become macerated.

■ Hydrogel dressings also come in a prepackaged, saturated gauze for wounds that require "dead space" to be filled. Follow the manufacturer's directions for usage.

Preventing pressure ulcers

■ Turn and reposition the patient every 1 to 2 hours, unless contraindicated. For a patient who can't turn himself or who is turned on a schedule, use a pressure-reducing device, such as air, gel, or a 4″ foam-mattress overlay. Low- or high-air-loss therapy may be indicated to reduce excessive pressure and promote evaporation of excess moisture. As appropriate, implement active or passive range-of-motion exercises to relieve pressure and promote circulation. To save time, combine these exercises with bathing, if applicable.

■ When turning the patient, lift him rather than slide him because sliding increases friction and shear. Use a turning sheet and get help from coworkers if necessary.

■ Use pillows to position your patient and increase his comfort. Also, eliminate sheet wrinkles, which could increase pressure and cause discomfort.

■ Post a turning schedule at the patient's bedside. Adapt position changes to his situation. Emphasize the importance of regular position changes to the patient and his family, and encourage their participation in treatment and prevention of pressure ulcers by having them perform a position change correctly after you've demonstrated how.

■ Avoid placing the patient directly on the trochanter. Instead, place him on his side, at about a 30-degree angle.

■ Except for brief periods, avoid raising the head of the bed more than 30 degrees to prevent shearing pressure.

■ Direct the patient confined to a chair or wheelchair to shift his weight every 15 minutes to promote blood flow to compressed tissues. Show a paraplegic patient how to shift his weight by doing push-ups in the wheelchair. If the patient needs your help, sit next to him and help him shift his weight to one buttock for 60 seconds; then repeat the procedure on the other side. Provide him with pressure-relieving cushions as appropriate. However, avoid seating the patient on a rubber or plastic doughnut, which can increase localized pressure at vulnerable points.

■ Adjust or pad appliances, casts, or splints as needed to ensure proper fit and avoid increased pressure and impaired circulation.

■ Tell the patient to avoid heat lamps and harsh soaps because they dry the skin. Applying lotion after bathing will help keep his skin moist. Also tell him to avoid vigorous massage because it can damage capillaries.

■ If the patient's condition permits, recommend a diet that includes adequate calories, protein, and vitamins. Dietary therapy may involve nutritional consultation, food supplements, enteral feeding, or total parenteral nutrition.

■ If diarrhea develops or if the patient is incontinent, clean and dry soiled skin. Then apply a protective moisture barrier to prevent skin maceration.

■ Make sure the patient, family members, and caregivers learn pressure ulcer prevention and treatment strategies so that they understand the importance of care, the choices that are available, the rationales for treatments, and their own role in selecting goals and shaping the patient's plan of care.

Special considerations

■ Avoid using elbow and heel protectors that fasten with a single narrow strap. The strap may impair neurovascular function in the involved hand or foot.

■ Avoid using artificial sheepskin. It doesn't reduce pressure, and it may create a false sense of security.

■ Repair of stage 3 and stage 4 ulcers may require surgical intervention — such as direct closure, skin grafting, and flaps — depending on the patient's needs.

■ Infection may cause foul-smelling drainage, persistent pain, severe erythema, induration, and elevated skin and body temperatures. Advancing infection or cellulitis can lead to septicemia. Severe erythema may signal worsening cellulitis, which indicates that the offending organisms have invaded the tissue and are no longer localized.

Documentation

Record the date and time of initial and subsequent treatments. Note the specific treatment given. Detail preventive strategies performed. Document the pressure ulcer's location and size (length, width, and depth); color and appearance of the wound bed; amount, odor, color, and consistency of drainage; and condition of the surrounding skin. Reassess pressure ulcers at least weekly.

Update the plan of care as needed. Note any change in the condition or size of the pressure ulcer and any elevation of skin temperature on the clinical record. Document when the doctor was notified of any pertinent abnormal observations. Record the patient's temperature daily on the graphic sheet to allow easy assessment of body temperature patterns.

Pulse oximetry

Performed intermittently or continuously, oximetry is a relatively simple procedure used to monitor arterial oxygen saturation noninvasively. Pulse oximeters usually denote arterial oxygen saturation values with the symbol SpO_2, whereas invasively measured arterial oxygen saturation values are denoted by the symbol SaO_2.

In this procedure, two diodes send red and infrared light through a pulsating arterial vascular bed, like the one in the fingertip. A photodetector slipped over the finger measures the transmitted light as it passes through the vascular bed, detects the relative amount of color absorbed by arterial blood, and calculates the exact mixed venous oxygen saturation without interference from surrounding venous blood, skin, connective tissue, or bone. Ear oximetry works by monitoring the transmission of light waves through the vascular bed of a patient's earlobe. Results will be inaccurate if the patient's earlobe is poorly perfused, as from a low cardiac output.

Equipment

Oximeter ◆ transducer (photodetector) for finger or ear probe ◆ alcohol pads ◆ nail polish remover, if necessary

Implementation

■ Explain the procedure to the patient.

Finger pulse oximetry

■ Select a finger for the test. Although the index finger is commonly used, a smaller finger may be selected if the patient's fingers are too large for the equipment. Make sure the patient isn't wearing false fingernails, and remove any nail polish from the test finger with nail polish remover. Place the transducer (photodetector) finger probe over the patient's finger so that light beams and sensors oppose each other and attach to the oximeter. If the patient has long fingernails, position the probe perpendicular to the finger, if possible, or clip the fingernail. Always position the patient's hand at heart level to eliminate venous pulsations and to promote accurate readings.

Age alert If you're testing a neonate or a small infant, wrap the probe around the foot so that light beams and detectors oppose each other. For a large infant, use a probe that fits on the great toe, and secure it to the foot.

■ Turn on the power switch. If the device is working properly, a beep will sound, a display will light momentarily, and the pulse searchlight will flash. The SpO_2 and pulse rate displays will show stationary zeros. After four to six heartbeats, the SpO_2 and pulse rate displays will supply information with each beat, and the pulse amplitude indicator will begin tracking the pulse.

Ear pulse oximetry

■ Using an alcohol pad, massage the patient's earlobe for 10 to 20 seconds. Mild erythema indicates adequate vascularization. Following the manufacturer's instructions, attach the ear probe to the patient's earlobe or pinna. Use the ear probe stabilizer for prolonged or exercise testing. Make sure you establish good contact on the ear; an unstable probe may set off the low-perfusion alarm. After the probe has been attached for a few seconds, a saturation reading and pulse waveform will appear on the oximeter's screen.

■ Leave the ear probe in place for 3 minutes or more, until readings stabilize at the highest point, or take three separate readings and average them, revascularizing the patient's earlobe each time.

■ After the procedure, remove the probe, turn off and unplug the unit, and clean the probe by gently rubbing it with an alcohol pad.

Special considerations

■ If oximetry has been performed properly, readings are typically accurate. However, certain factors may interfere with accuracy. For example, an elevated bilirubin level may falsely lower SpO_2 readings, while elevated carboxyhemoglobin or methemoglobin levels, such as occur in heavy smokers and urban dwellers, can cause a falsely elevated SpO_2 reading.

■ Certain intravascular substances, such as lipid emulsions and dyes, can also prevent accurate readings. Other factors that may interfere with accurate results include excessive light (for example, from phototherapy, surgical lamps, direct sunlight, and excessive ambient lighting), excessive patient movement, excessive ear pigment, hypothermia, hypotension, and vasoconstriction.

■ If the patient has compromised circulation in his extremities, you can place a photodetector across the bridge of his nose.

■ If SpO_2 is used to guide weaning of the patient from forced inspiratory oxygen, obtain arterial blood gas analysis occasionally to correlate SpO_2 readings with SaO_2 levels.

■ If an automatic blood pressure cuff is used on the same extremity that is used for measuring SpO_2, the cuff will interfere with SpO_2 readings during inflation.

■ If light is a problem, cover the probes; if patient movement is a problem, move the probe or select a different probe; and if ear pigment is a problem, reposition the probe, revascularize the site, or use a finger probe. (See *Diagnosing pulse oximeter problems,* page 406.)

■ Normal SpO_2 levels for ear and pulse oximetry are 95% to 100% for adults and 93.8% to 100% by 1 hour after birth for healthy, full-term neonates. Lower levels may indicate hypoxemia that warrants intervention. For such patients, follow facility policy or the doctor's orders, which may include increasing oxygen therapy. If SaO_2 levels decrease suddenly, you may need to

Diagnosing pulse oximeter problems

To maintain a continuous display of arterial oxygen saturation (SaO_2) levels, you'll need to keep the monitoring site clean and dry. Make sure the skin doesn't become irritated from adhesives used to keep disposable probes in place. You may need to change the site if this happens. Disposable probes that irritate the skin also can be replaced by nondisposable models that don't need tape.

Another common problem with pulse oximeters is the failure of the devices to obtain a signal. Your first reaction if this happens should be to check the patient's vital signs. If they're sufficient to produce a signal, check for the following problems.

Poor connection

See if the sensors are properly aligned. Make sure that the wires are intact and securely fastened and that the pulse oximeter is plugged into a power source.

Inadequate or intermittent blood flow to site

Check the patient's pulse rate and capillary refill time, and take corrective action if blood flow to the site is decreased. This may mean loosening restraints, removing tight-fitting clothes, taking off a blood pressure cuff, or checking arterial and I.V. lines. If none of these interventions works, you may need to find an alternate site. Finding a site with proper circulation may also prove challenging when a patient is receiving a vasoconstrictor.

Equipment malfunctions

Remove the pulse oximeter from the patient, set the alarm limits at 85% and 100%, and try the instrument on yourself or another healthy person. This will tell you if the equipment is working correctly.

---

resuscitate the patient immediately. Notify the doctor of any significant change in the patient's condition.

Documentation

Document the procedure, including the date, time, procedure type, oximetric measurement, and any action taken. Record reading in appropriate flowcharts if indicated.

Restraint application

Restraint application involves various soft restraints that limit movement to prevent the confused, disoriented, or combative patient from injuring himself or others. Vest and belt restraints, used to prevent falls from a bed or a chair, permit full movement of arms and legs. Limb restraints, used to prevent removal of supportive equipment — such

as I.V. lines, indwelling catheters, and nasogastric tubes — allow only slight limb motion. Like limb restraints, mitts prevent removal of supportive equipment, keep the patient from scratching rashes or sores, and prevent the combative patient from injuring himself or others. Body restraints, used to control the combative or hysterical patient, immobilize all or most of the body.

When soft restraints aren't sufficient and sedation is dangerous or ineffective, leather restraints can be used. Depending on the patient's behavior, leather restraints may be applied to all limbs (four-point restraints) or to one arm and one leg (two-point restraints). The duration of such restraint is governed by state law and facility policy.

Restraints must be used cautiously in seizure-prone patients because they increase the risk of fracture and trauma. Restraints can cause skin irritation and restrict blood flow, so they shouldn't be applied directly over wounds or I.V. catheters. Vest restraints should be used cautiously in patients with heart failure or a respiratory disorder. Such restraints can tighten with movement, further limiting circulation and respiratory function.

Equipment and preparation

For soft restraints
Restraint (vest, limb, mitt, belt, or body as needed) ◆ gauze pads, if needed

For leather restraints
Two wrist and two ankle leather restraints ◆ four straps ◆ key ◆ large gauze pads to cushion each extremity

Before entering the patient's room, make sure the restraints are the correct size, using the patient's build and weight as a guide. If you use leather restraints, make sure that the straps are unlocked and the key fits the locks.

Age alert For children, who typically are too small for standard restraints, use child restraints. (See *Types of child restraints,* page 408.)

Implementation

■ Obtain a doctor's order for the restraint, if required. However, never leave a confused or combative patient unattended or unrestrained while attempting to secure the order.

■ If necessary, obtain adequate assistance to restrain the patient before entering his room. Enlist the aid of several coworkers, and organize their effort, giving each person a specific task — for example, one person explains the procedure to the patient and applies the restraints while the others immobilize the patient's arms and legs.

■ Tell the patient what you're about to do, and describe the restraints to him. Assure him that they're being used to protect him from injury rather than to punish him.

Applying a vest restraint
■ Assist the patient to a sitting position if his condition permits. Then slip the vest over his gown. Crisscross the cloth flaps at the front, placing the V-shaped opening at the patient's throat. Never crisscross the flaps in the back because this may cause the patient to choke if he tries to squirm out of the vest.

■ Pass the tab on one flap through the slot on the opposite flap. Then adjust the vest for the patient's comfort. You should be able to slip your fist between the vest and the patient. Avoid wrapping the vest too tightly because it may restrict respiratory function.

■ Tie all restraints securely to the frame of the bed, chair, or wheelchair and out of the patient's reach. Use a bow or a knot that can be released quickly and easily in an emergency. (See *Knots for securing soft restraints,* page 409.) Never tie a regular knot to secure the straps. Leave 1″ to 2″ (2.5 to 5 cm) of slack in the straps to allow room for movement.

■ After applying the vest, check the patient's respiratory rate and breath sounds regularly. Watch for signs of respiratory distress. Also make sure the vest hasn't tightened with the patient's movement. Loosen the vest frequently, if possible, so the patient can stretch, turn, and breathe deeply.

Applying a limb restraint
■ Wrap the patient's wrist or ankle with gauze pads to reduce friction between the patient's skin and the restraint, helping to prevent irritation and skin breakdown. Then wrap the restraint around the gauze pads.

■ Pass the strap on the narrow end of the restraint through the slot in the broad end, and adjust for a snug fit. Or

Types of child restraints

You may need to restrain an infant or a child to prevent injury or to facilitate examination, diagnostic tests, or treatment. If so, follow these steps:

■ Provide a simple explanation, reassurance, and constant observation to minimize the child's fear.

■ Explain the restraint to the parents and enlist their help.

■ Reassure them that what you're doing won't hurt the child.

■ Make sure restraint ties or safety pins are secured outside the child's reach to prevent injury.

■ When using a mummy restraint, secure the infant's arms in proper alignment with the body to avoid dislocation and other injuries.

Vest

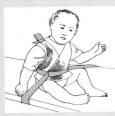

Elbow

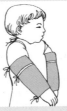

Mummy

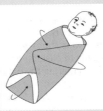

Belt

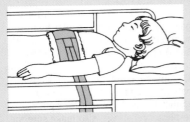

Limb

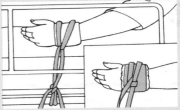

Crib with net

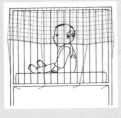

Mitt

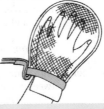

Restraining board

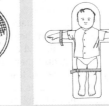

fasten the buckle or Velcro cuffs to fit the restraint. You should be able to slip one or two fingers between the restraint and the patient's skin. Avoid applying the restraint too tightly because it may impair circulation distal to the restraint.

■ Tie the restraint as mentioned earlier.

■ After applying limb restraints, watch for signs of impaired circulation in the extremity distal to the restraint. If the skin appears blue or feels cold, or if the patient complains of a tingling sensation or numbness, loosen the restraint. Perform range-of-motion (ROM) exercises regularly to stimulate circulation and prevent contractures and resultant loss of mobility.

Applying a mitt restraint

■ Wash and dry the patient's hands.

■ Roll up a washcloth or gauze pad, and place it in the patient's palm. Have him form a loose fist, if possible; then pull the mitt over it and secure the closure.

■ To restrict the patient's arm movement, attach the strap to the mitt and tie it securely, using a bow or a knot that can be released quickly and easily in an emergency.

■ When using mitts made of transparent mesh, check hand movement and skin color frequently to assess circulation. Remove the mitts regularly to stimulate circulation, and perform passive ROM exercises to prevent contractures.

Applying a belt restraint

■ Center the flannel pad of the belt on the bed. Then wrap the short strap of the belt around the bed frame and fasten it under the bed.

■ Position the patient on the pad. Then have him roll slightly to one side while you guide the long strap around his waist and through the slot in the pad.

Knots for securing soft restraints

When securing soft restraints, use knots that can be released quickly and easily, like those shown below. Remember, never secure restraints to the bed's side rails.

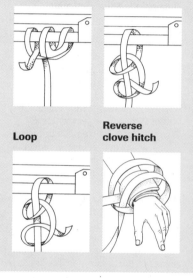

Magnus hitch   **Clove hitch**

Loop   **Reverse clove hitch**

■ Wrap the long strap around the bed frame and fasten it under the bed.

■ After applying the belt, slip your hand between the patient and the belt to ensure a secure but comfortable fit. A loose belt can be raised to chest level; a tight one can cause abdominal discomfort.

Applying a body restraint

■ Place the restraint flat on the bed, with arm and wrist cuffs facing down and the V at the head of the bed.

■ Place the patient in the prone position on top of the restraint.

■ Lift the V over the patient's head. Thread the chest belt through one of the loops in the V to ensure a snug fit.
■ Secure the straps around the patient's chest, thighs, and legs. Then turn the patient on his back.
■ Secure the straps to the bed frame to anchor the restraint. Then secure the straps around the patient's arms and wrists.

Applying leather restraints

■ Position the patient in supine position on the bed, with each arm and leg securely held down to minimize combative behavior and to prevent injury to the patient and others. Immobilize the patient's arms and legs at the joints — knee, ankle, shoulder, and wrist — to minimize his movement without exerting excessive force.
■ Apply large gauze pads to the patient's wrists and ankles to reduce friction between his skin and the leather, preventing skin irritation and breakdown.
■ Wrap the restraint around the gauze pads. Then insert the metal loop through the hole that gives the best fit. Apply the restraints securely but not too tightly to the two wrists and two ankles of the patient for four point restraints. Wrist restraints are generally smaller than ankle restraints. You should be able to slip one or two fingers between the restraint and the patient's skin. A tight restraint can compromise circulation; a loose one can slip off or move up the patient's arm or leg, causing skin irritation and breakdown.
■ Thread a strap through each of the metal loops on the restraints (there are four, two wrist and two ankle), close the metal loop, and secure the strap to the bed frame, out of the patient's reach.

■ Lock the restraint by pushing in the button on the side of the metal loop, and tug it gently to be sure it's secure. Once the restraint is secure, a coworker can release the arm or leg. Flex the patient's arm or leg slightly before locking the strap to allow room for movement and to prevent frozen joints and dislocations.
■ Place the key in an accessible location at the nurse's station.
■ After applying leather restraints, observe the patient regularly to give emotional support and to reassess the need for continued use of the restraint. Check his pulse rate and vital signs at least every 2 hours. Remove or loosen the restraints one at a time, every 2 hours, and perform passive ROM exercises if possible. Watch for signs of impaired peripheral circulation, such as cool, cyanotic skin. To unlock the restraint, insert the key into the metal loop, opposite the locking button. This releases the lock so the metal loop can be opened.

Special considerations

■ Because the authority to use restraints varies among facilities, follow facility policy. You may be able to apply restraints without a doctor's order in an emergency. Also, follow state regulations governing such restraints. For example, some states prohibit the use of four-point restraints. Additionally, some facilities may require that the family sign a consent form, indicating that restraints can be used if they're absolutely necessary.
■ When the patient is at high risk for aspiration, restrain him on his side. Never secure all four restraints to one side of the bed because the patient may fall out of bed.
■ When loosening restraints, have a coworker on hand to assist in restraining the patient, if necessary.

■ After assessing the patient's behavior and condition, you may decide to use a two-point restraint, which should restrain one arm and the opposite leg — for example, the right arm and the left leg. Never restrain the arm and leg on the same side because the patient may fall out of bed.

■ Don't apply a limb restraint above an I.V. site because the constriction may occlude the infusion or cause infiltration into surrounding tissue.

■ Never secure restraints to the side rails because someone might inadvertently lower the rail before noticing the attached restraint. This may jerk the patient's limb or body, causing him discomfort and trauma. Never secure restraints to the fixed frame of the bed if the patient's position is to be changed.

■ Don't restrain a patient in the prone position. This position limits his field of vision, intensifies feelings of helplessness and vulnerability, and impairs respiratory function, especially if he has been sedated.

■ Because the restrained patient has limited mobility, his nutrition, elimination, and positioning become your responsibility. To prevent pressure ulcers, reposition the patient regularly, and massage and pad bony prominences and other vulnerable areas.

■ Inspect the patient and the restraints every 15 to 30 minutes. Release the restraints every 2 hours; assess the patient's pulse and skin condition, and perform ROM exercises. Document all assessments and findings.

■ Excessively tight limb restraints can reduce peripheral circulation; tight vest restraints can impair respiratory function. Apply restraints carefully and check them regularly.

■ Skin breakdown can also occur under limb restraints. To prevent this, pad the patient's wrists and ankles, loosen or remove the restraints frequently, and provide regular skin care.

■ Long periods of immobility can predispose the patient to pneumonia, urine retention, constipation, and sensory deprivation. Reposition the patient, and attend to his elimination requirements as needed.

■ Some patients resist restraints by biting, kicking, scratching, or head butting, in the course of which they may injure themselves or others.

Documentation

Record the behavior that necessitated restraints, the time the restraints were applied and removed, and the type of restraints used.

Record vital signs, skin condition, respiratory status, peripheral circulation, and mental status.

Seizure management

Seizures are paroxysmal events associated with abnormal electrical discharges of neurons in the brain. Partial seizures are usually unilateral, involving a localized or focal area of the brain. Generalized seizures involve the entire brain. When a patient has a generalized seizure, nursing care aims to protect him from injury and prevent serious complications. Appropriate care also includes observation of seizure characteristics to help determine the area of the brain involved.

Patients considered at risk for seizures are those with a history of seizures and those with conditions that predispose them to seizures. These conditions include metabolic abnormalities, such as hypocalcemia, hypoglycemia, and pyridoxine deficiency; brain tumors or other space-occupying lesions; infections, such as meningitis, encephalitis, and brain abscess; traumatic injury, es-

Precautions for generalized seizures

By taking appropriate precautions, you can help protect a patient from injury, aspiration, and airway obstruction should he have a seizure. Plan your precautions using information obtained from the patient's history. What kind of seizure has the patient previously had? Is he aware of exacerbating factors? Sleep deprivation, missed doses of an anticonvulsant, and even upper respiratory tract infections can increase seizure frequency in some people who have had seizures. Was his previous seizure an acute episode, or did it result from a chronic condition?

Gather the equipment
Based on answers provided in the patient's history, you can tailor your precautions to his needs. Start by gathering the appropriate equipment, including a hospital bed with full-length side rails, commercial side rail pads or six bath blankets (four for a crib), adhesive tape, an oral airway, and oral or nasal suction equipment.

Bedside preparations
Carry out the precautions you think appropriate for the patient. Remember that a patient with preexisting seizures who is being admitted for a change in medication, treatment of an infection, or detoxification may have an increased risk of seizures.
■ Explain the reasons for the precautions to the patient.
■ To protect the patient's limbs, head, and feet from injury if he has a seizure while in bed, cover the side rails, headboard, and footboard with side rail pads or bath blankets. If you use blankets, keep them in place with adhesive tape. Make sure you keep the side rails raised while the patient is in bed to prevent falls. Keep the bed in a low position to minimize any injuries that may occur if the patient climbs over the side rails.
■ Place an airway at the patient's bedside, or tape it to the wall above the bed according to facility policy. Keep suction equipment nearby in case you need to establish a patent airway. Explain to the patient how the airway will be used.
■ If the patient has frequent or prolonged seizures, prepare an I.V. heparin lock to facilitate administration of emergency medications.

pecially if the dura mater was penetrated; ingestion of toxins, such as mercury, lead, or carbon monoxide; genetic abnormalities, such as tuberous sclerosis and phenylketonuria; perinatal injuries; and cerebrovascular accident. Patients at risk for seizures need precautionary measures to help prevent injury if a seizure occurs. (See *Precautions for generalized seizures*.)

Equipment

Oral airway ◆ suction equipment ◆ side rail pads ◆ seizure activity record ◆ optional: I.V. line and normal saline solution, oxygen as ordered, endotracheal intubation, dextrose 50% in water, 100-mg bolus of thiamine

Implementation

■ If you're with a patient when he experiences an aura, help him into bed, raise the side rails, and adjust the bed flat. Use side rail pads and blankets to pad the rails securely. If he's away from his room, lower him to the floor and place a pillow, blanket, or other soft material under his head to keep it from hitting the floor.
■ Stay with the patient during the seizure, and be ready to intervene if complications such as airway obstruc-

tion develop. If necessary, have another staff member obtain the appropriate equipment and notify the doctor of the obstruction.

■ Provide privacy, if possible.

■ Depending on facility policy, if the patient is in the beginning of the tonic phase of the seizure, you may insert an oral airway into his mouth so that his tongue doesn't block his airway. If an oral airway isn't available, don't try to hold his mouth open or place your hands inside because he may bite you. After the patient's jaw becomes rigid, don't force the airway into place because you could break his teeth or cause another injury. Some clinicians advocate waiting until the seizure subsides before inserting the airway.

■ Move hard or sharp objects out of the patient's way, and loosen his clothing.

■ Don't forcibly restrain the patient or restrict his movements during the seizure, because the force of his movements against restraints could cause muscle strain or even joint dislocation.

■ Continually assess the patient during the seizure. Observe the earliest sign, such as head or eye deviation, as well as how the seizure progresses, what form it takes, and how long it lasts. Document the act by writing on the hospital seizure activity record. Your description may help determine the seizure's type and cause.

■ If this is the patient's first seizure, notify the doctor immediately. If the patient has had seizures before, notify the doctor only if the seizure activity is prolonged or if the patient fails to regain consciousness. (See *Understanding status epilepticus*.)

■ If ordered, establish an I.V. line and infuse normal saline solution at a keep-vein-open rate.

■ If the seizure is prolonged and the patient becomes hypoxemic, administer oxygen as ordered. Some patients may require endotracheal intubation.

Understanding status epilepticus

Status epilepticus is a continuous seizure state, unless it's interrupted by emergency interventions; it can occur in all seizure types. The most life-threatening example is generalized tonic-clonic status epilepticus, a continuous generalized tonic-clonic seizure without intervening return of consciousness.

Status epilepticus, which is always an emergency, is accompanied by respiratory distress. It can result from abrupt withdrawal of an anticonvulsant, hypoxic or metabolic encephalopathy, acute head trauma, or septicemia secondary to encephalitis or meningitis.

Emergency treatment of status epilepticus usually consists of diazepam, phenytoin, or phenobarbital; dextrose 50% I.V. (when seizures are secondary to hypoglycemia); and thiamine I.V. (in the presence of chronic alcoholism or withdrawal).

■ If the patient is diabetic, administer 50 ml of dextrose 50% in water by I.V. push as ordered. If the patient is an alcoholic, a 100-mg bolus of thiamine may be ordered to stop the seizure.

■ After the seizure, turn the patient on his side and apply suction, if necessary, to facilitate drainage of secretions and maintain a patent airway. Insert an oral airway if needed.

■ Check for injuries.

■ Reorient and reassure the patient as necessary.

■ When the patient is comfortable and safe, document what happened during the seizure.

■ After the seizure, monitor vital signs and mental status every 15 to 20 minutes for 2 hours.

■ Ask the patient about his aura and activities preceding the seizure. The type of aura (auditory, visual, olfactory, gustatory, or somatic) helps pinpoint the site in the brain where the seizure originated.

Special considerations

■ Because a seizure commonly indicates an underlying disorder such as meningitis or a metabolic or electrolyte imbalance, a complete diagnostic workup will be ordered if the cause of the seizure isn't evident.
■ The patient who experiences a seizure may experience an injury, respiratory difficulty, and decreased mental capability. Common injuries include scrapes and bruises suffered when the patient hits objects during the seizure and traumatic injury to the tongue caused by biting. If you suspect a serious injury, such as a fracture or deep laceration, notify the doctor, and arrange for appropriate evaluation and treatment.
■ Changes in respiratory function include aspiration, airway obstruction, and hypoxemia. After the seizure, complete a respiratory assessment, and notify the doctor if you suspect a problem. Expect most patients to experience a postictal period of decreased mental status lasting 30 minutes to 24 hours. Reassure the patient that this doesn't indicate incipient brain damage.

Documentation

Document that the patient requires seizure precautions, and record all precautions taken. Record the date and the time the seizure began as well as its duration and any precipitating factors. Identify any sensation that may be considered an aura. If the seizure was preceded by an aura, have the patient describe what he experienced.

Record any involuntary behavior that occurred at the onset, such as lip smacking, chewing movements, or hand and eye movements. Describe

where the movement began and the parts of the body involved. Note any progression or pattern to the activity. Document whether the patient's eyes deviated to one side and whether the pupils changed in size, shape, equality, or reaction to light. Note if the patient's teeth were clenched or open. Record any incontinence, vomiting, or salivation that occurred during the seizure.

Note the patient's response to the seizure. Was the patient aware of what happened? Did he fall into a deep sleep after the seizure? Was he upset or ashamed? Also, document any medications given, any complications experienced during the seizure, and any interventions performed. Finally, record the patient's postseizure mental status.

Sequential compression therapy

Safe, effective, and noninvasive, sequential compression therapy helps prevent deep vein thrombosis (DVT) in surgical patients. This therapy massages the legs in a wavelike, milking motion that promotes blood flow and deters thrombosis.

Typically, sequential compression therapy complements other preventive measures, such as antiembolism stockings and anticoagulant therapy. Although patients at low risk for DVT may require only antiembolism stockings, those at moderate to high risk may require both antiembolism stockings and sequential compression therapy. These preventive measures are continued for as long as the patient remains at risk.

Both antiembolism stockings and sequential compression sleeves are commonly used preoperatively and postoperatively because blood clots tend to form during surgery. About 20% of blood clots form in the femoral vein. Sequential compression therapy counteracts blood stasis and coagulation changes, two of the three major factors that promote DVT. It reduces stasis by increasing peak blood flow velocity, helping to empty the femoral vein's valve cusps of pooled or static blood. Also, the compressions cause an anticlotting effect by increasing fibrinolytic activity, which stimulates the release of a plasminogen activator.

Equipment

Measuring tape and sizing chart for the brand of sleeves you're using ♦ pair of compression sleeves in correct size ♦ connecting tubing ♦ compression controller

Implementation

■ Explain the procedure to the patient to increase her cooperation.

Determining proper sleeve size
■ Before applying the compression sleeve, determine the proper size of sleeve that you need. Begin by washing your hands.
■ Then measure the circumference of the upper thigh while the patient rests in bed. Do this by placing the measuring tape under the thigh at the gluteal furrow (as shown below).

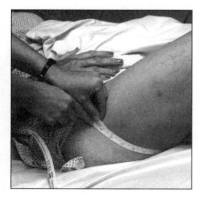

■ Hold the tape snugly, but not tightly, around the patient's leg. Note the exact circumference.
■ Find the patient's thigh measurement on the sizing chart, and locate the corresponding size of the compression sleeve.
■ Remove the compression sleeves from the package and unfold them.
■ Lay the unfolded sleeves on a flat surface with the cotton lining facing up (as shown below).

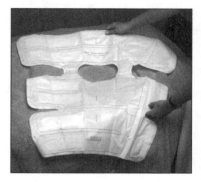

■ Notice the markings on the lining denoting the ankle and the area behind the knee at the popliteal pulse point. Use these markings to position the sleeves at the appropriate landmarks.

Applying the sleeves
■ Place the patient's leg on the lining of one of the sleeves. Position the back of the knee over the popliteal opening.
■ Make sure that the back of the ankle is over the ankle marking.
■ Starting at the side opposite the clear plastic tubing, wrap the sleeve snugly around the patient's leg.
■ Fasten the sleeve securely with the Velcro fasteners. For the best fit, first secure the ankle and calf sections and then the thigh.
■ The sleeve should fit snugly but not tightly. Check the fit by inserting two fingers between the sleeve and the patient's leg at the knee opening. Loosen

or tighten the sleeve by readjusting the Velcro fastener.

■ Using the same procedure, apply the second sleeve (as shown below).

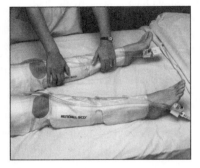

Operating the system

■ Connect each sleeve to the tubing leading to the controller. Both sleeves must be connected to the compression controller for the system to operate. Line up the blue arrows on the sleeve connector with the arrows on the tubing connectors, and firmly push the ends together. Listen for a click, signaling a firm connection. Make sure that the tubing isn't kinked.

■ Plug the compression controller into the proper wall outlet. Turn on the power.

■ The controller automatically sets the compression sleeve pressure at 45 mm Hg, which is the midpoint of the normal range (35 to 55 mm Hg).

■ Observe the patient to see how well she tolerates the therapy and the controller as the system completes its first cycle.

■ Check the AUDIBLE ALARM key. The green light should be lit, indicating that the alarm is working.

■ The compression sleeves should function continuously (24 hours/day) until the patient is fully ambulatory. Check the sleeves at least once each shift to ensure proper fit and inflation.

Removing the sleeves

■ You may remove the sleeves when the patient is walking, bathing, or leaving the room for tests or other procedures, as long as you reapply the sleeves immediately after the tests and procedures are over. To disconnect the sleeves from the tubing, press the latches on each side of the connectors, and pull the connectors apart.

■ Store the tubing and compression controller according to facility policy. This equipment isn't disposable.

Special considerations

■ The compression controller also has a mechanism to help cool the patient.

■ If you're applying only one sleeve — for example, if the patient has a cast — leave the unused sleeve folded in the plastic bag. Cut a small hole in the bag's sealed bottom edge, and pull the sleeve connector (the part that holds the connecting tubing) through the hole. Then you can join both sleeves to the compression controller.

■ If a malfunction triggers the instrument's alarm, you'll hear beeping. The system shuts off whenever the alarm is activated.

■ To respond to the alarm, remove the operator's card from the slot on the top of the compression controller.

■ Follow the instructions printed on the card next to the matching code. Don't use this therapy in patients with any of the following conditions:
-acute DVT (or DVT diagnosed within the past 6 months)
-severe arteriosclerosis or any other ischemic vascular disease
-massive edema of the legs resulting from pulmonary edema or heart failure
-any local condition that the compression sleeves would aggravate, such as dermatitis, vein ligation, gangrene, and recent skin grafting. A patient with a pronounced leg deformity also would

be unlikely to benefit from the compression sleeves.

Documentation

Document the procedure, the patient's response to and understanding of the procedure, and the status of the alarm and cooling settings.

Synchronized cardioversion

Used to treat tachyarrhythmias, cardioversion delivers an electric charge to the myocardium at the peak of the R wave. This causes immediate depolarization, interrupting reentry circuits and allowing the sinoatrial node to resume control. Synchronizing the electric charge with the R wave ensures that the current won't be delivered on the vulnerable T wave and thus won't disrupt repolarization.

Synchronized cardioversion is the treatment of choice for arrhythmias that don't respond to vagal massage or drug therapy, such as atrial tachycardia, atrial flutter, atrial fibrillation, and symptomatic ventricular tachycardia.

Cardioversion may be an elective or urgent procedure, depending on how well the patient tolerates the arrhythmia. For example, if the patient is hemodynamically unstable, he requires urgent cardioversion. Remember that, when preparing for cardioversion, the patient's condition can deteriorate quickly, necessitating immediate defibrillation.

Indications for cardioversion include stable paroxysmal atrial tachycardia, unstable paroxysmal supraventricular tachycardia, atrial fibrillation, atrial flutter, and ventricular tachycardia.

Equipment

Cardioverter-defibrillator ◆ conductive medium pads ◆ anterior, posterior, or transverse paddles ◆ electrocardiogram (ECG) monitor with recorder ◆ sedative ◆ oxygen therapy equipment ◆ airway ◆ handheld resuscitation bag ◆ emergency cardiac medication ◆ automatic blood pressure cuff (if available) ◆ pulse oximeter (if available)

Implementation

■ Explain the procedure to the patient, and make sure he has signed a consent form.

■ Check the patient's recent serum potassium and magnesium levels and arterial blood gas results. Also check recent digoxin levels. Although patients receiving digoxin may undergo cardioversion, they tend to require lower energy levels to convert. If the patient takes digoxin, withhold the dose on the day of the procedure.

■ Withhold all food and fluids for 6 to 12 hours before the procedure. If the cardioversion is urgent, withhold the previous meal.

■ Obtain a 12-lead ECG to serve as a baseline.

■ Check to see if the doctor has ordered administration of any cardiac drugs before the procedure. Also, verify that the patient has a patent I.V. site in case drug administration becomes necessary.

■ Connect the patient to a pulse oximeter and automatic blood pressure cuff, if available.

■ Consider administering oxygen for 5 to 10 minutes before the cardioversion to promote myocardial oxygenation. If the patient wears dentures, evaluate whether they support his airway or might cause an airway obstruction. If they might cause an obstruction, remove them.

■ Place the patient in the supine position, and assess his vital signs, level of consciousness (LOC), cardiac rhythm, and peripheral pulses.

■ Remove any oxygen delivery device just before cardioversion to avoid possible combustion.

■ Have emergency cardiac medication (epinephrine, lidocaine, and atropine) at the patient's bedside.

■ Administer a sedative as ordered. The patient should be heavily sedated but still able to breathe adequately.

■ Carefully monitor the patient's blood pressure and respiratory rate until he recovers.

■ Apply the ECG monitor with recorder and press the POWER button to turn on the cardioverter-defibrillator. Next, push the SYNC button to synchronize the machine with the patient's QRS complexes. Make sure the SYNC button flashes with each of the patient's QRS complexes. You should also see a bright green flag flash on the ECG monitor.

■ Turn the ENERGY SELECT dial to the ordered amount of energy. Advanced Cardiac Life Support protocols call for 50 to 360 joules for a patient with stable paroxysmal atrial tachycardia, 75 to 360 joules for a patient with unstable paroxysmal supraventricular tachycardia, 100 joules for a patient with atrial fibrillation, 50 joules for a patient with atrial flutter, 100 to 360 joules for a patient who has ventricular tachycardia with a pulse, and 200 to 360 joules for a patient with pulseless ventricular tachycardia.

■ Remove the paddles from the machine, and prepare them as you would if you were defibrillating the patient. Place the conductive medium pads or appropriate paddles in the same positions as you would to defibrillate.

■ Make sure everyone stands away from the bed; then push the discharge buttons. Hold the paddles in place and wait for the energy to be discharged — the machine has to synchronize the discharge with the QRS complex.

■ Check the waveform on the monitor. If the arrhythmia fails to convert, repeat the procedure two or three more times at 3-minute intervals. Gradually increase the energy level with each additional countershock.

■ After the cardioversion, frequently assess the patient's LOC and respiratory status, including airway patency, respiratory rate and depth, and the need for supplemental oxygen. Because the patient will be heavily sedated, he may require airway support with a hand-held rescusitation bag.

■ Record a postcardioversion 12-lead ECG, and monitor the patient's ECG rhythm for 2 hours. Check the patient's chest for electrical burns.

Special considerations

■ If the patient is attached to a bedside or telemetry monitor, disconnect the unit before cardioversion. The electric current it generates could damage the equipment.

■ Be aware that improper synchronization may result if the patient's ECG tracing contains artifact-like spikes, such as peaked T waves or bundle-branch blocks when the R' wave may be taller than the R wave.

■ Although the electric shock of cardioversion won't usually damage an implanted pacemaker, avoid placing the paddles directly over the pacemaker.

■ Common complications following cardioversion include transient, harmless arrhythmias such as atrial, ventricular, and junctional premature beats. Serious ventricular arrhythmias, such as ventricular fibrillation, may also occur. However, this type of arrhythmia is more likely to result from high amounts of electrical energy, digitalis toxicity, severe heart disease, electrolyte imbalance, or improper synchronization with the R wave.

Documentation

Document the procedure, including the voltage delivered with each attempt, rhythm strips before and after the procedure, and the patient's tolerance of the procedure.

Thoracic drainage

Thoracic drainage uses gravity and possibly suction to restore negative pressure and remove any material that collects in the pleural cavity. An underwater seal in the drainage system allows air and fluid to escape from the pleural cavity but doesn't allow air to reenter. The system combines drainage collection, water seal, and suction control into a single unit. (See *Disposable drainage systems.*)

Specifically, thoracic drainage may be ordered to remove accumulated air, fluids (blood, pus, chyle, serous fluids), or solids (blood clots) from the pleural cavity; to restore negative pressure in the pleural cavity; or to reexpand a partially or totally collapsed lung.

Equipment and preparation

Thoracic drainage system (Pleur-evac, Argyle, Ohio, or Thora-Klex systems, which can function as gravity draining systems or can be connected to suction to enhance chest drainage) ◆ sterile distilled water (usually 1 L) ◆ adhesive tape ◆ sterile clear plastic tubing ◆ two rubber-tipped Kelly clamps ◆ sterile 50-ml catheter-tip syringe ◆ suction source, if ordered ◆ optional: alcohol pad, lotion

Check the doctor's order to determine the type of drainage system to be used and specific procedural details. If appropriate, request the drainage system and suction system from the central supply department. Collect the appropriate equipment, and take it to the patient's bedside.

Implementation

■ Explain the procedure to the patient, and wash your hands.

■ Maintain sterile technique throughout the entire procedure and whenever you make changes in the system or al-

Disposable drainage systems

Commercially prepared disposable drainage systems combine drainage collection, water seal, and suction control in one unit (as shown here). These systems ensure patient safety with positive- and negative-pressure relief valves and have a prominent air-leak indicator. Some systems produce no bubbling sound.

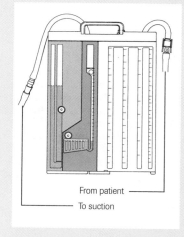

From patient
To suction

ter any of the connections to avoid introducing pathogens into the pleural space.

Setting up a commercially prepared disposable system

■ Open the thoracic drainage system, and place it on the floor in the rack that the manufacturer supplied, to avoid accidentally knocking it over or dislodging the components. After the system is prepared, it may be hung from the side of the patient's bed.

■ Remove the plastic connector from the short tube that is attached to the water-seal chamber. Using a sterile 50-ml catheter-tip syringe, instill sterile distilled water into the water-seal chamber until it reaches the 2-cm mark or the mark that the manufacturer specified. The Ohio and Thora-Klex systems are ready to use, but with the Pleur-evac and Thora-Klex system, 15 ml of sterile water may be added to help detect air leaks. Replace the plastic connector.

■ If suction is ordered, remove the cap (also called the muffler or atmosphere vent cover) on the suction-control chamber to open the vent. Next, instill sterile distilled water until it reaches the 20-cm mark or the ordered level, and recap the suction-control chamber.

■ Using the long tube, connect the patient's chest tube to the closed drainage collection chamber. Secure the connection with adhesive tape.

■ Connect the short tube on the drainage system to the suction source using the sterile clear plastic tubing, and turn on the suction. Gentle bubbling should begin in the suction chamber, indicating that the correct suction level has been reached.

Managing closed-chest underwater seal drainage

■ Monitor the character, consistency, and amount of drainage in the drainage collection chamber.

■ Mark the drainage level in the drainage collection chamber by noting the time and date at the drainage level on the chamber every 8 hours (or more often if there is a large amount of drainage).

■ Check the water level in the water-seal chamber every 8 hours. If necessary, carefully add sterile distilled water until the level reaches the 2-cm mark indicated on the water-seal chamber of the commercial system.

■ Check for fluctuation in the water-seal chamber as the patient breathes. Normal fluctuations of 2″ to 4″ (5 to 10 cm) reflect pressure changes in the pleural space during respiration. To check for fluctuation when a suction system is being used, momentarily disconnect the suction system so the air vent is opened, and observe for fluctuation.

■ Check for intermittent bubbling in the water-seal chamber. This occurs normally when the system is removing air from the pleural cavity. If bubbling isn't readily apparent during quiet breathing, have the patient take a deep breath or cough. Absence of bubbling indicates that the pleural space has sealed.

■ Check the water level in the suction-control chamber. Detach the chamber or bottle from the suction source; when bubbling ceases, observe the water level. If necessary, add sterile distilled water to bring the level to the 20-cm line or as ordered.

■ Check for gentle bubbling in the suction control chamber because it indicates that the proper suction level has been reached. Vigorous bubbling in this chamber increases the rate of water evaporation.

■ Periodically check that the air vent in the system is working properly. Occlusion of the air vent results in a buildup of pressure in the system that could cause the patient to develop a tension pneumothorax.

■ Coil the system's tubing, and secure it to the edge of the bed with a rubber band or tape. Avoid creating dependent loops, kinks, or pressure on the tubing. Avoid lifting the drainage system above the patient's chest because fluid may flow back into the pleural space.

■ Keep two rubber-tipped Kelly clamps at the patient's bedside, to clamp the chest tube if the commercially prepared system cracks or to locate an air leak in the system.

■ Encourage the patient to cough frequently and breathe deeply to help drain the pleural space and expand the lungs.

■ Tell him to sit upright for optimal lung expansion and to splint the insertion site while coughing to minimize pain.

■ Check the rate and quality of the patient's respirations, and auscultate his lungs periodically to assess air exchange in the affected lung. Diminished or absent breath sounds may indicate that the lung hasn't reexpanded.

■ Tell the patient to report any breathing difficulty immediately. Notify the doctor immediately if the patient develops cyanosis, rapid or shallow breathing, subcutaneous (S.C.) emphysema, chest pain, or excessive bleeding.

■ When clots are visible, you may be able to strip (or milk) the tubing, depending on facility policy. This procedure is controversial because it creates high negative pressure that could suck viable lung tissue into the drainage ports of the tube, with subsequent ruptured alveoli and pleural air leak. Strip the tubing only when clots are visible. Use an alcohol pad or lotion as a lubricant on the tube, and pinch it between

your thumb and index finger about 2″ (5 cm) from the insertion site. Using the other thumb and index finger, compress the tubing as you slide your fingers down the tube or use a mechanical stripper. After stripping, release the thumb and index finger, pinching the tube near the insertion site.

■ Check the chest tube dressing at least every 8 hours. Palpate the area surrounding the dressing for crepitus or S.C. emphysema, which indicates that air is leaking into the S.C. tissue surrounding the insertion site. Change the dressing, if necessary, or according to facility policy.

■ Encourage active or passive range-of-motion (ROM) exercises for the patient's arm or the affected side if he has been splinting the arm. Usually, the thoracotomy patient will splint his arm to decrease his discomfort.

■ Give ordered pain medication as needed to provide comfort and to help with deep breathing, coughing, and ROM exercises.

■ Remind the ambulatory patient to keep the drainage system below chest level and to be careful not to disconnect the tubing, to maintain the water seal. With a suction system, the patient must stay within range of the length of tubing attached to a wall outlet or portable pump.

Special considerations

■ Instruct staff and visitors to avoid touching the equipment, to prevent complications from separated connections.

■ If excessive continuous bubbling is present in the water-seal chamber, especially if suction is being used, rule out a leak in the drainage system. Try to locate the leak by clamping the tube momentarily at various points along its length. Begin clamping at the tube's proximal end, and work down toward the drainage system, paying special attention to the seal around the connections. If any connection is loose, push it back together and tape it securely. The bubbling will stop when a clamp is placed between the air leak and the water seal. If you clamp along the tube's entire length and the bubbling doesn't stop, the drainage unit may be cracked and need replacement.

■ If the commercially prepared drainage collection chamber fills, replace it: Double-clamp the tube close to the insertion site (use two clamps facing in opposite directions), exchange the system, remove the clamps, and retape the connection.

■ Never leave the tubes clamped for more than 1 minute, to prevent a tension pneumothorax, which may occur when clamping stops air and fluid from escaping.

■ If the commercially prepared system cracks, clamp the chest tube momentarily with the two rubber-tipped clamps at the bedside (placed there at the time of tube insertion). Place the clamps close to each other near the insertion site; they should face in opposite directions to provide a more complete seal. Observe the patient for altered respirations while the tube is clamped. Then replace the damaged equipment. (Prepare the new unit before clamping the tube.)

■ Instead of clamping the tube, you can submerge the distal end of the tube in a container of normal saline solution to create a temporary water seal while you replace the drainage system. Check facility policy for the proper procedure.

■ Tension pneumothorax may result from excessive accumulation of air, drainage, or both and eventually may exert pressure on the heart and aorta, causing a precipitous fall in cardiac output.

Documentation

Record the date and time thoracic drainage began, the type of system used, the amount of suction applied to the pleural cavity, the presence or absence of bubbling or fluctuation in the water-seal chamber, the initial amount and type of drainage, and the patient's respiratory status.

At the end of each shift, record how frequently the system is inspected and the chest tubes milked or stripped as well as the amount, color, and consistency of drainage; the presence or absence of bubbling or fluctuation in the water-seal chamber; the patient's respiratory status; the condition of the chest dressings; any pain medication given; and any complications and the nursing action taken.

Tracheal suction

Tracheal suction involves the removal of secretions from the trachea or bronchi by means of a catheter inserted through the mouth or nose, a tracheal stoma, a tracheostomy tube, or an endotracheal (ET) tube. In addition to removing secretions, tracheal suctioning stimulates the cough reflex. This procedure helps maintain a patent airway to promote optimal exchange of oxygen and carbon dioxide and to prevent pneumonia that results from pooling of secretions. Performed as frequently as the patient's condition warrants, tracheal suction calls for strict aseptic technique.

Equipment and preparation

Supplemental oxygen source (wall or portable unit such as a nasal cannula or aerosol source, and handheld resuscitation bag with a mask, 15-mm adapter, or a positive end–expiratory pressure [PEEP] valve, if indicated) ◆ wall or portable suction apparatus ◆ collection container ◆ connecting tube ◆ suction catheter kit (or a sterile suction catheter, one sterile glove, one clean glove, and a disposable sterile solution container) ◆ 1-L bottle of sterile water or normal saline solution ◆ sterile water-soluble lubricant (for nasal insertion) ◆ syringe for deflating cuff of ET or tracheostomy tube ◆ waterproof trash bag ◆ optional: sterile towel

Choose a suction catheter of appropriate size. The diameter should be no larger than half the inside diameter of the tracheostomy or ET tube, to minimize hypoxia during suctioning. (A #12 or #14 French catheter may be used for an 8-mm or larger tube.) Place the suction apparatus on the patient's overbed table or bedside stand. Position the table or stand on your preferred side of the bed to facilitate suctioning.

Attach the collection container to the suction unit and the connecting tube to the collection container. Label and date the normal saline solution or sterile water. Open the waterproof trash bag.

Implementation

■ Before suctioning, determine whether your facility requires a doctor's order and obtain one, if necessary.

■ Assess the patient's vital signs, breath sounds, and general appearance to establish a baseline for comparison after suctioning. Review the patient's arterial blood gas values and oxygen saturation levels if they're available. Evaluate the patient's ability to cough and deep-breathe because they'll help move secretions up the tracheobronchial tree. If you'll be performing nasotracheal suctioning, check the patient's history for a deviated septum, nasal polyps, nasal obstruction, nasal trauma, epistaxis, or mucosal swelling.

■ Wash your hands. Explain the procedure to the patient even if he's unresponsive. Tell him that suctioning usually causes transient coughing or gagging but that coughing helps remove the secretions. If the patient has been suctioned previously, summarize the reasons for suctioning. Continue to reassure the patient throughout the procedure to minimize anxiety, promote relaxation, and decrease oxygen demand.

■ Assemble all equipment, making sure the suction apparatus is connected to a collection container and connecting tube.

■ Unless contraindicated, place the patient in semi-Fowler's or high Fowler's position to promote lung expansion and productive coughing.

■ Remove the top from the normal saline solution or sterile water bottle.

■ Open the package containing the disposable sterile solution container.

■ Using strictly aseptic technique, open the suction catheter kit, and put on the gloves. If using individual supplies, open the suction catheter and the gloves, placing the clean glove on your nondominant hand and then the sterile glove on your dominant hand.

■ Using your nondominant (nonsterile) hand, pour the normal saline solution or sterile water into the solution container.

■ Place a small amount of sterile water-soluble lubricant on the sterile area. Lubricant may be used to facilitate passage of the catheter during nasotracheal suctioning.

■ Place a sterile towel over the patient's chest, if desired, to provide an additional sterile area.

■ Using your dominant (sterile) hand, remove the catheter from its wrapper. Keep it coiled so it can't touch a nonsterile object. Using your other hand to manipulate the connecting tubing, attach the catheter to the tubing (as shown on page 424).

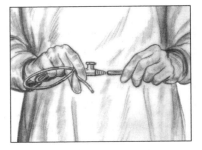

■ Using your nondominant hand, set the suction pressure according to facility policy. Typically, pressure may be set between 80 and 120 mm Hg. Higher pressures don't enhance secretion removal and may cause traumatic injury. Occlude the suction port to assess suction pressure (as shown below).

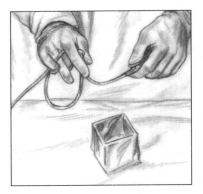

■ Dip the catheter tip in the saline solution to lubricate the outside of the catheter and reduce tissue trauma during insertion.
■ With the catheter tip in the sterile solution, occlude the control valve with the thumb of your nondominant hand. Suction a small amount of solution to lubricate the inside of the catheter, thus facilitating passage of secretions through it (as shown top right).

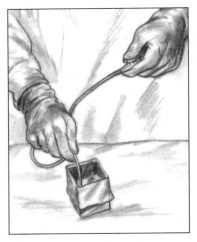

■ For nasal insertion of the catheter, lubricate the tip of the catheter with the sterile, water-soluble lubricant to reduce tissue trauma during insertion.
■ If the patient isn't intubated or is intubated but isn't receiving a supplemental oxygen source or aerosol, instruct him to take three to six deep breaths to help minimize or prevent hypoxia during suctioning.
■ If the patient isn't intubated but is receiving oxygen, evaluate his need for preoxygenation. If indicated, instruct him to take three to six deep breaths while using his supplemental oxygen source. (If needed, the patient may continue to receive supplemental oxygen during suctioning by leaving his nasal cannula in one nostril or by keeping the oxygen mask over his mouth.)
■ If the patient is being mechanically ventilated, preoxygenate him using a handheld resuscitation bag or the sigh mode on the ventilator. To use the resuscitation bag, set the oxygen flow meter at 15 L/minute, disconnect the patient from the ventilator, and deliver three to six breaths with the resuscitation bag (as shown top of next page).

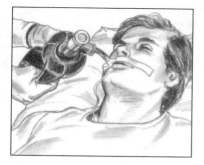

■ If the patient is being maintained on PEEP, evaluate the need to use a resuscitation bag with a PEEP valve.

■ To preoxygenate using the ventilator, first adjust the fraction of inspired oxygen (FIO_2) and tidal volume according to facility policy and patient need. Then, use the sigh mode on the ventilator, or manually deliver three to six breaths. If you have an assistant for the procedure, the assistant can manage the patient's oxygen needs while you perform the suctioning.

Nasotracheal insertion in a nonintubated patient

■ Disconnect the oxygen from the patient, if applicable.

■ Using your nondominant hand, raise the tip of the patient's nose to straighten the passageway and facilitate insertion of the catheter.

■ Insert the catheter into the patient's nostril while gently rolling it between your fingers to help it advance through the turbinates.

■ As the patient inhales, quickly advance the catheter as far as possible. To avoid oxygen loss and tissue trauma, don't apply suction during insertion.

■ If the patient coughs as the catheter passes through the larynx, briefly hold the catheter still, and then resume advancement when the patient inhales.

Nasotracheal insertion in an intubated patient

■ If you're using a closed system, see *Closed tracheal suctioning*, pages 426 and 427.

■ Using your nonsterile hand, disconnect the patient from the ventilator.

■ Using your sterile hand, gently insert the suction catheter into the artificial airway (as shown below). Advance the catheter, without applying suction, until you meet resistance. If the patient coughs, pause briefly and then resume advancement.

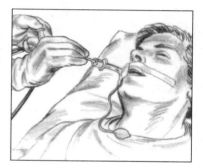

Suctioning the patient

■ After inserting the catheter, apply suction intermittently by removing and replacing the thumb of your nondominant hand over the control valve. Simultaneously use your dominant hand to withdraw the catheter, as you roll it between your thumb and forefinger. This rotating motion prevents the catheter from pulling tissue into the tube as it exits, thus avoiding tissue trauma. Never suction more than 10 seconds at a time to prevent hypoxia.

■ If the patient is intubated, use your nondominant hand to stabilize the tip of the ET tube, as you withdraw the catheter to prevent mucous membrane irritation or accidental extubation.

■ If applicable, resume oxygen delivery by reconnecting the source of oxygen or ventilation and hyperoxygenat-

Closed tracheal suctioning

The closed tracheal suction system can ease removal of secretions and reduce patient complications. Consisting of a sterile suction catheter in a clear plastic sleeve, the system permits the patient to remain connected to the ventilator during suctioning.

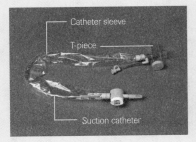

Catheter sleeve

T-piece

Suction catheter

As a result, the patient can maintain the tidal volume, oxygen concentration, and positive end-expiratory pressure delivered by the ventilator while being suctioned. In turn, this reduces the occurrence of suction-induced hypoxemia.

Another advantage of this system is a reduced risk of infection, even when the same catheter is used many times. Because the catheter remains in a protective sleeve, gloves aren't required. The caregiver doesn't need to touch the catheter, and the ventilator circuit remains closed.

Implementation

To perform the procedure, gather a closed suction control valve, a T-piece to connect the artificial airway to the ventilator breathing circuit, and a catheter sleeve that encloses the catheter and has connections at each end for the control valve and the T-piece. Then follow these steps:

■ Remove the closed suction system from its wrapping. Attach the control valve to the connecting tubing.

■ Depress the thumb suction control valve, and keep it depressed while setting the suction pressure to the desired level.

■ Connect the T-piece to the ventilator breathing circuit, making sure that the irrigation port is closed; then connect the T-piece to the patient's endotracheal or tracheostomy tube (as shown below).

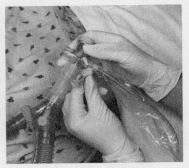

■ With one hand keeping the T-piece parallel to the patient's chin, use the thumb and index finger of the other hand to advance the catheter through the tube and into the patient's tracheobronchial tree (as shown below). It may be neces-

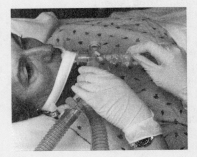

sary to gently retract the catheter sleeve as you advance the catheter.

■ While continuing to hold the T-piece and control valve, apply intermittent suction, and withdraw the catheter until it reaches its fully extended length in the sleeve. Repeat the procedure as necessary.

Closed tracheal suctioning *(continued)*

- After you've finished suctioning, flush the catheter by maintaining suction while slowly introducing normal saline solution or sterile water into the irrigation port.
- Place the thumb control valve in the OFF position.

- Dispose of and replace the suction equipment and supplies according to facility policy.
- Change the closed suction system every 24 hours to minimize the risk of infection.

ing the patient's lungs before continuing to prevent or relieve hypoxia.

- Observe the patient, and allow him to rest for a few minutes before the next suctioning. The timing of each suctioning and the length of each rest period depend on his tolerance of the procedure and the absence of complications. To enhance secretion removal, encourage the patient to cough between suctioning attempts.
- Observe the secretions. If they're thick, clear the catheter periodically by dipping the tip in the saline solution and applying suction. Normally, sputum is watery and tends to be sticky. Tenacious or thick sputum usually indicates dehydration. Watch for color variations. White or translucent color is normal; yellow indicates pus; green indicates retained secretions or *Pseudomonas* infection; brown usually indicates old blood; red indicates fresh blood; and a "red currant jelly" appearance indicates *Klebsiella* infection. When sputum contains blood, note whether it's streaked or well mixed. Also, indicate how often blood appeared. If the patient's heart rate and rhythm are being monitored, observe him for arrhythmias. If they occur, stop suctioning, and ventilate the patient.
- Patients who can't mobilize secretions effectively may need to perform tracheal suctioning after discharge.

After suctioning

- After suctioning, hyperoxygenate the patient being maintained on a ventilator using the handheld resuscitation bag or the ventilator's sigh mode, as described earlier.
- Readjust the FIO_2 and, for ventilated patients, the tidal volume to the ordered settings.
- After suctioning the lower airway, assess the patient's need for upper-airway suctioning. If the cuff of the ET or tracheostomy tube is inflated, suction the upper airway before deflating the cuff with a syringe. Always change the catheter and sterile glove before resuctioning the lower airway, to avoid introducing microorganisms into the lower airway.
- Discard the gloves and catheter in the waterproof trash bag. Clear the connecting tubing by aspirating the remaining saline solution or water. Discard and replace suction equipment and supplies according to facility policy. Wash your hands.
- Auscultate the lungs bilaterally and take vital signs, if indicated, to assess the procedure's effectiveness.

Special considerations

- Raising the patient's nose into the sniffing position helps align the larynx and pharynx and may facilitate passing the catheter during nasotracheal suctioning. If the patient's condition permits, have an assistant extend the patient's head and neck above his shoulders. The patient's lower jaw may need to be moved up and forward. If the patient is responsive, ask him to stick out his tongue so he doesn't swallow the catheter during insertion.

■ During suctioning, the catheter typically is advanced as far as the mainstem bronchi. However, because of tracheobronchial anatomy, the catheter tends to enter the right mainstem bronchi instead of the left. Using an angled catheter (such as a coudé) may help you guide the catheter into the left mainstem bronchus. Rotating the patient's head to the right seems to have a limited effect.

■ Studies show that instillation of normal saline solution into the trachea before suctioning may stimulate the patient's cough but doesn't liquefy his secretions. Keeping the patient adequately hydrated and using bronchial hygiene techniques seem to have a greater effect on mobilizing secretions.

■ In addition to the closed tracheal method, oxygen insufflation offers a new approach to suctioning. This method uses a double-lumen catheter that allows oxygen insufflation during suctioning.

■ Don't allow the collection container on the suction machine to become more than three-quarters full in order to avoid damaging the machine.

■ Assess the patient for complications. Because oxygen is removed along with secretions, the patient may experience hypoxemia and dyspnea. Anxiety may alter respiratory patterns. Cardiac arrhythmias can result from hypoxia and stimulation of the vagus nerve in the tracheobronchial tree. Tracheal or bronchial trauma can result from traumatic or prolonged suctioning.

■ Patients with compromised cardiovascular or pulmonary status are at risk for hypoxemia, arrhythmias, hypertension, or hypotension. Patients

with a history of nasopharyngeal bleeding, those who are taking an anticoagulant, those who recently have undergone a tracheostomy, and those who have a blood dyscrasia are at increased risk for bleeding as a result of suctioning.

■ Use caution when suctioning patients who have increased intracranial pressure because suction may further increase pressure.

■ If the patient experiences laryngospasm or bronchospasm (rare complications) during suctioning, disconnect the suction catheter from the connecting tubing, and allow the catheter to act as an airway. Discuss with the patient's doctor the use of a bronchodilator or lidocaine to reduce the risk of this complication.

Documentation

Record the date and time of the procedure; the technique used; the reason for suctioning; the amount, color, consistency, and odor (if any) of the secretions; any complications and the nursing action taken; and any pertinent data regarding the patient's subjective response to the procedure.

Transfusion of whole blood and packed cells

Whole blood transfusion replenishes both the volume and the oxygen-carrying capacity of the circulatory system by increasing the mass of circulating red blood cells (RBCs). Transfusion of packed RBCs, from which 80% of the plasma has been removed, restores only the oxygen-carrying capacity. After plasma is removed, the resulting component has a hematocrit of 65% to 80% and a usual volume of 300 to 350 ml. (Whole blood without the plasma removed has about a 38% hematocrit.) Each unit of whole blood or

RBCs contains enough hemoglobin to raise the hemoglobin level in an average-sized adult 1 g/L or by 3%. Both types of transfusion treat decreased hemoglobin levels and hematocrit. Whole blood is usually used only when decreased levels result from hemorrhage; packed RBCs are used when such depressed levels accompany normal blood volume to avoid possible fluid and circulatory overload. (See *Transfusing blood and selected components,* pages 430 to 435.) Whole blood and packed RBCs contain cellular debris, requiring in-line filtration during administration. (Washed packed RBCs, commonly used for patients previously sensitized to transfusions, are rinsed with a special solution that removes white blood cells and platelets, thus decreasing the chance of transfusion reaction.)

Depending on facility policy, two nurses may have to identify the patient and blood products before administering a transfusion to prevent errors and a potentially fatal reaction. If the patient is a Jehovah's Witness, a transfusion requires special written permission.

Equipment and preparation

Blood recipient set (170- to 260-micron filter and tubing with drip chamber for blood, or combined set) ◆ I.V. pole ◆ gloves ◆ gown ◆ face shield ◆ whole blood or packed RBCs ◆ 250 ml of normal saline solution ◆ venipuncture equipment, if necessary (should include 20G or larger catheter) ◆ optional: ice bag and warm compresses

Straight-line and Y-type blood administration sets are commonly used. The use of these filters can postpone sensitization to transfusion therapy.

Administer packed RBCs with a Y-type set. Using a straight-line set forces you to piggyback the tubing so that you can stop the transfusion, if necessary, but still keep the vein open. Piggybacking increases the chance of harmful microorganisms entering the tubing as you're connecting the blood line to the established line.

Multiple-lead tubing minimizes the risk of contamination, especially when transfusing multiple units of blood (a straight-line set would require multiple piggybacking). A Y-type set gives you the option of adding normal saline solution to packed cells — decreasing their viscosity — if the patient can tolerate the added fluid volume.

Avoid obtaining either whole blood or packed RBCs until you're ready to begin the transfusion. Prepare the equipment when you're ready to start the infusion.

Implementation

■ Explain the procedure to the patient. Make sure he has signed an informed consent form before any blood is transfused.
■ Record the patient's baseline vital signs.
■ Obtain whole blood or packed RBCs from the blood bank within 30 minutes of the transfusion start time. Check the expiration date on the blood bag, and observe for abnormal color, RBC clumping, gas bubbles, and extraneous material. Return outdated or abnormal blood to the blood bank.
■ Compare the name and number on the patient's wristband with those on the blood bag label. Check the blood bag identification number, ABO blood group, and Rh compatibility. Also, compare the patient's blood bank identification number, if present, with the number on the blood bag. Identification of blood and blood products is performed at the patient's bedside by two licensed professionals, according to facility policy.

(Text continues on page 434.)

Transfusing blood and selected components

Blood component	Indications
WHOLE BLOOD	
Complete (pure) blood *Volume: 500 ml*	■ To restore blood volume lost from hemorrhaging, trauma, or burns
PACKED RED BLOOD CELLS (RBCS)	
Same RBC mass as whole blood but with 80% of the plasma removed *Volume: 250 ml*	■ To restore or maintain oxygen-carrying capacity ■ To correct anemia and blood loss that occurs during surgery ■ To increase RBC mass
WHITE BLOOD CELLS (WBCS OR LEUKOCYTES)	
Whole blood with all the RBCs and about 80% of the supernatant plasma removed *Volume: usually 150 ml*	■ To treat sepsis that's unresponsive to antibiotics (especially if patient has positive blood cultures or a persistent fever exceeding 101° F [38.3° C]) and granulocytopenia (granulocyte count usually less than 500/µl)
LEUKOCYTE-POOR RBCS	
Same as packed RBCs with about 95% of the leukocytes removed *Volume: 200 ml*	■ Same as packed RBCs ■ To prevent febrile reactions from leukocyte antibodies ■ To treat immunocompromised patients

Crossmatching	Nursing considerations
■ ABO identical: Type A receives A; type B receives B; type AB receives AB; type O receives O. ■ Rh match necessary	■ Use a straight-line or Y-type I.V. set to infuse blood over 2 to 4 hours. ■ Avoid giving whole blood when the patient can't tolerate the circulatory volume. ■ Reduce the risk of a transfusion reaction by adding a microfilter to the administration set to remove platelets. ■ Warm blood if giving a large quantity.
■ Type A receives A or O. ■ Type B receives B or O. ■ Type AB receives AB, A, B, or O. ■ Type O receives O. ■ Rh match necessary	■ Use a straight-line or Y-type I.V. set to infuse blood over 2 to 4 hours. ■ Bear in mind that packed RBCs provide the same oxygen-carrying capacity as whole blood with less risk of volume overload. ■ Give packed RBCs as ordered to prevent potassium and ammonia buildup, which may occur in stored plasma. ■ Avoid administering packed RBCs for anemic conditions correctable by nutrition or drug therapy.
■ Same as packed RBCs ■ Compatibility with human leukocyte antigen (HLA) is preferable but not necessary unless patient is sensitized to HLA from previous transfusions ■ Rh match necessary	■ Use a straight-line I.V. set with a standard in-line blood filter to provide 1 unit daily for 5 days or until infection resolves. ■ As prescribed, premedicate with diphenhydramine. ■ Because a WBC infusion induces fever and chills, administer an antipyretic if fever occurs. Don't discontinue the transfusion; instead, reduce the flow rate as ordered for patient comfort. ■ Agitate container to prevent WBCs from settling, thus preventing the delivery of a bolus infusion of WBCs.
■ Same as packed RBCs ■ Rh match necessary	■ Use a straight-line or Y-type I.V. set to infuse blood over 1½ to 4 hours. ■ Use a 40-micron filter suitable for hard-spun, leukocyte-poor RBCs. ■ Other considerations are the same as those for packed RBCs.

(continued)

Transfusing blood and selected components *(continued)*

Blood component	Indications
PLATELETS	
Platelet sediment from RBCs or plasma *Volume: 35 to 50 ml/unit; 1 unit of platelets = 7 × 107 platelets*	■ To treat thrombocytopenia caused by decreased platelet production, increased platelet destruction, or massive transfusion of stored blood ■ To treat acute leukemia and marrow aplasia ■ To improve platelet count preoperatively in a patient whose count is 100,000/µl or less
FRESH FROZEN PLASMA (FFP)	
Uncoagulated plasma separated from RBCs and rich in coagulation factors V, VIII, and IX *Volume: 200 to 250 ml*	■ To expand plasma volume ■ To treat postoperative hemorrhage or shock ■ To correct an undetermined coagulation factor deficiency ■ To replace a specific factor when that factor alone isn't available ■ To correct factor deficiencies resulting from hepatic disease
ALBUMIN 5% (BUFFERED SALINE); ALBUMIN 25% (SALT POOR)	
A small plasma protein prepared by fractionating pooled plasma *Volume: 5% = 12.5 g/ 250 ml; 25% = 12.5 g/50 ml*	■ To replace volume lost because of shock from burns, trauma, surgery, or infections ■ To replace volume and prevent marked hemoconcentration ■ To treat hypoproteinemia (with or without edema)

Crossmatching	Nursing considerations
■ ABO compatibility unnecessary but preferable with repeated platelet transfusions ■ Rh match preferred	■ Use a component drip administration set to infuse 100 ml over 15 minutes. ■ As prescribed, premedicate with antipyretics and antihistamines if the patient's history includes a platelet transfusion reaction. ■ Avoid administering platelets when the patient has a fever. ■ Prepare to draw blood for a platelet count as ordered, 1 hour after the platelet transfusion to determine platelet transfusion increments. ■ Keep in mind that the doctor seldom orders a platelet transfusion for conditions in which platelet destruction is accelerated, such as idiopathic thrombocytopenic purpura and drug-induced thrombocytopenia.
■ ABO compatibility is unnecessary but is preferable with repeated platelet transfusions ■ Rh match preferred	■ Use a straight-line I.V. set, and administer the infusion rapidly. ■ Keep in mind that large-volume transfusions of FFP may require correction for hypocalcemia because citric acid in FFP binds calcium.
■ Unnecessary	■ Use a straight-line I.V. set with rate and volume dictated by the patient's condition and response. ■ Remember that reactions to albumin (fever, chills, nausea) are rare. ■ Avoid mixing albumin with protein hydrolysates and alcohol solutions. ■ Consider delivering albumin as a volume expander until the laboratory completes crossmatching for a whole blood transfusion. ■ Keep in mind that albumin is contraindicated in severe anemia and administered cautiously in cardiac and pulmonary disease because heart failure may result from circulatory overload.

(continued)

Transfusing blood and selected components *(continued)*

Blood component	Indications
FACTOR VIII (CRYOPRECIPITATE)	
Insoluble portion of plasma recovered from FFP *Volume: about 30 ml (freeze-dried)*	■ To treat a patient with hemophilia A ■ To control bleeding associated with factor VIII deficiency ■ To replace fibrinogen or deficient factor VIII
FACTORS II, VII, IX, X COMPLEX (PROTHROMBIN COMPLEX)	
Lyophilized, commercially prepared solution drawn from pooled plasma	■ To treat a congenital factor V deficiency and other bleeding disorders resulting from an acquired deficiency of factors II, VII, IX, and X

■ Put on gloves, a gown, and a face shield. Using a Y-type set, close all the clamps on the set. Then insert the spike of the line you're using for the normal saline solution into the bag of saline solution. Next, open the port on the blood bag, and insert the spike of the line you're using to administer the blood or cellular component into the port. Hang the bag of normal saline solution and blood or cellular component on the I.V. pole, open the clamp on the line of saline solution, and squeeze the drip chamber until it's half full. Then remove the adapter cover at the tip of the blood administration set, open the main flow clamp, and prime the tubing with saline solution.

■ If you're administering packed RBCs with a Y-type set, you can add saline solution to the bag to dilute the cells by closing the clamp between the patient and the drip chamber and opening the clamp from the blood. Then lower the blood bag below the saline container and let 30 to 50 ml of saline solution flow into the packed cells. Finally, close the clamp to the blood bag, rehang the bag, rotate it gently to mix the cells and saline solution, and close the clamp to the saline container.
■ If the patient doesn't have an I.V. line in place, perform a venipuncture, using a 20G or larger-diameter catheter. Avoid using an existing line if the needle or catheter lumen is smaller than

Crossmatching	Nursing considerations
■ ABO compatibility unnecessary but preferable	■ Use the administration set supplied by the manufacturer. Administer factor VIII with a filter. Standard dose recommended for treatment of acute bleeding episodes in hemophilia is 15 to 20 units/kg. ■ Half-life of factor VIII (8 to 10 hours) necessitates repeated transfusions at specified intervals to maintain normal levels.
■ ABO compatibility and Rh match unnecessary	■ Administer with a straight-line I.V. set, basing dose on desired factor level and patient's body weight. ■ Recognize that a high risk of hepatitis accompanies this type of transfusion. ■ Arrange to draw blood for a coagulation assay to be performed before administration and at suitable intervals during treatment. ■ Keep in mind that this type of transfusion is contraindicated when the patient has hepatic disease resulting in fibrinolysis and when the patient has disseminated intravascular coagulation and isn't undergoing heparin therapy.

20G. Central venous access devices also may be used for transfusion therapy.

■ If you're administering whole blood, gently invert the bag several times to mix the cells.

■ Attach the prepared blood administration set to the venipuncture device, and flush it with normal saline solution. Then close the clamp to the saline solution, and open the clamp between the blood bag and the patient. Adjust the flow rate to no greater than 5 ml/minute for the first 15 minutes of the transfusion so that you can observe the patient for a possible transfusion reaction.

■ If signs of a transfusion reaction develop, record vital signs, and stop the transfusion. Infuse saline solution at a moderately slow infusion rate, and notify the doctor at once. If no signs of a reaction appear within 15 minutes, adjust the flow clamp to the ordered infusion rate. A unit of RBCs may be given over 1 to 4 hours as ordered.

■ After completing the transfusion, put on gloves, and remove and discard the used infusion equipment. Then remember to reconnect the original I.V. fluid, if necessary, or discontinue the I.V. infusion.

■ Return the empty blood bag to the blood bank, and discard the tubing and filter.

■ Record the patient's vital signs.

Special considerations

■ Although some microaggregate filters can be used for up to 10 units of blood, always replace the filter and tubing if more than 1 hour elapses between transfusions. When administering multiple units of blood under pressure, use a blood warmer to avoid hypothermia. Blood components may be warmed to no more than 107.6° F (42° C).

■ For rapid blood replacement, you may need to use a pressure bag. Be aware that excessive pressure may develop, leading to broken blood vessels and extravasation, with hematoma and hemolysis of the infusing RBCs.

■ If the transfusion stops, take the following steps as needed:

– Check that the I.V. container is at least 3′ (0.9 m) above the level of the I.V. site.

– Make sure the flow clamp is open and that the blood completely covers the filter. If it doesn't, squeeze the drip chamber until it does.

– Gently rock the bag back and forth, agitating blood cells that may have settled.

– Untape the dressing over the I.V. site to check cannula placement. Reposition the cannula, if necessary.

– Flush the line with saline solution, and restart the transfusion. Using a Y-type set, close the flow clamp to the patient, and lower the blood bag. Next, open the saline clamp and allow some saline solution to flow into the blood bag. Rehang the blood bag, open the flow clamp to the patient, and reset the flow rate.

– If a hematoma develops at the I.V. site, immediately stop the infusion. Remove the I.V. cannula. Notify the doctor, and expect to place ice on the site intermittently for 8 hours; then apply warm compresses. Follow facility policy.

– If the blood bag empties before the next one arrives, administer normal saline solution slowly. If you're using a Y-type set, close the blood-line clamp, open the saline clamp, and let the saline run slowly until the new blood arrives. Decrease the flow rate or clamp the line before attaching the new unit of blood.

■ Despite improvements in cross-matching precautions, transfusion reactions can still occur. Unlike a transfusion reaction, an infectious disease transmitted during a transfusion may go undetected until days, weeks, or even months later, when it produces signs and symptoms. Measures to prevent disease transmission include laboratory testing of blood products and careful screening of potential donors, neither of which is guaranteed.

■ Hepatitis C accounts for most post-transfusion hepatitis cases. The tests that detect hepatitis B and hepatitis C can produce false-negative results and may allow some hepatitis cases to go undetected.

■ When testing for antibodies to human immunodeficiency virus (HIV), keep in mind that antibodies don't appear until 6 to 12 weeks after exposure. The estimated risk of acquiring HIV from blood products varies from 1 in 40,000 to 1 in 153,000.

■ Many blood banks screen blood for cytomegalovirus (CMV). Blood with CMV is especially dangerous for an immunosuppressed, seronegative patient. Blood banks also test blood for syphilis, but refrigerating blood virtually eliminates the risk of transfusion-related syphilis.

■ Circulatory overload and hemolytic, allergic, febrile, and pyogenic reactions can result from any transfusion. Coagulation disturbances, citrate intoxication, hyperkalemia, acid-base imbalance, loss of 2,3-diphosphoglycerate, ammonia intoxication, and hypothermia can result from massive transfusion.

Documentation

Record the date and time of the transfusion, the type and amount of transfusion product, the patient's vital signs, your check of all identification data, and the patient's response. Document any transfusion reaction and treatment.

Tube feedings

Tube feedings involve delivery of a liquid feeding formula directly to the stomach (known as gastric gavage), duodenum, or jejunum. Gastric gavage is typically indicated for a patient who can't eat normally because of dysphagia or oral or esophageal obstruction or injury. Gastric feedings also may be given to an unconscious or intubated patient or to a patient recovering from GI tract surgery who can't ingest food orally.

Duodenal or jejunal feedings decrease the risk of aspiration because the formula bypasses the pylorus. Jejunal feedings result in reduced pancreatic stimulation; thus, the patient may require an elemental diet.

Patients usually receive gastric feedings on an intermittent schedule. For duodenal or jejunal feedings, however, most patients seem to better tolerate a continuous slow drip.

Liquid nutrient solutions come in various formulas for administration through a nasogastric tube, small-bore feeding tube, gastrostomy or jejunostomy tube, percutaneous endoscopic gastrostomy or jejunostomy tube, or gastrostomy feeding button. Tube feeding is contraindicated in patients who have no bowel sounds or have a suspected intestinal obstruction.

Equipment and preparation

For gastric feedings
Feeding formula ◆ 120 ml of water ◆ gavage bag with tubing and flow regula-

tor clamp ◆ towel or linen-saver pad ◆ 60-ml syringe or barrel syringe ◆ stethoscope ◆ optional: infusion controller and gavage bag tubing set (for continuous administration) and adapter to connect gavage tubing to feeding tube

For duodenal or jejunal feedings
Feeding formula ◆ enteral administration set containing a gavage container, drip chamber, roller clamp or flow regulator, and tube connector ◆ I.V. pole ◆ 60-ml syringe with adapter tip ◆ water ◆ optional: volumetric pump administration set (for an enteral infusion pump) and Y-connector

A bulb syringe or large catheter-tip syringe may be substituted for a gavage bag after the patient demonstrates tolerance for a gravity drip infusion. The doctor may order an infusion pump to ensure accurate delivery of the prescribed formula.

Refrigerate formulas prepared in the dietary department or pharmacy. Refrigerate commercial formulas only after opening them. Check the date on all formula containers. Discard expired commercial formula. Use powdered formula within 24 hours of mixing. Always shake the container vigorously so the solution is thoroughly mixed.

Allow the formula to warm to room temperature before administering it. Cold formula can increase the chance of diarrhea. Never warm it over direct heat or in a microwave, because heat may curdle the formula or change its chemical composition. Also, hot formula may injure the patient.

Pour 60 ml of water into the graduated container. After closing the flow clamp on the administration set, pour the appropriate amount of formula into the gavage bag. Hang no more than a 4- to 6-hour supply at one time to prevent bacterial growth.

Open the flow clamp on the administration set to remove air from the lines. This keeps air from entering the patient's stomach and causing distention and discomfort.

Implementation

■ Provide privacy and wash your hands.

■ Inform the patient that he'll receive nourishment through the tube, and explain the procedure to him. If possible, give him a schedule of subsequent feedings.

■ If the patient has a nasal or oral tube, cover his chest with a towel or linen-saver pad to protect him and the bed linens from spills.

■ Assess the patient's abdomen for bowel sounds and distention.

Delivering a gastric feeding

■ Elevate the bed to semi-Fowler's or high Fowler's position to prevent aspiration by gastroesophageal reflux and to promote digestion.

■ Check placement of the feeding tube to ensure that it hasn't slipped out since the last feeding. Never give a tube feeding until you're certain the tube is properly positioned in the patient's stomach. Administering a feeding through a misplaced tube can cause the feeding formula to enter the patient's lungs.

■ To check tube patency and position, remove the cap or plug from the feeding tube, and use the syringe to inject 5 to 10 cc of air through the tube. At the same time, auscultate the patient's stomach with the stethoscope. Listen for a whooshing sound to confirm tube positioning in the stomach. Also, aspirate stomach contents to confirm tube patency and placement.

■ To assess gastric emptying, aspirate and measure residual gastric contents. Hold feedings if residual volume is greater than the predetermined amount specified in the doctor's order (usually 50 to 100 ml). Reinstill any aspirate obtained.

■ Connect the gavage bag tubing to the feeding tube. Depending on the type of tube used, you may need to use an adapter to connect the two.

■ If you're using a bulb or catheter-tip syringe, remove the bulb or plunger, and attach the syringe to the pinched-off feeding tube to prevent excess air from entering the patient's stomach, causing distention. If you're using an infusion controller, thread the tube from the formula container through the controller, according to the manufacturer's directions. Blue food dye can be added to the feeding to quickly identify aspiration. Purge the tubing of air, and attach it to the feeding tube.

■ Open the flow regulator clamp on the gavage bag tubing, and adjust the flow rate as appropriate. When using a bulb syringe, fill the syringe with formula and release the feeding tube to allow formula to flow through it. The height at which you hold the syringe determines the flow rate. When the syringe is three-quarters empty, pour more formula into it.

■ To prevent air from entering the tube and the patient's stomach, never allow the syringe to empty completely. If you're using an infusion controller, set the flow rate according to the manufacturer's directions. Always administer a tube feeding slowly — typically 200 to 350 ml over 15 to 30 minutes, depending on the patient's tolerance and the doctor's order — to prevent sudden stomach distention, which can cause nausea, vomiting, cramps, or diarrhea.

■ After administering the appropriate amount of formula, flush the tubing by adding about 60 ml of water to the gavage bag or bulb syringe, or manually flush it using a barrel syringe. This maintains the tube's patency by removing excess formula, which could occlude the tube.

■ If you're administering a continuous feeding, flush the feeding tube every 4 hours to help prevent tube occlusion. Monitor gastric emptying every 4 hours.

■ To discontinue gastric feeding (depending on the equipment you're using), close the regulator clamp on the gavage bag tubing, disconnect the syringe from the feeding tube, or turn off the infusion controller.

■ Cover the end of the feeding tube with its plug or cap to prevent leakage and contamination.

■ Leave the patient in semi-Fowler's or high Fowler's position for at least 30 minutes.

■ Rinse all reusable equipment with warm water. Dry it and store it in a convenient place for the next feeding. Change equipment every 24 hours or according to facility policy.

Delivering a duodenal or jejunal feeding

■ Elevate the head of the bed, and place the patient in low Fowler's position.

■ Open the enteral administration set and hang the gavage container on the I.V. pole.

■ If you're using a nasoduodenal tube, measure its length to check tube placement. Remember that you may not get any residual when you aspirate the tube.

■ Open the roller clamp and regulate the flow to the desired rate. To regulate the rate using a volumetric infusion pump, follow the manufacturer's directions for setting up the equipment. Most patients receive small amounts initially, with volumes increasing gradually once tolerance is established.

■ Flush the tube every 4 hours with water to maintain patency and provide hydration. A needle catheter jejunostomy tube may require flushing every 2 hours to prevent formula buildup inside the tube. A Y-connector may be useful for frequent flushing. Attach the continuous feeding tube to the main port and use the side port for flushes.

■ Change equipment every 24 hours or according to facility policy.

Special considerations

■ If the feeding solution doesn't initially flow through a bulb syringe, attach the bulb and squeeze it gently to start the flow. Then remove the bulb. Never use the bulb to force the formula through the tube.

■ If the patient becomes nauseated or vomits, stop the feeding immediately. He may vomit if his stomach becomes distended from overfeeding or delayed gastric emptying.

■ To reduce oropharyngeal discomfort from the tube, allow the patient to brush his teeth or care for his dentures regularly, and encourage frequent gargling. If the patient is unconscious, administer oral care swabs every 4 hours. Use petroleum jelly on dry, cracked lips. (*Note:* Dry mucous membranes may indicate dehydration, which requires increased fluid intake.) Clean the patient's nostrils with cotton-tipped applicators, apply lubricant along the mucosa, and assess the skin for signs of breakdown.

■ During continuous feedings, assess the patient frequently for abdominal distention. Flush the tubing by adding about 50 ml of water to the gavage bag or bulb syringe. This maintains the tube's patency by removing excess formula, which could occlude the tube.

■ If the patient develops diarrhea, administer small, frequent, less concentrated feedings, or administer bolus feedings over a longer time. Also, make sure that the formula isn't cold and that proper storage and sanitation practices have been followed. The loose stools associated with tube feedings make extra perineal skin care necessary. Giving paregoric, tincture of opium, or diphenoxylate hydrochloride may improve the condition. Changing to a formula with more fiber may eliminate liquid stools.

■ If the patient becomes constipated, the doctor may increase the fruit, vegetable, or sugar content of the formula. Assess the patient's hydration status because dehydration may produce constipation. Increase fluid intake as necessary. If the condition persists, administer an appropriate drug or enema as ordered.

■ Drugs can be administered through the feeding tube. Except for enteric-coated, time-released, or sustained-release medications, crush tablets or open and dilute capsules in water before administering them. Make sure you flush the tubing afterward to ensure full instillation of medication. Keep in mind that some drugs may change the osmolarity of the feeding formula and cause diarrhea.

■ Small-bore feeding tubes may kink, making instillation impossible. If you suspect this problem, try changing the patient's position, or withdraw the tube a few inches and restart. Never use a guide wire to reposition the tube.

■ Constantly monitor the flow rate of a blended or high-residue formula to determine if the formula is clogging the tubing as it settles. To prevent such clogging, squeeze the bag frequently to agitate the solution.

■ Collect blood samples as ordered. Hyperglycemia and diuresis may indicate an excessive carbohydrate level, which could lead to fatal hyperosmotic dehydration. Monitor blood glucose levels to assess glucose tolerance. (A serum glucose level of less than 200 mg/dl is considered stable.) Also monitor serum levels of electrolytes, blood urea nitrogen, and glucose as well as serum osmolality and other pertinent findings to determine the patient's response to therapy and to assess his hydration status.

■ Check the flow rate hourly to ensure correct infusion. (With an improvised administration set, use a time tape to record the rate because it's difficult to get precise readings from an irrigation container or enema bag.)

■ For duodenal or jejunal feeding, most patients tolerate a continuous drip better than bolus feedings. Bolus feedings can cause such complications as hyperglycemia and diarrhea.

■ Until the patient acquires a tolerance for the formula, you may need to dilute it to one-half or three-quarters strength to start, and increase it gradually. Patients who are under stress or who are receiving a steroid may experience a pseudodiabetic state. Assess them to determine the need for insulin.

⟲ *Patient teaching tips* Patient education for home tube feeding includes instructions on an infusion control device to maintain accuracy, use of the syringe or bag and tubing, care of the tube and insertion site, and formula mixing. Formula may be mixed in an electric blender according to package directions. Formula not used within 24 hours must be discarded. If the formula must hang for more than 8 hours, advise the patient to use a gavage or pump administration set with an ice pouch to decrease the incidence of bacterial growth. Tell him to use a new bag daily.

Teach family members which signs and symptoms to report to the doctor or home care nurse as well as measures to take in an emergency.

■ Erosion of esophageal, tracheal, nasal, and oropharyngeal mucosa can result if tubes are left in place for a long time. If possible, use smaller-lumen tubes to prevent such irritation. Check facility policy regarding the frequency of changing feeding tubes to prevent complications.

Managing tube feeding problems

Complications	Interventions
Aspiration of gastric secretions	■ Discontinue feeding immediately. ■ Perform tracheal suction of aspirated contents, if possible. ■ Notify the doctor. Prophylactic antibiotics and chest physiotherapy may be ordered. ■ Check tube placement before feeding to prevent complication.
Tube obstruction	■ Flush the tube with warm water. If necessary, replace the tube. ■ Flush the tube with 50 ml of water after each feeding to remove excess sticky formula, which could occlude the tube.
Oral, nasal, or pharyngeal irritation or necrosis	■ Provide frequent oral hygiene using mouthwash or lemon-glycerin swabs. Use petroleum jelly on cracked lips. ■ Change the tube's position. If necessary, replace the tube.
Vomiting, bloating, diarrhea, or cramps	■ Reduce the flow rate. ■ Administer metoclopramide to increase GI motility. ■ Warm the formula to prevent GI distress. ■ For 30 minutes after feeding, position the patient on his right side with his head elevated to facilitate gastric emptying. ■ Notify the doctor. He may want to reduce the amount of formula being given during each feeding.
Constipation	■ Provide additional fluids if the patient can tolerate them. ■ Administer a bulk-forming laxative. ■ Increase fruit, vegetable, or sugar content of the feeding.
Electrolyte imbalance	■ Monitor serum electrolyte levels. ■ Notify the doctor. He may want to adjust the formula content to correct the deficiency.
Hyperglycemia	■ Monitor blood glucose levels. ■ Notify the doctor of elevated levels. ■ Administer insulin, if ordered. ■ The doctor may adjust the sugar content of the formula.

■ With the gastric route, frequent or large-volume feedings can cause bloating and retention. Dehydration, diarrhea, and vomiting can cause metabolic disturbances. Cramping and abdominal distention usually indicate intolerance.
■ With the duodenal or jejunal route, clogging of the feeding tube is common. The patient may experience metabolic, fluid, and electrolyte abnormalities including hyperglycemia, hyperosmolar dehydration, coma, edema, hypernatremia, and essential fatty acid deficiency.
■ The patient also may experience dumping syndrome, in which a large amount of hyperosmotic solution in the duodenum causes excessive diffusion of fluid through the semipermeable membrane and results in diarrhea. In a patient with low serum albumin levels, these signs and symptoms may result from low oncotic pressure in the duodenal mucosa. (See *Managing tube feeding problems,* page 441.)

Documentation

On the intake and output sheet, record the date, volume of formula, and volume of water. In your notes, document abdominal assessment findings (including tube exit site, if appropriate); amount of residual gastric contents; verification of tube placement; amount, type, and time of feeding; and tube patency. Discuss the patient's tolerance of the feeding, including nausea, vomiting, cramping, diarrhea, and distention.

Note the result of blood and urine tests, hydration status, and any drugs given through the tube. Include the date and time of administration set changes, oral and nasal hygiene, and results of specimen collections.

Venipuncture

Performed to obtain a venous blood sample, venipuncture involves piercing a vein with a needle and collecting blood in a syringe or evacuated tube. Typically, venipuncture is performed using the antecubital fossa. If necessary, however, it can be performed on a vein in the wrist, the dorsum of the hand or foot, or another accessible location.

Equipment and preparation

Tourniquet ◆ gloves ◆ syringe or evacuated tubes and needle holder ◆ alcohol or povidone-iodine pads ◆ 20G or 21G needle for the forearm or 25G needle for the wrist, hand, and ankle, and for children ◆ color-coded collection tubes containing appropriate additives ◆ labels ◆ laboratory requests ◆ 2″ × 2″ gauze pads ◆ adhesive bandage ◆ optional: warm soaks

If you're using evacuated tubes, open the needle packet, attach the needle to its holder, and select the appropriate tubes. If you're using a syringe, attach the appropriate needle to it. Make sure you choose a syringe large enough to hold all the blood required for the test. Label all collection tubes with the patient's name and room number, the doctor's name, and the date and time of collection.

Implementation

■ Wash your hands thoroughly and put on gloves.
■ Tell the patient that you're about to collect a blood sample, and explain the procedure to ease his anxiety and ensure his cooperation. Ask him if he has ever felt faint, sweaty, or nauseated when having blood drawn.
■ If the patient is on bed rest, ask him to lie in a supine position, with his head slightly elevated and his arms at his sides. Ask the ambulatory patient to sit in a chair and support his arm securely on an armrest or a table.

Common venipuncture sites

The illustrations below show the anatomic locations of veins commonly used for venipuncture sites. The most commonly used sites are on the forearm, followed by those on the hand.

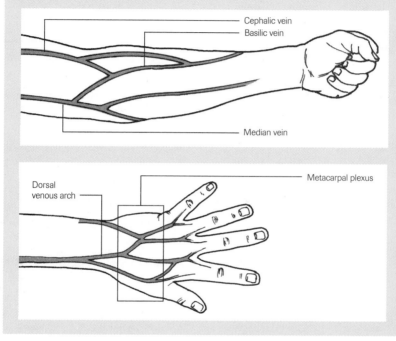

Cephalic vein
Basilic vein
Median vein
Dorsal venous arch
Metacarpal plexus

■ Assess the patient's veins to determine the best puncture site. (See *Common venipuncture sites*.) Observe the skin for the vein's blue color, or palpate the vein for a firm rebound sensation.
■ Tie a tourniquet 2″ (5.1 cm) proximal to the area chosen. By impeding venous return to the heart while still allowing arterial flow, a tourniquet produces venous dilation. If arterial perfusion remains adequate, you'll be able to feel the radial pulse. (If the tourniquet fails to dilate the vein, have the patient open and close his fist repeatedly. Then ask him to close his fist as you insert the needle and to open it again when the needle is in place.)

■ Clean the venipuncture site with an alcohol or a povidone-iodine pad. Don't wipe off the povidone-iodine with alcohol because alcohol cancels the effect of povidone-iodine. Wipe in a circular motion, spiraling outward from the site to avoid introducing potentially infectious skin flora into the vessel during the procedure. If you use alcohol, apply it with friction for 30 seconds or until the final pad comes away clean. Allow the skin to dry before performing venipuncture.
■ Immobilize the vein by pressing just below the venipuncture site with your thumb and drawing the skin taut.

■ Position the needle holder or syringe with the needle bevel up and the shaft parallel to the path of the vein and at a 30-degree angle to the arm. Insert the needle into the vein. If you're using a syringe, venous blood will appear in the hub; withdraw the blood slowly, pulling the plunger of the syringe gently to create steady suction until you obtain the required sample. Pulling the plunger too forcibly may collapse the vein. If you're using a needle holder and an evacuated tube, grasp the holder securely to stabilize it in the vein, and push down on the color-coded collection tube until the needle punctures the rubber stopper. Blood will flow into the tube automatically.

■ Remove the tourniquet as soon as blood flows adequately to prevent stasis and hemoconcentration, which can impair test results. If the flow is sluggish, leave the tourniquet in place longer, but always remove it before withdrawing the needle.

■ Continue to fill the required tubes, removing one and inserting another. Gently rotate each tube as you remove it, to help mix the additive with the sample.

■ After you've drawn the sample, place a gauze pad over the puncture site, and slowly and gently remove the needle from the vein. When using an evacuated tube, remove it from the needle holder to release the vacuum before withdrawing the needle from the vein.

■ Apply gentle pressure to the puncture site for 2 to 3 minutes or until bleeding stops. This prevents extravasation into the surrounding tissue, which can cause a hematoma.

■ After bleeding stops, apply an adhesive bandage.

■ If you used a syringe, transfer the sample to a collection tube. Detach the needle from the syringe, open the collection tube, and gently empty the sample into the tube, being careful to avoid foaming, which can cause hemolysis.

■ Finally, check the venipuncture site to see if a hematoma has developed. If it has, apply warm soaks to the site.

■ Discard syringes, needles, and used gloves in the appropriate containers.

Special considerations

■ Never collect a venous sample from an arm or a leg that is already being used for I.V. therapy or blood administration, because this may affect test results. Don't collect a venous sample from an infection site, because this may introduce pathogens into the vascular system. Likewise, avoid collecting blood from edematous areas, arteriovenous shunts, and sites of previous hematomas or vascular injury.

■ If the patient has large, distended, highly visible veins, perform venipuncture without a tourniquet to minimize the risk of hematoma formation. If the patient has a clotting disorder or is receiving anticoagulant therapy, maintain firm pressure on the venipuncture site for at least 5 minutes after withdrawing the needle, to prevent hematoma formation.

■ Avoid using veins in the patient's legs for venipuncture, if possible, because this increases the risk of thrombophlebitis.

■ Assess patient for complications. A hematoma at the needle insertion site is the most common complication of venipuncture. Infection may result from poor technique.

Documentation

Record the date, time, and site of the venipuncture; the name of the test; the time the sample was sent to the laboratory; the amount of blood collected; the patient's temperature; and any adverse reactions to the procedure.

8

Precautions
Preventing the spread of infection

Precaution principles

The Hospital Infection Control Practices Advisory Committee (HICPAC) of the Centers for Disease Control and Prevention (CDC) has developed the Guidelines for Isolation Precautions in Hospitals. These guidelines have two levels of precautions:

■ standard precautions
■ transmission-based precautions (which are further divided into airborne precautions, droplet precautions, and contact precautions).

Standard precautions

Standard precautions are designed to decrease the risk of transmission of microorganisms from both recognized and unrecognized sources of infection. They should be followed at all times and with every patient.

HICPAC and the CDC define the following materials as infectious, requiring you to observe standard precautions:

■ blood
■ body fluids, secretions, and excretions (except sweat)
■ nonintact skin
■ mucous membranes.

Standard precautions combine the major features of universal precautions, which were developed specifically to reduce the transmission of blood-borne pathogens, such as human immunodeficiency virus and hepatitis B virus (HBV), and body substance isolation, which was developed to decrease the risk of pathogen transmission from moist body surfaces. Because standard precautions reduce the risk of transmission of blood-borne pathogens and other pathogens, many patients with diseases or conditions that previously required category or disease-specific isolation precautions now only require standard precautions.

Implementation

■ Wash your hands immediately if they become contaminated with blood or body fluids, secretions, or excretions; also wash your hands before and after providing patient care and after removing gloves.

■ Use nonantimicrobial soap for routine hand washing.

■ Wear gloves if you will or could come in contact with blood, specimens, tissue, body fluid, secretions, excretions, or contaminated surfaces or objects.

■ Change your gloves between tasks and procedures on the same patient if you touch anything that might have a high concentration of microorganisms and between patient contacts to avoid cross-contamination. Vinyl and nitrile gloves are available for individuals who are allergic to latex.

■ Wear a gown, eye protection (goggles or glasses), and a mask during procedures — such as extubation, surgery, endoscopic procedures, and dialysis — that are likely to generate droplets of blood or body fluids, secretions, or excretions.

■ Carefully handle used patient care equipment soiled with blood, body fluids, secretions, or excretions, to prevent exposure to skin and mucous membranes, clothing contamination, and transfer of microorganisms to other patients and environments. Patient care equipment must be cleaned with a facility-approved disinfectant between patients. Discard disposable equipment appropriately.

■ Make sure that procedures for routine care, cleaning, and disinfection of environmental surfaces and equipment are followed.

■ Keep contaminated linens away from your body to prevent contamination and transfer of microorganisms. Place the linens in properly labeled containers, and make sure the linens are transported and processed according to facility policy.

■ Handle used needles and other sharps carefully. Don't bend, break, reinsert them into their original sheaths, or unnecessarily handle them. Immediately after use, discard them intact in an impervious disposal box. These measures reduce the risk of accidental injury and infection.

■ Use sharps with safety features whenever available.

■ Use mouthpieces, resuscitation bags, or other ventilation devices in place of mouth-to-mouth resuscitation whenever possible.

■ Place patients who can't maintain appropriate hygiene or who contaminate the environment in a private room. Notify infection control personnel.

■ If you have an exudative lesion, avoid direct patient contact until the condition has resolved and the employee health provider clears you.

■ Because precautions can't be specified for every clinical situation, use your judgment in individual cases. Refer to your facility's infection control manual or check with infection control personnel when you need more information.

■ If occupational exposure to blood is likely, get vaccinated with the HBV vaccine series.

Transmission-based precautions

Whenever a patient is known or suspected to be infected with highly contagious or epidemiologically important pathogens that are transmitted by air, droplet, or contact with dry skin or other contaminated surfaces, follow transmission-based precautions along with standard precautions. Examples of such pathogens include those that cause measles (air); influenza (droplet); and GI tract, respiratory tract, skin, and wound infections (contact). In fact, transmission-based precautions replace all older categories of isolation. One or more types of transmission-based precautions may be combined and followed when a patient has a disease with multiple routes of transmission.

Airborne precautions

Along with standard precautions, follow these precautions:

■ Place the patient in a private room that has monitored negative air pressure in relation to surrounding areas, 6 to 12 air exchanges per hour, and appropriate outdoor air discharge or high-efficiency filtration of room air. The room door should remain closed. If a private room isn't available, consult with infection control personnel. As an alternative, he may be placed in a room with a patient who has an active infection with the same microorganism.

■ Wear respiratory protection, such as a surgical mask or N-95 respirator (for tuberculosis [TB]), when entering the room of a patient with a known or suspected respiratory tract infection. Persons immune to measles and varicella don't need to wear respiratory protection when entering the room of a patient with these illnesses.

■ Limit patient transport and movement out of the room. If the patient must leave the room, have him wear a surgical mask.

Droplet precautions

In addition to standard precautions, follow these precautions:

■ Place the patient in a private room. If a private room isn't available, consult with infection control personnel. As an alternative, he may be placed in a room with a patient who has an active infection with the same microorganism. Special ventilation isn't necessary.

■ Wear a mask when working within 3 ft (0.9 m) of the infected patient. For a patient with known TB, it's necessary to wear an N-95 respirator. (See *N-95 respirator*.)

■ Instruct visitors to stay at least 3 ft away from the infected patient.

■ Limit movement of the patient from the room. If the patient must leave the room, have him wear a surgical mask.

N-95 respirator

You're required to wear a mask, called a respirator, when caring for a patient with known or suspected infectious pulmonary tuberculosis (TB). The specific type that the National Institute for Occupational Safety and Health and the Occupational Safety and Health Administration has approved for this purpose is the N-95 respirator. This type of respirator effectively protects and screens the wearer from at least 95% of particles the size of the TB droplet nuclei, as long as the respirator fits correctly and there's minimal face-seal leakage. Fit testing, which detects such leakage, is mandatory when a respirator is first given to an employee.

Contact precautions

In addition to standard precautions, follow these precautions:

■ Place the patient in a private room. If a private room isn't available, consult with infection control personnel. As an alternative, he may be placed in a room with a patient who has an active infection with the same microorganism.

■ Wear gloves whenever you enter the patient's room. Always change them after contact with infected material. Remove them before leaving the room.

Wash your hands immediately with an antimicrobial soap, or rub them with a waterless antiseptic. Then, avoid touching contaminated surfaces.

■ Wear a gown when entering the patient's room if you think your clothing will have extensive contact with him or anything in his room or if he has diarrhea or is incontinent. Remove the gown before leaving the room.

■ Limit the patient's movement from the room, and check with infection control personnel whenever he must leave it.

Recommended barriers to infection

The list here presents the minimum requirements for using gloves, gowns, masks, and eye protection to avoid coming in contact with and spreading pathogens. In addition to washing your hands thoroughly in all cases, refer to your facility guidelines and use your judgment when assessing the need for barrier protection in specific situations.

KEY

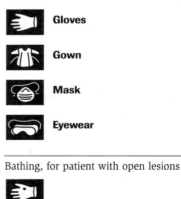

Gloves

Gown

Mask

Eyewear

Bathing, for patient with open lesions

if soiling likely

Bedding, changing visibly soiled

 if soiling likely

Bleeding or pressure application to control it

 if soiling likely

 if splattering likely

 if splattering likely

Blood glucose (capillary) testing

Cardiopulmonary resuscitation

 if splattering likely

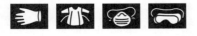 **if splattering likely**

if splattering likely

Central venous line insertion and vene-section

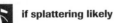

Chest drainage system change

 if splattering likely

 if splattering likely

 if splattering likely

Chest tube insertion or removal

 if soiling likely

 if splattering likely

 if splattering likely

Cleaning (feces, spilled blood or body substances, or surface contaminated by blood or body fluids)

if soiling likely

Colonoscopy, flexible sigmoidoscope

Coughing, frequent and forceful by pa-tient; direct contact with secretions

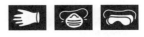

Dialysis, peritoneal (initiating acute treatment, performing an exchange, terminating acute treatment, dismantling tubing from cycler, discarding peritoneal drainage, irrigating peritoneal catheter, changing tubing, or assisting with insertion of acute peritoneal catheter outside sterile field)

 if splattering likely

 if splattering likely

Dressing change for burns

Dressing removal or change for wounds with little or no drainage

---

Dressing removal or change for wounds with large amounts of drainage

 if soiling likely

Emptying drainage receptacles, including suction containers, urine receptacles, bedpans, emesis basins

 if soiling likely

---

 if splattering likely

 if splattering likely

Enema

 if soiling likely

Fecal impaction, removal of

Fecal incontinence, placement of indwelling catheter for, and emptying bag of

 if splattering likely

I.V. or intra-arterial line (insertion, removal, tubing change at catheter hub)

Intubation or extubation

 if splattering likely

 if splattering likely

 if splattering likely

Invasive procedures (lumbar puncture, bone marrow aspiration, paracentesis, liver biopsy) outside the sterile field

---

Irrigation, wound

 if soiling likely

 if splattering likely

 if splattering likely

Nasogastric tube, insertion or irrigation

 if soiling likely

 if splattering likely

 if splattering likely

Ostomy care, irrigation, and teaching

 if soiling likely

Pelvic examination and Papanicolaou test

Postmortem care

 if soiling likely

Pressure ulcer care

Specimen collection (blood, stool, urine, sputum, wound)

Suctioning, nasotracheal or endotracheal

 if soiling likely

 if splattering likely

 if splattering likely

Suctioning, oral or nasal

Tracheostomy suctioning and cannula cleaning

if soiling likely

if splattering likely

if splattering likely

Tracheostomy tube change

if splattering likely

if splattering likely

Urine and stool testing

Wound packing

if soiling likely

Checklist of reportable diseases

Certain contagious diseases must be reported to local and state public health officials and, ultimately, to the CDC. Typically, these diseases fit one of two categories — those reported individually on definitive or suspected diagnosis and those reported by the number of cases per week. The most commonly

reported diseases include hepatitis, measles, viral meningitis, salmonellosis, shigellosis, syphilis, and gonorrhea.

In most states, the patient's primary care provider must report communicable diseases to health officials. In hospitals, the infection control practitioner or epidemiologist reports them. Therefore, you should know the reporting requirements and procedures. Fast, accurate reporting helps to identify and control infection sources, prevent epidemics, and guide public health policy.

The list here notes reportable diseases and conditions:

- acquired immunodeficiency syndrome
- amebiasis
- animal bites
- anthrax (cutaneous or pulmonary)
- aseptic meningitis
- botulism (food-borne, infant)
- brucellosis
- cholera
- diphtheria (cutaneous or pharyngeal)
- encephalitis (postinfectious or primary)
- gastroenteritis (institutional outbreaks)
- gonorrhea
- group A beta-hemolytic streptococcal infections (including scarlet fever)
- Guillain-Barré syndrome
- hepatitis A (include suspected source)
- hepatitis B (include suspected source)
- hepatitis C (include suspected source)
- hepatitis, unspecified (include suspected source)
- influenza
- legionellosis (Legionnaire's disease)
- leprosy
- leptospirosis
- malaria
- measles (rubeola)
- meningitis (specify etiology)
- meningococcal disease

- mumps
- pertussis
- plague (bubonic or pneumonic)
- poliomyelitis (spinal paralytic)
- psittacosis
- rabies
- Reye's syndrome
- rheumatic fever
- Rocky Mountain spotted fever
- rubella (congenital syndrome)
- rubella (German measles)
- salmonellosis (excluding typhoid fever)
- shigellosis
- smallpox
- staphylococcal infections (neonatal)
- syphilis (congenital less than 1 year)
- syphilis (primary or secondary)
- tuberculosis
- tetanus
- toxic shock syndrome
- trichinosis
- tularemia
- typhoid fever
- typhus (flea- and tick-borne)
- varicella (chickenpox)
- yellow fever.

Because disease reporting laws vary among states, the list isn't conclusive. Make sure that you verify the list of reportable diseases and conditions specific to your state with the infection control practitioner at your facility.

Basic procedures

Putting on and removing a gown

Handling isolation clothing properly is important for protecting yourself and avoiding contamination. Follow these steps when using a gown.

Implementation
- Put on the gown, and wrap it around the back of your uniform.
- Tie the strings or fasten the snaps or pressure-sensitive tabs at the neck.

- Make sure your clothing is completely covered; then secure the gown at the waist.
- Because the outside surfaces of this barrier clothing are contaminated, keep your gloves on when taking the clothing off.
- First, untie the waist strings of the gown; then untie the neck straps. Grasp the outside at the back of the shoulders, and pull it down over your arms, turning it inside out to contain pathogens as you remove it.
- Holding the gown well away from you, fold it inside out. Discard it in the laundry if it's cloth and in a trash container if it's paper.

Putting on and removing a mask

Wear a face mask to avoid inhaling airborne particles. Follow these steps when using a mask.

Implementation
- Place the mask snugly over your nose and mouth. Secure the ear loops, or tie the strings behind your head high enough so the mask won't slip off.
- If the mask has a metal strip, squeeze it to fit your nose firmly but comfortably. If you wear eyeglasses, tuck the mask under their lower edge.
- To remove your mask, untie it, holding it by the strings. Discard it in the trash container. (If the patient's disease is spread by airborne pathogens, consider removing the mask last.)

Removing contaminated gloves

To prevent the spread of pathogens from contaminated gloves to your skin surface, carefully follow these steps.

Implementation
- Using your nondominant hand, pinch the glove of the dominant hand

near the top, as shown below. Don't allow the glove's outer surface to buckle inward against your skin.

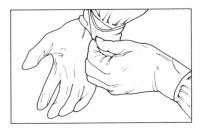

■ Pull downward so that the glove turns inside out as it comes off, as shown below. Keep the glove from your dominant hand in your nondominant hand after removing it.

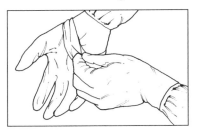

■ Now insert the first two fingers of your ungloved dominant hand under the edge of the nondominant glove, as shown below. Avoid touching the glove's outer surface or folding it against the wrist of your nondominant hand.

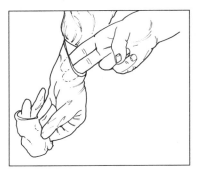

■ Pull downward so that the glove turns inside out as it comes off, as shown below. Continue pulling until the glove completely encloses the glove from your dominant hand and has its uncontaminated inner surface facing out.

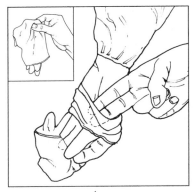

■ Discard your gloves in the appropriate trash container, and wash your hands.

Discarding contaminated equipment

To protect yourself and your patients from infection, observe precautions when disposing of soiled linens or dressings, used disposable equipment, and contaminated reusable equipment. Also, have a biohazard container available, as needed, to dispose of contaminated waste.

Keep in mind that regulations for contaminated-waste disposal vary from state to state and may change periodically.

Removing soiled linens

■ All linens used in patient care settings are considered soiled. Gloves are recommended when handling visibly soiled linen. If the bed linens are saturated with blood, feces, urine, or other body fluids, it's also recommended that you wear a gown.

■ Handle linens as little as possible and with minimum agitation to prevent contaminating yourself. If certain areas of the linens are heavily soiled, fold the fabric so that the soiled areas are on the inside of the folds. Then roll or fold the linens together in one bundle.

■ When carrying linens, carry them away from your body to avoid contaminating your clothes.

■ Bag the linens in the patient's room as soon as possible. Avoid placing them on chairs, tables, or the floor. Don't sort or rinse linens in patient care areas. Place soiled linens in leak-proof bags.

■ After you put the linens in the bag, close the bag securely. Then remove your gloves and wash your hands before carrying the bag to its appropriate destination.

Disposing of soiled dressings

■ Dispose of all wound dressings in a way that confines and contains any blood or body fluids present. Avoid touching soiled areas on the dressing.

■ Usually, you'll need to wear nonsterile gloves to handle and remove soiled dressings. If the wound is large and draining, however, you'll also need to wear a gown.

Large dressings

■ Immediately after removing a large dressing, fold it inward to enclose the soiled areas within the dressing.

■ Wrap the large dressing in the disposable linen-saver pad used during the dressing change.

■ Dispose of the dressing in a red-bagged biohazard container if the dressing is saturated with blood. Otherwise, it can be disposed of in the regular trash container.

■ Remove the gloves and wash your hands.

Small dressings

■ When removing a small dressing, enclose it in the disposable glove you used to remove the dressing. Holding the dressing in your gloved hand, pull the glove off with the inside out to contain the dressing inside it. Don't let your bare hand touch the dressing.

■ After you've sealed the dressing inside the disposable glove, discard both gloves and the dressing in the trash container in the patient's room.

Discarding disposable equipment

■ When disposing of a sharp object contaminated with potentially infectious materials, place it in an approved sharps container. Other contaminated disposable items should be placed in a red-bagged biohazard container if they're dripped with or covered in large amounts of blood. Items with small amounts of dried blood can be disposed of in the regular trash container.

■ When transporting a waste bag, hold it away from your body to prevent inadvertent injury from sharp objects that may protrude through the bag.

Disposing of body fluids

■ Check your facility's policy before handling infectious waste. Large amounts of secretions, excretions, or bulk blood may be carefully poured into a sanitary sewer. If fluids are poured into a hopper, it's required that you wear a splash guard as well as personal protective equipment.

9 Troubleshooting
Spotting and correcting equipment problems

I.V. equipment

Peripheral I.V. lines

Signs and symptoms	Possible causes	Interventions
LOCAL COMPLICATIONS		
Phlebitis ■ Tenderness at tip of and above venipuncture device ■ Redness at tip of catheter and along vein ■ Puffy area over vein ■ Vein hard on palpation ■ Possible fever	■ Poor blood flow around venipuncture device ■ Tip of catheter next to vessel wall ■ Friction from catheter movement in vein ■ Venipuncture device left in vein too long ■ Clotting at catheter tip (thrombophlebitis) ■ Drug or solution with high or low pH or high osmolarity	■ Remove the venipuncture device. ■ Apply warm soaks. Elevate the extremity if edema is present. ■ Notify the doctor if the patient has a fever. Document the patient's condition and your interventions. *Prevention* ■ Restart the infusion using a larger vein for an irritating solution, or restart with a smaller-gauge device to ensure adequate blood flow. ■ Use a filter to lower the risk of phlebitis. ■ Tape the device securely to prevent motion.
Extravasation ■ Swelling at and above I.V. site (may extend along entire limb) ■ Discomfort, burning, or pain at site (but may be painless) ■ Tight feeling at site ■ Decreased skin temperature around site ■ Blanching at site ■ Continuing fluid infusion even when vein is occluded (although rate may decrease) ■ Absent backflow of blood	■ Venipuncture device dislodged from vein or perforated vein	■ Remove the venipuncture device. Infiltrate site with antidote, if needed. ■ Apply ice (early) or warm soaks (later) to aid absorption. Elevate the limb. ■ Monitor the patient's pulse and capillary refill time. ■ Restart the infusion above the infiltration site or in another limb. ■ Document the patient's condition and your interventions. *Prevention* ■ Check the site often. ■ Don't obscure the area above the site with tape. ■ Teach the patient to observe the I.V. site, and advise him to report pain or swelling.
Catheter dislodgment ■ Catheter partly backed out of vein ■ Solution infiltrating	■ Loosened tape or tubing snagged in bed linens, resulting in partial retraction of catheter ■ Pulled out by confused patient	■ If no infiltration occurs, retape without pushing the catheter back into the vein. If pulled out, apply pressure to the I.V. site with a sterile dressing. *Prevention* ■ Tape the venipuncture device securely on insertion.

(continued)

Peripheral I.V. lines *(continued)*

Signs and symptoms	Possible causes	Interventions
LOCAL COMPLICATIONS *(continued)*		
Occlusion ■ No increase in flow rate when I.V. container is raised ■ Blood backflow in line ■ Discomfort at insertion site	■ I.V. flow interrupted ■ Saline lock not flushed ■ Blood backflow in line when patient walks ■ Line clamped too long	■ Use a mild flush injection. Don't force it. If unsuccessful, reinsert the I.V. line. *Prevention* ■ Maintain the I.V. flow rate. ■ Flush promptly after intermittent piggyback administration. ■ Have the patient walk with his arm folded to his chest to reduce the risk of blood backflow.
Vein irritation or pain at I.V. site ■ Pain during infusion ■ Possible blanching if vasospasm occurs ■ Red skin over vein during infusion ■ Rapidly developing signs of phlebitis	■ Solution with high or low pH or high osmolarity, such as 40 mEq/L of potassium chloride, phenytoin, and some antibiotics (vancomycin, erythromycin, and nafcillin)	■ Decrease the flow rate. ■ Try using an electronic flow device to achieve a steady flow. *Prevention* ■ Dilute the solutions before administration. For example, give antibiotics in a 250-ml solution rather than a 100-ml solution. ■ If long-term therapy of an irritating drug is planned, ask the doctor to use a central I.V. line.
Severed catheter ■ Leakage from catheter shaft	■ Catheter inadvertently cut by scissors ■ Reinsertion of needle into catheter	■ If a broken part is visible, attempt to retrieve it. If you're unsuccessful, notify the doctor. ■ If a portion of the catheter enters the bloodstream, place a tourniquet above the I.V. site to prevent progression of the broken part and immediately notify the doctor and radiology department. ■ Document the patient's condition and your interventions. *Prevention* ■ Don't use scissors around the I.V. site. ■ Never reinsert a needle into the catheter. ■ Remove an unsuccessfully inserted catheter and needle together.

Peripheral I.V. lines *(continued)*

Signs and symptoms	Possible causes	Interventions
LOCAL COMPLICATIONS *(continued)*		
Hematoma ■ Tenderness at venipuncture site ■ Bruised area around site ■ Inability to advance or flush I.V. site	■ Vein punctured through opposite wall at the time of insertion ■ Leakage of blood from needle displacement	■ Remove the venipuncture device. ■ Apply pressure and warm soaks to the affected area. ■ Recheck for bleeding. ■ Document the patient's condition and your interventions. ***Prevention*** ■ Choose a vein that can accommodate the size of the venipuncture device. ■ Release the tourniquet as soon as a successful insertion is achieved.
Venous spasm ■ Pain along vein ■ Flow rate sluggish when clamp is completely open ■ Blanched skin over vein	■ Severe vein irritation from irritating drugs or fluids ■ Administration of cold fluids or blood products ■ Very rapid flow rate (with fluids at room temperature)	■ Apply warm soaks over the vein and surrounding area. ■ Decrease the flow rate. ***Prevention*** ■ Use a blood warmer for blood or packed red blood cells.
Vasovagal reaction ■ Sudden collapse of vein during venipuncture ■ Sudden pallor, sweating, faintness, dizziness, and nausea ■ Decreased blood pressure	■ Vasospasm from anxiety or pain	■ Lower the head of the bed. ■ Have the patient take deep breaths. ■ Check the patient's vital signs. ***Prevention*** ■ To relieve the patient's anxiety, prepare him for the procedure. ■ Use a local anesthetic to prevent pain.
Thrombosis ■ Painful, reddened, and swollen vein ■ Sluggish or stopped I.V. flow	■ Injury to endothelial cells of vein wall, allowing platelets to adhere and thrombi to form	■ Remove the venipuncture device; restart the infusion in the opposite limb, if possible. ■ Apply warm soaks. ■ Watch for an I.V. therapy–related infection. ***Prevention*** ■ Use proper venipuncture techniques to reduce injury to the vein.

(continued)

Peripheral I.V. lines *(continued)*

Signs and symptoms	Possible causes	Interventions

LOCAL COMPLICATIONS *(continued)*

Signs and symptoms	Possible causes	Interventions
Thrombophlebitis ■ Severe discomfort at site ■ Reddened, swollen, and hardened vein	■ Thrombosis and inflammation	■ Follow the interventions for thrombosis. ***Prevention*** ■ Check the site frequently. Remove the venipuncture device at the first sign of redness and tenderness.
Nerve, tendon, or ligament damage ■ Extreme pain (similar to electrical shock when nerve is punctured), numbness, and muscle contraction ■ Delayed effects, including paralysis, numbness, and deformity	■ Improper venipuncture technique, resulting in injury to surrounding nerves, tendons, or ligaments ■ Tight taping or improper splinting with arm board	■ Stop the procedure. ***Prevention*** ■ Don't repeatedly penetrate tissues with the venipuncture device. ■ Don't apply excessive pressure when taping; don't encircle the limb with tape. ■ Pad arm boards and tape securing arm boards, if possible.

SYSTEMIC COMPLICATIONS

Signs and symptoms	Possible causes	Interventions
Circulatory overload ■ Discomfort ■ Neck vein engorgement ■ Respiratory distress ■ Increased blood pressure ■ Crackles ■ Increased difference between fluid intake and output	■ Roller clamp loosened to allow run-on infusion ■ Flow rate too rapid ■ Miscalculation of fluid requirements	■ Raise the head of the bed. ■ Administer oxygen, if needed. ■ Notify the doctor. ■ Give drugs as ordered. ***Prevention*** ■ Use a pump, controller, or rate minder for an elderly or compromised patient. ■ Recheck calculations of fluid requirements. ■ Monitor the infusion frequently.
Systemic infection (septicemia or bacteremia) ■ Fever, chills, and malaise for no apparent reason ■ Contaminated I.V. site, usually with no visible signs of infection at site	■ Failure to maintain aseptic technique during insertion or site care ■ Severe phlebitis, causing organism growth ■ Poor taping that permits the venipuncture device to move, introducing organisms into bloodstream	■ Notify the doctor. ■ Administer medications as prescribed. ■ Culture the site and device. ■ Monitor vital signs. ***Prevention*** ■ Use scrupulous aseptic technique when handling solutions and tubing, inserting venipuncture device, and discontinuing infusion.

Peripheral I.V. lines *(continued)*

Signs and symptoms	Possible causes	Interventions
SYSTEMIC COMPLICATIONS *(continued)*		
Systemic infection *(continued)*	■ Prolonged indwelling time ■ Compromised immune system	■ Secure all connections. ■ Change the I.V. solutions, tubing, and venipuncture device at the recommended times. ■ Use I.V. filters.
Speed shock ■ Flushed face, headache ■ Tightness in chest ■ Irregular pulse ■ Syncope ■ Rapid hypertension ■ Shock ■ Cardiac arrest	■ Too rapid injection of drug, causing plasma levels to become toxic ■ Improper administration of bolus infusion (especially additives)	■ Discontinue the infusion. ■ Begin an infusion of dextrose 5% in water at a keep-vein-open rate. ■ Notify the doctor. ***Prevention*** ■ Check the infusion guidelines before giving a drug. ■ Dilute the drug with a compatible solution.
Air embolism ■ Respiratory distress ■ Unequal breath sounds ■ Chest pain, dyspnea ■ Anxiety ■ Weak, rapid pulse ■ Increased central venous pressure ■ Decreased blood pressure ■ Altered consciousness	■ Solution container empty	■ Discontinue the infusion. ■ Place the patient in left lateral Trendelenburg's position to allow air to enter the right atrium and disperse through the pulmonary artery. ■ Administer oxygen. ■ Notify the doctor. ■ Document the patient's condition and your interventions. ***Prevention*** ■ Purge the tubing of air completely before starting an infusion. ■ Use the air-detection device on the pump or an air-eliminating filter proximal to the I.V. site. ■ Secure all connections.
Allergic reaction ■ Itching ■ Watery eyes and nose ■ Bronchospasm ■ Wheezing ■ Urticarial rash ■ Edema at I.V. site	■ Allergens such as medications	■ If a reaction occurs, stop the infusion immediately. ■ Maintain a patent airway. ■ Notify the doctor. ■ Administer an antihistaminic corticosteroid and antipyretic as ordered. ■ Give 0.2 to 0.5 ml of 1:1,000 aqueous epinephrine S.C. as ordered. Repeat at 3-minute intervals and as needed.

(continued)

Peripheral I.V. lines *(continued)*

Signs and symptoms	Possible causes	Interventions
SYSTEMIC COMPLICATIONS *(continued)*		
Allergic reaction *(continued)* ■ Anaphylactic reaction, which may occur within minutes or up to 1 hour after exposure (flushing, chills, anxiety, agitation, itching, palpitations, paresthesia, throbbing in ears, wheezing, coughing, seizures, cardiac arrest)		***Prevention*** ■ Obtain the patient's allergy history. Look for cross-allergies. ■ Assist with test dosing. ■ Monitor the patient carefully during the first 15 minutes of administration of a new drug.

Central venous lines

Signs and symptoms	Possible causes	Interventions
Pneumothorax, hemothorax, chylothorax, hydrothorax ■ Chest pain ■ Dyspnea ■ Cyanosis ■ Decreased breath sounds on affected side ■ With hemothorax, decreased hemoglobin levels because of blood pooling ■ Abnormal chest X-ray ■ Apprehension	■ Lung puncture by catheter during insertion or exchange over a guide wire ■ Large blood vessel puncture with bleeding inside or outside lung ■ Lymph node puncture with leakage of lymph fluid ■ Infusion of solution into chest area through infiltrated catheter	■ Notify the doctor. ■ Remove the catheter or assist with removal. ■ Administer oxygen as ordered. ■ Set up and assist with chest tube insertion. ■ Document all interventions. ***Prevention*** ■ Position the patient head-down with a rolled towel between his scapulae to dilate and expose the internal jugular or subclavian vein as much as possible during catheter insertion. ■ Assess the patient for early signs of fluid infiltration (swelling in the shoulder, neck, chest, and arm). ■ Ensure that the patient is immobilized and prepared for insertion. ■ Minimize the patient's activity after insertion, especially with a peripheral catheter.

Central venous lines *(continued)*

Signs and symptoms	Possible causes	Interventions
Air embolism ■ Respiratory distress ■ Chest pain ■ Unequal breath sounds ■ Weak, rapid pulse ■ Increased central venous pressure ■ Decreased blood pressure ■ Churning murmur over precordium ■ Alteration or loss of consciousness ■ Anxiety	■ Intake of air into central venous system during catheter insertion or tubing changes, or inadvertent opening, cutting, or breaking of catheter	■ Clamp the catheter immediately. ■ Place the patient in left lateral Trendelenburg's position so air can enter the right atrium and pulmonary artery. Make sure he remains in this position for 20 to 30 minutes. ■ Don't recommend Valsalva's maneuver because a large air intake worsens the condition. ■ Administer oxygen. ■ Notify the doctor. ■ Document your interventions. ***Prevention*** ■ Purge all air from the tubing before hookup. ■ Teach the patient to perform Valsalva's maneuver during catheter insertion and tubing changes. ■ Use air-eliminating filters or an infusion device with air-detection capability. ■ Use luer-lock tubing, tape the connections, or use locking devices for all connections.
Thrombosis ■ Edema at puncture site ■ Erythema ■ Ipsilateral swelling of arm, neck, and face ■ Pain along vein ■ Fever, malaise ■ Jugular vein distention	■ Sluggish flow rate ■ Composition of catheter material (polyvinyl chloride catheters are more thrombogenic) ■ Hematopoietic status of patient ■ Preexisting limb edema ■ Infusion of irritating solutions ■ Repeated or long-term use of same vein ■ Preexisting cardiovascular disease ■ Simultaneous administration of or inadequate flushing between incompatible medications	■ Notify the doctor. ■ Remove the catheter, if necessary. ■ Infuse a dose of heparin or a thrombolytic, if ordered. ■ Locally apply warm, wet compresses. ■ Don't use the limb on the affected side for subsequent venipuncture. ■ Verify thrombosis with diagnostic studies. ***Prevention*** ■ Maintain a steady flow rate with an infusion pump, or flush the catheter at regular intervals according to facility policy. ■ Use catheters made of less thrombogenic materials or catheters coated to prevent thrombosis. ■ Dilute irritating solutions.

(continued)

Central venous lines *(continued)*

Signs and symptoms	Possible causes	Interventions
Thrombosis *(continued)*		■ Use a 0.22-micron filter for infusions. ■ Ensure the compatibility of medications, and flush adequately.
Infection ■ Redness, warmth, tenderness, swelling at insertion or exit site ■ Possible exudate of purulent material ■ Local rash or pustules ■ Fever, chills, malaise ■ Leukocytosis ■ Nausea and vomiting ■ Elevated urine glucose level	■ Failure to maintain aseptic technique during catheter insertion or care ■ Failure to comply with dressing change protocol ■ Wet or soiled dressing remaining on site ■ Immunosuppression ■ Irritated suture line ■ Contaminated catheter or solution ■ Frequent opening of catheter or long-term use of single I.V. access site	■ Monitor temperatures frequently. ■ Monitor vital signs closely. ■ Culture the site. ■ Re-dress using aseptic technique. ■ Use an antibiotic ointment locally as needed. ■ Treat systemically with an antibiotic or an antifungal, depending on the culture results and the doctor's order. ■ Draw central and peripheral blood cultures; if the same organism appears in both, then the catheter is the primary source and should be removed. ■ If the cultures don't match but are positive, the catheter may be removed or the infection may be treated through the catheter. ■ Treat the patient with an antibiotic as ordered. ■ If the catheter is removed, culture its tip. ■ Document your interventions. ***Prevention*** ■ Maintain sterile technique using sterile gloves, masks, and gowns when appropriate. ■ Observe dressing-change protocols. ■ Teach the patient about restrictions on swimming, bathing, and other physical activities. (The doctor may allow these activities with adequate white blood cell count.) ■ Change a wet or soiled dressing immediately. ■ Change the dressing more frequently if the catheter is located in the femoral area or near a tracheostomy. Perform tracheostomy care after catheter care.

Central venous lines *(continued)*

Signs and symptoms	Possible causes	Interventions
Infection *(continued)*		■ Examine the solution for cloudiness and turbidity before infusing; check the fluid container for leaks. ■ Monitor the urine glucose level in patients receiving total parenteral nutrition (TPN); if greater than 2+, suspect early sepsis. ■ Use a 0.22-micron filter (or a 1.2-micron filter for three-in-one TPN solutions). ■ Change the catheter according to protocol. ■ Keep the system closed as much as possible.

Infusion control devices

When the alarm goes off, check for the following problems.

Problems	Interventions
Air in the line	While setting up, make sure all air is out of the line, including air trapped in Y-injection sites. Also, check that the connections are secure and the container is filled properly. Withdraw any air from a piggyback port with a syringe or an air-eliminating filter. A wet-air detector may give a false reading.
Infusion completed	Reset the pump as ordered or discontinue the infusion. A slow keep-vein-open rate will usually keep the I.V. line patent as long as enough fluid remains.
Empty container	Check for adequate fluid levels in the I.V. container, and have another container available before the last one runs out.
Low battery	Battery life varies; keep the machine plugged in on AC power as much as possible, especially while the patient is in bed. If the alarm goes off, plug in the machine immediately, or power may be lost for awhile (usually a half-hour to several hours).
Occlusion	Check that all clamps are open, look for kinked tubing, and check the patency of the venipuncture device.

(continued)

Infusion control devices *(continued)*

Problems	Interventions
Rate change	Check that the infusion control device displays the ordered rate. The patient or a family member may have tampered with the controls.
Open door	The door should be closed; it may not shut if the device isn't set up properly (for example, if the cassette isn't inserted all the way).
Malfunction	A mechanical failure usually must be handled by the biomedical engineering department or the manufacturer. Disconnect the infusion control device. Label it clearly with a sign that says BROKEN and indicate the specific problem.

I.V. flow rates

Problems and possible causes	Interventions
Flow rate too fast	
Clamp manipulated by patient or visitor	Instruct the patient not to touch the clamp, and place tape over it. Administer the I.V. solution with an infusion pump or a controller, if necessary.
Tubing disconnected from catheter	Using alcohol, wipe the distal end of the tubing with luer-lock connections. Then reinsert it firmly into the catheter hub, and apply tape at the connection site.
Change in patient position	Use an infusion pump or a controller to ensure the correct flow rate.
Bevel against vein wall (positional cannulation)	Manipulate the venipuncture device, and place a 2″ × 2″ gauze pad under or over the catheter hub to change the angle. Reset the flow clamp at the desired rate. If necessary, remove and reinsert the venipuncture device.
Flow clamp drifting from patient movement	Place tape below the clamp.
Flow rate too slow	
Venous spasm after insertion	Apply warm soaks over site.
Venous obstruction from bending arm	Secure the I.V. line with an arm board, if necessary.

I.V. flow rates *(continued)*

Problems and possible causes	Interventions
Flow rate too slow *(continued)*	
Pressure change (from decreased fluid in bottle)	Readjust the flow rate.
Elevated blood pressure	Readjust the flow rate. Use an infusion pump or a controller to ensure the correct rate.
Cold solution	Allow the solution to warm to room temperature before hanging the bag.
Change in solution viscosity from drug added	Readjust the flow rate.
I.V. container too low or patient's arm or leg too high	Hang the container higher, or remind the patient to keep his arm below heart's level.
Bevel against vein wall (positional cannulation)	Withdraw the needle slightly, or place a folded 2″ × 2″ gauze pad over or under the catheter hub to change the angle.
Excess tubing dangling below insertion site	Replace the tubing with a shorter piece, or tape the excess tubing to the I.V. pole below the flow clamp (making sure that the tubing isn't kinked).
Venipuncture device too small	Remove the venipuncture device in use and insert a larger-bore venipuncture device, or use an infusion pump.
Infiltration or clotted venipuncture device	Remove the venipuncture device in use, and insert a new one.
Kinked tubing	Check the tubing over its entire length, and unkink it.
Clogged filter	Remove the filter, and replace it with a new one.
Tubing compressed at clamped area	Massage or milk the tubing by pinching and wrapping it around a pencil four or five times. Then quickly pull the pencil out of the coiled tubing.

Infusion interruptions

When an infusion stops, systematically assess the I.V. system — from the patient to the fluid container — for potential trouble areas.

Check the I.V. site
Check for infiltration or phlebitis, which may slow or stop the flow rate.

Check for patency
Evaluate the I.V. device for patency, keeping in mind that several factors can affect it:

■ Increased blood pressure may stop the I.V. flow if the patient's limb is flexed or lying directly on the I.V. site. Reposition the patient's limb as necessary.

■ A blocked venipuncture device may be obstructed by the tip of the needle lying against the vein wall or a venous valve. Lift up or pull back the device to reestablish the I.V. flow.

■ A tourniquet effect — if the patient's arm is wrapped with tape — may reduce the I.V. flow rate. Taping the I.V. site too tightly can cause the same problem. Release or remove the tape. Then reapply the tape.

■ Smaller venipuncture devices may kink or fold, impeding the I.V. flow. Pull the device back to reestablish the flow.

■ Local edema or poor tissue perfusion from disease can block the venous flow. Move the I.V. line to an unaffected site.

■ Infusion of incompatible fluid or medication may cause a precipitate to form. This can block the I.V. tubing and venipuncture device and may even expose the patient to a life-threatening embolism. Always check the compatibility of all medications and the I.V. solution before administering them. Replace the venipuncture device if it's occluded.

Check the filter
Make sure that the in-line filter is the right size and type. I.V. fluids are usually run through a 0.22- or 0.45-micron filter to eliminate air and microorganisms from the system. Single-use filters shouldn't be used for in-line filtration — only for drawing up a medication or administering a bolus dose.

If you use the wrong size or type of filter, the solution may not pass through it. For example, drugs such as amphotericin B and lymphocyte immune globulin (Atgam) consist of molecules that are too large to pass through a 0.22-micron filter; they rapidly block the filter and stop the I.V. flow. If necessary, replace the filter.

Additionally, minute particles and microorganisms can block a filter that's used longer than recommended. Not only will the I.V. flow stop but also the patient may become exposed to bacterial toxins and sepsis. The interval between filter changes usually ranges from 24 to 48 hours, depending on the manufacturer's instructions. Change the filter, if necessary.

Check clamps
Make sure that the flow clamps are open. Check all clamps, including the roller clamp and any clamps on secondary sets such as a slide clamp on a filter. (A roller clamp may also become jammed if the roller is pushed up too far.)

Check tubing
Determine if the tubing is kinked or if the patient is lying on it. Also check whether the tubing remains crimped where a clamp was tightened around it. If so, gently squeeze the area between your fingers to round out the tubing to its original shape, or change the tubing altogether.

Check air vents
If you're using an evacuated glass container, you need an air vent to make the I.V. solution flow. Insert one as necessary. On a volume-control set, the air vent is usually located at the top of the calibrated chamber. If the solution flow

stops, check the patency of this vent and the position of the vent clamp. To check patency, follow the manufacturer's instructions.

Check fluid level

Observe the fluid level in the I.V. container. If it's empty, replace it as ordered. If the solution is cold, it may be causing venous spasm, thus decreasing the flow rate. Applying warm compresses can relieve venous spasm and thus increase the flow rate. Make sure other solutions are given at room temperature. Finally, check to see if the spike at the end of the administration set has been pushed far enough into the container to allow the solution to flow.

If you can't identify the problem with this series of checks, remove the I.V. line, and restart it at a different site. Also, be sure to document the episode in the patient's chart.

Vascular access ports

Problems and possible causes	Interventions
INABILITY TO FLUSH VASCULAR ACCESS PORT (V.A.P.) OR WITHDRAW BLOOD	
■ Kinked tubing or closed clamp	■ Check the tubing or clamp.
■ Catheter lodged against vessel wall	■ Reposition the patient. ■ Teach the patient to change his position to free the catheter from the vessel wall. ■ Raise the arm that's on the same side as the catheter. ■ Roll the patient to the opposite side. ■ Have the patient cough, sit up, or take a deep breath. ■ Infuse 10 ml of normal saline solution into the catheter. ■ Regain access to the catheter of the VAP using a new sterile needle.
■ Incorrect needle placement ■ Needle not advanced through septum	■ Regain access to the device. ■ Teach the home care patient to push down firmly on the noncoring needle in the septum and to verify needle position by aspirating for a blood return.
■ Clot formation	■ Assess patency by trying to flush the VAP while the patient changes position. ■ Notify the doctor, and obtain an order for a thrombolytic. ■ Teach the patient to recognize clot formation, to notify the doctor if it occurs, and to avoid forcibly flushing the VAP.

(continued)

Vascular access ports *(continued)*

Problems and possible causes	Interventions
INABILITY TO FLUSH V.A.P. OR WITHDRAW BLOOD *(continued)*	
■ Kinked catheter, catheter migration, port rotation	■ Notify the doctor immediately. ■ Tell the patient to notify the doctor if he has difficulty using the VAP.
INABILITY TO PALPATE THE V.A.P.	
■ Deeply implanted port	■ Note the portal chamber scar to locate the correct spot for palpation. ■ Use deep palpation technique. ■ Ask another nurse to locate the VAP. ■ Use a 1½″ or 2″ noncoring needle to gain access to the VAP.

Cardiovascular monitors and devices

Blood pressure readings

Problems and possible causes	Interventions
False-high reading Cuff too small	Make sure the cuff bladder is 20% wider than the circumference of the arm or leg being used for measurement.
Cuff wrapped too loosely, reducing its effective width	Tighten the cuff.
Slow cuff deflation, causing venous congestion in the arm or leg	Never deflate the cuff more slowly than 2 mm Hg per heartbeat.
Tilted mercury column	Read pressures with the mercury column vertical.
Poorly timed measurement — after patient has eaten, ambulated, appeared anxious, or flexed arm muscles	Postpone blood pressure measurement, or help the patient relax before taking pressure measurements.

Blood pressure readings *(continued)*

Problems and possible causes	Interventions
False-low reading	
Incorrect position of arm or leg	Make sure the arm or leg is level with the patient's heart.
Mercury column below eye level	Read the mercury column at eye level.
Failure to notice auscultatory gap (sound fades out for 10 to 15 mm Hg, then returns)	Estimate systolic pressure by palpation before actually measuring it. Then check this pressure against the measured pressure.
Inaudible low-volume sounds	Before reinflating the cuff, instruct the patient to raise his arm or leg to decrease venous pressure and amplify low-volume sounds. After inflating the cuff, tell the patient to lower his arm or leg. Then deflate the cuff and listen. If you still fail to detect low-volume sounds, chart the palpated systolic pressure.

Cardiac monitors

Problems and possible causes	Interventions
False-high-rate alarm	
Monitor interpreting large T waves as QRS complexes, which doubles the rate	Reposition the electrodes to the lead where the QRS complexes are taller than the T waves.
Skeletal muscle activity	Place the electrodes away from major muscle masses.
False-low-rate alarm	
Shift in electrical axis caused by patient movement, making QRS complexes too small to register	Reapply the electrodes. Set the gain so the height of the complex exceeds 1 mV.
Low amplitude of QRS complex	Increase the gain.
Poor electrode-skin contact	Reapply the electrodes.
Low amplitude	
Gain dial set too low	Increase the gain.

(continued)

Cardiac monitors *(continued)*

Problems and possible causes	Interventions
Low amplitude *(continued)* Poor contact between skin and electrodes, dried gel, broken or loose leadwires, poor connection between patient and monitor, malfunctioning monitor, physiologic loss of amplitude of QRS complex	Check the connections on all leadwires and the monitoring cable. Replace or reapply the electrodes as necessary.
Wandering baseline Poor electrode placement or contact with skin	Reposition or replace the electrodes.
Thoracic movement with respirations	Reposition the electrodes.
Artifact (waveform interference) Patient having seizures, chills, or anxiety	Notify the doctor, and treat the patient as ordered. Keep the patient warm, and reassure him.
Patient movement	Help the patient relax.
Electrodes applied improperly	Check the electrodes and reapply, if necessary.
Static electricity	Make sure the cables don't have exposed connectors. Change static-causing clothing.
Electrical short circuit in leadwires or cable	Replace the broken equipment. Use stress loops to apply the leadwires.
Interference from decreased room humidity	Regulate the humidity to 40%.
Broken leadwires or cable Tension on leadwires from repeated pulling	Replace and retape the leadwires, taping part of the wire into a loop. This absorbs tension that would otherwise tug at the ends of the wire.
Cables and leadwires cleaned with alcohol or acetone, causing brittleness	Clean the cable and leadwires with soapy water. *Don't let* the *cable ends get wet.* Replace the cable as necessary.

Cardiac monitors *(continued)*

Problems and possible causes	Interventions
60–cycle interference (fuzzy baseline)	
Electrical interference from other equipment in room	Attach the electrical equipment to a common ground, checking the plugs for loose prongs.
Patient's bed improperly grounded	Attach the bed ground to the room's common ground.
Skin excoriation under electrode	
Patient allergic to electrode adhesive	Remove the electrodes and apply hypoallergenic electrodes and tape.
Electrode remaining on skin too long	Remove the electrode, clean the site, and reapply the electrode at a new site.

Intra-aortic balloon pumps

When your patient undergoes intra-aortic balloon counterpulsation, you must respond immediately to equipment problems.

Problems and possible causes	Interventions
High gas leakage Balloon leakage or abrasion	Check for blood in the tubing. Stop pumping. Contact the doctor to remove the balloon.
Condensation in extension tubing, volume-limiter disk, or both	Remove the condensate from the tubing and the volume-limiter disk. Refill, autopurge, and resume pumping.
Kink in balloon catheter or tubing	Check the catheter and tubing for kinks and loose connections. Refill and resume pumping.
Tachycardia (rapid flow of helium causing insufficient fill pressure)	Change the wean control to 1:2, or operate in ON, or manual, mode. *Note:* Gas alarms are off in manual mode. Autopurge the balloon every 1 to 2 hours, and monitor the balloon pressure waveform closely.
Malfunctioning or loose volume-limiter disk	Replace or tighten the volume-limiter disk. Refill, autopurge, and resume pumping.

(continued)

Problems and possible causes	Interventions
High gas leakage *(continued)*	
System leak	Perform a leak test.
Balloon line block (automatic mode only)	
Kink in balloon catheter or tubing	Check the catheter and tubing for kinks. Refill and resume pumping.
Balloon catheter not unfurled; sheath or balloon positioned too high	Contact the doctor to verify placement; the balloon may have to be repositioned or inflated manually.
Condensation in tubing, volume-limiter disk, or both	Remove the condensate from the tubing and the volume-limiter disk. Refill, autopurge, and resume pumping.
Balloon too large for aorta	Decrease the volume-control percentage by one notch.
Malfunctioning volume-limiter disk or incorrect volume-limiter disk size	Replace the volume-limiter disk. Refill, autopurge, and resume pumping.
No electrocardiogram (ECG) trigger	
Inadequate signal	Adjust the ECG gain, and change the lead or the trigger mode.
Lead disconnected	Replace the lead.
Improper ECG input mode (skin or monitor) selected	Adjust the ECG input to the appropriate mode (skin or monitor). Apply new electrodes as needed.
No arterial pressure trigger	
Arterial line damped	Flush the line.
Arterial line open to atmosphere	Check the connections on the arterial pressure line.
Trigger mode change	
Trigger mode changed while pumping	Resume pumping.
Irregular heart rhythm	
Patient's rhythm is irregular (such as atrial fibrillation or ectopic beats)	Change to R or QRS sense, if necessary, to accommodate the irregular rhythm.

Intra-aortic balloon pumps *(continued)*

Problems and possible causes	Interventions
Erratic atrioventricular pacing	
Demand for paced rhythm occurs during atrioventricular sequential trigger mode	Change to the pacer reject trigger or QRS sense.
Noisy ECG signal	
Malfunctioning leads	Replace the leads; check the ECG cable and the electrodes.
Electrocautery in use	Switch to the arterial pressure trigger.
Internal trigger	
Trigger mode set on internal 80 beats/minute	Select an alternative trigger if the patient has a heartbeat or rhythm. *Caution:* Use an internal trigger only during cardiopulmonary bypass surgery or cardiac arrest.
Purge incomplete	
OFF button pressed during autopurge, interrupting purge cycle	Initiate autopurge again, or initiate pumping.
High fill pressure	
Malfunctioning volume-limiter disk	Replace the volume-limiter disk. Refill, autopurge, and resume pumping.
Occluded vent line or valve	Attempt to resume pumping. If this fails to correct the problem, contact the manufacturer.
No balloon drive	
No volume-limiter disk	Insert the volume-limiter disk, and lock it securely in place.
Tubing disconnected	Reconnect the tubing. Refill, autopurge, and pump.
Incorrect timing	
INFLATE and DEFLATE controls improperly set	Place the INFLATE and DEFLATE controls at set midpoints. Reassess the timing and readjust.
Low volume percentage	
Volume-control percentage not on 100%	Assess the cause of the decreased volume, and reset, if necessary.

Pacemakers

Life-threatening arrhythmias can result when the patient's pacemaker sends an impulse too weak to stimulate the heart (failure to capture). Furthermore, the pacemaker may fail to detect ventricular depolarization (failure to sense) or fail to send an impulse at all (failure to fire). Below are rhythm strips that compare these problems with a normal wave strip as well as lists of possible causes and interventions.

Normal
The location of the spike is your first clue that the pacemaker is functioning normally.

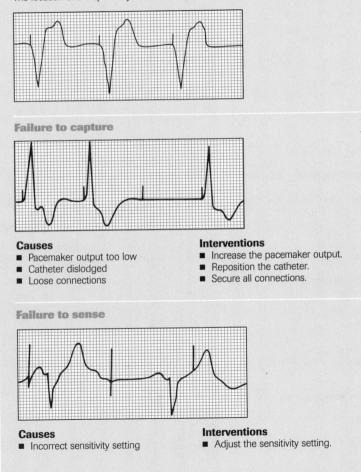

Failure to capture

Causes
- Pacemaker output too low
- Catheter dislodged
- Loose connections

Interventions
- Increase the pacemaker output.
- Reposition the catheter.
- Secure all connections.

Failure to sense

Causes
- Incorrect sensitivity setting

Interventions
- Adjust the sensitivity setting.

Pacemakers *(continued)*

Failure to fire

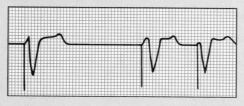

Causes
- Loose lead hookups
- Dead battery
- Malfunctioning pulse generator

Interventions
- Secure the lead hookups.
- Replace the battery.
- Replace the pulse generator.

Arterial lines

Problems	Possible causes	Interventions
Damped waveform Appearing as a small waveform with a slow rise in the anacrotic limb and a reduced or nonexistent dicrotic notch, a damped waveform may result from interference with the transmission of the physiologic signal to the transducer.	Air in the system	Check the system for air, paying particular attention to the tubing and the transducer's diaphragm. If you find air, aspirate it or force it from the system through a stopcock port. Never flush a fluid that contains air bubbles into a patient.
	Loose connection	Check and tighten all connections.
	Clotted catheter tip	Attempt to aspirate the clot. If you're successful, flush the line. If you're unsuccessful, avoid flushing the line: You could dislodge the clot.
	Catheter tip resting against arterial wall	Reposition the catheter by carefully rotating it or pulling it back slightly. Anticipate a possible change in the catheter placement site, and assist as appropriate.
	Kinked tubing	Unkink the tubing.
	Inadequately inflated pressure infuser bag	Inflate the pressure infuser bag to 300 mm Hg.

(continued)

Problems	Possible causes	Interventions
Drifting waveform Waveform floats above and below the baseline.	Temperature change in flush solution	Allow the temperature of the flush solution to stabilize before the infusion.
	Kinked or compressed monitor cable	Check the cable, and relieve the kink or compression.
Inability to flush the arterial line or to withdraw blood Activating the continuous flush device fails to move the flush solution, and blood can't be withdrawn from the stopcock.	Incorrectly positioned stopcocks	Properly reposition the stopcocks.
	Kinked tubing	Unkink the tubing.
	Inadequately inflated pressure infuser bag	Inflate the pressure infuser bag to 300 mm Hg.
	Clotted catheter tip	Attempt to aspirate the clot. If you're successful, flush the line. If you're unsuccessful, avoid flushing the line: You could dislodge the clot.
	Catheter tip resting against arterial wall	Reposition the catheter insertion area, and flush the catheter. Alternatively, reposition the catheter by carefully rotating it or pulling it back slightly.
	Position of insertion area	Check the position of the insertion area, and change it as indicated. For radial and brachial arterial lines, use an arm board to immobilize the area. With a femoral arterial line, keep the head of the bed at a 45-degree angle or less to prevent catheter kinking.
Artifact Waveform tracings follow an erratic pattern or fail to appear as a recognizable diagnostic pattern.	Electrical interference	Check the electrical equipment in the room.
	Patient movement	Ask the patient to lie quietly while you try to read the monitor.
	Catheter whip or fling (excessive catheter tip movement)	Shorten the tubing, if possible.

Arterial lines *(continued)*

Problems	Possible causes	Interventions
False-high pressure reading Arterial pressure exceeds the patient's normal pressure without a significant change in baseline clinical findings. Before responding to this high pressure, recheck the system to make sure that the reading is accurate.	Improper calibration	Recalibrate the system.
	Transducer positioned below phlebostatic axis	Relevel the transducer with the phlebostatic axis.
	Catheter kinked	Unkink the catheter.
	Clotted catheter tip	Attempt to aspirate the clot. If you're successful, flush the line. If you're unsuccessful, avoid flushing the line: You could dislodge the clot.
	Catheter tip resting against arterial line	Flush the catheter, or reposition it by carefully rotating it or pulling it back slightly.
	I.V. tubing too long	Shorten the tubing by removing the extension tubing (if used), or replace the administration set with a set that has shorter tubing.
	Small air bubbles in tubing close to patient	Remove the air bubbles.
False-low pressure reading Arterial pressure drops below the patient's normal pressure without a significant change in baseline clinical findings. Before responding to this low pressure, recheck the system to ensure that the reading is accurate.	Improper calibration	Recalibrate the system.
	Transducer positioned above level of the phlebostatic axis	Relevel the transducer with the phlebostatic axis.
	Loose connections	Check and tighten all connections.
	Catheter kinked	Unkink the catheter.
	Clotted catheter tip	Attempt to aspirate the clot. If you're successful, flush the line. If you're unsuccessful, avoid flushing the line: You could dislodge the clot.
	Catheter tip resting against arterial line	Reposition the catheter insertion area, and flush the catheter. Alternatively, reposition the catheter by carefully rotating it or pulling it back slightly.

(continued)

Arterial lines *(continued)*

Problems	Possible causes	Interventions
False-low pressure reading *(continued)*	I.V. tubing too long	Shorten the tubing by removing the extension tubing (if used), or replace the administration set with a set having shorter tubing.
	Large air bubble close to transducer	Reprime the transducer.
No waveform No waveform appears on the monitor.	No power supply	Turn on the power.
	Loose connections	Check and tighten all connections.
	Stopcocks turned off to patient	Position the stopcocks properly. Make sure that the transducer is open to the catheter.
	Transducer disconnected from monitor module	Reconnect the transducer to the monitor module.
	Occluded catheter tip	Attempt to aspirate the clot. If you're successful, flush the line. If you're unsuccessful, avoid flushing the line; you could dislodge the clot.
	Catheter tip resting against arterial wall	Flush the catheter, or reposition it by carefully rotating it or pulling it back slightly.

Arterial line, accidental removal of

If the patient removes his arterial line, he's in danger of hypovolemic shock from blood loss. Here's what to do.

Stanching blood flow

■ Apply direct pressure to the insertion site immediately, and send someone to call the doctor. Maintain firm, direct pressure on the insertion site for 5 to 10 minutes to encourage clot formation because arterial blood flows under extremely high intravascular pressure.

■ Check the patient's I.V. line and, if ordered, increase the flow rate temporarily to compensate for blood loss.

When the bleeding stops

■ Apply a sterile pressure dressing.

■ Reassess the patient's level of consciousness (LOC), and comfort and reassure him; losing large quantities of blood may have a significant psychological as well as physiologic impact.

■ Estimate the amount of blood loss from what you see and from changes in the patient's blood pressure and heart rate.

■ When the doctor arrives, help him to reinsert the catheter, ensuring that the patient's arm is immobilized and the tubing and catheter are secured.

■ Withdraw blood for a complete blood count and arterial blood gas analysis as ordered.

Ongoing care

■ Closely monitor the patient's vital signs, LOC, skin color, temperature, and circulation to the extremity.

■ Watch for further bleeding or hematoma.

■ Decrease the I.V. flow rate to the previous level after the patient's condition has stabilized.

Respiratory monitors and devices

Pulse oximeters

To maintain a continuous display of arterial oxygen saturation levels, keep the monitoring site clean and dry. Make sure the skin doesn't become irritated from the adhesives used to keep the disposable probes in place. You may need to change the site if this happens. Also, nondisposable probes that don't need tape can replace disposable probes that irritate the skin.

Another common problem with pulse oximeters is the failure of the devices to obtain a signal. Your first reaction if this happens should be to check the patient's vital signs. If they're sufficient to produce a signal, then check for problems, including poor connection, inadequate or intermittent blood flow to the site, and equipment malfunction.

Poor connection

Check to see if the sensors are properly aligned. Make sure that the wires are intact and securely fastened and that the pulse oximeter is plugged into a power source.

Inadequate or intermittent blood flow to the site

Check the patient's pulse rate and capillary refill time, and take corrective action if blood flow to the site is decreased. This may mean loosening restraints, removing tight-fitting clothes, taking off a blood pressure cuff, or checking arterial and I.V. lines. If none of these interventions works, you may need to find an alternate site. Finding a site with proper circulation may also prove challenging when a patient is receiving a vasoconstrictor.

Equipment malfunction

Remove the pulse oximeter from the patient, set the alarm limits at 90% and 100%, and try the instrument on yourself or another healthy person. This will tell you if the equipment is working correctly.

Sⅴo₂ monitors

During continuous mixed venous oxygen saturation (Sⅴo₂) monitoring, watch for signs of equipment malfunction so that you can distinguish them from changes in your patient's condition and thus respond appropriately. This chart identifies the common problems, their causes, and nursing interventions.

Problems and possible causes	Interventions
Low-intensity alarm sounds Inadequate blood flow past catheter tip	■ Look for and straighten any obvious kinks in the catheter. ■ Follow facility procedure to ensure patency of the distal lumen. ■ Check for proper connection between the optical module and the computer.
Damaged fiber-optic filaments	■ Replace the catheter.
Damped intensity Blood clot over catheter tip	■ Follow facility procedure to ensure patency of the distal lumen.
Wedging of catheter tip	■ Reposition the catheter.
Erratic intensity Blood clot over catheter tip	■ Follow facility procedure to ensure patency of the distal lumen.
Wedging of catheter tip	■ Reposition the catheter.
High-intensity alarm sounds Catheter tip pressing against vessel wall	■ Reposition the catheter, examine the pressure waveform to confirm proper position.
Catheter floating distally into wedge position	■ Check the balloon status and confirm the proper position by examining the pressure waveform. ■ Reposition the catheter as needed.
LOW-LIGHT message Poor concentration between catheter and optical module	■ Disconnect the catheter from the optical module, close the lid, and place the optical module out of direct light. If the LOW-LIGHT message disappears, the problem is the catheter. Check the connection, and reattach as needed.
Defective optical module	■ Replace the optical module.
Poor connection between optical module and computer	■ Check the connections, and reconnect as needed. Turn off the computer for a few seconds, and turn it back on. You'll hear two beeps if the computer is functional and the connections are secure.

S̄vo₂ monitors *(continued)*

Problems and possible causes	Interventions
LOW–LIGHT message *(continued)* Damaged fiber-optic filaments	■ Gently manipulate the catheter, particularly around the insertion site. If this doesn't solve the problem, replace the catheter.
CAL FAIL message Unsuccessful preinsertion calibration	■ Verify a correct attachment between the catheter and the optical module; then repeat calibration. ■ If the CAL FAIL message still appears, replace the optical module.
Dashes in oxygen saturation display Improper preinsertion calibration	■ Verify a correct attachment between the catheter and the optical module; then repeat calibration.
Optical module malfunction	■ If dashes continue to appear, replace the optical module; then repeat calibration.
Catheter damage	■ Gently manipulate the catheter. If the monitor doesn't compute a range, replace the catheter; then repeat calibration.
Catheter tip improperly positioned	■ Reposition the catheter.
Loss of electronic memory	■ Determine the cause of the power loss; then repeat calibration.

Ventilators

Most ventilators have alarms to warn you of hazardous situations — for instance, when inspiratory pressure rises too high or drops too low. Use the chart below to help you respond quickly and effectively to a ventilator alarm.

Problems and possible causes	Interventions
Low pressure Tube disconnected from ventilator	Reconnect the tube to the ventilator.
Endotracheal (ET) tube displaced above vocal cords or tracheostomy tube extubated	If extubation or displacement has occurred, open the patient's airway, manually ventilate the patient, and call the doctor.

(continued)

Ventilators *(continued)*

Problems and possible causes	Interventions
Low pressure *(continued)*	
Leaking tidal volume from low cuff pressure (from underinflated or ruptured ET cuff or leak in cuff or one-way valve)	Listen for a whooshing sound (an air leak) around the tube; check cuff pressure. If you can't maintain pressure, the doctor may insert a new tube.
Ventilator malfunction	Disconnect the patient from the ventilator, and manually ventilate him, if necessary. Get another ventilator.
Leak in ventilator circuitry (from loose connection or hole in tubing, loss of temperature-sensing device, or cracked humidification container)	Make sure all connections are intact. Check the humidification container and the tubing for holes or leaks and replace them, if necessary.
High pressure	
Increased airway pressure or decreased lung compliance caused by worsening disease	Auscultate the lungs for evidence of increasing lung consolidation, barotrauma, or wheezing. Call the doctor, if necessary.
Patient biting on ET tube	If needed, insert a bite block.
Secretions in airway	Suction or have the patient cough.
Condensation in large-bore tubing	Remove any condensation.
Intubation of right mainstem bronchus	Check the tube's position. If it has slipped, call the doctor; he may need to reposition it.
Patient coughing, gagging, or trying to talk	If the patient is fighting the ventilator in any way, he may need a sedative or a neuromuscular blocker. Administer the drug as ordered.
Chest-wall resistance	Reposition the patient if his position limits chest expansion. If ineffective, give him the prescribed analgesic.
Malfunctioning high-pressure relief valve	Have the faulty equipment replaced.
Bronchospasm, pneumothorax, or barotrauma	Assess the patient for the cause. Report the disorder to the doctor, and treat as ordered.

Ventilators *(continued)*

Problems and possible causes	Interventions
Spirometer or low exhaled tidal volume, or low exhaled minute volume	
Power interruption	Check all electrical connections.
Loose connection or leak in delivery system	Make sure all connections in the delivery system are secure; check for leaks.
Leaking cuff or inadequate cuff seal	Listen for a leak with a stethoscope. Reinflate the cuff according to facility policy. Replace the cuff, if necessary.
Leaking chest tube	Check all chest tube connections. Make sure the water seal is intact; then notify the doctor.
Increased airway resistance in patient on pressure-cycled ventilator	Auscultate the lungs for signs of airway obstruction, barotrauma, or lung consolidation.
Disconnected spirometer	Make sure the spirometer is connected.
Any change that sets off high- or low-pressure alarms and prevents delivery of full air volume	See the interventions for high- and low-pressure alarms.
Malfunctioning volume measuring device	Alert the respiratory therapist to replace the device.
High respiratory rate	
Anxious patient	Assess the patient for the cause. Dispel the patient's fears, if possible; sedate him, if necessary. Establish an effective means of communication.
Patient in pain	Position the patient comfortably. Administer a medication for pain as ordered.
Secretions in airway	Suction the patient.
Low positive end–expiratory pressure (PEEP)/continuous positive airway pressure	
Leak in system	Make sure all connections are secure. Check for holes in the tubing, and replace it, if necessary.
Mechanical failure of PEEP mechanism	Discontinue the PEEP, and call a respiratory therapist.

Endotracheal or tracheostomy tube, accidental removal of

If an endotracheal or tracheostomy tube is accidentally removed or if the patient deliberately removes it, immediately take the following steps.

Endotracheal tube

■ Remove any remaining part of the tube.
■ Ventilate the patient using common resuscitation techniques or a handheld resuscitation bag.
■ Send someone to notify the doctor.
■ Restrain the patient if he extubated himself.
■ Periodically check the tube's position and the condition of the tape holding it, after it's reinserted. For a secure fit, anchor the tape from the nape of the patient's neck to and around the tube.

Tracheostomy tube

■ Remove any remaining part of the tube.

■ Keep the stoma open with a Kelly clamp, and try to insert a new tube. If you can't get the tube in, insert a suction catheter instead, and thread the tube over the catheter.
■ Call a code if you can't establish an effective airway and you no longer detect a pulse. Then either ventilate with a face mask and resuscitation bag, or remove the Kelly clamp to close the stoma, and perform mouth-to-mouth resuscitation until the doctor arrives. If air leaks from the stoma, cover it with an occlusive dressing. *Note:* Don't leave the patient alone until you've established that he has an effective airway and can breathe comfortably.
■ When a new tracheostomy tube is in place and the patient can breathe more easily, provide him with supplemental humidified oxygen until he receives a full evaluation.
■ Monitor the patient's vital signs, skin color, and level of consciousness and, unless contraindicated, elevate the head of his bed.

Chest drains

Problems	Interventions
Patient rolling over on drainage tubing, causing obstruction	■ Reposition the patient, and remove any kinks in the tubing. ■ Auscultate for decreased breath sounds, and percuss for dullness, which indicates a fluid accumulation, or for hyperresonance, which indicates an air accumulation.
Dependent loops in tubing trapping fluids and preventing effective drainage	■ Make sure the chest drainage unit sits below the patient's chest level. If necessary, raise the bed slightly to increase the gravity flow. Remove any kinks in the tubing. ■ Monitor the patient for decreased breath sounds, and percuss for dullness.
No drainage appearing in collection chamber	■ If draining blood or other fluid, suspect a clot or obstruction in the tubing. Gently milk the tubing to expel the obstruction, if facility policy permits. ■ Monitor the patient for lung-tissue compression caused by accumulated pleural fluid.

Chest drains *(continued)*

Problems	Interventions
Substantial increase in bloody drainage, indicating possible active bleeding or drainage of old blood	■ Monitor the patient's vital signs. Look for an increased pulse rate, decreased blood pressure, and orthostatic changes that may indicate acute blood loss. ■ Measure drainage every 15 to 30 minutes to determine if it's occurring continuously or in one gush as a result of position changes.
No bubbling in suction-control chamber	■ Check for obstructions in the tubing. Make sure all connections are tight. ■ Check that the suction apparatus is turned on. Increase the suction slowly until you see gentle bubbling.
Loud, vigorous bubbling in suction-control chamber	■ Turn down the suction source until bubbling is just visible.
Constant bubbling in water-seal chamber	■ Assess the chest drainage unit and tubing for an air leak. ■ If an air leak isn't noted in the external system, notify the doctor immediately. Leaking and trapping of air in the pleural space can result in a tension pneumothorax.
Evaporation causing water level in suction-control chamber to drop below desired -20 cm H_2O	■ Using a syringe and needle, add water or normal saline solution through a resealable diaphragm on the back of the suction-control chamber.
Trouble breathing immediately after special procedure; chest drainage unit improperly placed on the patient's bed, interfering with drainage	■ Raise the head of the bed and reposition the unit so that gravity promotes drainage. ■ Perform a quick respiratory assessment, and take his vital signs. Make sure enough water is in the water-seal and suction-control chambers.
As bed lowers, chest drainage unit caught under bed; tubing comes apart and becomes contaminated	■ Clamp the chest tube proximal to the latex connecting tubing. ■ Irrigate the tubing, using the sealed jar of sterile water or normal saline solution kept at the patient's bedside. ■ Insert the distal end of the chest tube into the jar of fluid until the end is 2 to 4 cm below the top of the water. Unclamp the chest tube. ■ Have another nurse obtain a new closed chest drainage system, and set it up. ■ Attach the chest tube to the new unit.

GI tubes

Nasoenteric-decompression tubes

If your patient's nasoenteric-decompression tube appears to be obstructed, notify the doctor right away. He may order the following measures to restore patency quickly and efficiently:

■ First, disconnect the tube from the suction source, and irrigate with normal saline solution. Use gravity flow to help clear the obstruction, unless ordered otherwise.

■ If irrigation doesn't establish patency, the position of the tube against the gastric mucosa may be causing the obstruction. Gentle tugging may help. For a double-lumen tube, such as a Salem pump, irrigate the pigtail port (blue) with 10 to 30 cc of air to help move the tube away from the mucosa.

If these measures don't work, the tube may be kinked and may need additional manipulation. Before proceeding:

■ Never reposition or irrigate a nasoenteric-decompression tube (without a doctor's order) in a patient who has had GI surgery.

■ Avoid manipulating a tube in a patient who had the tube inserted during surgery because you may disturb new sutures.

■ Don't try to reposition the tube in a patient who was difficult to intubate (because of an esophageal stricture, for example).

T tubes

T tubes, typically inserted in the common bile duct after cholecystectomy, may become blocked by viscous bile or clots. Notify the doctor and take these steps while you wait for him to arrive:

■ Unclamp the T tube (if it was clamped before and after a meal), and connect the tube to a closed gravity-drainage system.

■ Inspect the tube carefully to detect any kinks or obstructions.

■ Irrigate the tube with normal saline solution, if ordered, and prepare the patient for direct X-ray of the common bile duct (cholangiography). Briefly describe these measures to the patient to reduce his apprehension and promote his cooperation.

Total parenteral nutrition setups

Problems and possible causes	Interventions
Clotted catheter Interrupted flow rate, hypoglycemia, no blood return	■ Reposition the patient on his side. Attempt to aspirate the clot. If the clot remains, use a thrombolytic, according to facility policy.
Dislodged catheter Catheter out of vein, anterior chest pain, neck pain	■ Place a sterile gauze pad on the site and apply pressure if the catheter is completely out. For partial displacement, call the doctor. ■ Prepare for X-ray and repositioning with a guide wire or for removal and replacement.

Total parenteral nutrition setups *(continued)*

Problems and possible causes	Interventions
Air embolism Chest pain, tachycardia, hypotension, fear, seizures, loss of consciousness, cardiac arrest	■ Clamp the catheter. ■ Place the patient in Trendelenburg's position on his left side. Give oxygen as ordered. ■ If cardiac arrest occurs, begin cardiopulmonary resuscitation.
Thrombosis Erythema, edema, or pain at insertion site or along vein; ipsilateral swelling of arm, neck, and face; tachycardia	■ Anticipate prompt catheter removal. ■ Administer heparin as ordered. ■ Prepare for a venous flow study as ordered.
Too-rapid infusion Nausea, headache, lethargy, hyperglycemia	■ Check the infusion rate. ■ Check the infusion pump.
Extravasation Swelling or pain around insertion site	■ Stop the infusion, and assess for cardiopulmonary abnormalities. ■ Take a chest X-ray, if needed.
Hypoglycemia Headache, sweating, dizziness, palpitations	■ Give dextrose I.V. (10% as an infusion, 50% as an I.V. bolus) as ordered. ■ Avoid abrupt increases or decreases in the total parenteral nutrition (TPN) flow rate; wean the patient slowly from TPN.
Cracked or broken tubing Fluid leakage	■ Apply a padded hemostat above the break to prevent air from entering the line.
Sepsis Fever, chills, leukocytosis, positive blood cultures, glucose intolerance	■ Remove the catheter, and culture the tip. ■ Give the appropriate antibiotic.

Tube feedings

Problems	Interventions
Tube obstruction or clogging	■ Flush the tube with warm water or cranberry juice. If necessary, replace the tube. ■ Flush the tube with 50 ml of water after each feeding to remove excess sticky formula, which could occlude the tube.
Aspiration of gastric secretions	■ Discontinue the feeding immediately. ■ Perform tracheal suction of the aspirated contents, if possible. ■ Notify the doctor. He may order a prophylactic antibiotic or chest physiotherapy. ■ Check the tube placement before the feeding to prevent complications.
Nasal or pharyngeal irritation or necrosis	■ Change the tube's position. If necessary, replace the tube. ■ Provide frequent oral hygiene using mouthwash or lemon-glycerin swabs. Use petroleum jelly on cracked lips.
Vomiting, bloating, diarrhea, or cramps	■ Reduce the flow rate. ■ As ordered, administer metoclopramide to increase GI motility. ■ Warm the formula. ■ Position the patient on his right side with his head elevated for 30 minutes after the feeding to facilitate gastric emptying. ■ Notify the doctor. He may reduce the amount of formula being given during each feeding.

Neurologic monitors

Damped ICP waveforms

An intracranial pressure (ICP) waveform that looks like the one shown below signals a problem with the transducer or monitor. Check for line obstruction, and determine if the transducer needs rebalancing.

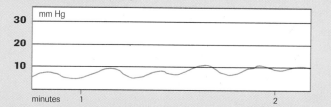

Problems	Interventions
Transducer or monitor needs recalibration	■ Turn the stopcock off to the patient. ■ Open the transducer's stopcock to air, and balance the transducer. ■ Recalibrate the transducer and monitor.
Air in line	■ Turn the stopcock off to the patient. ■ Using a syringe, flush the air out through an open stopcock port with sterile normal saline solution. *Note:* Never use heparin to flush the ICP line. You could accidentally inject some of the drug into the patient and cause bleeding. ■ Rebalance and recalibrate the transducer and monitor.
Loose connection in line	■ Check the tubing and stopcocks for moisture, which may indicate a loose connection. ■ Turn the stopcock off to the patient; then tighten all connections. ■ Make sure the tubing is long enough to allow the patient to turn his head without straining the tubing. This may prevent further problems.
Disconnection in line	■ Turn the stopcock off to the patient immediately. (Rapid cerebrospinal fluid loss through a ventricular catheter may allow the ICP to drop precipitously, causing a brain herniation.) ■ Replace the equipment to reduce the risk of infection.
Change in patient's position	■ Reposition the transducer's balancing port level with Monro's foramen. ■ Rebalance and recalibrate the transducer and monitor. *Remember:* Always balance and recalibrate at least once every 4 hours and whenever the patient is repositioned.
Tubing, catheter, or screw occluded with blood or brain tissue	■ Notify the doctor. He may want to irrigate the screw or catheter with a small amount (0.1 ml) of sterile normal saline solution. *Important:* Never irrigate the screw or catheter yourself.

10 Drug administration
Reviewing the methods

Administration guidelines

Precautions for drug administration

Whenever you administer any medication, observe the following precautions to ensure that you're giving the right drug in the right dose to the right patient.

Check the order
Check the order on the patient's medication record against the doctor's order.

Check the label
Check the label on the medication three times before administering it to a patient to ensure that you're administering the prescribed medication in the prescribed dose. Check it when you take the container from the shelf or drawer, right before pouring the medication into the medication cup or drawing it into the syringe, and before returning the container to the shelf or drawer. If you're administering a unit-dose medication, check the label for the third time immediately after pouring the medication and again before discarding the wrapper. (Remember, don't open a unit-dose medication until you're at the patient's bedside.)

Confirm the patient's identity
Before giving the medication, confirm the patient's identity by checking his name and the identification number on his wristband. Then make sure that you have the correct medication.

Always explain the procedure to the patient, and provide privacy.

Have a written order
Make sure you have a written order for every medication that's to be given. If the order is verbal, make sure the doctor signs for it within the specified time period.

Give labeled medication
Don't give medication from a poorly labeled or unlabeled container. Furthermore, don't attempt to label or reinforce drug labels yourself; a pharmacist must do that.

Monitor medication
Never give a medication that someone else has poured or prepared. Never allow your medication cart or tray out of your sight. Never return unwrapped or prepared medications to stock containers. Instead, dispose of them, and notify the pharmacy.

Respond to the patient's questions
If the patient questions you about his medication or the dosage, check his medication record again. If the medication is correct, reassure him that it's correct. Make sure you tell him about any changes in his medication or dosage. Instruct him, as appropriate, about possible adverse reactions, and encourage him to report any that he experiences.

Topical administration

Topical medications

Topical drugs, such as lotions and ointments, are applied directly to the patient's skin. They're commonly used for local, rather than systemic, effects. Typically, they must be applied two or three times per day for a full therapeutic effect.

Equipment
Patient's medication record and chart ◆ prescribed medication ◆ sterile tongue blades ◆ gloves ◆ sterile 4″ × 4″ gauze pads ◆ transparent semipermeable dressing ◆ adhesive tape ◆ solvent (such as cottonseed oil) ◆ optional: cotton-tipped applicators, cotton gloves, or terry cloth scuffs

Implementation

■ Explain the procedure to the patient because, after discharge, he may have to apply the medication by himself.

■ Wash your hands to prevent cross-contamination, and glove your dominant hand.

■ Help the patient to a comfortable position, and expose the area to be treated. Make sure the skin or mucous membrane is intact (unless the medication has been ordered to treat a skin lesion). Application of medication to broken or abraded skin may cause unwanted systemic absorption and result in further irritation.

■ If necessary, clean the skin of debris. You may have to change the glove if it becomes soiled.

To apply a paste, a cream, or an ointment

■ Open the container. Place the cap upside down to avoid contaminating its inner surface.

■ Remove a tongue blade from its sterile wrapper, and cover one end of it with medication from the tube or jar. Then transfer the medication from the tongue blade to your gloved hand.

■ Apply the medication to the affected area with long, smooth strokes that follow the direction of hair growth, as shown below.

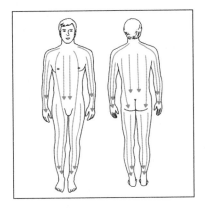

This technique avoids forcing medication into hair follicles, which can cause irritation and lead to folliculitis. Avoid excessive pressure when applying the medication because it could abrade the skin or cause patient discomfort.

■ When applying medication to the patient's face, use a cotton-tipped applicator for small areas such as under the eyes. For larger areas, use a sterile gauze pad, and follow the directions shown below.

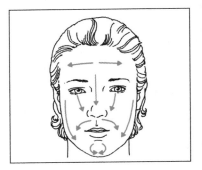

■ To prevent contamination of the medication, use a new sterile tongue blade each time you remove medication from the container.

To remove an ointment

■ Gently swab ointment from the patient's skin using a sterile 4″ × 4″ gauze pad saturated with a solvent such as cottonseed oil. Remove any remaining oil by wiping the area with a clean sterile gauze pad. Don't wipe too hard because you could irritate the skin.

To apply other topical medications

■ To apply a shampoo, follow package directions. Apply medication using your fingertips, or instruct the patient to do so, as shown at the top of the next page. Massage it into the scalp if appropriate.

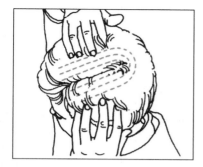

■ To apply an aerosol spray, shake the container, if indicated, to mix the medication. Hold the container 6″ to 12″ (15 to 30.5 cm) from the skin, or follow the manufacturer's recommendation. Spray the medication evenly over the treatment area to apply a thin film.

■ To apply a powder, dry the skin surface, and apply a thin layer of powder over the treatment area.

■ To protect applied medications and prevent them from soiling the patient's clothes, tape a sterile gauze pad or a transparent semipermeable dressing over the treated area. If you're applying topical medication to his hands, cover them with cotton gloves; to his feet, terry cloth scuffs.

■ Assess the patient's skin for signs of irritation, allergic reaction, or breakdown.

Special considerations

■ To prevent skin irritation from an accumulation of medication, always remove residue from previous applications before applying a new one.

■ Always wear gloves to prevent your skin from absorbing the medication.

■ Never apply ointment to the eyelids or ear canal unless ordered. The ointment may congeal and occlude the tear duct or ear canal.

■ Inspect the treated area frequently for any adverse or allergic reactions.

Transdermal medications

Given through an adhesive patch or measured dose of ointment applied to the skin, transdermal drugs deliver constant, controlled medication directly into the bloodstream for a prolonged systemic effect.

Medications available in transdermal form include nitroglycerin, which is used to control angina; scopolamine, which is used to treat motion sickness; estradiol, which is used for postmenopausal hormone replacement; clonidine, which is used to treat hypertension; and fentanyl, which is used to control chronic pain.

Nitroglycerin ointment dilates coronary vessels for 2 to 12 hours; a nitroglycerin patch can produce the same effect for as long as 24 hours.

The scopolamine patch can relieve motion sickness for as long as 72 hours. Transdermal estradiol lasts 72 hours to 1 week; clonidine, 7 days; and fentanyl, up to 72 hours.

Equipment

Patient's medication record and chart ◆ gloves ◆ prescribed medication (patch or ointment) ◆ application strip or measuring paper (for nitroglycerin ointment) ◆ adhesive tape ◆ optional: plastic wrap or semipermeable dressing (for nitroglycerin ointment)

Implementation

■ Wash your hands, and put on gloves.

■ Make sure that any previously applied medication has been removed from the skin.

■ Locate a new site for application, different from the previous site.

To apply transdermal ointment

■ Place the prescribed amount of ointment on the application strip or measuring paper, taking care not to get any on your skin.

■ Apply the strip to any dry, hairless area of the body. Don't rub the ointment into the skin.

■ Tape the application strip and ointment to the skin. If desired, cover the application strip with plastic wrap, and tape the wrap in place.

To apply a transdermal patch
■ Open the package and remove the patch.

■ Without touching the adhesive surface, remove the clear plastic backing.

■ Apply the patch to a dry, hairless area — behind the ear, for example, as with scopolamine. Avoid any area that may cause uneven absorption, such as skin folds or scars, or any irritated or damaged skin. Don't apply the patch below the elbow or knee.

After applying transdermal medications
■ Store the medication as ordered.

■ Instruct the patient to keep the area around the patch or ointment as dry as possible.

■ Wash your hands immediately after applying the patch or ointment.

Special considerations
■ Reapply daily transdermal medications at the same time every day to ensure a continuous effect, but alternate the application sites to avoid skin irritation.

■ Before applying nitroglycerin ointment, obtain the patient's baseline blood pressure. Obtain another blood pressure reading 5 minutes after applying the ointment. If the blood pressure has dropped significantly and the patient has a headache, notify the doctor immediately. If the blood pressure has dropped but the patient has no symptoms, instruct him to lie still until the blood pressure returns to normal.

■ Before reapplying nitroglycerin ointment, remove the plastic wrap, the application strip, and any ointment remaining on the skin at the previous site.

■ When applying a scopolamine patch, instruct the patient not to drive or operate machinery until his response to the drug has been determined.

■ If the patient is using a clonidine patch, encourage him to check with his doctor before using any over-the-counter cough preparations because they may counteract the effects of clonidine.

Nitroglycerin ointment

Unlike most topical medications, nitroglycerin ointment is used for its transdermal systemic effect. It's used to dilate the arteries and veins, thus improving cardiac perfusion in a patient with cardiac ischemia or angina pectoris.

Nitroglycerin ointment is prescribed by the inch, and comes with a rectangular piece of ruled paper to be used in applying the medication.

Equipment
Patient's medication record and chart ◆ ointment ◆ ruled paper ◆ plastic wrap or transparent semipermeable dressing ◆ adhesive tape ◆ sphygmomanometer ◆ optional: gloves

Implementation
■ Start by taking the patient's baseline blood pressure to compare it with later readings.

■ Put on gloves if you wish to avoid contact with the medication.

■ Squeeze the prescribed amount of ointment onto the ruled paper, as shown at the top of the next page.

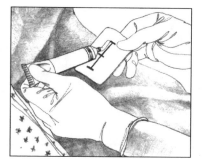

■ After measuring the correct amount of ointment, tape the paper, drug side down, directly to the skin. Some health care facilities require you to use the paper to apply the medication to the patient's skin, usually on the chest or arm. Spread a thin layer of ointment over a 3″ (7.6-cm) area.

Special considerations

■ For increased absorption, the doctor may request that you cover the site with plastic wrap or transparent semipermeable dressing, as shown below.

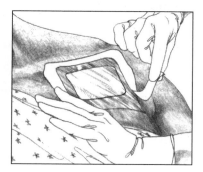

■ After 5 minutes, record the patient's blood pressure. If it has dropped significantly and he has a headache (from vasodilation of blood vessels in his head), notify the doctor immediately. He may reduce the dose.
■ If the patient's blood pressure has dropped but he has no adverse reac-

tions, instruct him to lie still until it returns to normal.

Eye medications

Eye medications — drop or ointments — serve diagnostic and therapeutic purposes. During an eye examination, eye medications can be used to anesthetize the eye, dilate the pupil, and stain the cornea to identify anomalies. Therapeutic uses include eye lubrication and treatment of such conditions as glaucoma and infections.

Equipment and preparation

Patient's medication record and chart ◆ prescribed eye medication ◆ sterile cotton balls ◆ gloves ◆ warm water or normal saline solution ◆ sterile gauze pads ◆ facial tissue ◆ optional: ocular dressing

Make sure the medication is labeled for opthalmic use. Then check the expiration date. Remember to date the container after first use.

Inspect ocular solutions for cloudiness, discoloration, and precipitation, but remember that some eye medications are suspensions and normally appear cloudy. Don't use any solution that appears abnormal.

Implementation

■ Make sure you know which eye to treat because different medications or doses may be ordered for each eye. Know that "OD" means right eye, "OS" means left eye, and "OU" means both eyes.
■ Put on gloves.
■ If the patient has an ocular dressing, remove it by pulling it down and away from his forehead. Avoid contaminating your hands.
■ To remove exudate or meibomian gland secretions, clean around the eye with sterile cotton balls or sterile gauze pads moistened with warm water or

normal saline solution. Have the patient close his eye; then gently wipe the eyelids from the inner to outer canthus. Use a fresh cotton ball or gauze pad for each stroke.

■ Have the patient sit or lie in the supine position. Instruct him to tilt his head back and toward his affected eye so that excess medication can flow away from the tear duct, minimizing systemic absorption through nasal mucosa.

■ Remove the dropper cap from the medication container, and draw the medication into it.

■ Before instilling eyedrops, instruct the patient to look up and away. This moves the cornea away from the lower lid and minimizes the risk of touching it with the dropper.

To instill eyedrops

■ Steady the hand that's holding the dropper by resting it against the patient's forehead. With your other hand, pull down the lower lid of the affected eye, and instill the drops in the conjunctival sac. Never instill eyedrops directly onto the eyeball.

⟳ *Patient teaching tips* When teaching elderly patients how to instill eyedrops, keep in mind that they may have difficulty sensing drops in the eye. Suggest chilling the medication slightly to enhance the sensation.

To apply eye ointment

■ Squeeze a small ribbon of medication on the edge of the conjunctival sac from the inner to the outer canthus, as shown at top right. Cut off the ribbon by turning the tube.

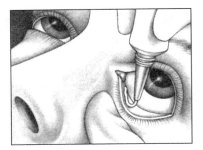

After instilling eyedrops or applying ointment

■ Instruct the patient to close his eyes gently, without squeezing the lids shut. If you instilled drops, tell him to blink. If you applied ointment, tell him to roll his eyes behind closed lids to help distribute the medication over the eyeball.

■ Use a clean facial tissue to remove any excess medication leaking from the eye. Use a fresh tissue for each eye to prevent cross-contamination.

■ Apply a new ocular dressing, if necessary.

■ Remove and discard gloves. Then wash your hands.

Special considerations

■ When administering an eye medication that may be absorbed systemically, press your thumb on the inner canthus for 1 to 2 minutes after instillation while the patient closes his eyes.

■ To maintain the drug container's sterility, never touch the tip of the dropper or bottle to the eye area. Discard any solution remaining in the dropper before returning it to the bottle. If the dropper or bottle tip has become contaminated, discard it, and use another sterile dropper.

Eye medication disks

Small and flexible, an eye medication disk is an oval disk that can release medication (such as pilocarpine) in the eye for up to 1 week. Floating between the eyelids and the sclera, the disk stays in the eye while the patient sleeps and even during swimming and other athletic activities. The disk frees the patient from having to remember to instill his eye medication. Eye moisture or contact lenses don't adversely affect the disk.

Equipment
Patient's medication record and chart ◆ prescribed eye medication ◆ sterile gloves

Implementation
■ Make sure you know which eye to treat because different medications or doses may be ordered for each eye.

To insert an eye medication disk
■ Insert the disk at bedtime to minimize initial blurring.
■ Wash your hands, and put on the sterile gloves.
■ Press your fingertip against the disk so that it sticks lengthwise across your fingertip.
■ Gently pull the patient's lower eyelid away from the eye, and place the disk in the conjunctival sac. It should lie horizontally, as shown below, not vertically. The disk will adhere to the eye naturally.

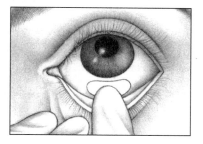

■ Pull the lower eyelid out, up, and over the disk. Tell the patient to blink several times. If the disk is still visible, pull lower lid out and over the disk again. Tell him that once the disk is in place, he can adjust its position by pressing his finger against his closed lid. Warn him not to rub his eye or move the disk across the cornea.
■ If the disk falls out, rinse the disk in cool water, and reinsert it. If the disk appears bent, replace it.
■ If both eyes are being treated with medication disks, replace both disks at the same time.
■ If the disk repeatedly slips out of position, reinsert it under the upper eyelid. To do this, gently lift and evert the upper eyelid, and insert the disk in the conjunctival sac. Then gently pull the lid back into position, and tell the patient to blink several times. The more he uses the disk, the easier it should be for him to retain it. If not, notify the doctor.

To remove an eye medication disk
■ To remove the disk with one finger, put on sterile gloves and evert the lower eyelid to expose the disk. Then use the forefinger of your other hand to slide the disk into the lid and out of the patient's eye. To use two fingers, evert the lower lid with one hand to expose the disk. Then pinch it with the thumb and forefinger of your other hand, and remove it.
■ If the disk is located in the upper eyelid, apply long circular strokes to the closed eyelid with your finger until you can see the disk in the corner of the eye. Then place your finger directly on the disk, move it to the lower sclera, and remove it as you would a disk located in the lower lid.

Special considerations

■ If the patient will continue therapy with an eye medication disk after discharge, teach him to insert and remove it himself. Have him demonstrate the techniques for you.

■ Explain that mild reactions are common but should subside within the first 6 weeks of use. Foreign-body sensation in the eye, mild tearing or redness, increased mucus discharge, eyelid redness, and itchiness can occur. Blurred vision, stinging, swelling, and headaches can occur with pilocarpine, specifically. Tell him to report persistent or severe signs or symptoms.

Eardrops

Eardrops may be instilled to treat infection and inflammation, to soften cerumen for later removal, to produce local anesthesia, or to facilitate removal of an insect trapped in the ear.

Equipment and preparation

Patient's medication record and chart ◆ prescribed eardrops ◆ light source ◆ facial tissue or cotton-tipped applicator ◆ optional: cotton ball, bowl of warm water

First, warm the medication to body temperature in the bowl of warm water or carry it in your pocket for 30 minutes before administration. If necessary, test the temperature of the medication by placing a drop on your wrist. (If the medication is too hot, it may burn the patient's eardrum.) To avoid injuring the ear canal, check the dropper before use to make sure it isn't chipped or cracked.

Implementation

■ Wash your hands.

■ Confirm the patient's identity by asking his name and checking the name, room number, and bed number on his wristband.

■ Have the patient lie on the side opposite the affected ear.

■ Straighten the patient's ear canal. For an adult, pull the auricle up and back.

 Age alert For an infant or child younger than age 3, gently pull the auricle down and back — the ear canal is straighter at this age.

■ Using a light source, examine the ear canal for drainage. If you find any, clean the canal with a facial tissue or cotton-tipped applicator because drainage can reduce the medication's effectiveness.

■ Compare the label on the eardrops with the order on the patient's medication record. Check the label again while drawing the medication into the dropper. Check the label for the final time before returning the eardrops to the shelf or drawer.

■ To avoid damaging the ear canal with the dropper, gently rest the hand holding the dropper against the patient's head. Straighten the patient's ear canal, and instill the ordered number of drops. To avoid patient discomfort, aim the dropper so that the drops fall against the sides of the ear canal, not on the eardrum. Hold the ear canal in position until you see the medication disappear down the canal. Lightly massage or apply gentle pressure to the targus of the ear after instilling the drops.

■ Instruct the patient to remain on his side for 5 to 10 minutes to allow the medication to run down into the ear canal.

■ Tuck the cotton ball (if ordered) loosely into the opening of the ear canal to prevent the medication from leaking out. Be careful not to insert it too deeply into the canal because doing so would prevent drainage of secretions and increase pressure on the eardrum.

■ Clean and dry the outer ear.

■ If ordered, repeat the procedure in the other ear after 5 to 10 minutes.
■ Assist the patient into a comfortable position.
■ Wash your hands.

Special considerations

■ Remember that some conditions make the normally tender ear canal even more sensitive, so be especially gentle when performing this procedure.
■ To prevent injury to the eardrum when inserting a cotton-tipped applicator make sure the cotton tip always remains in view. After applying eardrops to soften cerumen, irrigate the ear, as ordered, to facilitate its removal.
■ If the patient has vertigo, keep the side rails of his bed up, and assist him as necessary during the procedure. Also, move slowly and unhurriedly to avoid exacerbating his vertigo.
■ If necessary, teach the patient to instill the eardrops correctly so that he can continue treatment at home. Review the procedure, and let the patient try it himself while you observe.

Nasal medications

Nasal medications may be instilled by means of drops, a spray (using an atomizer), or an aerosol (using a nebulizer), most producing local rather than systemic effects. Drops can be directed at a specific area; sprays and aerosols diffuse medication throughout the nasal passages. Nasal medications include vasoconstrictors, antiseptics, anesthetics, and corticosteroids.

Equipment

Patient's medication record and chart ◆ prescribed medication ◆ emesis basin (for nose drops) ◆ facial tissues ◆ optional: pillow, piece of soft rubber or plastic tubing, gloves

Implementation

■ Wash your hands. Put on gloves, if necessary.

To instill nose drops

■ Draw some medication into the dropper.
■ To reach the ethmoidal and sphenoidal sinuses, have the patient lie on his back with his neck hyperextended and his head tilted back over the edge of the bed. Support his head with one hand to prevent neck strain.
■ To reach the maxillary and frontal sinuses, have the patient lie on his back with his head toward the affected side and hanging slightly over the edge of the bed. Ask him to rotate his head laterally after hyperextension, and support his head with one hand to prevent neck strain.
■ To relieve ordinary nasal congestion, help the patient to a reclining or supine position with his head tilted slightly toward the affected side. Aim the dropper upward, toward the patient's eye, rather than downward toward his ear.
■ Insert the dropper about $1/3''$ (8 mm) into the nostril. Make sure it doesn't touch the sides of the nostril to avoid contaminating the dropper or making the patient sneeze.
■ Instill the prescribed number of drops, observing the patient for any signs of discomfort.
■ Keep the patient's head tilted back for at least 5 minutes, and have him breathe through his mouth to prevent the drops from leaking out and to allow time for the medication to work.
■ Keep an emesis basin handy so that the patient can expectorate any medication that flows into the oropharynx and mouth. Wipe excess medication from the patient's face with facial tissues.

■ Instruct the patient not to blow his nose for several minutes after instillation.

■ Return the dropper to the bottle, and close it tightly.

To use a nasal spray

■ Have the patient sit upright with his head upright.

■ Remove the protective cap from the atomizer.

■ Occlude one of the patient's nostrils, and insert the atomizer tip about ½″ (1.3 cm) into the open nostril. Position the tip straight up toward the inner canthus of the eye.

■ Depending on the drug, have the patient hold his breath or inhale. Then squeeze the atomizer once quickly and firmly — just enough to coat the inside of the nose. Excessive force may propel the medication into the patient's sinuses and cause a headache. Repeat the procedure in the other nostril as ordered.

■ Tell the patient to keep his head tilted back for several minutes, to breathe slowly through his nose, and not to blow his nose, to ensure that the medication has time to work.

To use a nasal aerosol

■ Insert the medication cartridge according to the manufacturer's directions. Shake it well before each use, and remove the protective cap.

■ Hold the aerosol between your thumb and index finger (index finger on top of the cartridge).

■ Tilt the patient's head back slightly, and carefully insert the adapter tip in one nostril. Depending on the medication, tell the patient to hold his breath or inhale.

■ Press your fingers together firmly to release one measured dose of medication.

■ Shake the aerosol, and repeat the procedure to instill medication into the other nostril.

■ Remove the cartridge, and wash the nasal adapter daily in lukewarm water. Allow the adapter to dry before reinserting the cartridge.

■ Tell patient not to blow his nose for at least 2 minutes afterward.

Special considerations

🌀 *Age alert* For a child or an uncooperative patient, place a short piece of tubing on the dropper end to avoid damaging mucous membranes.

Vaginal medications

Vaginal medications include suppositories, creams, gels, and ointments. These medications can be inserted as topical treatment for infection (particularly *Trichomonas vaginalis* and candidal vaginitis) or inflammation, or as a contraceptive. Suppositories melt when they come in contact with the warm vaginal mucosa, and their medication diffuses topically — as effectively as creams, gels, and ointments.

Vaginal medications usually come with a disposable applicator that enables placement of medication in the anterior and posterior fornices. Vaginal administration is most effective when the patient can remain lying down afterward, to retain the medication.

Equipment

Patient's medication record and chart ◆ prescribed medication and applicator, if needed ◆ gloves ◆ water-soluble lubricant ◆ cotton balls ◆ soap and warm water ◆ small sanitary pad

Implementation

■ If possible, plan to give vaginal medications at bedtime, when the patient is recumbent.

■ Wash your hands, explain the procedure to the patient, and provide privacy.

■ Ask the patient to void.

■ Ask the patient if she would rather insert the medication herself. If so, provide appropriate instructions. If not, proceed with the following steps.

■ Help her into the lithotomy position.

■ Expose only the perineum.

To insert a suppository

■ Remove the suppository from the wrapper, and lubricate it with a water-soluble lubricant.

■ Put on gloves, and expose the vagina by spreading the labia.

■ If you see any discharge, wash the area with several cotton balls soaked in warm, soapy water. Clean each side of the perineum and then the center, using a fresh cotton ball for each stroke. While the labia are still separated, insert the suppository 3″ to 4″ (7.5 to 10 cm) into the vagina.

To insert an ointment, cream, or gel

■ Fit the applicator to the tube of medication, and gently squeeze the tube to fill the applicator with the prescribed amount of medication. Lubricate the applicator tip.

■ Put on gloves, and expose the vagina.

■ Insert the applicator about 2″ (5.1 cm) in the patient's vagina, and administer the medication by depressing the plunger on the applicator.

■ Instruct the patient to remain in a supine position with her knees flexed for 5 to 10 minutes, to allow the medication to flow into the posterior fornix.

After vaginal insertion

■ Remove and discard your gloves.

■ Wash the applicator with soap and warm water and store or discard it, as appropriate. Label it so it will be used only for the same patient.

■ To prevent the medication from soiling the patient's clothing and bedding, provide a sanitary pad.

■ Help the patient return to a comfortable position, and advise her to remain in bed as much as possible for the next several hours.

■ Wash your hands thoroughly.

Special considerations

■ Refrigerate vaginal suppositories that melt at room temperature.

■ If possible, teach the patient how to insert vaginal medication. She may have to administer it herself after discharge. Give her a patient-teaching sheet if one is available.

■ Instruct the patient not to wear a tampon after inserting vaginal medication because it will absorb the medication and decrease its effectiveness.

Respiratory administration

Handheld oropharyngeal inhalers

Handheld inhalers include the metered-dose inhaler or nebulizer, and the turbo-inhaler. These devices deliver topical medications to the respiratory tract, producing local and systemic effects. The mucosal lining of the respiratory tract absorbs the inhalant almost immediately. Examples of inhalants are bronchodilators, which are used to improve airway patency and facilitate mucus drainage, and mucolytics, which liquefy tenacious bronchial secretions.

Equipment

Patient's medication records and chart ◆ metered-dose inhaler or turbo-inhaler ◆ prescribed medications ◆ normal saline solution ♦ optional: spacer or extender

Implementation
To use a metered-dose inhaler
■ Shake the inhaler bottle. Remove the cap, and insert the stem into the small hole on the flattened portion of the mouthpiece, as shown below.

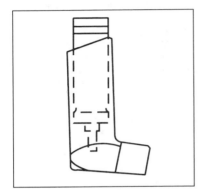

■ Have the patient exhale. Place the inhaler about 1″ (2.5 cm) in front of his open mouth.
■ As you push the bottle down against the mouthpiece, instruct the patient to inhale slowly through his mouth and to continue inhaling until his lungs feel full. Compress the bottle against the mouthpiece only once.
■ Remove the inhaler, and tell the patient to hold his breath for several seconds. Then instruct him to exhale slowly through pursed lips to keep the distal bronchioles open, allowing increased absorption and diffusion of the drug.
■ Have the patient gargle with tap water, if desired, to remove the medication from the mouth and back of the throat.
■ Have the patient wait 1 to 3 minutes before another inhalation is administered.

To use a turbo-inhaler
■ Hold the mouthpiece in one hand, and with the other hand, slide the sleeve away from the mouthpiece as far as possible, as shown below.

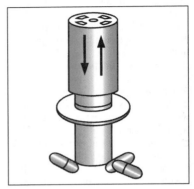

■ Unscrew the tip of the mouthpiece by turning it counterclockwise.
■ Press the colored portion of the medication capsule into the propeller stem of the mouthpiece. Screw the inhaler together again.
■ Holding the inhaler with the mouthpiece at the bottom, slide the sleeve all the way down and then up again to puncture the capsule and release the medication. Do this only once.
■ Have the patient exhale completely and tilt his head back. Instruct him to place the mouthpiece in his mouth, close his lips around it, and inhale once. Tell him to hold his breath for several seconds.
■ Remove the inhaler from the patient's mouth, and tell him to exhale as much air as possible.
■ Repeat the procedure until all the medication in the device is inhaled.
■ Have the patient gargle with normal saline solution, if desired.

To use a holding chamber (InspirEase)
■ Insert the inhaler into the mouthpiece of the holding chamber, and

shake the inhaler. Then place the mouthpiece into the opening of the holding device, and twist the mouthpiece to lock it in place.

■ Extend the holding device, have the patient exhale, and place the mouthpiece in his mouth.

■ Press down on the inhaler once. Then have the patient inhale slowly and deeply, collapsing the bag completely. If he breathes incorrectly, the bag will make a whistling sound. Tell the patient to hold his breath for 5 to 10 seconds and then exhale slowly into the bag. Then repeat the inhaling and exhaling steps.

■ Have the patient wait 1 to 2 minutes and then repeat the procedure, if ordered.

■ Disconnect the holding chamber from the mouthpiece, rinse both in lukewarm water, and allow them to air-dry.

Special considerations

■ Teach the patient how to use the inhaler so that he can continue treatments after discharge, if necessary. Explain that an overdose can cause the medication to lose its effectiveness. Tell him to record the date and time of each inhalation and his response.

■ Know that some oral respiratory drugs can cause restlessness, palpitations, nervousness, other systemic effects, and hypersensitivity reactions, such as rash, urticaria, and bronchospasm.

■ If the patient has heart disease, use caution when administering an oral respiratory drug because it can potentiate coronary insufficiency, cardiac arrhythmias, or hypertension. If paradoxical bronchospasm occurs, discontinue the drug, and call the doctor.

Enteral administration

Oral medications

Most drugs are administered orally because this route is usually the safest, most convenient, and least expensive. Drugs for oral administration are available in many forms, including tablets, enteric-coated tablets, capsules, syrups, elixirs, oils, liquids, suspensions, powders, and granules. Some require special preparation before administration, such as mixing with juice to make them more palatable.

Oral drugs are sometimes prescribed in higher dosages than their parenteral equivalents because after absorption through the GI system, the liver breaks them down before they reach the systemic circulation.

Equipment

Patient's medication record and chart ◆ prescribed medication ◆ optional: medication cup; appropriate vehicle (such as jelly or applesauce) for crushed pills commonly used with children or elderly patients, or juice, water, or milk for liquid medications; and crushing or cutting device

Implementation

■ Wash your hands.

■ Assess the patient's condition, including level of consciousness, swallowing ability, and vital signs as needed. Changes in his condition may warrant withholding medication.

■ Give the patient his medication and, as needed, liquid to aid swallowing, minimize adverse effects, or promote absorption. If appropriate, crush the medication to facilitate swallowing.

■ Stay with the patient until he has swallowed the drug. If he seems confused or disoriented, check his mouth to make sure he has swallowed it. Return and reassess the patient's response within 1 hour after giving the medication.

Special considerations
■ To avoid damaging or staining the patient's teeth, give acid or iron preparations through a straw. An unpleasant-tasting liquid can usually be made more palatable if taken through a straw because the liquid comes in contact with fewer taste buds.

■ If the patient can't swallow a whole tablet or capsule, ask the pharmacist if the drug is available in liquid form or if it can be administered by another route. If not, ask him if you can crush the tablet or open the capsule and mix it with food.

Drug delivery through a nasogastric tube or gastrostomy button

In addition to providing an alternate means of nourishment, the nasogastric (NG) tube allows direct instillation of medication into the GI system for patients who can't ingest it orally. The gastrostomy button, inserted into an established stoma, lies flush with the skin and receives a feeding tube.

Equipment and preparation
Patient's medication record and chart ♦ prescribed medication ♦ towel or linen-saver pad ♦ 50- or 60-ml piston-type catheter-tip syringe ♦ feeding tubing ♦ two 4″ × 4″ gauze pads ♦ stethoscope ♦ gloves ♦ diluent (juice, water, or a nutritional supplement) ♦ cup for mixing medication and fluid ♦ spoon ♦ 50-ml cup of water ♦ gastrostomy tube and funnel, if needed ♦ optional: pill-crushing equipment, clamp (if not already attached to tube)

Gather equipment for use at bedside. Liquids should be at room temperature to avoid abdominal cramping.

Make sure the cup, syringe, spoon, and gauze are clean.

Implementation
To give a drug through an NG tube
■ Wash your hands, and put on gloves.

■ Unpin the tube from the patient's gown. To avoid soiling the sheets during the procedure, fold back the bed linens, and drape the patient's chest with a towel or linen-saver pad.

■ Help the patient into Fowler's position, if her condition allows.

■ After unclamping the tube, auscultate the patient's abdomen about 3″ (7.6 cm) below the sternum, while you gently insert 10 cc of air into the tube with the 50- or 60-ml syringe. You should hear the air bubble entering the stomach. Gently draw back on the piston of the syringe. The appearance of gastric contents implies that the tube is patent and in the stomach.

■ If no gastric contents appear or if you meet resistance, the tube may be lying against the gastric mucosa. Withdraw the tube slightly, or turn the patient to free it.

■ Clamp the tube, detach the syringe, and lay the end of the tube on the 4″ × 4″ gauze pad.

■ If the medication is in tablet form, crush it before mixing with the diluent. (Make sure the particles are small enough to pass through the eyes at the distal end of the tube.) Open the capsules, and pour them into the diluent. Pour liquid medications into the diluent, and stir well.

■ Reattach the syringe, without the piston, to the end of the tube. Holding the tube upright at a level slightly above the patient's nose, open the clamp, and pour in the medication slowly and steadily, as shown at the top of the next page.

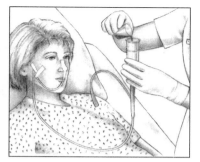

■ To prevent air from entering the patient's stomach, hold the tube at a slight angle, and add more medication before the syringe empties.
■ If the medication flows smoothly, slowly give the entire dose. If it doesn't flow, it may be too thick. If so, dilute it with water. If you suspect the tube placement is inhibiting the flow, stop the procedure, and reevaluate the placement.
■ Watch the patient's reaction, and stop immediately if she shows signs of discomfort.
■ As the last of the medication flows out of the syringe, start to irrigate the tube by adding 30 to 50 ml of water (15 to 30 ml for a child). Irrigation clears medication from the tube and reduces the risk of clogging.
■ When the water stops flowing, clamp the tube. Detach the syringe, and discard it properly.
■ Fasten the tube to the patient's gown, and make sure the patient is comfortable.
■ Leave the patient in Fowler's position, or on her right side with her head partially elevated, for at least 30 minutes to facilitate flow and prevent esophageal reflux.

To give a drug through a gastrostomy button
■ Assist the patient into an upright position.

■ Put on gloves, and open the safety plug on top of the device.
■ Attach the feeding tube set to the button.
■ Remove the piston from the catheter-tipped syringe, and insert the tip into the distal end of the feeding tube.
■ Pour the prescribed medication into the syringe and allow it to flow into the stomach.
■ After instilling all of the medication, pour 30 to 50 ml of water into the syringe, and allow it to flow through the tube.
■ When all water has been delivered, remove the feeding tube and replace the safety plug. Keep the patient in semi-Fowler's position for 30 minutes after giving the medication.

Special considerations
■ If you must give a tube feeding as well as instill medication, give the medication first to ensure that the patient receives it all.
■ If residual stomach contents exceed 100 ml, withhold the medication and feeding, and notify the doctor. Excessive contents may indicate intestinal obstruction or paralytic ileus.
■ If the NG tube is on suction, turn it off for 20 to 30 minutes after giving medication.

Buccal and sublingual medications

Certain drugs are given buccally (between the patient's cheek and teeth) or sublingually (under the patient's tongue) to bypass the digestive tract and facilitate their absorption into the bloodstream.

Drugs given buccally include erythrityl tetranitrate. Drugs given sublingually include ergotamine tartrate, erythrityl tetranitrate, isoproterenol hydrochloride, isosorbide dinitrate, and nitroglycerin.

When using either administration method, you must observe the patient carefully to ensure that he doesn't swallow the drug or suffer mucosal irritation.

Equipment

Patient's medication record and chart ◆ prescribed medication ◆ medication cup

Implementation

■ Wash your hands.
■ For buccal administration, place the tablet in the patient's buccal pouch, between the cheek and teeth.
■ For sublingual administration, place the tablet under the patient's tongue.
■ Instruct the patient to keep the medication in place until it dissolves completely to ensure absorption.
■ Caution him against chewing the tablet or touching it with his tongue, to prevent accidental swallowing.
■ Tell him not to smoke before the drug has dissolved because nicotine's vasoconstrictive effects slow absorption.

Special considerations

■ Don't give liquids because some buccal tablets may take up to 1 hour to be absorbed.
■ If the patient has angina, tell him to wet the nitroglycerin tablet with saliva and to keep it under his tongue until it's fully absorbed.

Rectal suppositories or ointment

A rectal suppository is a small, solid, medicated mass, usually cone-shaped, with a cocoa butter or glycerin base. It may be inserted to stimulate peristalsis and defecation or to relieve pain, vomiting, and local irritation. An ointment is a semisolid medication used to produce local effects. It may be applied externally to the anus or internally to the rectum.

Equipment and preparation

Patient's medication record and chart ◆ rectal suppository or tube of ointment and ointment applicator ◆ 4″ × 4″ gauze pads ◆ gloves ◆ water-soluble lubricant ◆ optional: bedpan

Store rectal suppositories in the refrigerator until needed to prevent softening and possible decreased effectiveness of the medication. A softened suppository is also difficult to handle and insert. To harden it again, hold the suppository (in its wrapper) under cold running water.

Implementation

■ Wash your hands.

To insert a rectal suppository

■ Place the patient on his left side in Sims' position. Drape him with the bedcovers, exposing only the buttocks. Put on gloves. Unwrap the suppository, and lubricate it with water-soluble lubricant.
■ Lift the patient's upper buttock with your nondominant hand to expose the anus.
■ Instruct the patient to take several deep breaths through his mouth to relax the anal sphincter and to reduce anxiety during drug insertion.
■ Using the index finger of your dominant hand, insert the suppository — tapered end first — about 3″ (7.6 cm) until you feel it pass the internal anal sphincter, as shown below.

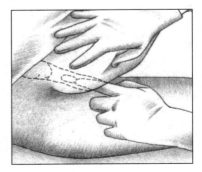

■ Direct the suppository's tapered end toward the side of the rectum so it touches the membranes.

■ Encourage the patient to lie quietly and, if applicable, to retain the suppository for the correct length of time. Press on the anus with a gauze pad, if necessary, until the urge to defecate passes.

■ Discard the used equipment.

To apply an ointment
■ For external application, wear gloves or use a gauze pad to spread medication over the anal area.

■ To apply internally, attach the applicator to the tube of ointment, and coat the applicator with water-soluble lubricant.

■ Expect to use about 1″ (2.5 cm) of ointment. To gauge how much pressure to use during application, try squeezing a small amount from the tube before you attach the applicator.

■ Lift the patient's upper buttock with your nondominant hand to expose the anus.

■ Tell the patient to take several deep breaths through his mouth to relax the anal sphincter and reduce discomfort during insertion. Then gently insert the applicator, directing it toward the umbilicus, as shown below.

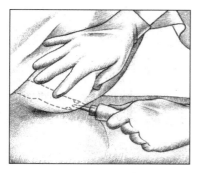

■ Squeeze the tube to eject medication.

■ Remove the applicator, and place a folded 4″ × 4″ gauze pad between the patient's buttocks to absorb excess ointment. Disassemble the tube and applicator. Recap the tube. Clean the applicator with soap and warm water. Remove and discard gloves. Then wash your hands thoroughly.

Special considerations
■ Because the intake of food and fluid stimulates peristalsis, a suppository for relieving constipation should be inserted about 30 minutes before mealtime to help soften the stool and facilitate defecation. A medicated retention suppository should be inserted between meals.

■ Tell the patient not to expel the suppository. If retaining it is difficult put him on a bedpan.

■ Make sure the patient's call button is handy, and watch for his signal because he may be unable to suppress the urge to defecate.

■ Inform the patient that the suppository may discolor his next bowel movement.

Parenteral administration

Subcutaneous injection

A subcutaneous (S.C.) injection allows slower, more sustained drug administration than intramuscular injection. Drugs and solutions for S.C. injections are injected through a relatively short needle, using meticulous sterile technique.

Equipment and preparation
Patient's medication record and chart ♦ prescribed medication ♦ needle of appropriate gauge and length ♦ gloves ♦ 1- to 3-ml syringe ♦ alcohol pads ♦ optional: antiseptic cleaner, filter needle, insulin syringe, insulin pump

Inspect the medication to make sure it isn't cloudy and doesn't contain precipitates.

Wash your hands. Select a needle of the proper gauge and length.

Age alert An average adult patient requires a 25G ⅝" needle; an infant, a child, or an elderly or thin patient usually requires a 25G to 27G ½" needle.

For single-dose ampules

Wrap the neck of the ampule in an alcohol pad, and snap off the top away from you. If desired, attach a filter needle to the needle, and withdraw the medication. Tap the syringe to clear air from it. Cover the needle with the needle sheath. Before discarding the ampule, check the label against the patient's medication record. Discard the filter needle and the ampule. Attach the appropriate needle to the syringe.

For single-dose or multidose vials

Reconstitute powdered drugs according to the label's instructions. Clean the vial's rubber stopper with an alcohol pad. Pull the syringe plunger back until the volume of air in the syringe equals the volume of drug to be withdrawn from the vial. Insert the needle into the vial. Inject the air, invert the vial, and keep the needle's bevel tip below the level of the solution as you withdraw the prescribed amount of medication. Cover the needle with the needle sheath. Tap the syringe to clear any air from it. Check the drug label against the patient's medication record before returning the multidose vial to the shelf or drawer or before discarding the single-dose vial.

Implementation

■ Select the injection site from those shown at top right, and tell the patient where you'll be giving the injection.

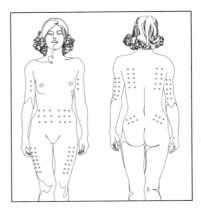

■ Put on gloves. Position and drape the patient, if necessary.

■ Clean the injection site with an alcohol pad. Loosen the protective needle cover.

■ With your nondominant hand, pinch the skin around the injection site firmly to elevate the S.C. tissue, forming a 1" (2.5-cm) fat fold, as shown below.

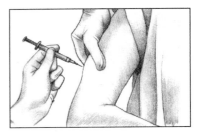

■ Holding the syringe in your dominant hand (while pinching the skin around the injection site with the index finger and thumb of your nondominant hand), grip the needle sheath between the fourth and fifth fingers of your nondominant hand, and pull back to uncover the needle. Don't touch the needle.

■ Position the needle with its bevel up.

■ Tell the patient she'll feel a prick as the needle is inserted. Insert the needle quickly in one motion at a 45- or 90-degree angle, as shown below, depending on needle length, medication, and the amount of S.C. tissue at the site. Some drugs, such as heparin, should always be injected at a 90-degree angle.

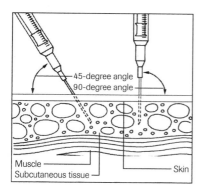

45-degree angle
90-degree angle

Muscle
Subcutaneous tissue — Skin

■ Release the skin to avoid injecting the drug into compressed tissue and irritating the nerves.
■ Pull the plunger back slightly to check for blood return. If none appears, slowly inject the drug. If blood appears upon aspiration, withdraw the needle, prepare another syringe, and repeat the procedure.
■ After injection, remove the needle at the same angle used for insertion. Cover the site with an alcohol pad and, if appropriate, massage the site gently.
■ Remove the alcohol pad, and check the injection site for bleeding or bruising.
■ Dispose of injection equipment according to facility policy. Don't recap the needle.

Special considerations
■ Don't aspirate for blood return when giving insulin or heparin. It isn't necessary with insulin and may cause a hematoma with heparin.

■ Repeated injections in the same site can cause lipodystrophy. A natural immune response, this complication can be minimized by rotating injection sites.

Intradermal injection

Used primarily for diagnostic purposes, as in allergy or tuberculin testing, an intradermal injection is administered in small amounts, usually 0.5 ml or less, into the outer layers of the skin. Because little systemic absorption takes place, this type of injection is used primarily to produce a local effect.

The ventral forearm is the most commonly used site because of its easy access and lack of hair. In extensive allergy testing, the outer aspect of the upper arms may be used as well as the area of the back between the scapulae.

Equipment
Patient's medication record and chart ◆ prescribed medication ◆ tuberculin syringe with a 26G or 27G ½″ to ⅝″ needle ◆ gloves ◆ alcohol pads ◆ marking pen

Implementation
■ Locate an injection site from those shown below, and tell the patient where you'll be giving the injection.

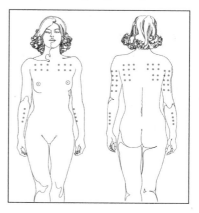

■ Instruct the patient to sit up and to extend and support her arm on a flat surface with the ventral forearm exposed.

■ Put on gloves.

■ With an alcohol pad, clean the surface of the ventral forearm about two or three fingerbreadths distal to the antecubital space. Make sure the test site is free from hair and blemishes. Allow the skin to dry completely before administering the injection.

■ While holding the patient's forearm in your hand, stretch the skin taut with your thumb.

■ With your free hand, hold the needle at a 15-degree angle to the patient's arm, with its bevel up.

■ Insert the needle about ⅛″ (3 mm) below the epidermis. Stop when the needle's bevel tip is under the skin, and inject the antigen slowly. You should feel some resistance as you do this, and a wheal should form as you inject the antigen, as shown below.

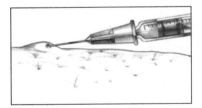

If no wheal forms, you have injected the antigen too deeply; withdraw the needle, and administer another test dose at least 2″ (5.1 cm) from the first site.

■ Withdraw the needle at the same angle at which it was inserted. Don't rub the site. This could irritate the underlying tissue, which may affect test results.

■ Circle each test site with a marking pen, and label each site according to the recall antigen given. Instruct the patient to refrain from washing off the circles until the test is completed.

■ Dispose of needles and syringes according to facility policy.

■ Remove and discard your gloves.

■ Assess the patient's response to the skin testing in 24 to 48 hours.

Special considerations

■ If the patient is hypersensitive to the test antigens, a severe anaphylactic response can result. Be prepared to give an immediate epinephrine injection and other emergency resuscitation procedures. Be especially alert after giving a test dose of penicillin or tetanus antitoxin.

Intramuscular injection

An intramuscular (I.M.) injection deposits medication deep into well-vascularized muscle for rapid systemic action and absorption of up to 5 ml.

Equipment and preparation

Patient's medication record and chart ◆ prescribed medication ◆ diluent or filter needle, if needed ◆ 3- to 5-ml syringe ◆ 20G to 25G 1″ to 3″ needle ◆ gloves ◆ alcohol pads ◆ marking pen

The prescribed medication must be sterile. The needle may be packaged separately or already attached to the syringe. Needles used for I.M. injections are longer than subcutaneous (S.C.) needles because they reach deep into the muscle. Needle length also depends on the injection site, the patient's size, and the amount of S.C. fat covering the muscle. A larger needle gauge accommodates viscous solutions and suspensions.

Check the drug for abnormal changes in color and clarity. If in doubt, ask the pharmacist.

Wipe the stopper of the vial with alcohol, and draw the prescribed amount of medication into the syringe.

Provide privacy, and explain the procedure to the patient. Position and drape him appropriately, making sure the site is well lit and exposed.

Implementation

■ Wash your hands, and select an appropriate injection site. Avoid any site that's inflamed, edematous, or irritated, or that contains moles, birthmarks, scar tissue, or other lesions. Dorsogluteal or ventrogluteal muscles are the most common sites, as shown below.

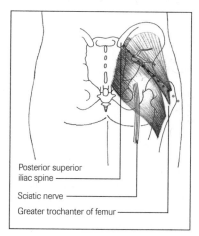

Posterior superior iliac spine —

Sciatic nerve —

Greater trochanter of femur —

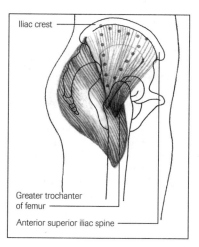

Iliac crest —

Greater trochanter of femur —

Anterior superior iliac spine —

■ The deltoid muscle may be used for injections of 2 ml or less, as shown below.

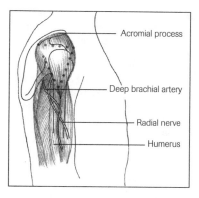

— Acromial process

— Deep brachial artery

— Radial nerve

— Humerus

■ The vastus lateralis is usually used in children; the rectus femoris may be used in infants, as shown below.

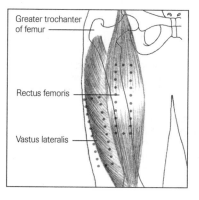

Greater trochanter of femur —

Rectus femoris —

Vastus lateralis —

■ Remember to rotate sites for patients who require repeated injections.
■ Position and drape the patient appropriately.
■ Loosen, but don't remove, the needle sheath.
■ Clean the site by moving an alcohol pad in circles increasing in diameter to about 2″ (5.1 cm). Allow the skin to dry; alcohol stings in the puncture.

■ Put on gloves. With the thumb and index finger of your nondominant hand, gently stretch the skin pulling it taut.

■ With the syringe in your dominant hand, remove the needle sheath with the free fingers of the other hand.

■ Position the syringe perpendicular to the skin surface and a couple of inches from the skin. Tell the patient that he'll feel a prick. Then quickly and firmly thrust the needle into the muscle.

■ Pull back slightly on the plunger to aspirate for blood. If none appears, inject the medication slowly and steadily to let the muscle distend gradually. You should feel little or no resistance. Gently but quickly, remove the needle at a 90-degree angle.

■ If blood appears, the needle is in a blood vessel. Withdraw it, prepare a fresh syringe, and inject another site.

■ Using a gloved hand, apply gentle pressure to the site with the used alcohol pad. Massage the relaxed muscle, unless contraindicated, to distribute the drug and promote absorption.

■ Inspect the site for bleeding or bruising. Apply pressure or ice as necessary.

■ Discard all equipment properly. Don't recap needles; put them in an appropriate biohazard container to avoid needle-stick injuries.

Special considerations

■ Some drugs are dissolved in oil to slow absorption. Mix them well before use.

■ Never inject into the gluteal muscles of a child who has been walking for less than a year.

■ If the patient must have repeated injections, consider numbing the area with ice before cleaning it. If you must inject more than 5 ml, divide the solution, and inject it at two sites.

■ Urge the patient to relax the muscles to reduce pain and bleeding.

■ I.M. injections can damage local muscle cells and elevate serum creatine kinase, which can be confused with the elevated levels that a myocardial infarction causes. Diagnostic tests can differentiate the two.

Z-track injection

The Z-track method of intramuscular injection prevents leakage, or tracking, into the subcutaneous (S.C.) tissue. Typically, it's used to administer drugs that irritate and discolor S.C. tissue — primarily iron preparations, such as iron dextran. It may also be used in elderly patients who have decreased muscle mass. Lateral displacement of the skin during the injection helps to seal the drug in the muscle.

This procedure requires careful attention to technique because leakage into S.C. tissue can cause patient discomfort and may permanently stain some tissues.

Equipment and preparation

Patient's medication record and chart ♦ two 20G 1″ to 3″ needles ♦ prescribed medication ♦ gloves ♦ 3- to 5-ml syringe ♦ alcohol pad

Wash your hands. Make sure the needle you're using is long enough to reach the muscle. As a rule of thumb, a 200-pound patient requires a 2″ needle; a 100-pound patient, a 1¼″ to 1½″ needle.

Attach one needle to the syringe, and draw up the prescribed medication. Then draw 0.2 to 0.5 cc of air (depending on facility policy) into the syringe. Remove the first needle, and attach the second to prevent tracking the medication through the S.C. tissue as the needle is inserted.

Implementation

■ Place the patient in the lateral position, exposing the gluteal muscle to be used as the injection site. The patient may also be placed in the prone position. Put on gloves.

■ Clean an area on the upper outer quadrant of the patient's buttock with an alcohol pad.

■ Displace the skin laterally by pulling it away from the injection site. To do so, place your finger on the skin surface, and pull the skin and S.C. layers out of alignment with the underlying muscle. In doing so, you should move the skin about 1″ (2.5 cm).

■ Insert the needle at a 90-degree angle in the site where you initially placed your finger, as shown below.

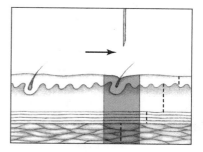

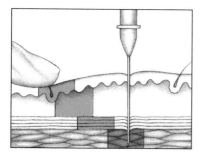

■ Aspirate for blood return; if none appears, inject the drug slowly, followed by the air. Injecting air after the drug helps clear the needle and prevents tracking the medication through S.C. tissues as the needle is withdrawn.

■ Wait 10 seconds before withdrawing the needle to ensure dispersion of the medication.

■ Withdraw the needle slowly. Then release the displaced skin and subcutaneous tissue to seal the needle track, as shown at top right.

■ Don't massage the injection site or allow the patient to wear a tight-fitting garment over the site because doing either could force the medication into S.C. tissue.

■ Encourage the patient to walk or move about in bed to facilitate absorption of the drug from the injection site.

■ Discard the needles and syringe in an appropriate biohazard container. Avoid needle-stick injuries by not recapping needles.

■ Remove and discard your gloves.

Special considerations

■ Never inject more than 5 ml of solution into a single site using the Z-track method. Alternate gluteal sites for repeat injections.

■ If the patient is on bed rest, encourage active range-of-motion (ROM) exercises, or perform passive ROM exercises to facilitate absorption from the injection site.

Drug infusion through a secondary I.V. line

A secondary I.V. line is a complete I.V. set connected to the lower Y-port (secondary port) of a primary line, instead of to the I.V. catheter or needle. It features an I.V. container, long tubing, and either a microdrip or a macrodrip system, and it can be used for continuous or intermittent drug infusion. When used continuously, it permits

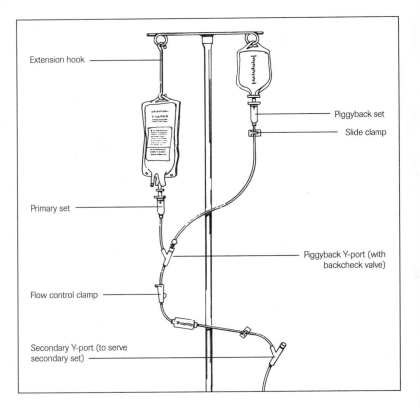

Extension hook

Piggyback set

Slide clamp

Primary set

Piggyback Y-port (with backcheck valve)

Flow control clamp

Secondary Y-port (to serve secondary set)

drug infusion and titration while the primary line maintains a constant total infusion rate.

A secondary I.V. line used only for intermittent drug administration is called a piggyback set. In this case, the primary line maintains venous access between drug doses. A piggyback set includes a small I.V. container, short tubing, and usually a macrodrip system, and it connects to the primary line's upper Y-port (piggyback port), as shown above.

Equipment and preparation

Patient's medication record and chart ◆ prescribed I.V. medication ◆ diluent, if necessary ◆ prescribed I.V. solution ◆ administration set with secondary injection port ◆ needleless adapter ◆ alcohol pads ◆ 1″ adhesive tape ◆ time tape ◆ labels ◆ infusion pump ◆ extension hook and solution for intermittent piggyback infusion

Wash your hands. Inspect the I.V. container for cracks, leaks, or contamination, and check compatibility with the primary solution. See if the primary line has a secondary injection port.

If necessary, add the drug to the secondary I.V. solution. To do so, remove any seals from the secondary container, and wipe the main port with an alcohol pad. Inject the prescribed medication and agitate the solution to mix the medication. Label the I.V. mixture. Insert the administration set spike. Open the flow clamp, and prime the line. Then close the flow clamp.

Some medications come in vials for hanging directly on an I.V. pole. In this case, inject diluent directly into the medication vial. Then spike the vial, prime the tubing, and hang the set.

Implementation

■ If the drug is incompatible with the primary I.V. solution, replace the primary I.V. solution with a fluid that's compatible with both solutions, and flush the line before starting the drug infusion.

■ Hang the container of the secondary set, and wipe the injection port of the primary line with an alcohol pad.

■ Insert the needleless adapter from the secondary line into the injection port, and tape it securely to the primary line.

■ To run the container of the secondary set by itself, lower the primary set's container with an extension hook. To run both containers simultaneously, place them at the same height.

■ Open the clamp, and adjust the drip rate. For continuous infusion, set the secondary solution to the desired drip rate; then adjust the primary solution to the desired total infusion rate.

■ For intermittent infusion, wait until the secondary solution is completely infused; then adjust the primary drip rate as required. If the secondary solution tubing is being reused, close the clamp on the tubing, and follow facility policy: Either remove the needleless adapter and replace it with a new one, or leave it taped in the injection port, and label it with the time it was first used. Leave the empty container in place until you replace it with a new dose of medication at the prescribed time. If the tubing won't be reused, discard it appropriately with the I.V. container.

Special considerations

■ If facility policy allows, use a pump for drug infusion. Put a time tape on the secondary container to help prevent an inaccurate administration rate.

■ When reusing secondary tubing, change it according to facility policy, usually every 48 to 72 hours. Inspect the injection port for leakage with each use; change it more often, if needed.

■ Except for lipids, don't piggyback a secondary I.V. line to a total parenteral nutrition line because it risks contamination.

I.V. bolus injection

The I.V. bolus injection method allows rapid I.V. drug administration to quickly achieve peak levels in the bloodstream. It may be used for drugs that can't be given I.M. because they're toxic or for a patient with reduced ability to absorb these drugs. Also, it may be used to deliver drugs that can't be diluted.

Bolus doses may be injected directly into a vein or through an existing I.V. line or implanted vascular access port (VAP).

Equipment and preparation

Patient's medication record and chart ◆ prescribed drug ◆ 20G needle and syringe ◆ diluent, if necessary ◆ tourniquet ◆ povidone-iodine pad ◆ alcohol pad ◆ sterile 2″ × 2″ gauze pad ◆ gloves ◆ adhesive bandage ◆ tape ◆ optional: winged-tip needle with catheter and second syringe (and needle) filled with normal saline solution, noncoring needle for VAP

Draw the drug into the syringe, and dilute it, if necessary.

Implementation

■ Wash your hands, and put on gloves.

To give direct injections

■ Select the largest vein suitable to dilute the drug and minimize irritation.

■ Apply a tourniquet above the site to distend the vein, and clean the site with an alcohol or povidone-iodine pad, working outward in a circle.

■ If you're using the needle of the drug syringe, insert it at a 30-degree angle with the bevel up. The bevel should reach 1/4" (6 mm) into the vein. Insert a winged-tip needle bevel up, tape the wings in place when you see blood return, and attach the syringe containing the drug.

■ Check for blood backflow.

■ Remove the tourniquet, and inject the drug at the ordered rate.

■ Check for blood backflow to ensure that the needle remained in place and all of the injected medication entered the vein.

■ For a winged-tip needle, flush the line with normal saline solution from the second syringe to ensure complete delivery.

■ Withdraw the needle, and apply pressure to the site with the sterile gauze pad for at least 3 minutes to prevent a hematoma.

■ Use an adhesive bandage when the bleeding stops.

To inject through an existing I.V. line

■ Check the compatibility of the medication.

■ Close the flow clamp, wipe the injection port with an alcohol pad, and inject the drug as you would a direct injection.

■ Open the flow clamp, and readjust the flow rate.

■ If the drug is incompatible with the I.V. solution, flush the line with normal saline solution before and after the injection.

To use a vascular access port

■ Wash your hands, put on gloves, and clean the site three times with an alcohol or povidone-iodine pad.

■ Palpate for the septum, anchor the port between your thumb and first two fingers of your nondominant hand, and give the injection.

Special considerations

■ If the existing I.V. line is capped, making it an intermittent infusion device, verify patency and placement of the device before injecting the medication. Then flush the device with normal saline solution, administer the medication, and follow with the appropriate flush.

■ Immediately report any signs of acute allergic reaction or anaphylaxis. If extravasation occurs, stop the injection, estimate the amount of infiltration, and notify the doctor.

■ When giving diazepam or chlordiazepoxide hydrochloride through a winged-tip needle or I.V. line, flush with bacteriostatic water to prevent precipitation.

Special administration

Epidural analgesics

When giving an epidural analgesic, the doctor injects or infuses it into the epidural space, thus into cerebrospinal fluid, so the medication can bypass the blood-brain barrier.

Epidural analgesia helps manage pain, including postoperative pain, and is especially useful for patients with cancer or degenerative joint disease.

Equipment and preparation

Patient's medication record and chart ◆ prescribed epidural solutions ◆ volume infusion device and epidural infusion tubing (depending on facility policy) ◆ transparent dressing or sterile gauze

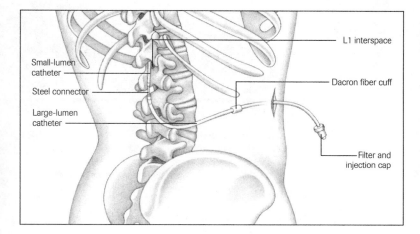

Small-lumen catheter

Steel connector

Large-lumen catheter

L1 interspace

Dacron fiber cuff

Filter and injection cap

pads ◆ epidural tray ◆ label for epidural infusion line ◆ silk tape

Make sure the pharmacy has been notified ahead of time regarding the medication order because epidural solutions require special preparation.

Implementation

■ Tell the patient he'll feel some pain as the catheter is inserted.

■ Put the patient on his side in the knee-chest position, or have him sit on the edge of the bed and lean over a bedside table.

■ After the catheter is in place, as shown above, prime the infusion device, confirm medication and infusion rate, and adjust the device.

■ After the infusion tubing is connected to the epidural catheter, connect the tubing to the infusion pump. Tape all connection sites, and apply a label that says EPIDURAL INFUSION.

■ Tell the patient to report any feeling of pain, which may require an increased infusion rate.

■ Change the dressing over the exit site every 24 to 48 hours or as specified.

Special considerations

■ After starting the infusion, assess the patient's respiratory rate and blood pressure every 2 hours for 8 hours, then every 4 hours for 8 hours, then once per shift unless ordered otherwise. Notify the doctor if the respiratory rate is below 10 breaths/minute or the systolic blood pressure is less than 90 mm Hg.

■ Assess the patient's sedation level, mental status, and pain relief every hour initially, then every 2 to 4 hours, until adequate pain control is achieved.

■ If the patient is receiving a local anesthetic, assess lower-extremity motor strength every 2 to 4 hours. If sensory and motor loss occurs, large motor nerve fibers have been affected, and dosage may need to be decreased.

■ The patient should always have a peripheral I.V. line open to allow administration of emergency drugs.

■ Don't give an analgesic by any other route because such administration increases the risk of respiratory depression.

11 Dosage calculations
Ensuring effective therapy

Calculating drug dosages

Reviewing ratios and proportions

A ratio is a mathematical expression of the relationship between two things. A proportion is a set of two equal ratios. A ratio may be expressed with a fraction, such as $\frac{1}{3}$, or with a colon, such as 1 : 3. When ratios are expressed as fractions in a proportion, their cross products are equal.

Proportion

$$\frac{2}{4} \diagdown\!\!\!\!\!\diagup \frac{5}{10}$$

Cross products

$2 \times 10 = 4 \times 5$

When ratios are expressed using colons in a proportion, the product of the means equals the product of the extremes.

Proportion

means
↓   ↓
3 : 30 :: 4 : 40
↑ extremes ↑

Product of means and extremes

$30 \times 4 = 3 \times 40$

Whether fractions or ratios are used in a proportion, they must appear in the same order on both sides of the equal sign. When the ratios are expressed as fractions, the units in the numerators must be the same, and the units in the denominators must be the same (although they don't have to be the same as the units in the numerators).

$$\frac{mg}{kg} = \frac{mg}{kg}$$

If the ratios in a proportion are expressed with colons, the units of the first term on the left side of the equal sign must be the same as the units of the first term on the right side. In other words, the units of the mean on one side of the equal sign must match the units of the extreme on the other side, and vice versa.

$$mg : kg :: mg : kg$$

Tips for simplifying dosage calculations

Incorporate units of measure into the calculation

Incorporating units of measure into your dosage calculation helps protect you from one of the most common dosage calculation errors — using the incorrect unit of measure. Simply keep in mind that the units of measure in the numerator and the denominator cancel each other out, leaving the correct unit of measure in the answer. The following example uses units of measure in calculating a drug with a usual dose of 4 mg/kg for a 55-kg patient.

1. State the problem as a proportion.

$$4 \text{ mg} : 1 \text{ kg} :: X : 55 \text{ kg}$$

2. Solve for X by applying the principle that the product of the means equals the product of the extremes.

$$1 \text{ kg} \times X = 4 \text{ mg} \times 55 \text{ kg}$$

3. Divide and cancel out the units of measure that appear in both the numerator and denominator.

$$X = \frac{4 \text{ mg} \times 55 \text{ kg}}{1 \text{ kg}}$$

$$X = 220 \text{ mg}$$

Check zeros and decimal places

Suppose you receive an order to administer 0.1 mg of epinephrine subcutaneously (S.C.), but the only epinephrine on hand is a 1-ml ampule that contains 1 mg of epinephrine. To calculate the volume for injection, use the ratio and proportion method.

1. State the problem as a proportion.

$$1 \text{ mg} : 1 \text{ ml} :: 0.1 \text{ mg} : X$$

2. Solve for X by applying the principle that the product of the means equals the product of the extremes.

$$1 \text{ ml} \times 0.1 \text{ mg} = 1 \text{ mg} \times X$$

3. Divide and cancel out the units of measure that appear in both the numerator and denominator, carefully checking the decimal placement.

$$\frac{1 \text{ ml} \times 0.1 \text{ mg}}{1 \text{ mg}} = X$$

$$0.1 \text{ ml} = X$$

Recheck calculations that seem unusual

If, for example, your calculation indicates that you should administer 25 tablets, you've probably made an error. Therefore, carefully recheck any figures that seem unusual. If you still have doubts, review your calculations with another health care professional.

Determining the number of tablets to administer

Calculating the number of tablets to administer lends itself to the use of ratios and proportions. To do the calculation, follow this process:
1. Set up the first ratio with the known tablet (tab) strength.
2. Set up the second ratio with the unknown quantity.

3. Use these ratios in a proportion.
4. Solve for X, applying the principle that the product of the means equals the product of the extremes.

For example, suppose a drug order calls for *100 mg propranolol P.O. q.i.d.,* but only 40-mg tablets are available. To determine the number of tablets to administer, follow these steps:
1. Set up the first ratio with the known tablet (tab) strength.

$$40 \text{ mg} : 1 \text{ tab}$$

2. Set up the second ratio with the desired dose and the unknown number of tablets.

$$100 \text{ mg} : X$$

3. Use these ratios in a proportion.

$$40 \text{ mg} : 1 \text{ tab} :: 100 \text{ mg} : X$$

4. Solve for X by applying the principle that the product of the means equals the product of the extremes.

$$1 \text{ tab} \times 100 \text{ mg} = 40 \text{ mg} \times X$$

$$\frac{1 \text{ tab} \times 100 \text{ mg}}{40 \text{ mg} \times X}$$

$$2\frac{1}{2} \text{ tab} = X$$

Determining the amount of liquid medication to administer

You can also use ratios and proportions to calculate the amount of liquid medication to administer. Simply follow the same four-step process used in determining the number of tablets to administer.

For example, a patient is to receive 750 mg of amoxicillin oral suspension. The label reads *amoxicillin (Amoxicillin trihydrate)* 250 mg/5 ml. The bottle contains 100 ml. To determine how many

milliliters of amoxicillin solution the patient should receive, follow these steps:
1. Set up the first ratio with the known liquid medication's strength.

$$250 \text{ mg} : 5 \text{ ml}$$

2. Set up the second ratio with the desired dose and the unknown quantity.

$$750 \text{ mg} : X$$

3. Use these ratios in a proportion.

$$250 \text{ mg} : 5 \text{ ml} :: 750 \text{ mg} : X$$

4. Solve for X by applying the principle that the product of the means equals the product of the extremes.

$$5 \text{ ml} \times 750 \text{ mg} = 250 \text{ mg} \times X$$

$$\frac{5 \text{ ml} \times 750 \text{ mg}}{250 \text{ mg}} = X$$

$$15 \text{ ml} = X$$

Administering drugs available in varied concentrations

Because drugs, such as epinephrine, heparin, and allergy serums, are available in varied concentrations, you must consider a drug's concentration when calculating a drug dosage. Otherwise, you could make a serious — even lethal — mistake. To avoid a dosage error, make sure that drug concentrations are part of the calculation.

For example, a drug order calls for *0.2 mg epinephrine S.C. stat.* The ampule is labeled as 1 ml of 1:1,000 epinephrine. To calculate the correct volume of drug to inject:
1. Determine the strength of the solution based on its unlabeled ratio.

$$1:1,000 \text{ epinephrine} = 1 \text{ g}/1,000 \text{ ml}$$

2. Set up a proportion with this information and the desired dose.

$$1 \text{ g} : 1,000 \text{ ml} :: 0.2 \text{ mg} : X$$

Before you can perform this calculation, however, you must convert grams to milligrams by using the conversion $1 \text{ g} = 1,000 \text{ mg}$.
3. Restate the proportion with the converted units, and solve for X.

$$1,000 \text{ mg} : 1,000 \text{ ml} :: 0.2 \text{ mg} : X$$

$$1,000 \text{ ml} \times 0.2 \text{ mg} = 1,000 \text{ mg} \times X$$

$$\frac{1,000 \text{ ml} \times 0.2 \text{ mg}}{1,000 \text{ mg}} = X$$

$$0.2 \text{ ml} = X$$

Calculating I.V. drip and flow rates

To compute the drip and flow rates, set up a fraction with the solution volume to be delivered over the prescribed duration. For example, if a patient is to receive 100 ml of solution within 1 hour, the fraction is:

$$\frac{100 \text{ ml}}{60 \text{ minutes}}$$

Next, multiply the fraction by the drip factor (the number of drops contained in 1 ml) to determine the drip rate (the number of drops per minute to be infused). The drip factor varies among I.V. sets and appears on the package containing the I.V. tubing administration set. Following the manufacturer's directions for drip factor is crucial. Standard sets have drip factors of 10, 15, or 20 gtt/ml. A microdrip (minidrip) set has a drip factor of 60 gtt/ml.

Use the following equation to determine the drip rate:

$$\frac{\text{total ml}}{\text{total minutes}} \times \text{drip factor} = \text{gtt/minute}$$

The equation applies to solutions that infuse over many hours or to such small-volume infusions as those used for antibiotics, which are given for less than 1 hour.

You can modify the equation by first determining the number of milliliters to be infused over 1 hour (the flow rate). Then, divide the flow rate by 60 minutes. Next, multiply the result by the drip factor to determine the number of drops per minute. You'll also use the flow rate when working with infusion pumps to set the number of milliliters to be delivered in 1 hour.

Quick calculations of drip rates

In addition to using the equation and its modified version, quicker computation methods exist. To administer solutions using a microdrip set, adjust the flow rate (ml/hour) to equal the drip rate (gtt/minute). Using the equation, divide the flow rate by 60 minutes and multiply by the drip factor, which also equals 60. Because the flow rate and drip factor are equal, the two arithmetic operations cancel each other out. For example, if the flow rate is 125 ml/hour, the equation would be:

$$\frac{125 \text{ ml}}{60 \text{ minutes}} \times 60 = \text{drip rate (125)}$$

Rather than spend the time solving the equation, you can simply use the number assigned to the flow rate as the drip rate. For sets that deliver 15 gtt/ml, the flow rate divided by 4 equals the drip rate. For sets with a drip factor of 10, the flow rate divided by 6 equals the drip rate.

To determine how many micrograms of a drug are in a milliliter of solution, use the following equation:

$$\text{mcg/ml} = \text{mg/ml} \times 1,000$$

To express drip rates in mcg/kg/minute, you must know the solution's concentration (mcg/ml), the patient's weight (kg), and the infusion rate (ml/hour):

$$\text{mcg/kg/min} = \frac{\text{mcg/ml} \times \text{ml/min}}{\text{body weight (kg)}}$$

To find ml/minute, divide ml/hour by 60.

You can also convert milliliters/hour from a dosage given in mcg/kg/min:

$$\text{ml/hr} = \frac{\text{wt (kg)} \times \text{mcg/kg/min}}{\text{mcg/ml}} \times 60$$

Dimensional analysis

Dimensional analysis (also known as factor analysis or factor labeling) is an alternative method of solving mathematical problems. It eliminates the need to memorize formulas and requires only one equation to determine an answer. To compare the ratio-and-proportion method and dimensional analysis at a glance, read the following problem and solutions.

The doctor prescribes *0.25 g streptomycin sulfate I.M.* The vial reads "2 ml = 1 g." How many milliliters should you administer?

Dimensional analysis

$$\frac{0.25 \text{ g}}{1} \times \frac{2 \text{ ml}}{1 \text{ g}} = 0.5 \text{ ml}$$

Ratio and proportion

$$1 \text{ g} : 2 \text{ ml} :: 0.25 \text{ g} : X$$

$$2 \text{ ml} \times 0.25 \text{ g} = 1 \text{ g} \times X$$

$$\frac{2 \text{ ml} \times 0.25 \cancel{g}}{1 \cancel{g}} = X$$

$$0.5 \text{ ml} = X$$

When using dimensional analysis, the problem solver arranges a series of ratios, called *factors*, in a single fractional equation. Each factor, written as a fraction, consists of two quantities and their units of measurement that are related to each other in a given problem. For instance, if 1,000 ml of a drug should be administered over 8 hours, the relationship between 1,000 ml and 8 hours is expressed by the fraction

$$\frac{1,000 \text{ ml}}{8 \text{ hours}}$$

When a problem includes a quantity and its unit of measurement that are unrelated to any other factor in the problem, they serve as the numerator of the fraction, and 1 (implied) becomes the denominator.

Some mathematical problems contain all of the information needed to identify the factors, set up the equation, and find the solution. Other problems require the use of a conversion factor. Conversion factors are equivalents (for example, 1 g = 1,000 mg) that the nurse can memorize or obtain from a conversion chart. Because the two quantities and units of measurement are equivalent, they can serve as the numerator or the denominator; thus, the conversion factor 1 g = 1,000 mg can be written in fraction form as:

$$\frac{1,000 \text{ mg}}{1 \text{ g}} \quad \text{or} \quad \frac{1 \text{ g}}{1,000 \text{ mg}}$$

The factors given in the problem plus any conversion factors necessary to solve the problem are called *knowns*. The quantity of the answer, of course, is *unknown*. When setting up an equation in dimensional analysis, work backward, beginning with the unit of measurement of the answer. After plotting all the knowns, find the solution by following this sequence:

1. Cancel similar quantities and units of measurement.
2. Multiply the numerators.
3. Multiply the denominators.
4. Divide the numerator by the denominator.

Mastering dimensional analysis can take practice, but you may find your efforts well rewarded. To understand more fully how dimensional analysis works, review the following problem and the steps taken to solve it.

The doctor prescribes X grains (gr) of a drug. The pharmacy supplies the drug in 300-mg tablets (tab). How many tablets should you administer?

1. Write down the unit of measurement of the answer, followed by an "equal to" symbol (=).

$$\text{tab} =$$

2. Search the problem for the quantity with the same unit of measurement (if one doesn't exist, use a conversion factor); place this in the numerator and its related quantity and unit of measurement in the denominator.

$$\text{tab} = \frac{1 \text{ tab}}{300 \text{ mg}}$$

3. Separate the first factor from the next with a multiplication symbol ($\times$).

$$\text{tab} = \frac{1 \text{ tab}}{300 \text{ mg}} \times$$

4. Place the unit of measurement of the denominator of the first factor in the numerator of the second factor. Search the problem for the quantity with the same unit of measurement (if one doesn't exist, as in this example, use a conversion factor). Place this in the numerator and its related quantity and unit of measurement in the denominator; follow with a multiplication symbol. Repeat this step until all known factors are included in the equation.

$$\text{tab} = \frac{1 \text{ tab}}{300 \text{ mg}} \times \frac{60 \text{ mg}}{1 \text{ gr}} \times \frac{10 \text{ gr}}{1}$$

Alternatively, you can treat the equation as a large fraction, using these steps:
1. First, cancel similar units of measurement in the numerator and the denominator (what remains should be what you began with — the unit of measurement of the answer; if not, recheck your equation to find and correct the error).
2. Multiply the numerators and then the denominators.

3. Divide the numerator by the denominator.

$$\text{tab} = \frac{1 \text{ tab}}{300 \text{ mg}} \times \frac{60 \text{ mg}}{1 \text{ gr}} \times \frac{10 \text{ gr}}{1}$$

$$= \frac{60 \times 10 \text{ tab}}{300}$$

$$= \frac{600 \text{ tab}}{300}$$

$$= 2 \text{ tablets}$$

Estimating body surface area in adults

Body surface area (BSA) is critical when calculating dosages for drugs such as chemotherapy that are extremely potent and need to be given in precise amounts. The nomogram shown here lets you plot the patient's height and weight to determine the BSA. To estimate the BSA of an adult patient, place a straightedge from the patient's height in the left-hand column to his weight in the right-hand column. The intersection of this line with the center scale reveals the BSA.

Estimating body surface area in children

Pediatric drug dosages should be calculated on the basis of body weight or body surface area (BSA). If your pediatric patient is average-sized, find his weight and corresponding BSA in the box. Otherwise, to use the nomogram, lay a straightedge on the correct height and weight points for your patient, and observe the point where it intersects on the surface area scale. Don't use drug dosages based on BSA in premature or full-term newborns; instead, use body weight.

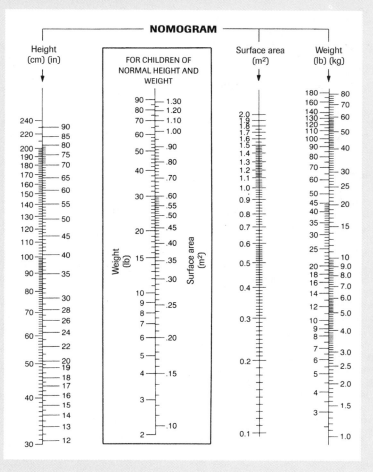

Administering drugs

Administering code drugs

adenosine
Indicated for patients with paroxysmal supraventricular tachycardia with atrioventricular node conduction

Dosage
Initially, 6 mg I.V. as a rapid bolus over 1 to 3 seconds; if there's no response in 1 to 2 minutes, 12 mg I.V.

Nursing considerations
■ Adverse effects, such as flushing, disappear quickly because the drug has a short half-life.
■ Follow each dose with a 20-ml flush of normal saline solution to ensure drug delivery.

amiodarone
Indicated for ventricular tachycardia, ventricular fibrillation, wide-complex tachycardia, paroxysmal supraventricular tachycardia, atrial tachycardia, and atrial fibrillation

Dosage
150 mg I.V. over 10 minutes followed by a 1 mg/minute infusion for 6 hours, and then 0.5 mg/minute to a maximum daily dose of 2 g

Nursing considerations
■ Administer through a central line whenever possible.
■ Monitor the patient for hypotension and bradycardia.

atropine sulfate
Indicated for sinus bradycardia with hemodynamic compromise and for ventricular asystole

Dosage
0.5 mg for bradycardia or 1 mg for asystole I.V. push over 1 to 2 minutes;

may be repeated every 3 to 5 minutes to a maximum of 2 mg

Nursing considerations
■ Monitor the patient for paradoxical initial bradycardia, especially if he's receiving 0.4 to 0.6 mg.
■ Monitor fluid intake and urine output.
■ Watch for tachycardia.

dobutamine hydrochloride
Indicated for patients with low cardiac output, hypotension, and pulmonary congestion

Dosage
Infuse 2.5 to 15 mcg/kg/minute; use the smallest effective dose, as indicated by hemodynamic values

Nursing considerations
■ Watch for reflex peripheral vasodilation.
■ Monitor heart rate closely; an increase of 10% or more may worsen myocardial ischemia.

dopamine hydrochloride
Indicated for patients with hypotension and bradycardia

Dosage
Initially, 1 to 5 mcg/kg/minute; titrated until the desired response is achieved

Nursing considerations
■ Drug effects vary with dosage: At 0.5 to 2 mcg/kg/minute, drug dilates renal and mesenteric vessels without increasing heart rate or blood pressure; at 2 to 10 mcg/kg/minute, it increases cardiac output without peripheral vasoconstriction; at over 10 mcg/kg/minute, it causes peripheral vasoconstriction.

epinephrine hydrochloride
Indicated for patients in cardiac arrest

Dosage

1 ml I.V. (10 ml of 1:10,000 solution), repeated every 3 to 5 minutes, if necessary

Nursing considerations

■ If I.V. line can't be established quickly, drug may be given endotracheally at 2 to 2½ times the I.V. dose.
■ Intracardiac injection is indicated only if venous and endotracheal routes are unavailable.

lidocaine hydrochloride

Indicated for patients with ventricular tachycardia (VT), ventricular ectopy, and ventricular fibrillation (VF); prophylactic administration in patients with uncomplicated myocardial infarction isn't recommended unless VT and VF persist after defibrillation and administration of epinephrine

Dosage

1 to 1.5 mg/kg I.V. bolus as a loading dose at 25 to 50 mg/minute; repeat bolus dose every 3 to 5 minutes until arrhythmias subside or adverse reactions develop, to a maximum of 3 mg/kg (300 mg over 1 hour); simultaneously, set up a continuous I.V. infusion at 1 to 4 mg/minute (Dilute 1 g of lidocaine in 250 ml of dextrose 5% in water for a 0.4% solution, or 4 mg/ml.)

Nursing considerations

■ For an elderly patient, a patient weighing less than 110 lb (50 kg), or a patient with heart failure or hepatic disease, administer half the bolus dose.
■ Drug improves response to defibrillation when the patient is in VF.
■ If an I.V. line can't be established quickly, the drug may be given endotracheally at 2 to 2½ times the I.V. dose.

magnesium sulfate

Indicated for treatment of ventricular fibrillation, ventricular tachycardia, or torsades de pointes

Dosage

1 to 6 g I.V. over several minutes, followed by continuous I.V. infusion of 3 to 20 mg/minute administered over 5 to 48 hours

Nursing considerations

■ Monitor serum magnesium levels.

nitroglycerin

Indicated for patients with heart failure associated with myocardial infarction and for patients with unstable angina

Dosage

5 mcg/minute I.V. infusion initially, increasing by 5 mcg/minute every 3 to 5 minutes until response occurs

Nursing considerations

■ Monitor the patient for hypotension, which could worsen myocardial ischemia.
■ Mean dosage range is 50 to 500 mcg/minute; however, most patients respond to 200 mcg/minute or less.
■ Because up to 80% of the drug binds to the plastic in normal I.V. administration sets, use the special I.V. tubing the manufacturer has supplied.

nitroprusside sodium

Indicated for patients with heart failure or in hypertensive crisis

Dosage

Dissolve 50 mg in 2 to 3 ml of dextrose 5% in water (D_5W); then mix with 250 to 1,000 ml of D_5W, depending on desired concentration; infuse at 0.3 to 10 mcg/kg/minute, titrating until the desired effect is achieved (The therapeutic dosage ranges from 0.5 to 8 mcg/kg/minute.)

Nursing considerations

■ Wrap the container in opaque material to prevent drug deterioration.

■ Monitor blood pressure with an intra-arterial line.

■ Large doses given at fast infusion rates increase the risk of cyanide toxicity. Measure cyanide levels and monitor for acidosis. If a toxic reaction is suspected, start treatment without the test results.

norepinephrine bitartrate
Indicated for patients with severe hypotension with low total peripheral resistance

Dosage

Mix 4 mg of norepinephrine bitartrate per 1,000 ml of dextrose 5% in water or normal saline solution to yield a 4 mcg/ml solution; initially, give 2 to 3 ml (8 to 12 mcg base)/minute I.V.; adjust flow to establish and maintain a low-normal blood pressure; average rate of maintenance infusion is 2 to 4 mcg/minute

Nursing considerations

■ Drug is contraindicated in patients with hypovolemia.

■ Monitor blood pressure with intra-arterial line because measurements with a standard cuff may be falsely low.

■ Cardiac output may increase or decrease, depending on vascular resistance, left ventricular function, and reflux response.

■ Avoid prolonged use; drug may cause ischemia of vital organs.

procainamide hydrochloride
Indicated for patients with ventricular arrhythmias, such as premature ventricular contractions or tachycardia, when lidocaine is contraindicated or ineffective

Dosage

100 ml by slow I.V. push every 5 minutes, no faster than 25 to 50 mg/minute, until arrhythmias disappear, adverse reactions develop, or 1 g has been given; when arrhythmias disappear, continuous I.V. infusion of 2 to 6 mg/minute

Nursing considerations

■ Lower the dosage for patients with renal failure.

■ Rapid infusion will cause acute hypotension.

■ Monitor electrocardiogram results carefully; if the QRS complex widens more than 50% or if the QT interval is prolonged, notify the doctor and discontinue the infusion as ordered.

vasopressin
Indicated for the treatment of adult shock-refractory ventricular fibrillation, asystole, or pulseless electrical activity

Dosage

40 units I.V., one time only

Nursing considerations

■ Use as an alternative to epinephrine.

verapamil hydrochloride
Indicated for patients with artrial fibrillation, atrial flutter, or multifocal atrial tachycardia; also used to help treat narrow QRS complex paroxysmal supraventricular tachycardia

Dosage

5 to 10 mg I.V. push over 2 minutes with electrocardiogram and blood pressure monitoring; if unresponsive, repeat dose in 30 minutes

Nursing considerations

■ Use cautiously and in lower doses for patients receiving a beta-adrenergic blocker.

■ Monitor the patient for hypotension, severe bradycardia, and heart failure.
■ Because verapamil may decrease myocardial contractility, it can aggravate heart failure in patients with severe left ventricular dysfunction.

A guide to equianalgesic doses

Narcotic agonists

The standard narcotic agonist dose, 10 mg of morphine sulfate I.M., is used to calculate equally effective (equianalgesic) doses of other narcotic agonists. This method is useful when a patient must be switched from one narcotic agonist to another with no change in dose effectiveness. This chart lists equianalgesic doses for selected narcotic agonists.

DRUG	DOSE
codeine	120 mg P.O.
fentanyl	0.1 to 0.2 mg I.M.
hydromorphone	1.5 mg I.M.
meperidine	75 to 100 mg I.M.
methadone	8 to 10 mg I.M.
morphine	10 mg I.M.
oxymorphone	1 to 1.5 mg I.M.

Mixed narcotic agonist-antagonists

This chart lists equianalgesic doses (based on the standard dose of 10 mg of morphine sulfate I.M.) for mixed narcotic agonist-antagonists.

DRUG	DOSE
buprenorphine	0.3 mg I.M.
butorphanol	2 mg I.M.
dezocine	10 mg I.M.
morphine	10 mg I.M.
nalbuphine	10 mg I.M.
pentazocine	30 mg I.M.

Critical elements of medication teaching

As a patient becomes more responsible for his own care, it's important that you supply him with all the information he needs to enable him to fully comply with his plan of treatment. Accurate written information is crucial for any patient, but it's especially so for young patients, elderly patients, and those with cognitive impairments. When preparing your written plan of medication teaching, include the following points:
■ name, dosage, and action of the drug
■ frequency and times of administration
■ special storage and preparation instructions
■ drugs (including over-the-counter products) and foods (including additives) to avoid
■ special comfort or safety measures and precautions
■ adverse effects and possible signs and symptoms of toxic reaction
■ warnings about discontinuing the medication.

12

Drug hazards
Recognizing and responding to them

Adverse or toxic drug reactions

Drug reactions and treatments

The key to treating toxic drug reactions successfully is quickly and accurately identifying the drug, then immediately beginning the appropriate treatment.

Managing toxic drug reactions

Toxic reactions and clinical effects	Interventions	Selected causative drugs
Anemia, aplastic ■ Bleeding from mucous membranes, ecchymoses, petechiae ■ Fatigue, pallor, progressive weakness, shortness of breath, tachycardia (progresses to heart failure) ■ Fever, oral and rectal ulcers, sore throat without characteristic inflammation	■ Stop drug, if possible. ■ Order vigorous supportive care, including transfusions, neutropenic isolation, antibiotics, and oxygen. ■ Colony-stimulating factors may be given. ■ For severe cases, a bone marrow transplant may be needed.	■ altretamine ■ aspirin (long-term) ■ carbamazepine ■ chloramphenicol ■ co-trimoxazole ■ ganciclovir ■ Gold salts ■ hydrochlorothiazide ■ mephenytoin ■ methimazole ■ penicillamine ■ Phenothiazines ■ phenylbutazone ■ propylthiouracil ■ triamterene ■ zidovudine
Anemia, hemolytic ■ Chills, fever, back and abdominal pain (hemolytic crisis) ■ Jaundice, malaise, splenomegaly ■ Signs of shock	■ Stop drug. ■ Order supportive care, including transfusions and oxygen. ■ Consider obtaining a blood sample for Coombs' test.	■ carbidopa-levodopa ■ levodopa ■ mefenamic acid ■ methyldopa ■ Penicillins ■ phenazopyridine ■ primaquine ■ quinidine ■ quinine ■ Sulfonamides
Bone marrow toxicity (agranulocytosis) ■ Enlarged lymph nodes, spleen, and tonsils ■ Septicemia, shock ■ Progressive fatigue and weakness, then sudden overwhelming infection with chills, fever, headache, and tachycardia ■ Pneumonia	■ Stop drug. ■ Begin antibiotic therapy while awaiting blood culture and sensitivity results. ■ Order supportive therapy, including neutropenic isolation, warm saline gargles, and oral hygiene.	■ Angiotensin-converting enzyme inhibitors ■ aminoglutethimide ■ carbamazepine ■ chloramphenicol ■ clomipramine ■ co-trimoxazole ■ flucytosine

Managing toxic drug reactions *(continued)*

Toxic reactions and clinical effects	Interventions	Selected causative drugs
Bone marrow toxicity (agranulocytosis) *(continued)* ■ Ulcers in the colon, mouth, and pharynx		■ Gold salts ■ penicillamine ■ Phenothiazines ■ phenylbutazone ■ phenytoin ■ procainamide ■ propylthiouracil ■ Sulfonylureas
Bone marrow toxicity (thrombocytopenia) ■ Fatigue, weakness, lethargy, malaise ■ Hemorrhage, loss of consciousness, shortness of breath, tachycardia ■ Sudden onset of ecchymoses or petechiae; large blood-filled bullae in the mouth	■ Stop drug or reduce dosage. ■ Order corticosteroids and platelet transfusions. ■ Consider ordering platelet-stimulating factors.	■ anistreplase ■ ciprofloxacin ■ cisplatin ■ colfosceril ■ etretinate ■ floxuridine ■ flucytosine ■ ganciclovir ■ Gold salts ■ heparin ■ Interferons alfa-2a and alpha-2b ■ lymphocyte immune globulin ■ methotrexate ■ penicillamine ■ procarbazine ■ quinidine ■ quinine ■ Tetracyclines ■ valproic acid
Cardiomyopathy ■ Acute hypertensive reaction ■ Atrial and ventricular arrhythmias ■ Chest pain ■ Heart failure ■ Chronic cardiomyopathy ■ Pericarditis-myocarditis syndrome	■ Discontinue drug, if possible. ■ Closely monitor the patient receiving concurrent radiation therapy. ■ Institute cardiac monitoring at earliest sign of problems. ■ If the patient is receiving doxorubicin, limit cumulative dose to less than 500 mg/m^2.	■ cyclophosphamide ■ cytarabine ■ daunorubicin ■ doxorubicin ■ idarubicin ■ mitoxantrone

(continued)

Managing toxic drug reactions *(continued)*

Toxic reactions and clinical effects	Interventions	Selected causative drugs
Dermatologic toxicity ■ May vary from phototoxicity to acneiform eruptions, alopecia, exfoliative dermatitis, lupus erythematosus-like reactions, toxic epidermal necrolysis	■ Stop drug. ■ Order topical antihistamines and analgesics.	■ Androgens ■ Barbiturates ■ Corticosteroids ■ Cephalosporins ■ Gold salts ■ hydralazine ■ Interferons ■ Iodides ■ Penicillins ■ pentamidine ■ phenolphthalein ■ Phenothiazines ■ phenylbutazone ■ procainamide ■ Psoralens ■ Quinolones ■ Sulfonamides ■ Sulfonylureas ■ Tetracyclines ■ Thiazides
Hepatotoxicity ■ Abdominal pain, hepatomegaly ■ Abnormal levels of alanine aminotransferase, aspartate aminotransferase, serum bilirubin, and lactate dehydrogenase ■ Bleeding, low-grade fever, mental changes, weight loss ■ Dry skin, pruritus, rash ■ Jaundice	■ Reduce dosage or stop drug. ■ Order monitoring of vital signs, blood levels, weight, intake and output, and fluids and electrolytes. ■ Promote rest. ■ Perform hemodialysis, if needed. ■ Order symptomatic care: vitamins A, B complex, D, and K; potassium for alkalosis; salt-poor albumin for fluid and electrolyte balance; neomycin for GI flora; stomach aspiration for blood; reduced dietary protein; and lactulose for blood ammonia.	■ amiodarone ■ asparaginase ■ carbamazepine ■ chlorpromazine ■ chlorpropamide ■ cytarabine ■ dantrolene ■ erythromycin estolate ■ ifosfamide ■ isoniazide ■ ketoconazole ■ leuprolide ■ methotrexate ■ methyldopa ■ mitoxantrone ■ niacin ■ phenobarbital ■ plicamycin ■ Quinolones ■ sulindac
Nephrotoxicity ■ Altered creatinine clearance (decreased or increased)	■ Reduce dosage or stop drug.	■ Aminoglycosides ■ Cephalosporins

Managing toxic drug reactions *(continued)*

Toxic reactions and clinical effects	Interventions	Selected causative drugs
Nephrotoxicity *(continued)* ■ Blurred vision, dehydration (depending on part of kidney affected), edema, mild headache, pallor ■ Casts, albumin, or red or white blood cells in urine ■ Dizziness, fatigue, irritability, slowed mental processes ■ Electrolyte imbalance ■ Elevated blood urea nitrogen level ■ Oliguria	■ Perform hemodialysis, if needed. ■ Order monitoring of vital signs, weight changes, and urine volume. ■ Give symptomatic care: fluid restriction and loop diuretics to reduce fluid retention, I.V. solutions to correct electrolyte imbalance.	■ cisplatin ■ Contrast media ■ Corticosteroids ■ cyclosporine ■ gallium ■ Gold salts (parenteral) ■ Nitrosoureas ■ Nonsteroidal anti-inflammatory drugs ■ penicillin ■ pentamidine isethionate ■ plicamycin ■ Vasopressors or vasoconstrictors
Neurotoxicity ■ Akathisia ■ Bilateral or unilateral palsies ■ Muscle twitching, tremor ■ Paresthesia ■ Seizures ■ Strokelike syndrome ■ Unsteady gait ■ Weakness	■ Notify the doctor as soon as changes appear. ■ Reduce dosage or stop drug. ■ Monitor carefully for changes in the patient's condition. ■ Order symptomatic care. Remain with the patient, reassure him, and protect him during seizures. Provide a quiet environment, draw shades, and speak in soft tones. Maintain the airway, and ventilate the patient as needed.	■ Aminoglycosides ■ cisplatin ■ cytarabine ■ isoniazid ■ nitroprusside ■ polymyxin B injection ■ Vinca alkaloids
Ocular toxicity ■ Acute glaucoma ■ Blurred, colored, or flickering vision ■ Cataracts ■ Corneal deposits ■ Diplopia ■ Miosis ■ Mydriasis ■ Optic neuritis ■ Scotomata ■ Vision loss	■ Notify the doctor as soon as changes appear. ■ Stop drug if possible. (Some oculotoxic drugs used to treat serious conditions may be given again at a reduced dosage after the eyes are rested and have returned to near normal.) ■ Monitor carefully for changes in symptoms.	■ amiodarone ■ Antibiotics such as chloramphenicol ■ Anticholinergics ■ Cardiac glycosides ■ chloroquine ■ clomiphene ■ Corticosteroids ■ cyclophosphamide ■ cytarabine ■ ethambutol

(continued)

Managing toxic drug reactions *(continued)*

Toxic reactions and clinical effects	Interventions	Selected causative drugs
Ocular toxicity *(continued)*	■ Treat effects symptomatically.	■ hydroxychloroquine ■ lithium carbonate ■ methotrexate ■ Phenothiazines ■ quinidine ■ quinine ■ rifampin ■ tamoxifen ■ Vinca alkaloids
Ototoxicity ■ Ataxia ■ Hearing loss ■ Tinnitus ■ Vertigo	■ Notify the doctor as soon as changes appear. ■ Stop drug or reduce dosage. ■ Monitor carefully for symptomatic changes.	■ Aminoglycosides ■ Antibiotics, such as colistimethate sodium, erythromycin, gentamicin, kanamycin, and streptomycin ■ chloroquine ■ cisplatin ■ Loop diuretics ■ minocycline ■ quinidine ■ quinine ■ Salicylates ■ vancomycin
Pseudomembranous colitis ■ Abdominal pain ■ Colonic perforation ■ Fever ■ Hypotension ■ Severe dehydration ■ Shock ■ Sudden, copious diarrhea (watery or bloody)	■ Discontinue drug and order another antibiotic, such as vancomycin or metronidazole. ■ Maintain fluid and electrolyte balance. ■ Check serum electrolyte levels daily. If pseudomembranous colitis is mild, order an ion exchange resin. ■ Monitor vital signs and hydration status. ■ Immediately report signs of shock to doctor. ■ Observe for signs of hypokalemia, especially malaise and weak, rapid, irregular pulse.	■ Antibiotics

Drug dosages in patients with renal failure

Impaired renal function can modify a drug's bioavailability, distribution,

pharmacologic action, and elimination. Therefore, drug dosages must be evaluated and adjusted, as needed, to avoid accidental overdose.

Adjusting drug dosages in renal failure

To prevent an accidental drug overdose in a patient with renal failure, adjust dosages according to the severity of renal impairment, as shown in the chart below. (Note: "GFR" refers to glomerular filtration rate.)

Drug	Mild renal impairment (GFR > 50 ml/ minute)		Moderate renal impairment (GFR 10 to 50 ml/minute)		Severe renal impairment (GFR < 10 ml/ minute)	
	% of normal dose	Interval	% of normal dose	Interval	% of normal dose	Interval
acetaminophen	100%	q 4 hr	100%	q 6 hr	100%	q 8 hr
acetazolamide	100%	q 6 hr	100%	q 12 hr	Avoid	Avoid
acetohexamide	100%	q 12 hr	Avoid	Avoid	Avoid	Avoid
acyclovir	100%	q 8 hr	100%	q 24 hr	100%	q 48 hr
allopurinol	75%	q 8 hr	75%	q 8 hr	50%	q 8 hr
amantadine	100%	q 24 to 48 hr	100%	q 48 to 72 hr	100%	q 7 days
amikacin	60% to 90%	q 12 hr	30% to 70%	q 12 to 18 hr	20% to 30%	q 24 to 48 hr
amoxicillin	100%	q 6 hr	100%	q 8 to 12 hr	100%	q 24 hr
amphotericin B	100%	q 24 hr	100%	q 24 hr	100%	q 24 to 36 hr
ampicillin	100%	q 6 hr	100%	q 6 to 12 hr	100%	q 12 to 24 hr
aspirin	100%	q 4 hr	100%	q 4 to 6 hr	Avoid	Avoid
atenolol	100%	q 24 hr	50%	q 48 hr	30% to 50%	q 96 hr

(continued)

Drug	Mild renal impairment (GFR > 50 ml/ minute)		Moderate renal impairment (GFR 10 to 50 ml/minute)		Severe renal impairment (GFR < 10 ml/ minute)	
	% of normal dose	Interval	% of normal dose	Interval	% of normal dose	Interval
azathioprine	100%	q 24 hr	75%	q 24 hr	50%	q 36 hr
betaxolol	100%	q 24 hr	100%	q 24 hr	50%	q 24 hr
bleomycin	100%	Varies	75%	Varies	50%	Varies
captopril	100%	q 8 to 12 hr	75%	q 12 to 18 hr	50%	q 24 hrs
carbamazepine	100%	q 6 to 8 hr	100%	q 6 to 8 hr	75%	q 6 to 8 hr
carbenicillin	100%	q 8 to 12 hr	100%	q 12 to 24 hr	100%	q 24 to 48 hr
cefaclor	100%	q 8 hr	50% to 100%	q 6 hr	33%	q 6 hr
cefadroxil	100%	q 12 hr	100%	q 12 to 24 hr	100%	q 24 to 48 hr
cefonicid	50%	q 24 hr	10% to 50%	q 24 hr	10%	q 24 hr to 5 days
cefotaxime	100%	q 6 to 8 hr	100%	q 8 to 12 hr	100%	q 24 hr
cefoxitin	100%	q 8 hr	100%	q 8 to 12 hr	100%	q 24 to 48 hr
cephalexin	100%	q 8 hr	100%	q 12 hr	100%	q 12 hr
cephalothin	100%	q 6 hr	100%	q 6 to 8 hr	100%	q 12 hr
cephapirin	100%	q 6 hr	100%	q 6 to 8 hr	100%	q 12 hr
cephradine	100%	q 6 hr	50% to 100%	q 6 hr	25%	q 6 to 12 hr
chloral hydrate	100%	At bed-time	Avoid	Avoid	Avoid	Avoid

Adjusting drug dosages in renal failure *(continued)*

Drug	Mild renal impairment (GFR > 50 ml/minute)		Moderate renal impairment (GFR 10 to 50 ml/minute)		Severe renal impairment (GFR < 10 ml/minute)	
	% of normal dose	Interval	% of normal dose	Interval	% of normal dose	Interval
chlorpropamide	50%	q 24 hr	Avoid	Avoid	Avoid	Avoid
chlorthalidone	100%	q 24 hr	100%	q 24 hr	Avoid	Avoid
cimetidine	100%	q 6 hr	100%	q 8 hr	100%	q 12 hr
ciprofloxacin	100%	q 12 hr	100%	q 12 to 24 hr	100%	q 24 hr
cisplatin	100%	Varies	75%	Varies	50%	Varies
clofibrate	100%	q 6 to 12 hr	100%	q 12 to 18 hr	Avoid	Avoid
clonidine	100%	b.i.d.	100%	b.i.d.	50% to 75%	b.i.d.
colchicine	100%	Varies	50%	Varies	25%	Varies
cyclophosphamide	100%	q 24 hr	100%	q 24 hr	75%	q 24 hr
diflunisal	100%	q 12 hr	50%	q 12 hr	50%	q 12 hr
digitoxin	100%	q 24 hr	100%	q 24 hr	50% to 75%	q 24 hr
digoxin	100%	q 24 hr	100%	q 36 hr	100%	q 48 hr
diphenhydramine	100%	q 6 hr	100%	q 6 to 8 hr	100%	q 8 to 12 hr
disopyramide	100%	q 8 hr	100%	q 12 to 24 hr	100%	q 24 to 40 hr
doxycycline	100%	q 24 hr	100%	q 24 hr	100%	q 24 hr
efamandole	100%	q 6 hr	100%	q 6 to 8 hr	100%	q 8 hr
ethacrynic acid	100%	q 8 to 12 hr	100%	q 8 to 12 hr	Avoid	Avoid

(continued)

Drug	Mild renal impairment (GFR > 50 ml/ minute)		Moderate renal impairment (GFR 10 to 50 ml/minute)		Severe renal impairment (GFR < 10 ml/ minute)	
	% of normal dose	Interval	% of normal dose	Interval	% of normal dose	Interval
ethambutol	100%	q 24 hr	100%	q 24 to 36 hr	100%	q 48 hr
ethosuximide	100%	q 12 hr	100%	q 12 hr	75%	q 12 hr
flucytosine	100%	q 12 hr	100%	q 16 hr	100%	q 24 hr
ganciclovir	100%	q 12 hr	100%	q 24 hr	100%	q 24 hr
gemfibrozil	100%	b.i.d.	50%	b.i.d.	25%	b.i.d.
gentamicin	60% to 90%	q 8 to 12 hr	30% to 70%	q 12 hr	20% to 30%	q 24 hr
guanethidine	100%	q 24 hr	100%	q 24 hr	100%	q 24 to 36 hr
hydralazine	100%	q 8 hr	100%	q 8 hr	100%	q 8 to 16 hr or q 12 to 24 hr
hydroxyurea	100%	Varies	50%	Varies	20%	Varies
isoniazid	100%	q 24 hr	100%	q 24 hr	66% to 75%	q 24 hr
kanamycin	60% to 90%	q 8 to 12 hr	30% to 70%	q 12 hr	20% to 30%	q 24 hr
ketorolac	100%	p.r.n.	50%	p.r.n.	Avoid	Avoid
lincomycin	100%	q 6 hr	100%	q 12 hr	100%	q 24 hr
lisinopril	100%	q 24 hr	50%	q 24 hr	25%	q 24 hr
lithium carbonate	100%	t.i.d. to q.i.d.	50% to 75%	t.i.d. to q.i.d	25% to 50%	t.i.d. to q.i.d.
loracarbef	100%	q 12 to 24 hr	50%	q 12 to 24 hr	100%	q 3 to 5 days

Adjusting drug dosages in renal failure *(continued)*

Drug	Mild renal impairment (GFR > 50 ml/minute)		Moderate renal impairment (GFR 10 to 50 ml/minute)		Severe renal impairment (GFR <10 ml/minute)	
	% of normal dose	Interval	% of normal dose	Interval	% of normal dose	Interval
lorazepam	100%	t.i.d. to q.i.d.	100%	t.i.d. to q.i.d.	50%	t.i.d. to q.i.d.
meperidine	100%	Varies	75%	Varies	Avoid	Avoid
meprobamate	100%	q 6 hr	100%	q 9 to 12 hr	100%	q 12 to 18 hr
methadone	100%	q 6 to 8 hr	100%	q 6 to 8 hr	50% to 75%	q 6 to 8 hr
methotrexate	100%	Varies	50%	Varies	Avoid	Avoid
methyldopa	100%	q 6 hr	100%	q 8 to 18 hr	100%	q 12 to 24 hr
metoclopramide	100%	Varies	75%	Varies	50%	Varies
metronidazole	100%	q 8 hr	100%	q 8 to 12 hr	100%	q 12 to 24 hr
mexiletine	100%	q 12 hr	100%	q 12 hr	50% to 75%	q 12 hr
mezlocillin	100%	q 4 to 6 hr	100%	q 6 to 8 hr	100%	q 8 hr
mitomycin	100%	Varies	100%	Varies	75%	Varies
moricizine	100%	q 8 hr	100%	q 8 hr	100%	q 8 hr
nadolol	100%	q 24 hr	50%	q 24 hr	25%	q 24 hr
nalidixic acid	100%	q.i.d.	Avoid	Avoid	Avoid	Avoid
neostigmine	100%	q 24 hr	50%	q 24 hr	25%	q 24 hr
netilmicin	60% to 90%	q 8 to 12 hr	30% to 70%	q 12 hr	20% to 30%	q 24 hr
nicotinic acid	100%	t.i.d.	50%	t.i.d.	25%	ti.d.

(continued)

Adjusting drug dosages in renal failure *(continued)*

Drug	Mild renal impairment (GFR > 50 ml/minute)		Moderate renal impairment (GFR 10 to 50 ml/minute)		Severe renal impairment (GFR < 10 ml/minute)	
	% of normal dose	Interval	% of normal dose	Interval	% of normal dose	Interval
nitrofurantoin	100%	q.i.d.	Avoid	Avoid	Avoid	Avoid
oxazepam	100%	q.i.d.	100%	q.i.d.	75%	q.i.d.
penicillin G	100%	q 6 to 8 hr	100%	q 8 to 12 hr	Avoid over 10 million U/day	q 12 to 16 hr
pentamidine isethionate (parenteral)	100%	q 24 hr	100%	q 24 to 36 hr	100%	q 48 hr
phenobarbital	100%	t.i.d.	100%	t.i.d.	100%	q 12 to 16 hr
phenylbutazone	100%	t.i.d. to q.i.d.	100%	t.i.d. to q.i.d.	Avoid	Avoid
piperacillin	100%	q 4 to 6 hr	100%	q 6 to 8 hr	100%	q 8 hr
plicamycin	100%	Varies	75%	Varies	50%	Varies
primidone	100%	q 8 hr	100%	q 8 to 12 hr	50%	q 12 to 24 hr
probenecid	100%	q.i.d.	Avoid	Avoid	Avoid	Avoid
procainamide	100%	q 4 hr	100%	q 6 to 12 hr	100%	q 8 to 24 hr
propoxyphene	100%	q 4 hr	100%	q 4 hr	Avoid	Avoid
reserpine	100%	q 24 hr	100%	q 24 hr	Avoid	Avoid
spironolactone	100%	q 6 to 12 hr	100%	q 12 to 24 hr	Avoid	Avoid
streptomycin	100%	q 24 hr	100%	q 24 to 72 hr	100%	q 72 to 96 hr

Adjusting drug dosages in renal failure *(continued)*

Drug	Mild renal impairment (GFR > 50 ml/minute)		Moderate renal impairment (GFR 10 to 50 ml/minute)		Severe renal impairment (GFR < 10 ml/minute)	
	% of normal dose	Interval	% of normal dose	Interval	% of normal dose	Interval
streptozocin	100%	Varies	75%	Varies	50%	Varies
sulfamethoxazole	100%	q 12 hr	100%	q 18 hr	100%	q 24 hr
sulfisoxazole	100%	q 6 hr	100%	q 8 to 12 hr	100%	q 12 to 24 hr
sulindac	100%	b.i.d.	100%	b.i.d.	50%	b.i.d.
terbutaline	100%	t.i.d.	50%	t.i.d.	Avoid	Avoid
thiazides	100%	Daily to b.i.d.	100%	Daily to b.i.d.	Avoid	Avoid
ticarcillin	100%	q 8 to 12 hr	100%	q 12 to 24 hr	100%	q 24 to 48 hr
tobramycin	60% to 90%	q 8 to 12 hr	30% to 70%	q 12 hr	20% to 30%	q 24 hr
triamterene	100%	q 12 hr	100%	q 12 hr	Avoid	Avoid
trimethoprim	100%	q 12 hr	100%	q 18 hr	100%	q 24 hr
vancomycin	100%	q 1 to 3 days	100%	q 3 to 10 days	100%	q 10 days
vidarabine	100%	Continuous infusion	100%	Continuous infusion	75%	Continuous infusion

Reversing anaphylaxis

Anaphylaxis — the sudden, extreme reaction to a foreign antigen — requires immediate treatment. Generally, the faster the onset of symptoms, the more severe the reaction. This chart lists drugs useful in reversing anaphylactic reactions.

Drug and dosage	Action	Nursing considerations
Aminophylline (Aminophyllin) Severe anaphylaxis I.V.: 5 to 6 mg/kg as loading dose, followed by 0.4 to 0.9 mg/kg/hour by infusion.	■ Causes bronchodilation ■ Stimulates respiratory drive ■ Dilates constricted pulmonary arteries ■ Causes diuresis ■ Strengthens cardiac contractions ■ Increases vital capacity ■ Causes coronary vasodilation	■ Monitor blood pressure, pulse, and respirations. ■ Monitor intake and output, hydration status, and aminophylline and electrolyte levels. ■ Monitor the patient for arrhythmias. ■ Use an I.V. controller to reduce the risk of overdose. ■ Maintain serum levels at 10 to 20 mcg/ml.
Cimetidine (Tagamet) Severe anaphylaxis (experimental use in refractory cases) I.V.: 600 mg diluted in dextrose 5% in water (D_5W) and administered over 20 minutes.	■ Competes with histamine for histamine$_2$-receptor sites ■ Prevents laryngeal edema	■ Be aware that this drug is incompatible with aminophylline. ■ Reduce the dosage for patients with impaired renal or hepatic function.
Diphenhydramine (Benadryl) Mild anaphylaxis P.O.: 25 to 100 mg t.i.d. I.V.: 25 to 50 mg q.i.d.	■ Competes with histamine for histamine$_1$-receptor sites ■ Prevents laryngeal edema ■ Controls localized itching	■ Administer I.V. doses slowly to avoid hypotension. ■ Monitor the patient for hypotension and drowsiness. ■ Give fluids as needed. Drug causes dry mouth.
Epinephrine (Adrenalin) Severe anaphylaxis (drug of choice) Initial infusion: 0.2 to 0.5 mg (0.2 to 0.5 ml of 1:1,000 strength diluted in 10 ml of normal saline solution) given I.V. slowly over 5 to 10 minutes followed by continuous infusion.	*Alpha-adrenergic effects* ■ Increases blood pressure ■ Reverses peripheral vasodilation and systemic hypotension ■ Considered the drug of choice for treating anaphylaxis ■ Decreases angioedema and urticaria	■ Select a large vein for infusion. ■ Use an infusion controller to regulate drip rate. ■ Check blood pressure and heart rate frequently. ■ Monitor the patient for arrhythmias. ■ Check the solution strength, dosage, and label before administration.

Reversing anaphylaxis *(continued)*

Drug and dosage	Action	Nursing considerations
Epinephrine *(continued)* Continuous infusion: 1 to 4 mcg/minute (mix 1 ml of 1:1,000 epinephrine in 250 ml of D_5W to get a concentration of 4 mcg/ml).	■ Improves coronary blood flow by raising diastolic pressure ■ Causes peripheral vaso-constriction *Beta-adrenergic effects* ■ Causes bronchodila-tion ■ Causes positive ino-tropic and chronotropic cardiac activity ■ Decreases synthesis and release of chemical mediators	■ Watch for signs of extravasation at the infusion site. ■ Monitor intake and output. ■ Assess the color and tempera-ture of the extremities.
Hydrocortisone (Solu-Cortef) Severe anaphylaxis I.V.: 100 to 200 mg q 4 to 6 hour.	■ Prevents neutrophil and platelet aggregation ■ Inhibits the synthesis of mediators ■ Decreases capillary permeability	■ Monitor fluid and electrolyte balance, intake and output, and blood pressure closely. ■ Keep the patient on a prophy-lactic ulcer and antacid regimen.

Recognizing common adverse reactions in elderly patients

Elderly patients are especially suscepti-ble to adverse reactions, such as urti-caria, impotence, incontinence, GI up-set, and rashes. Less common adverse reactions — such as anxiety, confusion, and forgetfulness — may be mistaken for typical elderly behaviors. Because the reactions described below are seri-ous, you need to know how to recog-nize and deal with them.

Altered mental status
Agitation or confusion may result from use of an anticholinergic, a diuretic, an antihypertensive, or an antidepressant. Paradoxically, an antidepressant can cause depression.

Anorexia
Anorexia is a warning sign of a toxic reaction, especially from a cardiac gly-coside such as digoxin. Cardiac glyco-sides have a narrow therapeutic win-dow.

Blood disorders
If the patient is taking an anticoagu-lant, watch for signs of easy bruising or bleeding, such as excessive bleeding after tooth brushing. Such signs may signal thrombocytopenia or blood dys-crasias. Other drugs that may cause these reactions include antineoplastics such as methotrexate, antibiotics such as nitrofurantoin, and anticonvulsants such as valproic acid and phenytoin. Tell your patient to report easy bruising immediately.

Dehydration

If the patient is taking a diuretic, watch for dehydration and electrolyte imbalance. Monitor blood levels of the drug, and give the patient a potassium supplement. Many drugs, such as anticholinergics, cause dry mouth. Suggest sucking on sugarless candy for relief.

Orthostatic hypotension

Marked by light-headedness or faintness and unsteady footing, orthostatic hypotension can occur with the use of a sedative, an antidepressant, an antihypertensive, or an antipsychotic. To prevent falls, warn the patient not to sit up or get out of bed too quickly, and to call for help with walking if he feels dizzy or faint.

Tardive dyskinesia

Characterized by abnormal tongue movements, lip pursing, grimacing, blinking, and gyrating motions of the face and extremities, tardive dyskinesia can be triggered by the use of a psychotropic drug, such as haloperidol or chlorpromazine.

Identifying the most dangerous drugs

Almost any drug can cause an adverse reaction in some patients, but the following drugs cause about 90% of all reported reactions.

Anticoagulants

■ heparin
■ warfarin

Antimicrobials

■ Cephalosporins
■ Penicillins
■ Sulfonamides

Bronchodilators

■ Sympathomimetics
■ theophylline

Cardiac drugs

■ Antihypertensives
■ digoxin
■ Diuretics
■ quinidine

Central nervous system drugs

■ Analgesics
■ Anticonvulsants
■ Neuroleptics
■ Sedative-hypnotics

Diagnostic agents

■ X-ray contrast media

Hormones

■ Corticosteroids
■ Estrogens
■ insulin

Reporting reactions to the FDA

Drug manufacturers monitor adverse drug reactions and report them to the Food and Drug Administration (FDA). That's the law.

The FDA also wants to hear from nurses whose patients have experienced serious reactions associated with drugs — especially drugs that have been on the market for 3 years or less. After all, you and your colleagues are the ones most likely to see the reactions, so you can give the best clinical descriptions. Unlike the manufacturers, though, you aren't required by law to make a report.

What constitutes a serious reaction? According to the FDA, it's one that:
■ is life-threatening.
■ causes death.
■ leads to or prolongs hospitalization.
■ results in permanent or severe disability.

The FDA also wants to know about drugs that don't produce a therapeutic response. It doesn't need to hear about inappropriate drug use, prescriber errors, or administration errors. (However, the United States Pharmacopeia does want to know about medication errors — especially those caused by sound-alike or look-alike drug names. See your hospital pharmacist for more information.)

You can submit a report to the FDA even when you aren't sure whether your patient's reaction was serious or when you suspect, but you don't know for certain, that a reaction is the result of a drug.

To file a report, use the MEDWATCH form, which should be available in your pharmacy. When you fill it out, be as complete as possible. You don't have to include the patient's name or initials, but you should be able to identify the patient if the FDA requests follow-up information.

Approximately 60,000 reports on adverse reactions are collected annually; more than 400,000 are currently in the FDA's database. This translates into improved patient safety because the more reports that are submitted, the more information the FDA has to alert health care professionals to these adverse reactions.

What JCAHO requires

To meet standards set by the Joint Commission on Accreditation of Healthcare Organizations (JCAHO), a hospital must have an adverse drug reaction reporting program in place. The hospital's pharmacy and therapeutics committee is required to review "all significant untoward drug reactions" to ensure quality patient care.

What's a "significant" reaction? According to JCAHO, it's one in which:
■ the drug suspected of causing the reaction must be discontinued.
■ the patient requires treatment with another drug, such as an antihistamine, a steroid, or epinephrine.

■ the patient's hospital stay is prolonged — for example, because surgery had to be delayed or more diagnostic tests had to be done.

Why is such a reporting program important? For one thing, the quality of care improves when you know which patients are at higher risk for an adverse drug reaction and which drugs are most likely to cause these reactions. You'll be more alert for the early signs and symptoms of problems, and you'll be prepared to intervene before things get out of hand.

Second, the hospital will get more mileage out of its health care dollars because the lengthy stays and extra treatments associated with adverse drug reactions will be decreased.

Third, reducing the drug-induced injuries will decrease the number of malpractice lawsuits brought against the hospital and staff. That saves money, time, and aggravation.

Managing I.V. extravasation

Extravasation is the leakage of infused solution from a vein into surrounding tissue. The result of a needle puncturing the vessel wall or leakage around a venipuncture site, extravasation causes local pain and itching, edema, blanching, and decreased skin temperature in the affected extremity. Extravasation of I.V. solution may be referred to as infiltration because the fluid infiltrates the tissues.

Extravasation of a small amount of isotonic fluid or nonirritating drug usually causes only minor discomfort. Treatment involves routine comfort measures, such as the application of warm compresses. However, extravasation of some drugs can severely damage tissue through irritative, sclerotic, vesicant, corrosive, or vasoconstrictive action. In these cases, emergency measures must be taken to minimize tissue damage and necrosis, prevent the need for skin grafts or, rarely, avoid amputation.

Equipment and preparation
Three 25G ⁵⁄₈″ needles ♦ antidote for extravasated drug in appropriate syringe ♦ 5-ml syringe ♦ three tuberculin syringes ♦ alcohol pad or gauze pad soaked in antiseptic cleaning agent ♦ 4″ × 4″ gauze pad ♦ cold and warm compresses

Optional: anti-inflammatory drug ♦ 8.4% sodium bicarbonate ♦ normal saline solution

Attach one 25G ⁵⁄₈″ needle to the syringe containing the antidote. Connect the two remaining needles to two tuberculin syringes. Then fill the remaining tuberculin syringe with the anti-inflammatory drug, if needed.

Implementation
Hospital policy dictates extravasation treatment steps, which may include some or all of these steps:
■ Stop the infusion, and remove the I.V. needle unless you need the route to infiltrate the antidote. Carefully estimate the amount of extravasated solution, and notify the doctor.
■ Disconnect the tubing from the I.V. needle. Attach the 5-ml syringe to the needle and try to withdraw 3 to 5 ml of blood to remove any medication or blood in the tubing or needle and to provide a path to the infiltrated tissues.
■ Clean the area around the I.V. site with an alcohol pad or 4″ × 4″ gauze pad soaked in an antiseptic agent. Then insert the needle of the empty tuberculin syringe into the subcutaneous tissue around the site, and gently aspirate as much solution as possible from the tissue.

■ Instill the prescribed antidote into the subcutaneous tissue around the site. Then, if ordered, slowly instill an anti-inflammatory drug subcutaneously to help reduce the inflammation and edema.
■ If ordered, instill the prescribed antidote through the I.V. needle.
■ Apply cold compresses to the affected area for 24 hours, or apply an ice pack for 20 minutes every 4 hours, to cause vasoconstriction that may localize the drug and slow cell metabolism. After 24 hours, apply warm compresses, and elevate the affected extremity to reduce discomfort and promote fluid reabsorption. If the extravasated drug is a vasoconstrictor, such as norepinephrine or metaraminol bitartrate, apply warm compresses only.
■ Continuously monitor the I.V. site for signs of abscess or necrosis.

Special considerations
■ If you're administering a potentially tissue-damaging drug by I.V. bolus or push, first start an I.V. infusion, preferably with normal saline solution. Infuse a small amount of this solution, and check for signs of infiltration before injecting the drug.
■ Know the antidote (if any) for an I.V. drug that can cause tissue necrosis, in case extravasation occurs. Make sure you're familiar with your hospital's policy regarding the administration of such drugs and their antidotes.
■ Tell the patient to report any discomfort at the I.V. site. During infusion, frequently check the site for signs of infiltration.

Antidotes for extravasation

Antidote	Dose	Extravasated drug
Ascorbic acid injection	50 mg	■ dactinomycin
Edetate calcium disodium (calcium EDTA)	150 mg	■ cadmium ■ copper ■ manganese ■ zinc
Hyaluronidase 15 units/ml Mix a 150-U vial with 1 ml normal saline solution for injection. Withdraw 0.1 ml, and dilute with 0.9 ml of the normal saline solution to get 15 U/ml.	0.2 ml injected subcutaneously five times around site of extravasation	■ aminophylline ■ Calcium solutions ■ Contrast media ■ Dextrose solutions (concentrations of 10% or more) ■ nafcillin ■ Potassium solutions ■ Total parenteral nutrition solutions ■ vinblastine ■ vincristine ■ vindesine
Hydrocortisone sodium succinate 100 mg/ml Usually followed by topical application of hydrocortisone cream 1%	50 to 200 mg or 25 to 50 mg/ml of extravasate injected locally around site of extravasation	■ doxorubicin ■ vincristine
Phentolamine Dilute 5 to 10 mg with 10 ml of sterile normal saline solution for injection.	5 to 10 ml in 10 ml of normal saline solution injected locally around site of extravasation	■ dobutamine ■ dopamine ■ epinephrine ■ metaraminol bitartrate ■ norepinephrine
Sodium bicarbonate 8.4%	5 ml injected locally around site of extravasation	■ carmustine ■ daunorubicin ■ doxorubicin ■ vinblastine ■ vincristine
Sodium thiosulfate 10% Dilute 4 ml with 6 ml of sterile water for injection.	10 ml injected locally around site of extravasation	■ cisplatin ■ dactinomycin ■ mechlorethamine ■ mitomycin

Drug overdoses

General guidelines

If your patient has signs of an acute toxic reaction, institute advanced life support measures as indicated. Administer the prescribed antidote, if available, and institute measures to block absorption and speed elimination of the drug. Consult with a regional poison control center for additional information about treatment of specific toxins. The steps below outline how to manage an acute overdose of ingested systemic drugs.

Starting advanced life support
■ Establish and maintain an airway. This is usually done by inserting an oropharyngeal or endotracheal airway.
■ If the patient isn't breathing, start ventilation with a bag-valve mask until a mechanical ventilator is available. Check pulse oximetry results or arterial blood gas levels, and administer oxygen as needed.
■ Maintain circulation. Start an I.V. infusion, and obtain laboratory specimens to check for toxic drug levels as well as electrolyte and glucose levels as indicated. If patient has hypotension, administer fluids and a vasopressor such as dopamine (Intropin). If the patient has hypertension, prepare to administer an antihypertensive (usually a beta-adrenergic blocker if a catecholamine was ingested). Prepare to treat arrhythmias as indicated for the specific toxin.
■ Protect the patient from injury, and monitor him for seizures. Observe him, and provide supportive care. Prepare to administer diazepam, lorazepam, or phenytoin.

Administering the antidote
The antidote is administered as soon as possible. Administer the prescribed antidote, which depends on the type of drug the patient has taken.

Blocking drug absorption
■ Gastric emptying is effective up to 2 hours after drug ingestion. Two methods are used: syrup of ipecac for a conscious patient whose condition isn't expected to deteriorate and gastric lavage for a comatose patient or one who doesn't respond to syrup of ipecac.
■ Adsorption with activated charcoal is used in place of emesis or lavage if the drug is well adsorbed by activated charcoal or after emesis or lavage to adsorb co-ingestants if the primary toxin isn't well adsorbed by activated charcoal.
■ A cathartic may be given to speed transit of the poison through the GI tract. Whole-bowel irrigation with a balanced polyethylene glycol and electrolyte solution may be ordered if a sustained-release product was ingested.

Speeding drug elimination
■ Gastric dialysis uses timed doses of activated charcoal for 1 to 2 days. The charcoal binds to the drug, thus facilitating its removal in feces.
■ Diuresis is effective for some drug overdoses. Forced diuresis uses furosemide and an osmotic diuretic, alkaline diuresis uses I.V. sodium bicarbonate, and acid diuresis uses oral or I.V. ascorbic acid or ammonium chloride.
■ Peritoneal dialysis and hemodialysis are occasionally used for severe overdose.

Managing an acute toxic reaction

If your patient has signs of an acute toxic reaction, institute advanced life support measures as indicated. Administer the prescribed antidote, if available, and take steps to block absorption and speed elimination of the drug. Consult with a regional poison control center for information on how to treat ingestion of a specific toxin.

Managing poisoning or overdose

Antidote and indications	Dosages	Nursing considerations
acetylcysteine (Mucomyst, Mucosil, Parvolex) ■ Treatment of acetaminophen toxicity	■ Adults and children: 140 mg/kg P.O. initially, followed by 70 mg/kg every 4 hours for 17 doses (total of 1,330 mg/kg)	■ Use cautiously in an elderly or debilitated patient and in a patient with asthma or severe respiratory insufficiency. ■ Don't use with activated charcoal. ■ Don't combine with amphotericin B, ampicillin, chymotrypsin, erythromycin lactobionate, hydrogen peroxide, oxytetracycline, tetracycline, iodized oil, or trypsin. Administer separately.
activated charcoal (Actidose-Aqua, Charcoaid, CharcoCaps, Liqui-Char) ■ Treatment of poisoning or overdose with most orally administered drugs, except caustic agents and hydrocarbons	■ Adults: initially, 1 g/kg (30 to 100 g) P.O., or 5 to 10 times the amount of poison ingested as a suspension in 180 to 240 ml of water ■ Children ages 1 to 12: 20 to 50 g P.O. as single dose ■ Children younger than age 1: 1 g/kg P.O. as single dose	■ Don't give to a semiconscious or unconscious patient. ■ If possible, administer within 30 minutes of poisoning. Administer larger dose if the patient has food in his stomach. ■ Don't give with syrup of ipecac because charcoal inactivates ipecac. If a patient needs syrup of ipecac, give charcoal after he has finished vomiting. ■ Don't give in ice cream, milk, or sherbet because these foods reduce the adsorption capacities of charcoal. ■ The powder form is the most effective; mix it with tap water to form a thick syrup. You may add a small amount of fruit juice or flavoring to make the syrup more palatable. ■ You may need to repeat the dose if the patient vomits shortly after administration.
aminocaproic acid (Amicar) ■ Antidote for alteplase, anistreplase, streptokinase, or urokinase toxicity	■ Adults: 4 to 5 g I.V. in 1st hour, followed by 1 g/hour until bleeding is controlled; not to exceed 30 g daily	■ Use cautiously with oral contraceptives and estrogens because they may increase the risk of hypercoagulability. ■ For infusion, dilute solution with sterile water for injection, normal saline solution, dextrose 5% in water (D_5W), or lactated Ringer's solution. ■ Monitor coagulation studies, heart rhythm, and blood pressure.

(continued)

Managing poisoning or overdose *(continued)*

Antidote and indications	Dosages	Nursing considerations
amyl nitrite ■ Antidote for cyanide poisoning	■ Adults: 0.2 or 0.3 ml by inhalation for 30 to 60 seconds every 5 minutes until patient regains consciousness	■ Amyl nitrite is effective within 30 seconds, but its effects last only 3 to 5 minutes. ■ To administer, wrap an ampule in a cloth and crush. Hold it near the patient's nose and mouth so that he can inhale the vapor. ■ Monitor the patient for orthostatic hypotension. ■ The patient may experience headache after administration.
atropine sulfate ■ Antidote for anticholinesterase toxicity and organophosphate poisoning	■ Adults: initially, 1 to 2 mg by direct I.V. injection, then 2 mg every 5 to 60 minutes until symptoms subside; in severe cases, initial dose may be as much as 6 mg every 4 to 60 minutes, as needed (administer over 1 to 2 minutes)	■ Atropine sulfate is contraindicated for a patient with glaucoma, myasthenia gravis, obstructive uropathy, or unstable cardiovascular status. ■ Monitor intake and output to assess the patient for urine retention.
botulism antitoxin, trivalent equine ■ Treatment of botulism	■ Adults and children: 2 vials I.V.; dilute antitoxin 1:10 in D_5W, $D_{10}W$, or normal saline solution before administration; give first 10 ml of diluted solution over 5 minutes; after 15 minutes, you may increase rate	■ Obtain an accurate patient history of allergies, especially to horses, and of reactions to immunizations. ■ Test the patient for sensitivity (against a control of normal saline solution in opposing extremity) before administration. Read the results after 5 to 30 minutes. A wheal indicates a positive reaction, requiring patient desensitization. ■ Keep epinephrine 1:1,000 available in case of an allergic reaction.
deferoxamine mesylate (Desferal) ■ Adjunctive treatment of acute iron intoxication	■ I.V. 15 mg/kg/hour maximum total of 90 mg/hour over 8 hours; maximum of three 8-hour doses except in severe cases *For patients in shock* ■ Initial 1 g followed by two 500-mg doses 4 hours apart, at a rate of 15 mg/kg/hour.	■ Don't administer the drug to a patient with severe renal disease or anuria. Use cautiously in a patient with impaired renal function. ■ Keep epinephrine 1:1,000 available in case of an allergic reaction. ■ Use I.M. route if possible. Use I.V. route only when the patient is in shock.

Managing poisoning or overdose *(continued)*

Antidote and indications	Dosages	Nursing considerations
deferoxamine mesylate (Desferal) *(continued)*		■ To reconstitute for I.M. administration, add 2 ml of sterile water for injection to each ampule. Make sure the drug dissolves completely. To reconstitute for I.V. administration, dissolve as for I.M. use but in normal saline solution, D$_5$W, or lactated Ringer's solution. ■ Monitor intake and output carefully. Warn the patient that his urine may turn red. ■ Reconstituted solution can be stored for up to 1 week at room temperature. Protect it from light.
digoxin immune Fab (ovine) (Digibind) ■ Treatment of potentially life-threatening digoxin or digitoxin intoxication	■ Adults and children: give I.V. over 30 minutes or as a bolus if cardiac arrest is imminent; dosage varies according to amount of drug ingested; average dose is 10 vials (400 mg), but if toxic reaction resulted from acute digoxin ingestion and neither serum digoxin level nor estimated ingestion amount is known, increase dose to 20 vials (760 mg) ■ Package inserts or reference books contain charts and formulas to calculate dose based on number of tablets ingested or serum digoxin level.	■ Use cautiously in a patient who is allergic to ovine proteins because the drug is derived from digoxin-specific antibody fragments obtained from immunized sheep. Perform a skin test before administering. ■ Use only for a patient in shock or cardiac arrest with ventricular arrhythmias, such as ventricular tachycardia or fibrillation; with progressive bradycardia, such as severe sinus bradycardia; or with second- or third-degree atrioventricular block who are unresponsive to atropine. ■ Infuse through a 0.22-micron membrane filter, if possible. ■ Refrigerate powder for reconstitution. If possible, use the reconstituted drug immediately, although you may refrigerate it for up to 4 hours. ■ Drug interferes with digoxin immunoassay measurements, resulting in misleading standard serum digoxin levels until the drug is cleared from the body (about 2 days). ■ Total serum digoxin levels may rise after administration of this drug, reflecting fat-bound (inactive) digoxin. ■ Monitor potassium levels closely.

(continued)

Antidote and indications	Dosages	Nursing considerations
edetate calcium disodium (Calcium Disodium Versenate, Calcium EDTA) edetate calcium disodium (Calcium Disodium Versenate, Calcium EDTA) ■ Treatment of lead poisoning in patients with blood levels > 50 µg/dl	*For blood levels of 51 to 100 µg/dl* ■ Adults and children: 1 g/m², I.M. or I.V. daily for 3 to 5 days. For I.V. infusion, dilute in D_5W or normal saline solution and give over 8 to 12 hours. *For blood levels > 100 µg/dl* ■ Adults and children: 1.5 g/m², I.M. or I.V. daily for 3 to 5 days, usually with dimercaprol. For I.V. infusion, dilute in D_5W or normal saline solution and administer over 1 to 2 hours. If necessary, repeat course 2 to 3 weeks later.	■ Don't give to a patient with severe renal disease or anuria. ■ Avoid using I.V. route in a patient with lead encephalopathy because intracranial pressure may increase; use I.M. route. ■ Avoid rapid infusion; I.M. route is preferred, especially for children. ■ If giving a high dose, give with dimercaprol to avoid a toxic reaction. ■ Give plenty of fluids to facilitate lead excretion, except in patients with lead encephalopathy. ■ Before giving the drug, obtain baseline intake and output, urinalysis, blood urea nitrogen, and serum alkaline phosphatase, calcium, creatinine, and phosphorus levels. Then monitor these values on 1st, 3rd, and 5th days of treatment. Monitor electrocardiogram results periodically. ■ If procaine hydrochloride has been added to I.M. solution to minimize pain, watch for local reaction.
methylene blue ■ Treatment of cyanide poisoning	■ Adults and children: 1 to 2 mg/kg of 1% solution by direct I.V. injection over several minutes; may repeat dose in 1 hour	■ Don't give to a patient with severe renal impairment or a hypersensitivity to the drug. ■ Use with caution in glucose-6-phosphate dehydrogenase deficiency; may cause hemolysis. ■ Avoid extravasation; S.C. injection may cause necrotic abscesses. ■ Warn the patient that methylene blue will discolor his urine and stools and stain his skin. Hypochlorite solution rubbed on skin will remove stains.
naloxone hydrochloride (Narcan) ■ Treatment of respiratory depression caused by opioids	*For respiratory depression caused by opioid ingestion* ■ Adults: 0.4 to 2 mg I.V., S.C., or I.M.; may repeat every 2 to 3 minutes, as needed	■ Use cautiously in a patient with cardiac irritability or narcotic addiction. ■ Monitor respiratory depth and rate. Be prepared to provide oxygen, ventilation, and other resuscitative measures.

Managing poisoning or overdose *(continued)*

Antidote and indications	Dosages	Nursing considerations
naloxone hydrochloride (Narcan) *(continued)* ■ Treatment of postoperative narcotic depression ■ Treatment of asphyxia neonatorum	*For postoperative narcotic depression* ■ Adults: 0.1 to 0.2 mg I.V. every 2 to 3 minutes, as needed ■ Children: 0.01 mg/kg I.V., I.M., or S.C.; repeat as necessary every 2 to 3 minutes; if the patient doesn't improve with initial dose he may need up to 10 times this dose (0.1 mg/kg) *For asphyxia neonatorum* ■ Neonates: 0.01 mg/kg I.V. into umbilical vein; repeat every 2 to 3 minutes for three doses, if necessary	■ If neonatal concentration (0.02 mg/ml) isn't available, dilute adult concentration (0.4 mg) by mixing 0.5 ml with 9.5 ml of sterile water or normal saline solution. ■ Respiratory rate increases within 2 minutes. Effects last 1 to 4 hours. ■ Duration of narcotic may exceed that of naloxone, causing the patient to relapse into respiratory depression. ■ You may administer drug by continuous I.V. infusion to control adverse effects of epidurally administered morphine. ■ You may see "overshoot" effect — the patient's respiratory rate after receiving drug exceeds his rate before respiratory depression occurred. ■ Naloxone is the safest drug to use when the cause of respiratory depression is uncertain. ■ This drug doesn't reverse respiratory depression caused by diazepam. ■ Although generally believed ineffective in treating respiratory depression caused by nonopioids, naloxone may reverse coma induced by alcohol intoxication, according to recent reports.
pralidoxime chloride (Protopam Chloride) ■ Antidote for organophosphate poisoning and cholinergic overdose	■ Adults: I.V. infusion of 1 to 2 g in 100 ml of normal saline solution over 15 to 30 minutes (If the patient has pulmonary edema, administer by slow I.V. push over 5 minutes. Repeat in 1 hour if weakness persists. If the patient needs additional doses, administer them cautiously. If I.V. administration isn't possible, give I.M. or S.C., or 1 to 3 g P.O. every 5 hours.) ■ Children: 20 to 40 mg/kg I.V.	■ Don't give to a patient poisoned with carbaryl (Sevin), a carbamate insecticide, because it increases the toxic effects of carbaryl. ■ Use with caution in a patient with renal insufficiency, myasthenia gravis, asthma, or peptic ulcer. ■ Use in a hospitalized patient only; have respiratory and other supportive equipment available. ■ Administer the antidote as soon as possible after poisoning. Treatment is most effective if started within 24 hours of exposure. ■ Before administering, suction secretions and make sure airway is patent. ■ Dilute the drug with sterile water without preservatives. Give atropine along with pralidoxime.

(continued)

Managing poisoning or overdose *(continued)*

Antidote and indications	Dosages	Nursing considerations
pralidoxime chloride (Protopam Chloride) *(continued)*		■ If the patient's skin was exposed, remove his clothing and wash his skin and hair with sodium bicarbonate, soap, water, and alcohol as soon as possible. He may need a second washing. When washing the patient, wear protective gloves and clothes to avoid exposure. ■ Observe the patient for 48 to 72 hours after he ingested poison. Delayed absorption may occur. Watch for signs of rapid weakening in the patient with myasthenia gravis being treated for overdose of cholinergic drugs. He may pass quickly from cholinergic crisis to myasthenic crisis and require more cholinergic drugs to treat the myasthenia. Keep edrophonium available.
protamine sulfate ■ Treatment of heparin overdose	■ Adults: usually 1 mg for every 78 to 95 units of heparin, based on coagulation studies; dilute to 1% (10 mg/ml) and give by slow I.V. injection over 1 to 3 minutes; don't exceed 50 mg in 10 minutes	■ Use cautiously after cardiac surgery. ■ Administer slowly to reduce adverse reactions. Have equipment available to treat shock. ■ Monitor the patient continuously, and check vital signs frequently. ■ Watch for spontaneous bleeding (heparin "rebound"), especially in patients undergoing dialysis and in those who have had cardiac surgery. ■ Protamine sulfate may act as an anticoagulant in extremely high doses.
syrup of ipecac ■ Induction of vomiting in poisoning	■ Adults: 15 ml P.O., followed by 200 to 300 ml of water ■ Children older than age 1: 15 ml P.O., followed by 200 ml of water ■ Children younger than age 1: 5 to 10 ml P.O., followed by 100 to 200 ml of water or milk; repeat dose once after 20 minutes, if necessary	■ Syrup of ipecac is contraindicated for a semicomatose, an unconscious, or a severely inebriated patient and for a patient with seizures, shock, or absent gag reflex. ■ Don't give after ingestion of petroleum distillates or volatile oils because of the risk of aspiration pneumonitis. Don't give after ingestion of caustic substances such as lye because further injury can result.

Managing poisoning or overdose *(continued)*

Antidote and indications	Dosages	Nursing considerations
syrup of ipecac *(continued)*		■ Before giving, make sure you have ipecac syrup, not ipecac fluid extract (14 times more concentrated, and deadly). ■ If two doses don't induce vomiting, consider gastric lavage. ■ If the patient also needs activated charcoal, give charcoal after he has vomited, or charcoal will neutralize the emetic effect. ■ Suggest to parents of children over age 1 that they keep 1 oz (30 ml) of syrup of ipecac available.

Acetaminophen overdose

With an acute acetaminophen overdose, plasma levels of 300 µg/ml 4 hours after ingestion or 50 µg/ml 12 hours after ingestion are associated with hepatotoxicity. Signs and symptoms of overdose include cyanosis, anemia, jaundice, skin eruptions, fever, emesis, central nervous system (CNS) stimulation, delirium, and methemoglobinemia progressing to CNS depression, coma, vascular collapse, seizures, and death. Acetaminophen poisoning develops in stages:

■ *stage 1 (12 to 24 hours after ingestion)* — nausea, vomiting, diaphoresis, anorexia
■ *stage 2 (24 to 48 hours after ingestion)* — clinically improved but elevated liver function test results
■ *stage 3 (72 to 96 hours after ingestion)* — peak hepatotoxicity
■ *stage 4 (7 to 8 days after ingestion)* — recovery.

To treat acetaminophen toxicity, immediately induce emesis with syrup of ipecac if the patient is conscious or with gastric lavage if he's comatose or doesn't respond to syrup of ipecac. Administer activated charcoal via a nasogastric tube and oral acetylcysteine. Monitor laboratory results and vital signs closely. Provide symptomatic and supportive measures, including respiratory support and correction of fluid and electrolyte imbalances.

Oral acetylcysteine, a specific antidote for acetaminophen poisoning, is most effective if started within 12 hours after ingestion but can help if started as late as 24 hours after ingestion. Administer an oral loading dose of acetylcysteine, 140 mg/kg of body weight, followed by oral maintenance doses, 70 mg/kg of body weight every 4 hours for an additional 17 doses. Doses vomited within 1 hour of administration must be repeated. Remove charcoal by lavage before administering acetylcysteine because it may interfere with this antidote's absorption. Acetylcysteine minimizes hepatic injury by supplying sulfhydryl groups that bind with acetaminophen metabolites.

Also, hemodialysis may help remove acetaminophen from the body, and cimetidine has been used investigationally to block acetaminophen's metabolism to toxic intermediates. Determine plasma acetaminophen levels at least 4 hours after overdose. If they indicate hepatotoxicity, perform liver function tests every 24 hours for at least 96 hours.

Analeptic overdose (amphetamines, cocaine)

Individual responses to overdose with analeptics vary widely. Toxic doses also vary, depending on the drug and the route of ingestion.

Signs and symptoms of overdose include restlessness, tremor, hyperreflexia, tachypnea, confusion, aggressiveness, hallucinations, and panic; fatigue and depression usually follow the excitement stage. Other effects include arrhythmias, shock, altered blood pressure, nausea, vomiting, diarrhea, and abdominal cramps; seizures and coma usually precede death.

Treat overdose symptomatically and supportively: If oral ingestion is recent (within 4 hours), use gastric lavage or syrup of ipecac to empty the stomach and reduce further absorption. Follow with activated charcoal. Monitor vital signs and fluid and electrolyte balance. If the drug was smoked or injected, focus on enhancing drug elimination and providing supportive care. Administer a sedative if needed. Urine acidification may enhance excretion. A saline cathartic (magnesium citrate) may hasten GI evacuation of unabsorbed sustained-release drug.

Anticholinergic overdose

Signs and symptoms of anticholinergic overdose include such peripheral effects as dilated, nonreactive pupils; blurred vision; flushed, hot, dry skin;

dry mucous membranes; dysphagia; decreased or absent bowel sounds; urine retention; hyperthermia; tachycardia; hypertension; and increased respiratory rate.

Treatment is primarily symptomatic and supportive as needed. If the patient is alert, induce emesis (or use gastric lavage), and follow with a saline cathartic and activated charcoal to prevent further drug absorption. In severe cases, physostigmine may be administered to block central antimuscarinic effects. Give fluids as needed to treat shock. If urine retention occurs, catheterization may be necessary.

Anticoagulant overdose

Signs and symptoms of oral anticoagulant overdose vary with severity. They may include internal or external bleeding or skin necrosis, but the most common sign is hematuria.

If patient develops an excessively prolonged prothrombin time, elevated International Normalized Ratio, or minor bleeding, anticoagulant therapy must be stopped; withholding one or two doses may be adequate in some cases. Other measures to control bleeding include oral or I.V. phytonadione (vitamin K_1) and, for severe hemorrhage, fresh frozen plasma or whole blood. Menadione (vitamin K_3) isn't as effective. Use of phytonadione may interfere with subsequent oral anticoagulant therapy.

Antihistamine overdose

Drowsiness is the most common sign of antihistamine overdose. Seizures, coma, and respiratory depression may occur with severe overdose. Certain histamine antagonists, such as diphenhydramine, also block cholinergic receptors and produce modest anticholinergic signs and symptoms, such as dry mouth, flushed skin, fixed and dilated pupils, and GI symptoms, especially in children. Phenothiazine-type antihistamines such as promethazine also block dopamine receptors. Patient may experience movement disorders mimicking Parkinson's disease.

Treat overdose with gastric lavage followed by activated charcoal. Syrup of ipecac generally isn't recommended because acute dystonic reactions may increase the risk of aspiration. Also, phenothiazine-type antihistamines may have antiemetic effects. Treat hypotension with fluids or a vasopressor, and treat seizures with phenytoin or diazepam. Watch for arrhythmias, and treat accordingly.

Barbiturate overdose

A barbiturate overdose can cause unsteady gait, slurred speech, sustained nystagmus, somnolence, confusion, respiratory depression, pulmonary edema, areflexia, and coma. Typical shock syndrome with tachycardia and hypotension, jaundice, hypothermia followed by fever, and oliguria may occur.

To treat barbiturate overdose, maintain and support ventilation and pulmonary function as necessary; support cardiac function and circulation with a vasopressor and I.V. fluids as needed. If the patient is conscious and the gag reflex is intact, induce emesis (if ingestion was recent) by administering syrup of ipecac. If emesis is contraindicated, perform gastric lavage while a cuffed endotracheal tube is in place, to prevent aspiration. Then administer activated charcoal and saline cathartic. Measure intake and output, vital signs, and laboratory parameters; maintain body temperature. The patient should

be rolled from side to side every 30 minutes to avoid pulmonary congestion.

Alkalinization of urine may be helpful in removing the drug from the body; hemodialysis may be useful in severe overdose.

Benzodiazepine overdose

Benzodiazepine overdose can produce somnolence, confusion, coma, hypoactive reflexes, dyspnea, labored breathing, hypotension, bradycardia, slurred speech, and unsteady gait or impaired coordination.

Treatment of overdose involves supporting blood pressure and respiration until drug effects subside and monitoring vital signs. Mechanical ventilatory assistance via an endotracheal tube may be required to maintain a patent airway and support adequate oxygenation. Flumazenil, a specific benzodiazepine antagonist, may be useful. Use I.V. fluids or a vasopressor, such as dopamine and phenylephrine, to treat hypotension as needed. If the patient is conscious and his gag reflex is intact, induce emesis (if ingestion was recent) by administering syrup of ipecac. If emesis is contraindicated, perform gastric lavage while a cuffed endotracheal tube is in place, to prevent aspiration. After emesis or lavage, administer activated charcoal with a cathartic as a single dose. Dialysis is of limited value.

CNS depressant overdose

Signs of central nervous system (CNS) depressant overdose include prolonged coma, hypotension, hypothermia followed by fever, and inadequate ventilation even without significant respiratory depression. Absence of pupillary reflexes, dilated pupils, loss of deep tendon reflexes, tonic muscle spasms, and apnea may also occur.

Treatment of overdose involves supporting respiratory and cardiovascular function; mechanical ventilation may be necessary. Maintain adequate urine output with adequate hydration while avoiding pulmonary edema. Empty gastric contents by inducing emesis. For lipid-soluble drugs such as glutethimide, charcoal and resin hemoperfusion are effective in removing the drug; hemodialysis and peritoneal dialysis are of minimal value. Because glutethimide is stored in fat tissue, blood levels commonly show large fluctuations with worsening of symptoms.

Digoxin overdose

Signs and symptoms of digoxin overdose are primarily related to the GI, cardiovascular, and central nervous systems. Severe overdose may cause hyperkalemia, which may develop rapidly and result in life-threatening cardiac effects. Cardiac signs of digoxin toxicity may occur with or without other signs of toxic reaction and commonly precede other toxic effects. Because cardiotoxic effects also can occur with heart disease, determining whether these effects result from an underlying heart disease or digoxin toxicity may be difficult. Digoxin has caused almost every kind of arrhythmia; various combinations of arrhythmias may occur in the same patient. Patients with chronic digoxin toxicity commonly have ventricular arrhythmias, atrioventricular (AV) conduction disturbances, or both. Patients with digoxin-induced ventricular tachycardia have a high mortality because ventricular fibrillation or asystole may result.

If toxicity is suspected, the drug should be discontinued and serum drug level measurements obtained. Usually, the drug takes at least 6 hours to be distributed between plasma and tissue and reach equilibrium; plasma levels drawn earlier may show higher digoxin levels than those present after the drug is distributed into the tissues.

Other treatment measures include inducing emesis immediately, performing gastric lavage, and administering activated charcoal to reduce absorption of the remaining drug. Multiple doses of activated charcoal (such as 50 g every 6 hours) may help reduce further absorption, especially of any drug undergoing enterohepatic recirculation. Some clinicians advocate administering cholestyramine if digoxin was recently ingested; however, this may not be useful if the patient ingested a life-threatening amount. Any interacting drugs probably should be discontinued.

Ventricular arrhythmias may be treated with I.V. potassium (replacement doses; but not in patients with significant AV block), I.V. phenytoin, I.V. lidocaine, or I.V. propranolol. Refractory ventricular tachyarrhythmias may be controlled with overdrive pacing. Procainamide may be used for ventricular arrhythmias that don't respond to the above treatments. For severe AV block, asystole, and hemodynamically significant sinus bradycardia, atropine restores a normal rate.

Administration of digoxin-specific antibody fragments (digoxin immune Fab [Digibind]) treats life-threatening digoxin toxicity. Each 40 mg of digoxin immune Fab binds about 0.6 mg of digoxin in the bloodstream. The complex is then excreted in the urine, rapidly decreasing serum levels and, therefore, cardiac drug concentrations.

Iron supplement overdose

Iron supplements represent a major source of poisoning, especially in small children. In fact, as little as 1 g of ferrous sulfate can kill an infant. Signs and symptoms of poisoning result from iron's acute corrosive effects on the GI mucosa as well as the adverse metabolic effects caused by iron overload. These signs and symptoms may occur within the first 10 to 60 minutes of ingestion or may be delayed several hours. Four stages of acute iron poisoning have been identified.

The first findings reflect acute GI irritation and include epigastric pain, nausea, and vomiting. Diarrhea may be green, followed by tarry stools and then melena. Hematemesis may be accompanied by drowsiness, lassitude, shock, and coma. Local erosion of the stomach and small intestine may further enhance the absorption of iron. If death doesn't occur in the first phase, a second phase of apparent recovery may last 24 hours.

A third phase, which can occur 4 to 48 hours after ingestion, is marked by central nervous system abnormalities, metabolic acidosis, hepatic dysfunction, renal failure, and bleeding diathesis. This phase may progress to circulatory failure, coma, and death. If the patient survives, the fourth phase consists of late complications of acute iron intoxication and may occur 2 to 6 weeks after overdose. Severe gastric scarring, pyloric stenosis, or intestinal obstruction may be present.

Patients who develop vomiting, diarrhea, leukocytosis, or hyperglycemia and have an abdominal X-ray positive for iron within 6 hours of ingestion are likely to be at risk for a serious toxic reaction. Empty the stomach by inducing emesis with syrup of ipecac, and perform gastric lavage.

If patients have had multiple episodes of vomiting or if the vomitus contains blood, avoid ipecac and perform lavage. Some clinicians add sodium bicarbonate to the lavage solution to convert ferrous iron to ferrous carbonate, which is poorly absorbed. Disodium phosphate has also been used; however, some children may develop life-threatening hyperphosphatemia or hypocalcemia. Other possible treatments include lavage with normal saline solution, administration of a saline cathartic, surgical removal of tablets, and chelation therapy with deferoxamine mesylate. Hemodialysis is of little value. Supportive treatment includes monitoring acid-base balance, maintaining a patent airway, and controlling shock and dehydration with appropriate I.V. therapy.

NSAID overdose

Signs and symptoms of nonsteroidal anti-inflammatory drug (NSAID) overdose include dizziness, drowsiness, paresthesia, vomiting, nausea, abdominal pain, headache, sweating, nystagmus, apnea, and cyanosis.

To treat an ibuprofen overdose, empty the stomach at once by inducing emesis with syrup of ipecac or gastric lavage. Administer activated charcoal by nasogastric tube. Provide symptomatic and supportive measures, including respiratory support and correction of fluid and electrolyte imbalances. Monitor laboratory tests and vital signs closely. Alkaline diuresis may enhance renal excretion. Dialysis is of minimal value because ibuprofen is strongly protein-bound.

Opiate overdose

Rapid I.V. administration of opiates may result in overdose because of a 30-minute delay in maximum central nervous system (CNS) effect. The most common signs of morphine overdose are respiratory depression with or without CNS depression and miosis (pinpoint pupils). Other acute toxic effects include hypotension, bradycardia, hypothermia, shock, apnea, cardiopulmonary arrest, circulatory collapse, pulmonary edema, and seizures.

To treat acute overdose, establish adequate respiratory exchange via a patent airway and ventilation as needed; then administer a narcotic antagonist (naloxone) to reverse respiratory depression. (Because the duration of action of morphine is longer than that of naloxone, repeated doses of naloxone are necessary.) Naloxone shouldn't be given unless clinically significant respiratory or cardiovascular depression is present. Monitor vital signs closely.

If the patient presents within 2 hours of an oral overdose, empty the stomach immediately by inducing emesis with syrup of ipecac or using gastric lavage. Use caution to avoid risk of aspiration. Administer activated charcoal via a nasogastric tube to remove more drug.

Provide symptomatic and supportive treatment (continued respiratory support and correction of fluid or electrolyte imbalance). Monitor laboratory parameters, vital signs, and neurologic status closely.

Phenothiazine overdose

Phenothiazine overdose can cause central nervous system depression, which is characterized by deep, unarousable sleep and possible coma, hypotension or hypertension, extrapyramidal symptoms, abnormal involuntary muscle movements, agitation, seizures, arrhythmias, electrocardiogram changes, hypothermia or hyperthermia, and autonomic nervous system dysfunction.

Treatment is symptomatic and supportive, including maintaining vital signs, a patent airway, stable body temperature, and fluid and electrolyte balance. Don't induce vomiting; phenothiazines inhibit the cough reflex, so aspiration may occur. Use gastric lavage and then activated charcoal and saline cathartics. Dialysis doesn't help. Regulate body temperature as needed. Treat hypotension with I.V. fluids: Don't give epinephrine. Treat seizures with parenteral diazepam or barbiturates, arrhythmias with parenteral phenytoin, and extrapyramidal reactions with benztropine or parenteral diphenhydramine.

Salicylate overdose

Signs and symptoms of salicylate overdose include metabolic acidosis with respiratory alkalosis, hyperpnea, and tachypnea due to increased carbon dioxide production and direct stimulation of the respiratory center.

To treat the overdose, empty the patient's stomach immediately by inducing emesis with syrup of ipecac if the patient is conscious, or by performing gastric lavage. Administer activated charcoal via a nasogastric tube. Provide symptomatic and supportive measures (respiratory support and correction of fluid and electrolyte imbalances). Closely monitor laboratory values and vital signs. Enhance renal excretion by administering sodium bicarbonate to alkalinize urine. Use a cooling blanket or sponging if the patient's rectal temperature is above 104° F (40° C). Hemodialysis is effective in removing aspirin but is used only in those with severe poisoning or in those at risk for pulmonary edema.

Tricyclic antidepressant overdose

Tricyclic antidepressant overdose is commonly life-threatening, particularly when combined with alcohol. The first 12 hours after ingestion are a stimulatory phase, characterized by excessive anticholinergic activity (agitation, irritation, confusion, hallucinations, hyperthermia, parkinsonian symptoms, seizures, urine retention, dry mucous membranes, pupillary dilation, constipation, and ileus). This phase precedes central nervous system (CNS) depressant effects, including hypothermia, decreased or absent reflexes, sedation, hypotension, cyanosis, and cardiac irregularities, including tachycardia, conduction disturbances, and quinidine-like effects on the electrocardiogram.

The severity of an overdose is best indicated by a widening of the QRS complex, which usually represents severe toxic reaction; obtaining serum measurements usually isn't helpful. Metabolic acidosis may follow hypotension, hypoventilation, and seizures.

Treatment is symptomatic and supportive, including maintaining a patent airway, stable body temperature, and fluid and electrolyte balance. Induce emesis if the patient is conscious; follow with gastric lavage and activated charcoal to prevent further absorption. Dialysis is of little use. Treat seizures with parenteral diazepam or phenytoin, arrhythmias with parenteral phenytoin or lidocaine, and acidosis with sodium bicarbonate. Don't give barbiturates;

they may enhance CNS and respiratory depressant effects.

Dangers of uncontrolled I.V. flow

Let's suppose that you're caring for a patient who is receiving a drug through an electronic infusion device. His gown needs changing, but it doesn't have sleeve snaps. So you have to deactivate the device, clamp and remove the tubing, remove the fluid bag from the I.V. pole, and pull the I.V. bag and tubing through the sleeve — a tiresome job.

Actually, the task is more than tiresome: It's dangerous. In one documented case, a nurse deactivated the infusion device and her patient died. Either she didn't secure the roller clamp correctly or it malfunctioned, causing rapid, uncontrolled drug flow into the patient.

No standards

No standards exist for I.V. devices and sets, so many systems don't have free-flow protection. Because safer systems are more expensive, hospitals may use them only in labor and delivery units or critical areas, or to give drugs with narrow therapeutic windows. This increases your risk for error because you may get used to using the safer equipment and mistake one system for another.

To protect your patients and yourself, be extremely careful when using infusion sets — especially if you're unfamiliar with a hospital's equipment because you're floating to a temporary assignment. This will have to do until free-flow protected equipment becomes the standard.

Interactions

Compatibility of drugs combined in a syringe

KEY

Y = compatible for at least 30 minutes

P = provisionally compatible; administer within 15 minutes

$P_{(5)}$ = provisionally compatible; administer within 5 minutes

N = not compatible

* = conflicting data (A blank space indicates no available data.)

	atropine sulfate	butorphanol tartrate	chlorpromazine HCl	cimetidine HCl	codeine phosphate	dexamethasone sodium phosphate	dimenhydrinate	diphenhydramine HCl	droperidol	fentanyl citrate	glycopyrrolate	heparin Na	hydromorphone HCl	hydroxyzine HCl	meperidine HCl	metoclopramide HCl
atropine sulfate		Y	P	Y			P	P	P	P	Y	$P_{(5)}$	Y	Y	P	P
butorphanol tartrate	Y		Y	Y			N	Y	Y	Y				Y	Y	Y
chlorpromazine HCl	P	Y		N			N	P	P	P	Y	N	Y	P	P	P
cimetidine HCl	Y	Y	N					Y	Y	Y	Y	Y	Y	Y	Y	
codeine phosphate											Y			Y		
dexamethasone sodium phosphate								N*					N	N*		Y
dimenhydrinate	P	N	N					P	P	P	N	$P_{(5)}$	Y	N	P	P
diphenhydramine HCl	P	Y	P	Y		N*	P		P	P	Y	N		Y	P	P
droperidol	P	Y	P	Y			P	P		P	Y	N		P	P	P
fentanyl citrate	P	Y	P	Y			P	P	P		$P_{(5)}$		Y	P	P	P
glycopyrrolate	Y		Y	Y	Y	N	N	Y	Y				Y	Y	Y	
heparin Na	$P_{(5)}$		N	Y			$P_{(5)}$		N	$P_{(5)}$					N	Y
hydromorphone HCl	Y		Y	Y		N*	Y	Y		Y	Y			Y		
hydroxyzine HCl	Y	Y	P	Y	Y		N	P	P	P	Y		Y		P	P
meperidine HCl	P	Y	P	Y			P	P	P	P	Y	N		P		P
metoclopramide HCl	P	Y	P			Y	P	Y	P	P		Y		P	P	
midazolam HCl	Y	Y	Y	Y			N	Y	Y	Y	Y		Y	Y	Y	Y
morphine sulfate	P	Y	P	Y			P	P	P	P	Y	N*		P	N	P
nalbuphine HCl	Y		Y				Y	Y		Y				Y		
pentazocine lactate	P	Y	P	Y			P	P	P	P	N	N	Y	P	P	P
pentobarbital Na	P	N	N	N			N	N	N	N	N		Y	N	N	
perphenazine	Y	Y	Y	Y			Y	Y	Y	Y				Y	Y	P
phenobarbital Na											$P_{(5)}$					
prochlorperazine edisylate	P	Y	P	Y			N	P	P	P	Y		N*	P	P	P
promazine HCl	P		P	Y			N	P	P	P	Y			P	P	P
promethazine HCl	P	Y	P	Y			N	P	P	P	Y	N	Y	P	P	P
ranitidine HCl	Y		N*		Y	Y	Y		Y	Y			Y	N	Y	Y
scopolamine HBr	P	Y	P	Y			P	P	P	P	Y		Y	P	P	P
secobarbital Na			N									N				
sodium bicarbonate												N				N
thiethylperazine maleate		Y												Y		
thiopental Na			N				N	N				N			N	

midazolam HCl	morphine sulfate	nalbuphine HCl	pentazocine lactate	pentobarbital Na	perphenazine	phenobarbital Na	prochlorperazine edisylate	promazine HCl	promethazine HCl	ranitidine HCl	scopolamine HBr	secobarbital Na	sodium bicarbonate	thiethylperazine maleate	thiopental Na	
Y	P	Y	P	P	Y		P	P	P	Y	P					atropine sulfate
Y	Y		Y	N	Y		Y		Y		Y			Y		butorphanol tartrate
Y	P		P	N	Y		P	P	P	N*	P				N	chlorpromazine HCl
Y	Y	Y	Y	N	Y		Y	Y	Y		Y	N				cimetidine HCl
																codeine phosphate
										Y						dexamethasone sodium phosphate
N	P		P	N	Y		N	N	N	Y	P				N	dimenhydrinate
Y	P	Y	P	N	Y		P	P	P	Y	P				N	diphenhydramine HCl
Y	P	Y	P	N	Y		P	P	P		P					droperidol
Y	P		P	N	Y		P	P	P	Y	P					fentanyl citrate
Y	Y	Y	N	N			Y	Y	Y	Y	Y	N	N		N	glycopyrrolate
	N*		N			$P_{(5)}$			N							heparin Na
Y			Y	Y			N*		Y	Y	Y			Y		hydromorphone HCl
Y	P	Y	P	N	Y		P	P	P	N	P					hydroxyzine HCl
Y	N		P	N	Y		P	P	P	Y	P				N	meperidine HCl
Y	P		P		P		P	P	P	Y	P		N			metoclopramide HCl
	Y	Y		N	N		N	Y	Y	N	Y			Y		midazolam HCl
Y			P	N*	Y		P*	P	P*	Y	P				N	morphine sulfate
Y				N			Y		N*	Y	Y			Y		nalbuphine HCl
	P			N	Y		P	Y	Y	Y	P					pentazocine lactate
N	N*	N	N		N		N	N	N	N	P		Y		Y	pentobarbital Na
N	Y		Y	N			Y		Y	Y	Y			N		perphenazine
										N						phenobarbital Na
N	P*	Y	P	N	Y			P	P	Y	P				N	prochlorperazine edisylate
Y	P		Y	N			P		P		P					promazine HCl
Y	P*	N*	Y	N	Y		P	P		Y	P				N	promethazine HCl
N	Y	Y	Y	N	Y	N	Y		Y		Y			Y		ranitidine HCl
Y	P	Y	P	P	Y		P	P	P	Y					Y	scopolamine HBr
																secobarbital Na
			Y												N	sodium bicarbonate
Y		Y			N					Y						thiethylperazine maleate
	N			Y			N		N		Y		N			thiopental Na

I.V. compatibilty

KEY

- Compatible
- [4] Compatible only for hours indicated
- Incompatible
- [?] Questionable compatibility
- Data unavailable

	acyclovir	amikacin	amino acid injection	aminophylline	amphotericin B	ampicillin	bretylium	calcium gluconate	cefazolin	cefoxitin	ceftazidime	cimetidine	ciprofloxacin	clindamycin	dexamethasone sodium phosphate	dextrose 5% in water (D₅W)	D₅W in lactated Ringer's solution	D₅W in normal saline solution	diazepam	diphenhydramine	dobutamine	dopamine	epinephrine	erythromycin lactobionate	esmolol	fluconazole	furosemide	gentamicin	heparin sodium
acyclovir		4				4			4	4	4	4			4	4				4				4				4	4
amikacin	4		24	8			24	8	48		24	48	48	4	24	24	24		4			24			24	24	72	24	
amino acid injection		24		24				24	24	24	24	24	2	24					24		24	24	24	4		24	24	8	24
aminophylline		8	24			48						48		24	24	24	24									24	24		72
amphotericin B															24												?		24
ampicillin	4							48				?		24		24	48	48				24			24	24		72	4
bretylium		24						48				24				24	24	24		?	48		24						
calcium gluconate		24	24			48			3			2			24	24	24				3				72				
cefazolin	4	8	24					3			?		48		24	24	24								24	24			6
cefoxitin	4	48	24								24		24	24	24	24										24		48	8
ceftazidime	4		24									24	48		24		24								24		72		6
cimetidine	4	24	24	48		?		2			24		24	48	48	48	4	4			24	24	24	24	72	24	6
ciprofloxacin	48	2					2			24					24	24	24										48		
clindamycin	4	48	24			24			48	48	48	24			24	24	24								24			24	24
dexamethasone sodium phosphate	4	4		24							24					24										24	72		6
dextrose 5% in water (D₅W)	24		24	24		24	24	24	24	48		24								24	24	24		24	24	24	
D₅W in lactated Ringer's solution	24		24			48	24	24		48		24							24	48	24		24		24		24
D₅W in normal saline solution	24		24			48	24	24	24	48		24							24	48	24		24		24		24
diazepam		24								4																	
diphenhydramine	4	24							4	24					24								24		24		?
dobutamine		24			?				24			24	24	24					24	24			24				
dopamine		24				48						24	48	48		24			24				24		6	24
epinephrine	24	24					3				24			24	24	24			24					4	4
erythromycin lactobionate	4		4	24		24						24			24						24				24		
esmolol		24		24	24	24		24			24	24		24							24		24			24	24
fluconazole	72	24		?				24	24		24			24	24					24	24	24					72	24
furosemide	24	24	72		72		72					72			72	24	24	24			4					4			4
gentamicin	4	8						24	24	48	24	24								6				24	72		
heparin sodium	4		24		24	4		6	8	6	6	24	6		24					?	24	4		24	24	4		
hydrocortisone sodium succinate	4	24	24	24	24	?					24	4	48	24	48		24		18	4		24	24	?		?
insulin (regular)		24		2	48		2	24		24									24		2	2
isoproterenol		24		3				24			24	24	24		24									24
lactated Ringer's solution	4	24				48	24	24	24			48	24						24	48	24	18	24	24	24	24	
lidocaine		24	24			24	24				24	24		24	24	24			24	24				72		24
methylprednisolone sodium succinate	4		24	?				24		24		?		?					18							?
metronidazole	12		48		?			72	24	72	48	24							?		24	72		24	48
mezlocillin		?								24											
morphine	?	4			4		4	4	4	4		4	4						24	24	4	4	8	24	?	4
multiple vitamin infusion	4	?		24		24	24	24			24		24	24	24					24			24		24
nafcillin	4		24	24								24		24						24	24			
norepinephrine		24	24								24					24	4	24	4		24	
normal saline solution		24		24	8	48	24	24	24	24	48		24						24	48	24	22	24	24	24	
ondansetron	4					4	4	4	4		4	4	48		48	4			4		4	4
oxytocin												6							4
penicillin G potassium	4	8	24								24		24	24	24		24			24	24		?
phenytoin																			24	24
phytonadione	24	24		3					24								3				4
piperacillin	4	?									24	48	24	24					24	72		6
potassium chloride	4	4	4	4		4	48	4			24	24	24	4	24	24	4	?	24	4		24	24	4		24
procainamide			24								24					24				24	4
ranitidine	4	24	12	24		?	24	?	?		24	?	24	48		?	1	48	48	24	24	24	4	72	24	24
sodium bicarbonate	4	24		24	24	?	48		24	6		24	4	24		24		24			72	24
thiamine											24	24	24	
ticarcillin	4										24						6
tobramycin	4		24			1		24		24	48		24	48			24	24	72
vancomycin	4	24	24					24			24						24	24
verapamil		24				48	48	24	24		24	24	24	24	24	24	24		24	24	24	24	?	24	24
vitamin B complex with C					4			4	4	24		48			24	4			4	4		4	24	24

	hydrocortisone sodium succinate	insulin (regular)	isoproterenol	lactated Ringer's solution	lidocaine	methylprednisolone sodium succinate	metronidazole	mezlocillin	morphine	multiple vitamin infusion	nafcillin	norepinephrine	normal saline solution	ondansetron	oxytocin	penicillin G potassium	phenytoin	phytonadione	piperacillin	potassium chloride	procainamide	ranitidine	sodium bicarbonate	thiamine	ticarcillin	tobramycin	vancomycin	verapamil	vitamin B complex with C
acyclovir	4			4		4			?	4	4					4			4			4	4		4	4	4		
amikacin	24			24			12		4				24	24	4	8		24		4		24	24				24	24	
amino acid injection	24	24	24			24	24		?		?	24	24			24		24	24	?	4	12				24	24		
aminophylline	24			24	24	?	48					24		24					4			24	24						
amphotericin B	24																					24							
ampicillin	?	2				?			4	24			8					3		4		?	?						4
bretylium		48	3	48	24						48								48	24	24	48					48		
calcium gluconate			24	24							48			24						4					1		48	4	
cefazolin		2		24				72		4	24			24	4						?						24	4	
cefoxitin		24		24				24		4	24			24	4							24			24		24	24	
ceftazidime								72		4	24			24	4						?	6						24	
cimetidine		24	24		24	24			4				48	4	24		24		24			4	1				24	24	48
ciprofloxacin				48	24		48									24	24		24					24			24	24	
clindamycin	24			24		24	24		4	24			24	4		24		48	24		?	24			48		24	24	
dexamethasone sodium phosphate	4								4					4					4			24	4				24	4	
dextrose 5% in water (D5W)	48		24		24		?		24	24	24			48	6	24			24	24	24	48	24	24	24	24	24	24	24
D5W in lactated Ringer's solution	24		24		24				24					24					24		24				24			24	
D5W in normal saline solution	24		24		24	?			24	24			48			24			24	24			24	24		48		24	
diazepam																							?						24
diphenhydramine	24								4				24			24				4	1							24	
dobutamine		24	24	24					24				24	24					?	24	48							24	
dopamine	18			48	24	18	?		24				48							24	48							24	4
epinephrine	4			24					4				4	24				3		4	24							24	4
erythromycin lactobionate				18					4	24			22									24	24					24	
esmolol	24	24		24				24	8			24	24	24			24	24		24	24		24			24	24	24	
fluconazole	24			24				72	24		24				4		24	24		72	24		4				24	24	
furosemide	?			24	72				?				4	24							4		72	72		72		?	4
gentamicin		2		24			24	4	24				24	4						24			24				24	24	
heparin sodium	?	2	24		24	?	48						4	4	?		4	6	24	4	24	24		6			24	24	
hydrocortisone sodium succinate		4	4	24		?	48	4			24	4					4	24		4	24							24	
insulin (regular)	4			24					24			2							4		24	3		2	2	2	48	4	
isoproterenol	4			24							24										24							24	
lactated Ringer's solution	24		24		24	?		72		24	24						24		24	24					24	24	24	24	
lidocaine		24		24					4		48		24								24	24	24					48	
methylprednisolone sodium succinate	?		?			24			4				?			24				?		48	2					24	?
metronidazole	48					24			4	48			4				48								48				
mezlocillin				72					4							48													
morphine	4	24			4	4	4	4		4	24	4		1	4			4	4		4			4	4	4	24	4	
multiple vitamin infusion				24			48		4				24							24			24						?
nafcillin				24	48				24				24						24		?		24						
norepinephrine	24		24		24	?		48	4	24	24	24		48		24			24	24	24	48	24	24	24	48	24	24	
normal saline solution	4												48							4	4		4		4	4			
ondansetron		2							1						48					4			24					24	4
oxytocin				24		24	48		4				24							?		24						24	
penicillin G potassium																						24						48	
phenytoin	4			24					4				24							4			24						4
phytonadione	24			24					4				24							24	4							24	
piperacillin		4		24		?			4	24		24	4	4	?		4	24			4	48	24				24		
potassium chloride	4			24							24								4			4	24				48	24	
procainamide		24	24		24	48			4				?	48	4		24		4	48	24				24	24	24		
ranitidine	24	3		24	2				24	24		24		24		24	24	24	24								?		?
sodium bicarbonate			24							24																			
thiamine		2		24					4				24	4						24								24	
ticarcillin		2		24			48		4				48							24								24	
tobramycin		2		24					4				24	4						24	?							24	
vancomycin	24	48	24	24	48	24			24	24			24	24		24	24	48		24	24	48			24	24	24		24
verapamil		4			?				4		?		4				4		4			24		?				24	
vitamin B complex with C																													

Drug combinations

Drugs can interact to produce undesirable, even hazardous, effects. Such interactions can decrease therapeutic efficacy or cause toxic reaction.

Dangerous effects of drug combinations

If possible, avoid administering the drug combinations shown below to prevent dangerous drug interactions.

Drug	Interacting drug	Possible effect
Aminoglycosides amikacin gentamicin kanamycin neomycin netilmicin streptomycin tobramycin	Parenteral cephalosporins ■ ceftazidime ■ ceftizoxime ■ cephalothin	Possible enhanced nephrotoxicity
	Loop diuretics ■ bumetanide ■ ethacrynic acid ■ furosemide	Possible enhanced ototoxicity
Amphetamines amphetamine benzphetamine dextroamphetamine methamphetamine	Urine alkalinizers ■ potassium citrate ■ sodium acetate ■ sodium bicarbonate ■ sodium citrate ■ sodium lactate ■ tromethamine	Decreased urinary excretion of amphetamine
Angiotensin-converting enzyme (ACE) inhibitors captopril enalapril lisinopril benazepril fosinopril ramipril quinapril	indomethacin Nonsteroidal anti-inflammatory drugs (NSAIDs)	Decreased or abolished effectiveness of antihypertensive action of ACE inhibitors
Barbiturate anesthetics methohexital thiopental	Opiate analgesics	Enhanced central nervous system and respiratory depression

Dangerous effects of drug combinations *(continued)*

Drug	Interacting drug	Possible effect
Barbiturates amobarbital aprobarbital butabarbital mephobarbital pentobarbital phenobarbital primidone secobarbital	valproic acid	Increased serum barbiturate levels
Beta-adrenergic blockers acebutolol atenolol betaxolol carteolol esmolol levobunolol metoprolol nadolol penbutolol pindolol propranolol timolol	verapamil	Enhanced pharmacologic effects of both beta-adrenergic blockers and verapamil
carbamazepine	erythromycin	Increased risk of carbamazepine toxicity
carmustine	cimetidine	Enhanced risk of bone marrow toxicity
ciprofloxacin	Antacids that contain magnesium or aluminum hydroxide, iron supplements, sucralfate, multivitamins that contain iron or zinc	Decreased plasma levels and effectiveness of ciprofloxacin
clonidine	Beta-adgrenergic blockers	Enhanced rebound hypertension following rapid clonidine withdrawal
cyclosporine	carbamazepine, isoniazid, phenobarbital, phenytoin, rifabutin, rifampin	Reduced plasma levels of cyclosporine

(continued)

Dangerous effects of drug combinations *(continued)*

Drug	Interacting drug	Possible effect
Cardiac glycosides	Loop and thiazide diuretics	Increased risk of cardiac arrhythmias due to hypokalemia
	Thiazide-like diuretics	Increased therapeutic or toxic effects
digoxin	amiodarone	Decreased renal clearance of digoxin
	quinidine	Enhanced clearance of digoxin
	verapamil	Elevated serum digoxin levels
dopamine	phenytoin	Hypertension and bradycardia
epinephrine	Beta-adgrenergic blockers	Increased systolic and diastolic pressures; marked decrease in heart rate
erythromycin	astemizole	Increased risk of arrhythmia
	carbamazepine	Decreased carbamazepine clearance
	theophylline	Decreased hepatic clearance of theophylline
ethanol	disulfiram furazolidone metronidazole	Acute alcohol intolerance reaction
furazolidone	Amine-containing foods Anorexiants	Inhibits monoamine oxidase (MAO), possibly leading to hypertensive crisis
heparin	Salicylates NSAIDs	Enhanced risk of bleeding
levodopa	furazolidone	Enhanced toxic effects of levodopa
lithium	Thiazide diuretics NSAIDs	Decreased lithium excretion
meperidine	MAO inhibitors	Cardiovascular instability and increased toxic effects

Dangerous effects of drug combinations *(continued)*

Drug	Interacting drug	Possible effect
methotrexate	probenecid	Decreased methotrexate elimination
	Salicylates	Increased risk of methotrexate toxicity
MAO inhibitors	Amine-containing foods Anorexiants meperidine	Risk of hypertensive crisis
Nondepolarizing muscle relaxants	Aminoglycosides Inhaled anesthetics	Enhanced neuromuscular blockade
Potassium supplements	potassium-sparing diuretics	Increased risk of hyperkalemia
quinidine	amiodarone	Increased risk of quinidine toxicity
Sympathomimetics	MAO inhibitors	Increased risk of hypertensive crisis
Tetracyclines	Antacids containing magnesium, aluminum, or bismuth salts Iron supplements	Decreased plasma levels and effectiveness of tetracyclines
theophylline	carbamazepine	Reduced theophylline levels
	cimetidine	Increased theophylline levels
	ciprofloxacin	Increased theophylline levels
	erythromycin	Increased theophylline levels
	phenobarbital	Reduced theophylline levels
	rifampin	Reduced theophylline levels
warfarin	testosterone	Possible enhanced bleeding caused by increased hypoprothrombinemia
	Barbiturates carbamazepine	Reduced effectiveness of warfarin

(continued)

Dangerous effects of drug combinations *(continued)*

Drug	Interacting drug	Possible effect
warfarin *(continued)*	amiodarone Cephalosporins (certain ones) chloral hydrate cholestyramine cimetidine clofibrate co-trimoxazole dextrothyroxine disulfiram	Increased risk of bleeding
	erythromycin glucagon metronidazole phenylbutazone quinidine quinine Salicylates sulfinpyrazone Thyroid drugs Tricyclic antidepressants	Increased risk of bleeding
	ethchlorvynol glutethimide griseofulvin	Decreased pharmacologic effect
	rifampin trazodone	Decreased risk of bleeding
	methimazole propylthiouracil	Increased or decreased risk of bleeding

Drug-tobacco interactions

Smoking — or living and working in a smoke-filled environment — can affect a patient's drug therapy, especially if he's taking one of the drugs listed here. If your patient is using any of these drugs, monitor plasma drug levels closely, and watch for possible adverse reactions.

Ascorbic acid (vitamin C)
Possible effects
■ Low serum vitamin C levels
■ Decreased oral absorption of vitamin C

Nursing considerations
■ Tell the patient to increase his vitamin C intake.

Chlordiazepoxide hydrochloride, chlorpromazine hydrochloride, diazepam
Possible effects
■ Increased drug metabolism, which results in reduced plasma levels
■ Decreased sedative effects

Nursing considerations
■ Watch for a decrease in the drug's effectiveness.
■ Adjust the patient's drug dosage, if ordered.

Propoxyphene hydrochloride
Possible effect
■ Increased drug metabolism and diminished analgesic effects

Nursing considerations
■ Watch for a decrease in the drug's effectiveness.

Propranolol hydrochloride
Possible effects
■ Increased metabolism, which decreases drug's effectiveness
■ Reduced drug effectiveness (Smoking increases heart rate, stimulates catecholamine release from the adrenal medulla, raises arterial blood pressure, and increases myocardial oxygen consumption.)

Nursing considerations
■ Monitor the patient's blood pressure and heart rate.
■ To reduce drug and smoking interaction, the doctor may order a selective beta-adrenergic blocker, such as atenolol.

Oral contraceptives containing estrogen and progestogen
Possible effects
■ Increased risk of adverse reactions, such as headache, dizziness, depression, libido changes, migraine, hypertension, edema, worsening of astigmatism or myopia, nausea, vomiting, and gallbladder disease.

Nursing considerations
■ Inform the patient of increased risk of myocardial infarction and cerebrovascular accident.

■ Suggest that the patient stop smoking or use a different birth control method.

Theophylline
Possible effects
■ Increased theophylline metabolism (due to induction of liver microsomal enzymes)
■ Lower plasma theophylline levels

Nursing considerations
■ Monitor plasma theophylline levels, and watch for decreased therapeutic effect.
■ Increase drug dosage, if ordered.

Selected drug-food interactions

acebutolol hydrochloride (Sectral): Food in general. *Slightly decreases drug absorption and peak levels.*

amiloride hydrochloride (Midamor): Potassium-rich diet. *May rapidly increase serum potassium levels.*

antihypertensives: Licorice. *Decreases antihypertensive effect.*

bacampicillin hydrochloride (Spectrobid powder for oral suspension): Food in general. *Decreases drug absorption.*

buspirone hydrochloride (BuSpar): Food in general. *May decrease presystemic drug clearance.*
   Grapefruit juice. *May increase serum drug levels.*

caffeine (NoDoz): Caffeine-containing beverages and food. *May cause sleeplessness, irritability, nervousness, and rapid heartbeat.*

calcium glubionate (Neo-Calglucon syrup): Large quantities bran, cereals (whole grain), dairy products, rhubarb, spinach. *Interferes with calcium absorption.*

captopril (Capoten): Food in general. *Reduces drug absorption by 30% to 40%.*

cefuroxime axetil (Ceftin tablets): Food in general. *Increases drug absorption.*

choline and magnesium salicylate (Trilisate): Food that lowers urinary pH. *Decreases urinary salicylate excretion, and increases plasma levels.*

Food that raises urinary pH. *Enhances renal salicylate clearance, and diminishes plasma salicylate concentration.*

demeclocycline hydrochloride (Declomycin): Dairy products, food in general. *Interferes with absorption of oral forms of demeclocycline.*

dextroamphetamine sulfate (Dexedrine elixir): Fruit juice. *Lowers blood drug levels and efficacy.*

dicumarol: Diet high in vitamin K. *Decreases prothrombin time.*

digoxin (Lanoxin tablets, Lanoxicaps): Food high in bran fiber. *May reduce bioavailability of oral digoxin.*

Food in general. *Slows drug absorption rate.*

dyclonine hydrochloride (Dyclone 0.5% and 1% topical solutions, USP): Food in general. *Topical anesthesia may impair swallowing, enhancing risk of aspiration; food shouldn't be ingested for 60 minutes.*

erythromycin base (Eryc, PCE Dispertab tablets): Food in general. *Optimum blood levels are obtained on a fasting stomach; administration is preferable 30 minutes before or 2 hours after meals.*

estramustine phosphate sodium (Emcyt): Dairy products, calcium-rich foods. *Impairs drug absorption.*

etodolac (Lodine): Food in general. *Reduces peak levels by about 50%, and increases time to peak levels by 1.4 to 3.8 hours.*

etretinate (Tegison capsules): Dairy products, high lipid diet. *Increases drug absorption.*

famotidine (Pepcid oral suspension): Food in general. *Slightly increases bioavailability.*

felodipine (Plendil): Grapefruit juice. *Increases bioavailability more than twofold.*

fenoprofen calcium (Nalfon pulvules and tablets): Dairy products, food in general. *Delays and diminishes peak blood levels.*

ferrous sulfate (Feosol, Slow FE): Dairy products, eggs. *Inhibits iron absorption.*

fluoroquinolone antibiotics, such as ciprofloxacin (Cipro), norfloxacin (Noroxin), ofloxacin (Floxin): Food in general (particularly dairy products). *May decrease absorption of oral fluoroquinolones.*

flurbiprofen (Ansaid): Food in general. *Alters rate of absorption but not extent of drug availability.*

fosinopril sodium (Monopril): Food in general. *May slow rate but not extent of drug absorption.*

glipizide (Glucotrol): Food in general. *Delays absorption by about 40 minutes.*

hydralazine hydrochloride (Apresoline tablets): Food in general. *Increases plasma levels.*

hydrochlorothiazide (Esidrix, HydroDIURIL): Food in general. *Enhances GI drug absorption.*

ibuprofen (Advil, Children's Advil suspension, Motrin, Nuprin, Children's Motrin suspension, Rufen): Food in general. *Reduces rate but not extent of absorption.*

isotretinoin (Accutane): Dairy products, food in general. *Increases absorption of oral isotretinoin.*

isradipine (DynaCirc): Food in general. *Significantly increases time to peak by about 1 hour with no effect on bioavailability.*

ketoprofen (Orudis capsules): Food in general. *Slows absorption rate and delays and reduces peak levels.*

levodopa-carbidopa (Sinemet tablets): High-protein diet. *May impair levodopa absorption.*
   Food in general. *Increases the extent of availability and peak levels of sustained-release levodopa-carbidopa.*

levothyroxine sodium (Synthroid injection): Soybean formula (infants). *May cause excessive fecal loss.*

lidocaine hydrochloride (Xylocaine): Food in general. *Topical anesthesia may impair swallowing, enhancing risk of aspiration; avoid food ingestion for 60 minutes.*

liotrix (Thyrolar): Soybean formula (infants). *May cause excessive fecal loss.*

lovastatin (Mevacor): Grapefruit juice. *Increases serum levels.*

meclofenamate (Meclomen): Food in general. *Decreases rate and extent of drug absorption.*

methenamine mandelate (Mandelamine granules): Food that raises urinary pH. *Reduces essential antibacterial activity.*

methotrexate sodium (Rheumatrex): Food in general. *Delays absorption and reduces peak levels of oral methotrexate sodium.*

minocycline hydrochloride (Minocin): Dairy products. *Slightly decreases peak plasma levels and delays them by 1 hour.*

misoprostol (Cytotec): Food in general. *Diminishes maximum plasma concentrations.*

monoamine oxidase (MAO) inhibitors, such as isocarboxazid (Marplan tablets), phenelzine sulfate (Nardil), or tranylcypromine sulfate (Parnate tablets); drugs that also inhibit MAO, such as amphetamines, furazolidone (Furoxone), isoniazid (Laniazid), or procarbazine (Matulane capsules): Anchovies, avocados, bananas, beans (broad, fava), beer (including alcohol-free and reduced-alcohol), caviar, cheese (especially aged, strong, unpasteurized), chocolate, sour cream, canned figs, pickled herring, liver, liqueurs, meat extracts, meat prepared with tenderizers, raisins, sauerkraut, sherry, soy sauce, red wine, yeast extract, yogurt. *Can cause hypertensive crisis.*

moricizine hydrochloride (Ethmozine): Food in general. *Administration 30 minutes after a meal delays rate but not extent of drug absorption.*

nifedipine (Procardia XL tablets): Food in general. *Slightly alters early rate of drug absorption.*
   Grapefruit juice. *May increase bioavailability and drug levels.*

nitrofurantoin (Macrodantin capsules): Food in general. *Increases drug bioavailability.*

pancrelipase (Cotazym capsules): Food with a pH greater than 5.5. *Dissolves protective enteric coating.*

pentoxifylline (Trental): Food in general. *Delays drug absorption but doesn't affect total absorption.*

phenytoin (Dilantin): Charcoal-broiled meats. *May decrease blood drug levels.*

polyethylene glycol electrolyte solution (GoLYTELY, NuLYTELY): Food in general. *For best results, no solid food should be consumed for 3 to 4 hours before drinking solution.*

propafenone hydrochloride (Rythmol): Food in general. *Increased peak blood levels and bioavailability in a single-dose study.*

propranolol hydrochloride (Inderal): Food in general. *Increases bioavailability of oral propranolol.*

ramipril (Altace): Food in general. *Reduces rate but not extent of drug absorption.*

salsalate (Disalcid, Mono-Gesic, Salflex): Food that lowers urinary pH. *Decreases urinary excretion, and increases plasma levels.*

Food that raises urinary pH. *Increases renal clearance and urinary excretion of salicylic acid.*

selegiline hydrochloride (Eldepryl): Food with high concentration of tyramine. *May precipitate hypertensive crisis if daily dosage exceeds recommended maximum.*

sodium fluoride (Luride): Dairy products. *Form calcium fluoride, which is poorly absorbed.*

sulindac (Clinoril tablets): Food in general. *Slightly delays peak plasma levels of biologically active sulfide metabolite.*

tetracycline hydrochloride (Achromycin V): Dairy products, food in general. *Interferes with absorption of oral tetracycline.*

theophylline (Quibron-T Dividose, Quibron-T/SR Dividose, Respbid, Slo-Bid Gyrocaps, Theo-Dur, Theo-24, Theolair-SR, Theo-X, Uniphyl): Caffeine-containing beverages, chocolate, cola. *Large quantities increase adverse effects of theophylline.*

High-lipid diet. *Reduces plasma levels and delays time of peak plasma levels.*

Charcoal-broiled foods, especially meats; cruciferous (cabbage family) vegetables; and high-protein and low-carbohydrate diets. *Large quantities may increase hepatic metabolism of theophylline.*

tolmetin sodium (Tolectin): Dairy products. *Decreased total tolmetin bioavailability by 16%.*

Food in general. *Decreases total tolmetin bioavailability by 16% and reduces peak plasma levels by 50%.*

trazodone hydrochloride (Desyrel): Food in general. *May affect bioavailability, including amount of drug absorbed and peak plasma levels.*

triazolam (Halcion): Grapefruit juice. *May increase serum levels.*

verapamil hydrochloride (Calan SR, Isoptin SR): Food in general. *Decreases bioavailability but narrows peak and trough ratio.*

warfarin sodium (Coumadin, Panwarfin): Diet high in vitamin K. *Decreases prothrombin time.*

Charcoal-broiled meats. *May decrease blood drug levels.*

Drug-alcohol interactions

Drug-alcohol interactions are more than just potentiated central nervous system depression. Combined with nonsteroidal anti-inflammatory drugs, alcohol is highly irritating to the stomach; combined with some diuretics and cardiac medications, it may cause a steep drop in blood pressure.

Effects of mixing drugs and alcohol

Drug	Effects
■ Analgesics ■ Anxiolytics ■ Antidepressants ■ Antihistamines ■ Antipsychotics ■ Hypnotics	Deepened central nervous system (CNS) depression
■ Monoamine oxidase inhibitors	Deepened CNS depression; possible hypertensive crisis with certain types of beer and wine containing tyramine (Chianti, Alicante)
■ Oral antidiabetics	Disulfiram-like effects (facial flushing, headache), especially with chlorpropamide; inadequate food intake may trigger increased antidiabetic activity
■ Cephalosporins ■ metronidazole ■ disulfiram	Facial flushing, headache

Compatibility of drugs with tube feedings

Some feeding formulas such as Ensure may break down chemically when combined with a drug such as Dimetapp Elixir. Increased formula viscosity — and a clogged tube — can occur from giving Klorvess, Neo-Calglucon Syrup, or Phenergan Syrup with a feeding formula.

Drug preparations such as ferrous sulfate or potassium chloride liquids are incompatible with some formulas, causing clumping and other problems when mixed in a tube. Still other combinations may alter the bioavailability of some drugs, such as phenytoin.

To avoid incompatibility problems, follow these guidelines:

■ Never add a drug to a feeding formula container.

■ Always check the compatibility of an ordered drug and the feeding formula before administering.

■ Infuse 30 ml of water before and after giving a single drug dose through the tube.

■ Flush the feeding tube with 5 ml of water between drug doses if you're giving more than one drug.

■ Dilute highly concentrated liquids with 60 ml of water before giving.

■ Instill drugs in liquid form when possible. If you must crush a tablet, crush it into fine dust and dissolve it in warm water. (Never crush and liquefy enteric-coated tablets or timed-release capsules.)

■ Time drug and formula administration intervals appropriately; you may need to withhold tube feeding and supply medication by mouth to an empty stomach or with food.

Drug interference with test results

Drugs can interfere with the results of blood or urine tests in two ways. A drug in a blood or urine specimen may interact with the chemicals used in the laboratory test, causing a false result. Alternatively, a drug may cause a physiologic change in the patient, resulting in an actual increased or decreased blood or urine level of the substance being tested. This chart identifies drugs that can cause these two types of interference in some common blood and urine tests.

Test and drugs causing chemical interference	Drugs causing physiologic interference	
	Increase test values	Decrease test values
Alkaline phosphatase ■ albumin ■ Fluorides	■ Anticonvulsants ■ Hepatotoxic drugs ■ ticlopidine	■ clofibrate ■ Estrogens ■ Vitamin D ■ Zinc salts
Ammonia, blood	■ acetazolamide ■ ammonium chloride ■ asparaginase ■ Barbiturates ■ Diuretics, loop and thiazide ■ ethanol	■ kanamycin, oral ■ lactulose ■ neomycin, oral ■ Potassium salts ■ Tetracyclines
Amylase, serum ■ Chloride salts ■ Fluorides	■ asparaginase ■ Cholinergic agents ■ Contraceptives, oral ■ Contrast media with iodine ■ Drugs inducing acute pancreatitis: azathioprine, corticosteroids, loop and thiazide diuretics ■ methyldopa ■ Narcotics	■ somatostatin
Aspartate aminotransferase ■ erythromycin ■ methyldopa	■ Cholinergic agents ■ Hepatotoxic drugs ■ Opium alkaloids	■ interferon ■ naltrexone
Bilirubin, serum ■ ascorbic acid ■ dextran ■ epinephrine ■ pindolol ■ propanolol ■ levodopa ■ theophylline	■ Hemolytic agents ■ Hepatotoxic drugs ■ methyldopa ■ rifampin	■ Barbiturates ■ Sulfonamides

Drug interference with test results *(continued)*

Test and drugs causing chemical interference	Drugs causing physiologic interference	
	Increase test values	**Decrease test values**
Blood urea nitrogen ■ chloral hydrate ■ chloramphenicol ■ streptomycin	■ Anabolic steroids ■ Nephrotoxic drugs ■ pentamidine	■ Tetracyclines
Calcium, serum ■ aspirin ■ heparin ■ hydralazine ■ sulfisoxazole	■ Calcium salts ■ Diuretics, loop and thiazide ■ lithium ■ Thyroid hormones ■ Vitamin D ■ Anabolic steroids	■ acetazolamide ■ Anticonvulsants ■ calcitonin ■ cisplatin ■ Contraceptives, oral ■ Corticosteroids ■ Laxatives ■ Magnesium salts ■ plicamycin
Chloride, serum	■ acetazolamide ■ Androgens ■ Diuretics ■ Estrogens ■ Nonsteroidal anti-inflammatory drugs (NSAIDs)	■ Corticosteroids ■ Diuretics, loop and thiazide ■ Laxatives
Cholesterol, serum ■ Androgens ■ aspirin ■ Corticosteroids ■ Nitrates ■ Phenothiazines ■ Vitamin D	■ alcohol ■ Beta-adrenergic blockers ■ Contraceptives, oral ■ Corticosteroids ■ cyclosporine ■ Diuretics, thiazide ■ Phenothiazines ■ Sulfonamides ■ ticlopidine	■ Androgens ■ captopril ■ chlorpropamide ■ cholestyramine ■ clofibrate ■ colestipol ■ haloperidol ■ neomycin, oral
Creatine kinase	■ aminocaproic acid ■ amphotericin B ■ chlorthalidone ■ ethanol (long-term use) ■ gemfibrozil	■ Not applicable

(continued)

Drug interference with test results *(continued)*

Test and drugs causing chemical interference	Drugs causing physiologic interference	
	Increase test values	**Decrease test values**
Creatinine, serum ■ cefoxitin ■ cephalothin ■ flucytosine	■ cimetidine ■ flucyxtosine ■ Nephrotoxic drugs	■ Not applicable
Glucose, serum ■ acetaminophen ■ ascorbic acid (urine) ■ Cephalosporins (urine)	■ Antidepressants, tricyclic ■ Beta-adrenergic blockers ■ Corticosteroids ■ cyclosporine ■ dextrothyroxine ■ diazoxide ■ Diuretics, loop and thiazide ■ epinephrine ■ Estrogens ■ isoniazid ■ lithium ■ Phenothiazines ■ phenytoin ■ Salicylates ■ somatostatin	■ acetaminophen ■ Anabolic steroids ■ clofibrate ■ disopyramide ■ ethanol ■ gemfibrozil ■ Monoamine oxidase inhibitors ■ pentamidine
Magnesium, serum	■ lithium ■ Magnesium salts	■ albuterol ■ Aminoglycosides ■ amphotericin B ■ Calcium salts ■ cisplatin ■ Cardiac glycosides ■ Diuretics, loop and thiazide ■ ethanol
Phosphates, serum	■ Vitamin D (excessive amounts)	■ Antacids, phosphate-binding ■ lithium ■ mannitol
Potassium, serum	■ aminocaproic acid ■ Angiotensin-converting enzyme (ACE) inhibitors ■ Antineoplastics ■ cyclosporine ■ Diuretics, potassium-sparing	■ Aminoglycosides ■ ammonium chloride ■ amphotericin B ■ Corticosteroids ■ Diuretics, potassium-wasting ■ glucose

Drug interference with test results *(continued)*

Test and drugs causing chemical interference	Drugs causing physiologic interference	
	Increase test values	**Decrease test values**
Potassium, serum *(continued)*	■ isoniazid ■ lithium ■ mannitol ■ succinylcholine	■ insulin ■ Laxatives ■ Penicillins, extended-spectrum ■ Salicylates
Protein, serum	■ Anabolic steroids ■ Corticosteroids ■ phenazopyridine	■ Contraceptives, oral ■ Estrogens ■ Hepatotoxic drugs
Protein, urine ■ Aminoglycosides ■ Cephalosporins ■ Contrast media ■ magnesium sulfate ■ miconazole ■ nafcillin ■ phenazopyridine ■ Sulfonamides ■ tolbutamide ■ tolmetin	■ ACE inhibitors ■ Cephalosporins ■ Contrast media with iodine ■ Corticosteroids ■ nafcillin ■ Nephrotoxic drugs ■ Sulfonamides	■ Not applicable
Prothrombin time	■ Anticoagulants ■ asparaginase ■ aspirin ■ azathioprine ■ Certain cephalosporins ■ chloramphenicol ■ cholestyramine ■ colestipol ■ cyclophosphamide ■ Hepatotoxic drugs ■ propylthiouracil ■ quinidine ■ quinine ■ Sulfonamides	■ Anabolic steroids ■ Contraceptives, oral ■ Estrogens ■ Vitamin K
Sodium, serum	■ carbamazepine ■ clonidine ■ diazoxide ■ Estrogens	■ ammonium chloride ■ carbamazepine ■ desmopressin ■ Diuretics

(continued)

Drug interference with test results *(continued)*

Test and drugs causing chemical interference	Drugs causing physiologic interference	
	Increase test values	**Decrease test values**
Sodium, serum *(continued)*	■ guanabenz ■ guanadrel ■ guanethidine ■ methyldopa ■ NSAIDs ■ Steroids	■ lithium ■ lypressin ■ vasopressin ■ vincristine
Uric acid, serum ■ ascorbic acid ■ caffeine ■ hydralazine ■ isoniazid ■ levodopa ■ theophylline	■ acetazolamide ■ cisplatin ■ cyclosporine ■ diazoxide ■ Diuretics ■ epinephrine ■ ethambutol ■ ethanol ■ levodopa ■ niacin ■ phenytoin ■ propranolol ■ spironolactone	■ acetohexamide ■ allopurinol ■ clofibrate ■ Contrast media with iodine ■ diflunisal ■ Glucose infusions ■ guaifenesin ■ Phenothiazines ■ phenylbutazone ■ Salicylates (small doses) ■ Uricosuric agents

Drug additives

Drugs with ethanol additives

Many oral liquid drug preparations contain ethanol, which produces a slight sedative effect but isn't harmful to most patients and can in fact be beneficial. However, ingesting ethanol can be undesirable and even dangerous in some circumstances. The list below identifies generic drugs that commonly contain ethanol. (Note that some manufacturers of these drugs also produce ethanol-free [alcohol-free] formulations. Check with your pharmacist for more information.)

■ acetaminophen, acetaminophen with codeine elixir
■ bitolterol mesylate
■ brompheniramine maleate elixir
■ butabarbital sodium
■ chlorpheniramine maleate elixir
■ chlorpromazine hydrochloride
■ clemastine fumarate
■ co-trimoxazole
■ cyproheptadine hydrochloride
■ dexchlorpheniramine maleate
■ dextroamphetamine sulfate
■ diazepam
■ diazoxide
■ digoxin
■ dihydroergotamine mesylate injection
■ diphenhydramine hydrochloride
■ epinephrine
■ ergoloid mesylates
■ esmolol hydrochloride
■ ferrous sulfate elixirs
■ fluphenazine hydrochloride
■ hydromorphone hydrochloride cough syrup
■ hyocyamine sulfate

- indomethacin suspension
- isoetharine mesylate
- isoproterenol hydrochloride
- mesoridazine besylate
- methadone hydrochloride oral solution
- methdilazine hydrochloride
- methyldopa suspension
- minocycline hydrochloride
- molindone hydrochloride
- nitroglycerin infusion
- nystatin
- opium alkaloids hydrochlorides
- oxycodone hydrochloride
- paramethadione
- pentobarbital sodium elixir, pentobarbital sodium injection
- perphenazine
- phenobarbital injection
- phenytoin sodium injection
- promethazine hydrochloride
- pyridostigmine bromide
- thioridazine hydrochloride
- thiothixene hydrochloride
- trimeprazine tartrate
- trimethoprim
- tripelennamine hydrochloride
- triprolidine hydrochloride

Drugs with sulfite additives

Used as a drug preservative, sulfites can cause allergic reactions in certain patients. The list below identifies generic drugs that commonly contain sulfites. (A pharmacist can provide definitive information on brand-name drugs.)

- amikacin sulfate
- aminophylline
- amrinone lactate
- atropine sulfate with meperidine hydrochloride
- betamethasone sodium phosphate
- bupivacaine hydrochloride and epinephrine 1:200,000
- carisoprodol with aspirin and codeine phosphate
- chlorpromazine, chlorpromazine hydrochloride
- dexamethasone acetate, dexamethasone sodium phosphate
- diphenhydramine hydrochloride
- dobutamine hydrochloride
- dopamine hydrochloride
- epinephrine, epinephrine bitartrate, epinephrine bitartrate with pilocarpine hydrochloride, epinephrine hydrochloride
- etidocaine hydrochloride with epinephrine bitartrate 1:200,000
- heparin calcium, heparin sodium
- hydralazine hydrochloride
- hydrocortisone sodium phosphate
- hyoscyamine sulfate
- imipramine hydrochloride
- influenza virus vaccine
- isoetharine hydrochloride, isoetharine mesylate
- isoproterenol hydrochloride, isoproterenol sulfate
- lidocaine hydrochloride with epinephrine hydrochloride
- mafenide acetate
- metaraminol bitartrate
- methotrimeprazine hydrochloride
- methyldopa; methyldopate hydrochloride
- metoclopramide hydrochloride
- orphenadrine citrate, orphenadrine hydrochloride
- oxycodone hydrochloride with acetaminophen
- pentazocine hydrochloride, pentazocine hydrochloride with acetaminophen
- perphenazine
- phenylephrine hydrochloride
- procainamide hydrochloride
- procaine hydrochloride
- prochlorperazine, prochlorperazine edisylate, prochlorperazine maleate
- promazine hydrochloride
- propoxycaine hydrochloride with procaine hydrochloride 2% and levonordefrin 1:20,000
- ritodrine hydrochloride

- scopolamine hydrobromide with phenylephrine hydrochloride 10%
- tetracycline hydrochloride 0.22% topical
- theophylline
- thiethylperazine maleate
- trifluoperazine hydrochloride
- tubocurarine chloride

Drugs with tartrazine additives

Also known as FD&C Yellow No. 5, tartrazine is a dye used as an additive in certain drugs. It can provoke a severe allergic reaction in some people, especially those who are also allergic to aspirin. The list below identifies some drugs containing tartrazine. (However, not all dosage forms contain the dye. Check with your pharmacist for more information.)

- benzphetamine hydrochloride (Didrex tablets)
- butabarbital sodium (Butisol elixir and tablets)
- carisoprodol (Rela)
- chlorphenesin carbonate (Maolate)
- chlorprothixene (Taractan)
- clindamycin hydrochloride (Cleocin capsules)
- desipramine hydrochloride (Norpramin)
- dextroamphetamine sulfate (Dexedrine elixir, spansule, and tablets)
- dextrothyroxine hydrochloride (Choloxin)
- fluphenazine hydrochloride (Prolixin)
- haloperidol (Haldol tablets)
- hydralazine hydrochloride (Apresoline tablets)
- hydromorphone hydrochloride (Dilaudid cough syrup)
- imipramine (Janimine, Tofranil-PM)
- mepenzolate bromide (Cantil tablets)
- methamphetamine hydrochloride (Desoxyn Gradumets)
- methenamine hippurate (Hiprex tablets)
- methylsergide maleate (Sansert tablets)
- niacin (Nicolar)
- paramethadione (Paradione)
- penicillin G potassium (Pentids syrup, Pentids 400 syrup, Pentids 800)
- penicillin V potassium (Veetids 125 oral solution)
- pentobarbital sodium (Nembutal Sodium)
- procainamide hydrochloride (Pronestyl)
- promazine hydrochloride (Sparine)
- rauwolfia serpentina (Raudixin).

How aging increases the risk of drug hazards

The physiologic changes of aging make older adult patients more susceptible to drug-induced illnesses, adverse effects, toxicity, and interactions than younger adults. Other conditions common to many older adult patients also increase the risk of these problems.

To help prevent these problems or detect them early, check the patient's history for the following risk factors when developing your teaching plan:

- altered mental status
- financial problems
- frail health
- history of allergies
- history of previous adverse effects
- multiple chronic illnesses
- patient is a woman
- patient lives alone
- polypharmacy or complex medication regimens.
- poor nutritional status
- renal failure
- small build
- treatment by several doctors.

Substance abuse

Acute toxic reactions

Treatment of substance abuse is a long-term process beset with relapses. You need to understand the signs and symptoms of a toxic reaction before you can take steps to help the patient recover from his addiction.

Managing acute toxicity

Substance	Signs and symptoms	Interventions
alcohol (ethanol) ■ Beer and wine ■ Distilled spirits ■ Other preparations, such as cough syrup, aftershave, or mouthwash	■ Ataxia ■ Seizures ■ Coma ■ Hypothermia ■ Alcohol breath odor ■ Respiratory depression ■ Bradycardia ■ Hypotension ■ Nausea and vomiting	■ Induce vomiting or perform gastric lavage if ingestion occurred in the previous 4 hours. Give activated charcoal and a saline cathartic. ■ Start I.V. fluid replacement and administer dextrose 5% in water, thiamine, B-complex vitamins, and vitamin C to prevent dehydration and hypoglycemia and to correct nutritional deficiencies. ■ Pad bed rails and apply cloth restraints to protect the patient from injury. ■ Give an anticonvulsant such as diazepam to control seizures. ■ Watch the patient for signs and symptoms of withdrawal, such as hallucinations and alcohol withdrawal delirium. If these occur, consider giving chlordiazepoxide or benzodiazepines. ■ Auscultate the patient's lungs frequently to detect crackles or rhonchi, possibly indicating aspiration pneumonia. If you note these breath sounds, consider antibiotics. ■ Monitor the patient's neurologic status and vital signs every 15 minutes until his condition is stable. Assist with dialysis if his vital functions are severely depressed.
Amphetamines ■ Amphetamine sulfate (Benzedrine): bennies, greenies, cartwheels	■ Dilated reactive pupils ■ Altered mental status (from confusion to paranoia) ■ Hallucinations ■ Tremors and seizure activity	■ If the drug was taken orally, induce vomiting or perform gastric lavage; give activated charcoal and a sodium or magnesium sulfate cathartic. ■ Lower the patient's urine pH to 5 by adding ammonium chloride or ascorbic acid to his I.V. solution. ■ Force diuresis by giving the patient mannitol.

(continued)

Managing acute toxicity *(continued)*

Substance	Signs and symptoms	Interventions
Amphetamines *(continued)* ■ Dextroamphetamine sulfate (Dexedrine): dexies, hearts, oranges ■ Methamphetamine: speed, meth, crystal	■ Hyperactive deep tendon reflexes ■ Exhaustion ■ Coma ■ Dry mouth ■ Shallow respirations ■ Tachycardia ■ Hypertension ■ Hyperthermia ■ Diaphoresis	■ Give a short-acting barbiturate such as pentobarbital to control stimulant-induced seizures. ■ Restrain the patient, especially if he's paranoid or hallucinating, so he doesn't injure himself or others. ■ Give haloperidol I.M. or I.V. to treat agitation or assaultive behavior. ■ Give an alpha-adrenergic blocker such as phentolamine for hypertension. ■ Watch for cardiac arrhythmias. If these develop, consider propranolol or lidocaine to treat tachyarrhythmias or ventricular arrhythmias, respectively. ■ Treat hyperthermia with tepid sponge baths or a hypothermia blanket. ■ Provide a quiet environment to avoid overstimulation. ■ Be alert for signs and symptoms of withdrawal, such as abdominal tenderness, muscle aches, and long periods of sleep. ■ Observe suicide precautions, especially if the patient shows signs of withdrawal.
Antipsychotics ■ Chlorpromazine (Thorazine) ■ Phenothiazines ■ Thioridazine (Mellaril)	■ Constricted pupils ■ Photosensitivity ■ Extrapyramidal effects (dyskinesia, opisthotonos, muscle rigidity, ocular deviation) ■ Dry mouth ■ Decreased level of consciousness (LOC) ■ Decreased deep tendon reflexes ■ Seizures ■ Hypothermia or hyperthermia ■ Dysphagia ■ Respiratory depression ■ Hypotension ■ Tachycardia	■ Expect to perform gastric lavage if the patient ingested the drug within the past 6 hours. (Don't induce vomiting because phenothiazines have an antiemetic effect.) Consider activated charcoal and a cathartic. ■ Give diphenhydramine to treat extrapyramidal effects. ■ Give physostigmine salicylate to reverse anticholinergic effects in severe cases. ■ Replace fluids I.V. to correct hypotension; monitor the patient's vital signs often. ■ Monitor his respiratory rate, and give supplemental oxygen to treat respiratory depression. ■ Give an anticonvulsant such as diazepam or a short-acting barbiturate such as pentobarbital sodium to control seizures. ■ Keep the patient's room dark to avoid exacerbating his photosensitivity.

Substance	Signs and symptoms	Interventions
Anxiolytic sedative-hypnotics ■ Benzodi-azepines (Ativan, Valium, Librium, Xanax)	■ Confusion ■ Drowsiness ■ Stupor ■ Decreased reflexes ■ Seizures ■ Coma ■ Shallow respirations ■ Hypotension	■ Induce vomiting or perform gastric lavage; consider activated charcoal and a cathartic. ■ Give supplemental oxygen to correct hypoxia-induced seizures. ■ Replace fluids I.V. to correct hypotension; monitor the patient's vital signs often. ■ For benzodiazepine overdose, or to reverse the effect of benzodiazepine-induced sedation or respiratory depression, give flumazenil (Romazicon).
Barbiturate sedative-hypnotics ■ Amobarbital sodium (Amytal): blue angels, blue devils, blue birds ■ Phenobarbital (Luminal): phennies, purple hearts, goofballs ■ Secobarbital sodium (Seconal): reds, red devils	■ Poor pupil reaction to light ■ Nystagmus ■ Depressed LOC (from confusion to coma) ■ Flaccid muscles and absent reflexes ■ Hyperthermia or hypothermia ■ Cyanosis ■ Respiratory depression ■ Hypotension ■ Blisters or bullous lesions	■ Induce vomiting or perform gastric lavage if the patient ingested the drug within 4 hours; consider activated charcoal and a saline cathartic. ■ Maintain his blood pressure with I.V. fluid challenges and vasopressors. ■ If the patient has taken a phenobarbital overdose, give sodium bicarbonate I.V. to alkalinize his urine and speed the drug's elimination. ■ Apply a hyperthermia or hypothermia blanket to help return the patient's temperature to normal. ■ Prepare your patient for hemodialysis or hemoperfusion if toxic reaction is severe. ■ Perform frequent neurologic assessments, and check your patient's pulse rate, temperature, skin color, and reflexes often. ■ Notify the doctor if you see signs of respiratory distress or pulmonary edema. ■ Watch for signs and symptoms of withdrawal, such as hyperreflexia, tonic-clonic seizures, and hallucinations. Provide symptomatic relief of withdrawal symptoms. ■ Protect the patient from injuring himself.

(continued)

Substance	Signs and symptoms	Interventions
cocaine ■ Cocaine hydro-chloride: crack, freebase	■ Dilated pupils ■ Confusion ■ Alternating euphoria and apprehension ■ Hyperexcitability ■ Visual, auditory, and olfactory hallucinations ■ Spasms and seizures ■ Coma ■ Tachypnea ■ Hyperpnea ■ Pallor or cyanosis ■ Respiratory arrest ■ Tachycardia ■ Hypertension or hypotension ■ Fever ■ Nausea and vomiting ■ Abdominal pain ■ Perforated nasal septum or mouth sores	■ Calm the patient by talking to him in a quiet room. ■ If cocaine was ingested, induce vomiting or perform gastric lavage; give activated charcoal followed by a saline cathartic. ■ Give the patient a tepid sponge bath, and administer an antipyretic to reduce fever. ■ Monitor his blood pressure and heart rate. Expect to give propranolol for symptomatic tachycardia. ■ Administer an anticonvulsant such as diazepam to control seizures. ■ Scrape the inside of his nose to remove residual amounts of the drug. ■ Monitor his cardiac rate and rhythm—ventricular fibrillation and cardiac standstill can occur as a direct cardiotoxic result of cocaine ingestion. Defibrillate the patient, and initiate cardiopulmonary resuscitation, if indicated.
Hallucinogens ■ Lysergic acid diethylamide (LSD): hawk, acid, sunshine ■ Mescaline (peyote): mese, cactus, big chief	■ Dilated pupils ■ Intensified perceptions ■ Agitation and anxiety ■ Synesthesia ■ Impaired judgment ■ Hyperactive movement ■ Flashback experiences ■ Hallucinations ■ Depersonalization ■ Moderately increased blood pressure ■ Increased heart rate ■ Fever	■ Reorient the patient repeatedly to time, place, and person. ■ Restrain the patient to protect him from injuring himself and others. ■ Calm the patient by talking to him in a quiet room. ■ If the drug was taken orally, induce vomiting or perform gastric lavage; give activated charcoal and a cathartic. ■ Give diazepam I.V. to control seizures.

Managing acute toxicity *(continued)*

Substance	Signs and symptoms	Interventions
Narcotics ■ Codeine ■ Heroin: junk, smack, H, snow ■ Hydromorphone hydrochloride (Dilaudid): D, lords ■ Morphine: Mort, M, monkey, Emma	■ Constricted pupils ■ Depressed LOC (but the patient is usually responsive to persistent verbal or tactile stimuli) ■ Seizures ■ Hypothermia ■ Slow, deep respirations ■ Hypotension ■ Bradycardia ■ Skin changes (pruritus, urticaria, flushed skin)	■ Give naloxone until the drug's central nervous system depressant effects are reversed. ■ Replace fluids I.M. to increase circulatory volume. ■ Correct hypothermia by applying extra blankets; if the patient's body temperature doesn't increase, use a hyperthermia blanket. ■ Reorient the patient often. ■ Auscultate the lungs often for crackles, possibly indicating pulmonary edema. (Onset may be delayed.) ■ Administer oxygen via nasal cannula, mask, or mechanical ventilation to correct hypoxemia from hypoventilation. ■ Monitor cardiac rate and rhythm, being alert for atrial fibrillation. (This should resolve when hypoxemia is corrected.) ■ Be alert for signs of withdrawal, such as piloerection (goose flesh), diaphoresis, and hyperactive bowel sounds. ■ Institute safety measures to prevent patient injury.
phencyclidine (PCP) ■ Angel dust, peace pill, hog	■ Blank stare ■ Nystagmus ■ Amnesia ■ Decreased awareness of surroundings ■ Recurrent coma ■ Violent behavior ■ Hyperactivity ■ Seizures ■ Gait ataxia ■ Muscle rigidity ■ Drooling ■ Hyperthermia ■ Hypertensive crisis ■ Cardiac arrest	■ If the drug was taken orally, induce vomiting or perform gastric lavage; instill and remove activated charcoal repeatedly. ■ Acidify the patient's urine with ascorbic acid to increase drug excretion. ■ Expect to continue to acidify urine for 2 weeks because signs and symptoms may recur when fat cells release PCP stores. ■ Give diazepam and haloperidol to control agitation or psychotic behavior. ■ Institute safety measures to protect the patient from injury. ■ Administer diazepam to control seizures. ■ Institute seizure precautions. ■ Provide a quiet environment and dimmed light. ■ Give propranolol for hypertension and tachycardia, and give nitroprusside for severe hypertension. ■ Closely monitor urine output and serial renal function tests. Rhabdomyolysis, myoglobinuria, and renal failure may occur in severe intoxication. ■ If renal failure develops, prepare the patient for hemodialysis.

13

Complications
Spotting and correcting life-threatening conditions

Air embolism

Air embolism refers to the migration of a bolus of gas from the systemic circulation into the microvasculature. Obstruction occurs when the gas reaches the capillary system. Besides impairing blood flow, an air embolus causes a physiologic response as fibrin, platelets, and red blood cells congregate at the occlusion site. This further restricts blood flow and contributes to an inflammatory vasospasm of the affected vessel.

Arterial air emboli may lodge in the small vessels supplying major organs or peripheral circulation. Venous air emboli commonly occlude pulmonary blood flow; they may also obstruct arterial circulation if the patient has an intracardiac defect or a microvascular shunt between arterioles and venules of the lungs.

Causes

A bolus of air may enter the bloodstream during positive-pressure ventilation if the patient has a lung tear, or when air enters an artery or vein through an I.V. cannula during insertion, maintenance, or removal of the line. Air emboli have also been associated with oral-vaginal sex, laser surgery, and pneumoperitoneum, and as a complication of needle biopsies and pregnancy. Air emboli also result from rapid decompression following underwater diving.

Venous air emboli may occur as a complication of surgery or blunt or penetrating trauma to the head, neck, chest, heart, or abdomen.

Signs and symptoms

The first sign of a venous air embolism may be cardiopulmonary collapse, especially in the presence of a rapid infusion of a large volume of air.

If the embolus moves into the arterial circulation, central nervous system and cardiac symptoms may develop. The patient may complain of dyspnea, vertigo, anxiety, or impending doom. He may also experience a "gasp" reflex (cough, short exhalation, and prolonged inhalation).

Other signs include tachycardia, tachypnea, and elevated central venous and pulmonary artery pressures. Electrocardiogram results show ST-segment changes reflecting ischemia. A transient churning heart murmur has been noted. Hypotension and decreased peripheral vascular resistance indicate progressive shock. Crepitus occasionally is palpable, and wheezes and crackles may be auscultated when pulmonary edema is present.

Treatment

Treatment aims to promote reabsorption of trapped air, and mitigate life-threatening signs and symptoms. In the event of cardiac arrest, cardiopulmonary resuscitation (CPR) is initiated immediately. External cardiac massage improves circulation and may help break up large right ventricular bubbles, increasing blood flow to the pulmonary vasculature.

An air embolus may be removed through a central venous catheter or by needle aspiration. Bubble size may be reduced by administering 100% oxygen (which reduces the amount of nitrogen in the bubble) or by administering hyperbaric oxygen; the latter approach also may improve signs and symptoms by oxygenating ischemic tissue.

Nursing interventions

■ Preventing air embolism is the key to nursing care. Make sure that all air is purged from catheters and I.V. lines before connecting them.

■ Keep closed systems as airtight as possible; tape all tubing connections, or use luer-lock devices for all connections.

■ Place the patient in the Trendelenburg position when inserting all central venous line catheters. Have the patient perform Valsalva's maneuver during catheter insertion and tubing changes.

■ Position the patient on his left side in the Trendelenburg position so air can enter the right atrium and be dispersed by the pulmonary artery.

■ Initiate CPR immediately if cardiac collapse occurs.

Atelectasis

In atelectasis, alveolar clusters (lobules) or lung segments fail to expand completely during respiration, causing part or all of the affected lung to collapse. Because the collapsed lung tissue is effectively isolated from gas exchange, unoxygenated blood is shunted and passes unchanged through these tissues, producing hypoxia.

Causes
Atelectasis can result from bronchial occlusion by mucus plugs — a problem for patients with chronic obstructive pulmonary disease, bronchiectasis, or cystic fibrosis. Atelectasis may also result from occlusion caused by foreign bodies, bronchogenic cancer, or inflammatory lung disease.

Other causes include idiopathic respiratory distress syndrome of the neonate, oxygen toxicity, and pulmonary edema.

External compression, which inhibits full lung expansion, or any condition that makes deep breathing painful also may cause atelectasis. Compression or pain may result from upper abdominal surgical incisions, rib fractures, pleuritic chest pain, tight chest dressings, or obesity (which elevates the diaphragm and reduces tidal volume).

Lung collapse or reduced expansion may accompany prolonged immobility or mechanical ventilation; central nervous system depression eliminates periodic sighing and predisposes the patient to progressive atelectasis.

Signs and symptoms
Clinical effects vary with the causes of lung collapse, the degree of hypoxia, and the underlying disease. If atelectasis affects a small lung area, symptoms may be minimal and transient; however, if atelectasis affects a large area, symptoms may be severe and may include dyspnea, anxiety, and pleuritic chest pain.

Inspection may disclose decreased chest wall movement, cyanosis, diaphoresis, and substernal or intercostal retractions. Palpation may reveal decreased fremitus and mediastinal shift to the affected side. Percussion may disclose dullness or flatness over lung fields. Auscultation, crackles during the last part of inspiration and decreased (or absent) breath sounds with major lung involvement; auscultation may also disclose tachycardia.

A chest X-ray is the primary diagnostic tool. Other diagnostic tests include bronchoscopy to rule out an obstructing neoplasm or a foreign body, arterial blood gas (ABG) analysis to detect respiratory acidosis and hypoxemia resulting from atelectasis, and pulse oximetry, which may show deteriorating arterial oxygen saturation levels.

Treatment
Incentive spirometry, chest percussion, postural drainage, mucolytics, and frequent coughing and deep-breathing exercises may improve oxygenation. If these measures fail, bronchoscopy may help remove secretions. Humidity and a bronchodilator can improve mucociliary clearance and dilate the airways.

To minimize the risk of atelectasis after thoracic and abdominal surgery, the patient requires an analgesic to facilitate deep breathing. If the patient has atelectasis secondary to an obstructing neoplasm, he may need surgery or radiation therapy.

Nursing interventions

■ Offer reassurance and emotional support because the patient may be frightened by his limited ability to breathe.

■ Encourage the patient recovering from surgery to perform coughing and deep-breathing exercises and incentive spirometry every 1 to 2 hours while splinting the incision. Encourage these procedures in any patient who is at high risk for atelectasis.

■ Assess breath sounds and respiratory status frequently. Report any changes immediately; monitor pulse oximetry readings and ABG values for evidence of hypoxia.

■ *Gently* reposition the patient often, and help him walk as soon as possible. Administer adequate analgesics to control pain.

■ If the patient is receiving mechanical ventilation, maintain tidal volume at 10 to 15 cc/kg of body weight to ensure adequate lung expansion. Use the ventilator's sigh mechanism, if appropriate, to intermittently increase tidal volume at the rate of 10 to 15 sighs per hour.

■ Humidify inspired air, and encourage adequate fluid intake to mobilize secretions. Use postural drainage and chest percussion to remove secretions. Suction as needed.

■ Administer sedatives cautiously because they depress respirations and the cough reflex and also suppress sighs.

Bone marrow suppression

Bone marrow suppression is characterized by reduced numbers of hematopoietic (blood-forming) stem cells in the bone marrow. Impaired hematopoiesis leads to reduced numbers of peripheral blood leukocytes and neutrophils (neu-tropenia), thrombocytes (thrombocytopenia), and erythrocytes (anemia).

Causes

Many chemotherapeutic agents injure the rapidly proliferating stem cells. Other drugs, such as sulfa compounds, anticonvulsants, and immunosuppressants, also may suppress bone marrow.

Radiation to large marrow-bearing areas — such as the pelvis, ribs, spine, and sternum — may produce significant and permanent bone marrow damage. Bone marrow suppression and depressed peripheral blood cell counts occur in patients with tumor replacement of the bone marrow (leukemia, myeloma, or metastatic deposits from solid tumors). Additional causes of bone marrow suppression include autoimmune disorders, certain congenital disorders, and exposure to pesticides, benzene-containing solvents, and other toxins.

Signs and symptoms

Clinical effects of bone marrow suppression are related to its severity. A patient with neutropenia is at risk for infection from bacteria, viruses, or fungi. He may exhibit fever, chills, malaise, or other localized signs of infection.

Thrombocytopenia is associated with bleeding (especially from the gums and nose), bruising, petechiae, ecchymoses, hematuria, and possibly hematochezia. Spontaneous bleeding is likely to occur if the platelet count drops below 20,000/mm^3.

Signs and symptoms of anemia include fatigue, weakness, pallor, tachycardia, exertional dyspnea, and headache.

Treatment

Improved antimicrobial therapy has dramatically reduced morbidity and mortality of patients with neutropenia. Chemotherapy-induced neutropenia can be reduced by use of myeloid growth factors (granulocyte colony-stimulating

Nursing interventions in bone marrow suppression

This chart summarizes essential nursing interventions for patients experiencing anemia, neutropenia, or thrombocytopenia.

Condition	Interventions
Anemia (Hemoglobin <14 g/dl in males; <12 g/dl in females) (Severe anemia hemoglobin <8 g/dl)	■ Monitor complete blood count (CBC) at least daily. ■ Monitor the patient for signs of inadequate oxygenation, such as pallor, tachypnea, and increased capillary refill time. ■ Teach the patient about nutritional supplementation (such as iron or folic acid). ■ Assess the patient for source of blood loss, if applicable. ■ Teach the patient energy conservation measures. ■ Teach the patient to avoid driving or participating in hazardous activities if dizziness is present. ■ Teach the patient to change positions slowly to avoid syncopal episodes. ■ Administer transfusions of packed red blood cells as ordered. Monitor the patient for transfusion reactions. ■ Administer recombinant erythropoetin or other blood replacement alternatives, as ordered.
Neutropenia (Neutrophil count <1,500/mm³) (Severe neutropenia <500/mm³)	■ Monitor the patient's temperature and vital signs. Report fever > 101.3° F (38.5° C). ■ Monitor CBC and blood chemistries. ■ Assess the patient for localized signs of infection. ■ Assess the patient for symptoms of sepsis. ■ Obtain cultures of blood, urine, throat, sputum, and stool as ordered (blood cultures with temperature spike > 101.3° F). ■ Avoid invasive procedures or rectal manipulation. ■ Avoid contact with persons with viral or bacterial infections. ■ Administer broad-spectrum antibiotics as indicated. ■ Teach the patient or the caregiver rationale for use of hematopoietic growth factors and self-administration, if indicated. ■ Teach proper storage and precautions for hematopoietic growth factors.
Thrombocytopenia (Platelet count <100,000/mm³) (Severe thrombocytopenia platelet count <20,000/mm³)	■ Teach the patient to avoid injury and sharp objects. ■ Teach the patient to avoid straining or Valsalva's maneuver. ■ Avoid invasive procedures (such as I.M. injections, enemas, or suppositories). ■ Apply direct pressure for 5 minutes to needle puncture sites. ■ Assess the patient for signs of bleeding, increased petechiae, or increased bruising.

Condition	Interventions
Thrombocytopenia *(continued)*	■ Monitor the patient for signs of internal bleeding (such as blood in stool and hematuria) and signs and symptoms of intracranial bleeding (such as headache, restlessness, decreased level of consciousness, pupillary changes, and seizures). ■ Administer platelet transfusions as ordered. ■ Monitor the patient for transfusion reactions. Check posttransfusion platelet count.

Nursing interventions in bone marrow suppression *(continued)*

factor [filgrastim] or granulocyte-macrophage colony-stimulating factor [sargramostim]).

Removal of the offending agents in patients with drug-induced thrombocytopenia or proper treatment of the underlying cause (when possible) is essential. A corticosteroid or lithium carbonate or folate may be used to increase platelet production. Platelet transfusions may be used to stop episodic abnormal bleeding caused by a low platelet count; however, if platelet destruction results from an immune disorder, platelet infusions may have only a minimal effect and may be reserved for life-threatening bleeding.

Recombinant erythropoietin may help improve anemia due to chronic disease or renal dysfunction. Packed red blood cells and platelets are administered to support the patient until bone marrow function recovers.

Nursing interventions
Nursing interventions for the patient with bone marrow suppression are summarized in *Nursing interventions in bone marrow suppression.*

Brain herniation

Brain herniation results from distortion and displacement of brain tissue through a natural opening in the intracranial cavity.

Three types of brain herniation syndromes exist: cingulate, central, and transtentorial. *Cingulate herniation* occurs across the midline where the hemisphere is distorted beneath the cerebellar falx. Few symptoms are associated with this type of herniation because it rarely occurs in isolation. *Central herniation* occurs when the medial aspects of the temporal lobe, the diencephalon, and the midbrain are pushed downward into the posterior fossa. In *transtentorial herniation,* the most common type of brain herniation, the medial aspect of the temporal lobe is pushed over the tentorium. Signs and symptoms reflect pressure on the midbrain and surrounding structures.

Causes
Brain herniation results from space-occupying lesions, cerebral edema due to trauma or stroke, or hydrocephalus. It can also be caused by excessive drainage of cerebrospinal fluid (CSF) from a ventricular catheter or a lumbar puncture.

Signs and symptoms
Signs and symptoms vary with the type of herniation. General early signs include decreasing level of conscious-

ness, pupillary abnormalities, impaired motor function, and impaired brain stem reflexes. Signs of central herniation include small reactive pupils (early phase), roving eye movements with loss of upward gaze, intermittent agitation and drowsiness progressing to stupor, contralateral hemiparesis, and Cheyne-Stokes respirations. Signs of transtentorial herniation include ipsilateral pupil dilation, paralysis of eye movements, restlessness progressing to loss of consciousness, contralateral hemiparesis, decorticate or decerebrate posturing, and bilateral Babinski's sign. Altered vital signs become evident late in the syndrome, such as widening pulse pressure and bradycardia.

Treatment

If herniation results from a space-occupying lesion such as a hematoma or tumor, surgical removal of the lesion will relieve the pressure and allow adjacent structures to resume their normal shape. If herniation is related to increased intracranial pressure (ICP) resulting from cerebral edema, treatment involves reducing the edema using an osmotic diuretic or a corticosteroid, CSF drainage, hyperventilation and, in extreme cases, barbiturate therapy. Maintenance of temperature control and normal fluid balance also are important. In some situations, such as cerebral edema resulting from traumatic injury, the patient may have an ICP monitor in place to help guide treatment.

Nursing interventions

■ Perform neurologic assessment at least hourly.
■ Institute precautionary measures to decrease ICP, including maintaining the head of the bed at 15 to 30 degrees to promote venous drainage. Position the patient in a neutral position, avoiding extreme hip and neck flexion.

■ Institute seizure precautions, and assess the patient frequently for signs of seizures.
■ Monitor vital signs frequently to ensure adequate cerebral perfusion.
■ If the patient has undergone a craniotomy for a hematoma or tumor, provide postoperative craniotomy care.
■ Observe the patient carefully for other postoperative complications, such as infection, thrombophlebitis, or diabetes insipidus.

Cardiac tamponade

In cardiac tamponade, a rapid unchecked rise in intrapericardial pressure impairs diastolic filling of the heart. The increased pressure usually results from blood or fluid accumulation in the pericardial sac. If fluid accumulates rapidly, as little as 250 ml can create an emergency situation. Gradual fluid accumulation, as in pericardial effusion associated with cancer, may not produce immediate signs and symptoms because the fibrous wall of the pericardial sac can stretch to accommodate as much as 1 to 2 L of fluid.

Causes

Cardiac tamponade may be idiopathic (Dressler's syndrome), or it may result from effusion (in cancer, bacterial infection, tuberculosis and, rarely, acute rheumatic fever), hemorrhage from trauma, hemorrhage from nontraumatic causes (with pericarditis), acute myocardial infarction, chronic renal failure during dialysis, drug reaction, or a connective tissue disorder.

Signs and symptoms

Cardiac tamponade classically produces increased venous pressure with neck vein distention, reduced arterial blood pressure, muffled heart sounds on auscultation, and paradoxical pulse (an abnormal inspiratory drop in systemic blood pressure greater than 15 mm Hg).

Cardiac tamponade may also cause dyspnea, diaphoresis, pallor or cyanosis, anxiety, tachycardia, narrowed pulse pressure, restlessness, and hepatomegaly, but the lung fields will be clear. The patient typically sits upright and leans forward.

Chest X-rays show a slightly widened mediastinum and enlarged cardiac silhouette. Electrocardiography is done to rule out other cardiac disorders. Pulmonary artery pressure monitoring detects increases in right atrial pressure, right ventricular diastolic pressure, and central venous pressure (CVP). Echocardiography records pericardial effusion with signs of right ventricular and atrial compression.

Treatment

The goal of treatment is to relieve intrapericardial pressure and cardiac compression by removing accumulated blood or fluid. Pericardiocentesis (needle aspiration of the pericardial cavity) or surgical creation of an opening dramatically improves systemic arterial pressure and cardiac output with the aspiration of as little as 25 ml of fluid.

In a hypotensive patient, trial volume loading with normal saline solution I.V. with albumin — and perhaps an inotropic drug such as dopamine — is necessary to maintain cardiac output. Depending on the cause of tamponade, additional treatment may be needed.

Nursing interventions

■ Infuse I.V. solutions and inotropic drugs (such as dopamine), as ordered, to maintain the patient's blood pressure.

■ Administer oxygen therapy as needed.

■ Prepare the patient for pericardiocentesis, thoracotomy, or central venous line insertion as indicated.

■ Check for signs of increasing tamponade, increasing dyspnea, and arrhythmias.

■ Watch for a decrease in CVP and a concomitant rise in blood pressure following treatment, which indicate relief of cardiac compression.

■ Monitor respiratory status for signs of respiratory distress, such as severe tachypnea or changes in level of consciousness.

Disseminated intravascular coagulation

Also known as consumption coagulopathy or defibrination syndrome, disseminated intravascular coagulation (DIC) complicates conditions that accelerate clotting — thereby causing small vessel occlusion, organ necrosis, depletion of circulating clotting factors and platelets, and activation of the fibrinolytic system — which can provoke severe hemorrhage.

Clotting in the microcirculation usually affects the kidneys and extremities but can occur in the brain, lungs, pituitary and adrenal glands, and GI mucosa. Other conditions — such as vitamin K deficiency, hepatic disease, and anticoagulant therapy — can cause similar hemorrhage.

Although usually acute, DIC may be chronic in cancer patients. The prognosis depends on early detection and treatment, the severity of the hemorrhage, and treatment of the underlying condition.

Causes

DIC results when tissue factor, a lipoprotein that helps initiate blood coagulation, is introduced into the bloodstream due to pathologic states such as infections, obstetric complications, neoplastic disease, and disorders that produce necrosis. Other causes include heatstroke, shock, poisonous snakebite, cirrhosis, fat embolism, incompatible blood transfusion, cardiac arrest, surgery necessitating cardiopulmonary bypass, giant hemangioma, severe venous thrombosis, and purpura fulminans.

Signs and symptoms
The most significant sign of DIC is abnormal bleeding *without* an accompanying history of hemorrhagic disorder. Principle signs of such bleeding include cutaneous oozing, petechiae, ecchymoses, and hematomas caused by bleeding into the skin. Bleeding from sites of surgical or invasive procedures and from the GI tract are equally significant indications, as are acrocyanosis and signs of acute tubular necrosis.

Related signs and symptoms and other possible effects include nausea, vomiting, dyspnea, oliguria, seizures, coma, shock, failure of major organ systems, and severe muscle, back, and abdominal pain.

The following initial laboratory findings suggest a tentative diagnosis of DIC: decreased platelet count, reduced fibrinogen levels, prolonged prothrombin time, prolonged partial thromboplastin time, and increased fibrin degradation products.

Treatment
Successful management of DIC requires prompt recognition and adequate treatment of the underlying disorder. If the patient isn't actively bleeding, supportive care alone may reverse DIC. However, active bleeding may require administration of blood, fresh frozen plasma, platelets, or packed red blood cells.

Heparin therapy is controversial but is usually mandatory if thrombosis occurs. Such drugs as antithrombin III and gabexate are being considered for use as antithrombins to inhibit the clotting cascade.

Nursing interventions
■ Administer prescribed analgesics for pain as needed.

■ Administer oxygen therapy as ordered.

■ To prevent clots from dislodging and causing fresh bleeding, don't vigorously rub these areas when washing. If bleeding occurs, use pressure, cold compresses, and topical hemostatic agents to control it.

■ After giving an I.V. injection or removing a catheter or needle, apply pressure to the injection site for at least 10 minutes. Alert other staff members to the patient's tendency to hemorrhage. Limit venipunctures whenever possible.

■ Protect the patient from injury. Enforce complete bed rest during bleeding episodes. If the patient is very agitated, pad the bed rails.

■ Reposition the patient every 2 hours, and provide meticulous skin care to prevent skin breakdown.

■ If the patient can't tolerate activity because of blood loss, provide frequent rest periods.

■ Monitor intake and output hourly. Watch for transfusion reactions and signs of fluid overload.

■ Weigh dressings and linens, and record drainage. Weigh the patient daily.

■ Watch for bleeding from the GI and genitourinary tracts. If you suspect intra-abdominal bleeding, measure the patient's abdominal girth at least every 4 hours, and observe closely for signs of shock.

■ Monitor the results of serial blood studies.

■ Test all stools and urine for occult blood.

■ Inform the family of the patient's progress, and provide emotional support and encouragement.

Hyperglycemic crisis

Diabetic ketoacidosis (DKA) and hyperosmolar hyperglycemic nonketotic syndrome (HHNS) are acute complications of hyperglycemic crisis that may occur in a diabetic patient. They require quick and effective treatment to prevent coma and, possibly, death. DKA usually occurs in patients with type 1 diabetes; in fact, DKA may be the first sign of previously unrecognized diabetes. HHNS usually occurs in patients with type 2 diabetes but may also occur in patients whose insulin tolerance is stressed and in those who have undergone certain therapeutic procedures, such as peritoneal dialysis, hemodialysis, total parenteral nutrition, or tube feedings.

Causes

Acute insulin deficiency (absolute in DKA; relative in HHNS) precipitates both conditions. Causes include illness trauma, stress, infection, and failure to take insulin (*only* in a patient with DKA).

Signs and symptoms

Signs and symptoms of DKA and HHNS result primarily from soaring blood glucose levels and include fluid loss, dehydration, shock, coma and, possibly, death. Acetone breath, dehydration, Kussmaul's respirations, and a weak, rapid pulse are evident in patients with DKA. Polyuria, thirst, neurologic abnormalities, and stupor are seen in the patient with HHNS. Keep in mind that the patient with DKA also shows evidence of metabolic acidosis. Acidosis may start a cycle that leads to additional tissue breakdown, followed by more ketosis, more acidosis, and eventually shock, coma, and death.

Treatment

Both DKA and HHNS are treated with fluid and electrolyte replacement and supportive care. Normal or half-normal saline solution is given I.V. at 1 L/hour until blood pressure is stabilized and urine output reaches 60 ml/hour. Then regular insulin is started, initially as an I.V. bolus dose, followed by continuous infusion. The rate is adjusted until the patient's serum glucose levels decrease by 80 to 100 mg/dl/hour.

When renal blood flow and urine output are established, potassium is given I.V. If acidosis is severe (pH less than 7.1), sodium bicarbonate may also be infused.

Nursing interventions

■ When you recognize the signs and symptoms of DKA or HHNS, notify the doctor immediately and prepare the patient for transfer to the intensive care unit.

■ Monitor the patient's vital signs, level of consciousness, electrocardiogram results, and arterial blood gas, electrolyte, glucose, and osmolarity levels frequently, as ordered. Also check the patient's urine for ketones.

■ Begin I.V. fluid replacement therapy as soon as possible.

■ Expect to administer an injection of regular insulin immediately — either I.M. or I.V. — followed by a continuous I.V. insulin drip.

■ Provide supportive care as indicated by the patient's condition.

■ Prepare to administer potassium replacements as ordered.

Hypertensive crisis

Hypertensive crisis refers to a severe, life-threatening form of hypertension. It's classified according to the degree of organ damage apparent when the patient comes in for treatment.

Hypertensive emergency, the more critical crisis level, develops over hours to days and is accompanied by signs of imminent or progressive end-organ damage. Severely elevated diastolic blood pressure must be reduced within minutes to an hour to prevent or reduce irreversible organ damage. Hypertensive urgency, a less critical crisis level, develops over several days to weeks and is characterized by severely elevated diastolic blood pressure, but without evidence of end-organ damage.

Causes
Hypertensive crisis is caused by conditions or circumstances that elevate cardiac output, such as increased circulating volume due to primary aldosteronism or eclampsia; it's also caused by conditions that increase peripheral vascular resistance, such as excessive vasoconstriction due to catecholamine release accompanying pheochromocytoma, blockage of some antihypertensives by monoamine oxidase (MAO) inhibitors, or release of angiotensin into circulation (as in renal disease).

Other causes of hypertensive crisis include acute aortic dissection, coarctation of the aorta, acute left-sided heart failure and pulmonary edema, renal artery stenosis, thyroid crisis, hypercalcemia, and adrenocortical disorders.

Signs and symptoms
Patients in hypertensive emergency generally have a diastolic blood pressure of 120 mm Hg or greater, with evidence of incipient or progressive end-organ damage. Patients with hypertensive urgency may have an elevated diastolic blood pressure reading (100 to 120 mm Hg), but with no evidence of concomitant end-organ damage.

Signs and symptoms may be absent in early stages of either hypertensive state. The patient may experience vague discomfort and fatigue or such neurologic signs as dizziness or occipital or anterior headache. In later stages of hypertensive crisis, particularly in hypertensive emergency, the patient may exhibit signs related to organs, tissues, or body systems affected:
- *eyes* — retinal changes, including arterial narrowing or papilledema, decreased acuity, and nystagmus
- *neurologic* — slow responses, decreased level of consciousness (LOC), cranial nerve abnormality, changes in deep tendon reflexes, nausea, vomiting, seizures, throbbing suboccipital or anterior headache, muscle weakness, and altered speech
- *renal* — oliguria, hematuria, azotemia, palpable enlarged kidneys, costovertebral angle tenderness
- *cardiopulmonary* — angina; cool, pale skin; shift in point of maximum impulse; third and fourth heart sounds; left ventricular heave; jugular vein distention; and adventitious breath sounds such as basilar crackles.

Diagnostic tests (X-rays, electrocardiogram, computed tomography scan, urinalysis, and blood work) may determine the underlying cause.

Treatment
The priority for treating a patient with hypertensive crisis is lowering blood pressure rapidly but cautiously, to avoid sharply reducing perfusion of organs that have accommodated to higher pressures.

Some patients may require surgery to correct the underlying cause of hypertension, but most are treated conservatively with an oral or parenteral antihypertensive. For patients with hypertensive emergency, blood pressure is reduced rapidly over a few minutes to an hour; for those with hypertensive urgency, it's reduced gradually, over several hours to 24 hours.

Medical therapy is directed at reducing systemic vascular resistance or reducing circulating volume as appropriate.

Nursing interventions

■ The most important nursing responsibilities are accurately assessing the patient's blood pressure, detecting possible causes of the hypertension, and preventing or detecting end-organ damage.

■ After medication therapy is initiated, monitor blood pressure every 5 to 15 minutes, depending on the medication used.

■ If mechanical or arterial line blood pressure readings are used, check their accuracy with cuff pressures at least once every 4 hours.

■ Administer medications according to protocols to maintain blood pressure within a designated parameter and avoid insufficient or excessive reduction of blood pressure.

■ Assess pulses, skin color, and temperature in all extremities. Note pulse deficits; differences in rate, rhythm, and quality; bruits; or edema.

■ Monitor cardiac rhythm and assess trends. Report results of 12-lead ECG monitoring, and assess them for changes from the baseline.

■ Perform neurologic and visual checks at least once every 4 hours to determine adequate cerebral and ocular circulation. Note any changes in LOC, sensory motor changes, dizziness, visual status, and ocular fundus changes.

■ Monitor the patient closely for signs of cardiac decompensation with pulmonary edema and chest pain, which might signal the onset of angina or myocardial infarction.

■ Teach the patient to avoid stress, sudden movement, straining, and Valsalva's maneuver, to prevent sudden changes in blood pressure.

■ Monitor renal status, including hourly intake and output.

■ Administer an analgesic or sedative, as ordered, for possible headache secondary to medication therapy or chest pain. Institute other measures to control pain and anxiety (such as a quiet environment, distraction, guided imagery, and massage), to increase relaxation and comfort and relieve stress.

■ Monitor the patient carefully when desired blood pressure control is attained and he's weaned from parenteral therapy to oral maintenance therapy.

■ Address the patient's and family's anxiety, and explain the situation and all therapy as thoroughly as possible.

■ Assess the patient's knowledge of and compliance with the antihypertensive regimen. Plan interventions, as needed, to educate the patient and promote proper blood pressure control.

Hypoglycemia

Hypoglycemia, which is an abnormally low blood glucose level, can be dangerous. It occurs when glucose burns up too rapidly, when the glucose release rate falls behind tissue demands, or when too much insulin enters the bloodstream.

Hypoglycemia may be classified as reactive or fasting. *Reactive hypoglycemia* results from a reaction to a meal or administration of too much insulin.

Fasting hypoglycemia causes discomfort during periods of abstinence from food, for example in the early morning hours before breakfast.

Causes

Reactive hypoglycemia may occur in several forms. In a diabetic patient, it may result from administration of too much insulin or, less commonly, too much of an oral antidiabetic. In a mildly diabetic patient (or one in the early stages of diabetes mellitus), reactive hypoglycemia may result from delayed and excessive insulin production after carbohydrate ingestion.

Similarly, a nondiabetic patient may suffer reactive hypoglycemia from a sharp increase in insulin output after a meal. Sometimes called postprandial hypoglycemia, this form usually disappears when the patient eats something sweet.

In some patients, reactive hypoglycemia may have no known cause or may result from hyperalimentation due to gastric dumping syndrome or from impaired glucose tolerance.

Fasting hypoglycemia usually results from an excess of insulin or insulin-like substances, or from a decrease in counterregulatory hormones. It also may be exogenous (such as from alcohol or drug ingestion) or endogenous (such as from organic problems).

Other endocrine causes include destruction of the pancreatic islet cells, adrenocortical insufficiency, and pituitary insufficiency. Nonendocrine causes include severe liver disease, such as hepatitis, liver cancer, cirrhosis, and liver congestion associated with heart failure.

Signs and symptoms

Reactive and fasting hypoglycemia cause fatigue, malaise, nervousness, irritability, trembling, tension, headache, hunger, diaphoresis, and rapid heart rate.

Fasting hypoglycemia also may cause central nervous system (CNS) disturbances, such as altered level of consciousness, blurry or double vision, confusion, motor weakness, hemiplegia, seizures, or coma.

Age alert In infants and children, signs and symptoms are vague. A neonate's refusal to feed may be the primary clue to underlying hypoglycemia. Associated effects include tremors, twitching, weak or high-pitched cry, diaphoresis, limpness (or weakness), seizures, and coma.

Treatment

Reactive hypoglycemia requires dietary modification to help delay glucose absorption and gastric emptying. Usually, this includes small, frequent, high-protein meals with added fiber and avoidance of simple carbohydrates. The patient also may receive an anticholinergic to slow gastric emptying and intestinal motility and to inhibit vagal stimulation of insulin release.

For fasting hypoglycemia, surgery and drug therapy may be required. For patients with insulinoma, removal of the tumor is the treatment of choice. Drug therapy may include a nondiuretic thiazide, such as diazoxide, to inhibit insulin secretion, streptozocin and hormones such as a glucocorticoid, and long-acting glycogen.

Age alert For neonates who have hypoglycemia, a hypertonic solution of dextrose 10% in water, calculated at 5 to 10 ml/kg of body weight, administered I.V. over 10 minutes and followed by 4 to 8 mg/kg/minute for maintenance should correct a severe hypoglycemic state. To reduce the chance of hypoglycemia in high-risk neonates, feedings of either breast milk or a solution of dextrose 5% to 10% in water should begin as soon after birth as possible.

For severe hypoglycemia (producing confusion or coma), initial treatment is usually I.V. administration of bolus of

25 or 50 g of glucose as a 50% solution. This is followed by a constant infusion of glucose until the patient can eat a meal. A patient who experiences adrenergic reactions without CNS symptoms may receive oral carbohydrates; parenteral therapy isn't required.

Nursing interventions
■ Administer medications as ordered.
■ Avoid delays in meal times, and provide a proper diet.
■ Correct hypoglycemic episodes quickly. Measure the patient's blood glucose level to verify the presence and severity of hypoglycemia before taking steps to correct it.
■ Monitor I.V. infusion of hypertonic glucose, circulatory overload, and cellular dehydration.
■ Measure blood glucose levels as ordered.
■ Assess the effects of drug therapy, and watch for adverse reactions.

Hypovolemic shock

Potentially life-threatening hypovolemic shock stems from reduced intravascular blood volume, which leads to decreased cardiac output and inadequate tissue perfusion. The subsequent tissue anoxia prompts a shift in cellular metabolism from aerobic to anaerobic pathways, thus resulting in an accumulation of lactic acid, which produces metabolic acidosis. Without immediate treatment, hypovolemic shock can cause adult respiratory distress syndrome, acute tubular necrosis and renal failure, disseminated intravascular coagulation, and multisystem organ dysfunction syndrome.

Causes
Hypovolemic shock usually results from acute blood loss — that is, about 20% of total volume. Massive blood loss may result from GI bleeding, internal or external hemorrhage, or any condition that reduces circulating intravascular volume or other body fluids.

Other causes include intestinal obstruction, peritonitis, acute pancreatitis, ascites, and dehydration from excessive perspiration, severe diarrhea or protracted vomiting, diabetes insipidus, diuresis, and inadequate fluid intake.

Signs and symptoms
The patient's history will include conditions that reduce blood volume, such as GI hemorrhage, trauma, and severe diarrhea and vomiting. A patient with cardiac disease may report anginal pain.

Inspection may reveal pale skin, decreased sensorium, and rapid, shallow respirations. Urine output usually falls below 25 ml/hour. Palpation may disclose rapid, thready peripheral pulses and cold, clammy skin. Auscultation of blood pressure usually detects a mean arterial pressure below 60 mm Hg and a narrowing pulse pressure.

Laboratory findings may include low hematocrit; decreased hemoglobin level and red blood cell and platelet counts; elevated serum potassium, sodium, lactate dehydrogenase, creatinine, and blood urea nitrogen levels; increased urine specific gravity (greater than 1.020) and urine osmolality; decreased urine creatinine levels; decreased pH and partial pressure of arterial oxygen; and increased partial pressure of arterial carbon dioxide .

X-rays, gastroscopy, aspiration of gastric contents through a nasogastric tube, and tests for occult blood identify internal bleeding sites. Coagulation studies may detect coagulopathy from disseminated intravascular coagulation.

Treatment

Emergency treatment relies on prompt and adequate blood and fluid replacement to restore intravascular volume and to raise blood pressure and maintain it above 60 mm Hg. Rapid infusion of normal saline or lactated Ringer's solution and, possibly, albumin or other plasma expanders may expand volume adequately until packed cells can be matched.

Treatment also may include application of a pneumatic antishock garment, in severe cases, or an intra-aortic balloon pump and ventricular assist device. Other measures include administration of oxygen, control of bleeding, administration of dopamine or another inotropic drug and, possibly, surgery. (To be effective, dopamine and other inotropic drugs must be used with vigorous fluid resuscitation.)

Nursing interventions

■ Check for a patent airway and adequate circulation. If the patient experiences cardiac or respiratory arrest, start cardiopulmonary resuscitation.
■ Begin an I.V. infusion with normal saline or lactated Ringer's solution.
■ Monitor the patient's central venous pressure, right atrial pressure, pulmonary artery pressure, pulmonary artery wedge pressure (PAWP), and cardiac output at least once hourly or as ordered.
■ Monitor urine output hourly; if output falls below 30 ml/hour in an adult, increase the fluid infusion rate, but watch for signs of fluid overload such as elevated PAWP. Notify the doctor if urine output doesn't increase.
■ Obtain arterial blood gas (ABG) samples as ordered. Administer oxygen by face mask or an established airway to ensure adequate tissue oxygenation. Adjust the oxygen flow rate as ABG measurements indicate.

■ Record blood pressure, pulse and respiratory rates, and peripheral pulse rates every 15 minutes until stable. Monitor cardiac rhythm continuously.
■ Notify the doctor and increase the infusion rate if the patient experiences a progressive drop in blood pressure accompanied by a thready pulse.
■ Obtain a complete blood count, electrolyte levels, typing and crossmatching, and coagulation studies, as ordered.
■ During therapy, assess skin color and temperature, and note any changes.
■ Watch for signs of impending coagulopathy.

Paralytic ileus

Paralytic ileus is a physiologic form of intestinal obstruction that may develop in the small bowel after abdominal surgery. It causes decreased or absent intestinal motility that usually recovers spontaneously after 2 to 3 days.

Causes

This condition can develop as a response to trauma, toxemia, or peritonitis, or as a result of electrolyte deficiencies, especially hypokalemia, and the use of certain drugs, such as ganglionic blockers and anticholinergics. It also can result from vascular causes, such as thrombosis or embolism. Excessive air swallowing may contribute to it, but paralytic ileus brought on by this factor alone seldom lasts more than 24 hours.

Signs and symptoms

Clinical effects of paralytic ileus include severe abdominal distention, extreme distress and, possibly, vomiting. The patient may be severely constipated or may pass flatus and small, liquid stools.

Treatment

Paralytic ileus lasting longer than 48 hours requires nasogastric (NG) intubation for decompression and suctioning.

When paralytic ileus results from surgical manipulation of the bowel, treatment may also include a cholinergic, such as neostigmine or bethanechol.

Nursing interventions

■ Encourage early postoperative movement and ambulation.

■ Assess patient for nausea and vomiting. Inspect the abdomen for signs of distention.

■ Auscultate for bowel sounds, noting any passage of flatus or stool.

■ Monitor patients receiving a cholinergic for possible paradoxical adverse effects, such as intestinal cramps and diarrhea.

■ Prepare for NG intubation and suctioning, if indicated.

■ Provide fastidious mouth and nose care if the patient has vomited or has undergone decompression by intubation.

■ Assess patient for signs of dehydration.

■ Monitor fluid and electrolyte balance closely.

■ Maintain the patient on nothing by mouth as ordered. Provide I.V. fluid replacement therapy.

■ Monitor intake and output. Irrigate the decompression tube with normal saline solution.

■ Keep the patient in Fowler's position as much as possible to promote pulmonary ventilation and ease respiratory distress.

■ Check frequently for return of bowel sounds and peristalsis (passage of flatus and mucus through the rectum).

Pneumothorax

Pneumothorax is characterized by an accumulation of air or gas between the parietal and visceral pleurae. The amount of air or gas trapped in the intrapleural space determines the degree of lung collapse. The most common types of pneumothorax are open, closed, and tension. Many factors contribute to pneumothorax. If left untreated, extensive pneumothorax and tension pneumothorax can lead to fatal pulmonary and circulatory collapse.

Causes

Open pneumothorax can be caused by penetrating chest injury, (such as a gunshot or knife wound), insertion of a central venous catheter, chest surgery, transbronchial or closed pleural biopsy, or thoracentesis. *Closed pneumothorax* can be caused by blunt chest trauma, air leakage (from ruptured, congenital blebs adjacent to the visceral pleural space), rupture of emphysematous bullae, barotrauma from mechanical ventilation, tubercular or cancerous lesions that erode into the pleural space, or interstitial lung disease. *Tension pneumothorax* can be caused by a penetrating chest wound treated with an airtight dressing, lung or airway puncture by a fractured rib, mechanical ventilation, high-level positive end-expiratory pressure causing alveolar blebs to rupture, or chest tube occlusion or malfunction.

Signs and symptoms

The patient history reveals sudden, sharp, pleural pain. The patient may report that chest movement, breathing, and coughing exacerbate the pain. He may also report shortness of breath.

Inspection reveals asymmetrical chest wall movement with overexpansion and rigidity on the affected side.

The patient may appear cyanotic. If he has tension pneumothorax, he may have distended neck veins and pallor, and he may exhibit anxiety.

Palpation may reveal crackling beneath the skin, indicating subcutaneous emphysema and decreased vocal fremitus. If the patient has tension pneumothorax, palpation may disclose tracheal deviation away from the affected side and a weak and rapid pulse. Percussion may demonstrate hyperresonance on the affected side, and auscultation may disclose decreased or absent breath sounds over the collapsed lung. The patient may also be hypotensive. Spontaneous pneumothorax that releases only a small amount of air into the pleural space may not cause any signs or symptoms.

Treatment

Chest X-rays confirm the diagnosis. Other supportive diagnoses include early decline in pulse oximetry and hypoxemia, and respiratory acidosis, as revealed by arterial blood gas studies. Treatment is conservative (bed rest, oxygen administration, aspiration of air with a large bore needle and, possibly, Heimlich valve insertion) for patients with spontaneous pneumothorax and no signs of increased pleural pressure, lung collapse less than 30%, and no dyspnea or other indications of physiologic compromise.

For patients with lung collapse of more than 30%, treatment to reexpand the lung includes placing a thoracostomy tube in the second or third intercostal space in the midclavicular line. The tube is then connected to underwater seal or low-pressure suction.

Recurring spontaneous pneumothorax requires thoracotomy and pleurectomy. Traumatic and tension pneumothorax require chest tube drainage; traumatic pneumothorax may also re-

quire surgical repair. An analgesic may be prescribed.

Nursing interventions

■ Listen to the patient's fears and concerns. Offer reassurance as appropriate.
■ Keep the patient as comfortable as possible, and administer an analgesic, if necessary.
■ Position the patient to comfort; many patients with pneumothorax feel most comfortable sitting upright.
■ Monitor for complications signaled by pallor, gasping respirations, and chest pain.
■ Carefully monitor vital signs at least once every hour for indications of shock, increasing respiratory distress, or mediastinal shift. Auscultate breath sounds over both lungs.
■ Make sure the suction set-up is functioning appropriately. Monitor patient for signs of tension pneumothorax. If he doesn't have a chest tube to suction, monitor him for recurrence of pneumothorax and recollapse of the lung.

Septic shock

Usually caused by a bacterial infection, septic shock causes inadequate blood perfusion and circulatory collapse. Unless treated promptly (preferably before symptoms fully develop), it progresses to multisystem organ dysfunction syndrome or death within a few hours in up to 80% of cases. Septic shock usually occurs in hospitalized patients, especially men older than age 40 and women ages 25 to 45.

Causes

Many gram-positive and gram-negative bacteria, as well as actinomyces, can cause septic shock. Preexisting infections caused by viruses, rickettsiae, chlamydiae, and protozoa may be complicated by septic shock. Other predisposing factors include immunodeficiency, advanced age, trauma, burns, diabetes mellitus, cirrhosis, and disseminated intravascular coagulation.

Signs and symptoms

Clinical effects of septic shock vary according to the stage of the shock, the organism causing it, and the age of the patient. Early signs and symptoms include oliguria, sudden fever (over 101° F [38.3° C]), chills, nausea, vomiting, diarrhea, and prostration. Late signs and symptoms include restlessness, apprehension, irritability, thirst due to reduced cerebral tissue perfusion, hypothermia, anuria, tachycardia, and tachypnea.

Age alert Hypotension, altered level of consciousness, and hyperventilation may be the only signs of septic shock in infants and elderly patients.

Treatment

The first goal of treatment is to monitor and reverse shock through volume expansion. I.V. fluids are administered, and a pulmonary artery catheter is inserted. Whole blood or plasma may be administered to raise the pulmonary artery wedge pressure (PAWP) to a satisfactory level. An I.V. antibiotic is given, and a urinary catheter is inserted to monitor hourly output. Mechanical ventilation may be necessary.

If shock persists after fluid infusion, a vasopressor is given to help the patient maintain adequate blood perfusion. Other treatments include I.V. bicarbonate to correct acidosis.

Nursing interventions

■ Remove any I.V., intra-arterial, or urinary drainage catheters, and send them to the laboratory to culture for causative organisms.
■ Start an I.V. infusion of normal saline solution or lactated Ringer's solution.
■ Administer an antibiotic I.V. to achieve effective blood levels rapidly. Monitor serum drug levels.
■ Measure hourly urine output. Watch for signs of fluid overload such as an increase in PAWP.
■ If urine output is less than 30 ml/hour, increase the fluid infusion rate. Notify the doctor if urine output doesn't improve. A diuretic may be ordered to increase renal blood flow and urine output.
■ Monitor arterial blood gas (ABG) studies. Administer oxygen by face mask or airway. Adjust oxygen flow rate according to ABG measurements.
■ If the patient's blood pressure drops below 80 mm Hg, increase the oxygen flow rate and notify the doctor immediately.
■ Record the patient's blood pressure, pulse and respiratory rates, and peripheral pulses every 5 minutes until his condition is stabilized. Record hemodynamic pressure readings every 15 minutes. Monitor cardiac rhythm continuously.
■ Provide emotional support to the patient and his family.
■ Document the occurrence of a nosocomial infection, and report it to the infection-control nurse.

Spinal cord compression

Compression of the spinal cord results in multiple disturbances that affect the individual's ability to perform activities of daily living. The onset and severity of symptoms vary with the etiology of the compression; onset may be acute (traumatic injury) or insidious (tumor growth). Outcome depends on the nature of the compression and how promptly the diagnosis is made.

Causes

Traumatic injuries are the most common cause of spinal cord compression. Hyperflexion injuries usually result from sudden deceleration, most commonly affecting the cervical region. Hyperextension injuries tend to cause more damage because the spine swings through a larger arc, making cord compression more likely. Rotational injuries result from extreme lateral flexion. Compression injuries result from extreme vertical pressure, usually caused by a long fall.

Spinal cord tumors are less common than other types of tumors. They usually are benign, located in the thoracic region, and extradural.

Signs and symptoms

Clinical effects of spinal cord compression are related to the level of the injury. Generally, sudden and complete compression causes loss of movement, spinal reflexes, and pain sensation below the level of the lesion. Bowel and bladder dysfunction also may occur, along with an inability to perspire below the level of the lesion. Incomplete, acute traumatic compression may result in any combination of these symptoms. (For more information see, *Functional loss from spinal cord injury.*)

With spinal cord tumors, the location of symptoms is also related to the level of the lesion. Pain is the most common initial symptom, along with coldness and numbness. Motor weakness usually occurs along with sensory loss. Loss of sphincter control may occur; bladder control usually is affected before bowel control.

Treatment

For traumatic injury, treatment begins with immediate stabilization followed by the basic goals of decompression, realignment, and further stabilization. Specific treatment depends on the type of injury and may be surgical, nonsurgical, or a combination. If surgery is indicated, it's usually to decrease compression and stabilize the spine.

Treatment of spinal tumors — which may include radiation, chemotherapy, and surgery — depends on the tumor type and location, and rapidity of onset of the symptoms.

Nursing interventions

■ With traumatic injuries, perform physical assessments with each vital sign assessment and each time the patient is moved.
■ Pay special attention to respiration status, especially with a cervical lesion; frequently measure vital capacity and tidal volume.
■ Maintain a patent airway and suction as needed; frequently perform chest physiotherapy.
■ Instruct the patient to cough and deep-breathe every 2 hours.
■ Provide range-of-motion exercises and encourage patient participation as much as function allows.
■ Reposition the patient every 2 hours, and provide meticulous skin care.
■ Administer an analgesic and muscle relaxant as ordered.
■ Monitor intake and output to assess fluid balance. Ensure adequate oral intake.
■ Provide emotional support and encouragement to the patient and his family. Help enhance the patient's capabilities.
■ Assist with arrangements and follow-up for rehabilitation.

Functional loss from spinal cord injury

Functional losses from spinal cord injury include variable losses of motor function, deep tendon reflexes, sensory function, respiratory function, and bowel and bladder function, depending on which vertebral level is affected.

Level C1 to C4
■ Complete loss of motor function below neck
■ No reflux loss
■ Loss of sensory function in neck and below
■ Loss of involuntary and voluntary respiratory function
■ Loss of bowel and bladder control

Level C5
■ Loss of all motor function below upper shoulders
■ Loss of deep tendon reflexes in biceps
■ Loss of sensation below clavicle and in most of chest, abdomen, and upper and lower extremities
■ Phrenic nerve is intact but not intercostal and abdominal muscles
■ Loss of bowel and bladder control

Level C6
■ Loss of all function below shoulders; no elbow, forearm, or hand control
■ Loss of deep tendon reflexes in biceps
■ Loss of sensation below clavicle and in most of chest, abdomen, and upper and lower extremities
■ Phrenic nerve is intact but not intercostal and abdominal muscles
■ Loss of bowel and bladder control

Level C7
■ Loss of motor control to portions of arms and hands
■ Loss of deep tendon reflexes in triceps
■ Loss of sensation below clavicle and in portions of arms and hands

■ Phrenic nerve is intact but not intercostal and abdominal muscles
■ Loss of bowel and bladder function

Level C8
■ Loss of motor control to portions of arms and hands
■ Loss of deep tendon reflexes in triceps
■ Loss of sensation below chest and in portions of hands
■ Phrenic nerve is intact but not intercostal and abdominal muscles
■ Loss of bowel and bladder function

Level T1 to T6
■ Loss of all motor function below midchest region, including trunk muscles
■ No reflex loss
■ Loss of sensation below midchest area
■ Phrenic nerve functions independently
■ Some impairment of intercostal and abdominal muscles
■ Loss of bowel and bladder function

Level T6 to T12
■ Loss of motor control below waist
■ No reflux loss
■ Loss of all sensation below waist
■ No interference with respiratory function
■ Impairment of abdominal muscles leading to diminished cough
■ Loss of bowel and bladder control

Lever L1 to L3
■ Loss of most of leg and pelvis control
■ Loss of knee-jerk reflex
■ Loss of sensation to portions of lower legs, feet, and ankles
■ No interference with respiratory function
■ Loss of bowel and bladder control

Level L3 to L4
■ Loss of control of portions of lower legs, ankles, and feet

(continued)

Functional loss from spinal cord injury *(continued)*

- Loss of knee-jerk reflex
- Loss of sensation to portions of lower legs, feet, and ankles
- No interference with respiratory function
- Loss of bowel and bladder control

Level L4 to L5
- Varying extent of motor control loss
- Loss of ankle jerk reflex (S1, S2)

- Loss of sensation in upper legs and portions of lower legs (lumbar sensory nerves) and in lower legs, feet, and perineum (sacral sensory nerves)
- No interference with respiratory function
- Possible impairment of bowel and bladder control

Syndrome of inappropriate antidiuretic hormone secretion

Syndrome of inappropriate antidiuretic hormone (SIADH) secretion is marked by excessive release of antidiuretic hormone (ADH), which disturbs fluid and electrolyte balance. Such disturbances result from an inability to excrete dilute urine, retention of free water, expansion of extracellular fluid volume, and hyponatremia. The syndrome occurs secondary to diseases that affect the osmoreceptors of the hypothalamus.

Causes
Most commonly, SIADH results from oat-cell carcinoma of the lung, which secretes excessive ADH or vasopressor-like substances. Other neoplastic diseases (such as pancreatic and prostatic cancer, Hodgkin's disease, and thymoma) may also trigger SIADH.

Additional causes include central nervous system disorders, pulmonary disorders, positive-pressure ventilation, drugs, and such miscellaneous conditions as myxedema or psychosis.

Signs and symptoms
SIADH may produce weight gain despite appetite loss, nausea and vomiting, muscle weakness, restlessness

and, possibly, seizures and coma. Edema is rare unless water overload exceeds 4 L, because much of the free water excess exists within cellular boundaries.

A complete medical history revealing positive-water balance may suggest SIADH. Serum osmolality less than 280 mOsm/kg of water and serum sodium level less then 123 mEq/L confirm it. Supportive laboratory values include high urine sodium secretion (more than 20mEq/L) without a diuretic. Other diagnostic studies show normal renal function and no evidence of dehydration.

Treatment
Treatment begins with restricted fluid intake (17 to 34 oz [503 to 1,005.5 ml]/day). With severe water intoxication, administration of 200 to 300 ml of 3% to 5% sodium chloride solution may be needed to raise the serum sodium level. If fluid restriction is ineffective, demeclocycline or lithium may be given to help block renal response to ADH. When possible, treatment should include correcting the root cause of SIADH. If it's related to cancer, surgery, irradiation, or chemotherapy may relieve the water retention.

Nursing interventions

■ Restrict fluids, and provide comfort measures for thirst, including ice chips, mouth care, lozenges, and staggered water intake.

■ Reduce unnecessary environmental stimuli, and orient the patient as needed.

■ Provide a safe environment for the patient with an altered level of consciousness (LOC). Take seizure precautions as needed.

■ Monitor the patient's serum osmolality and serum and urine sodium levels.

■ Closely monitor and record intake and output, vital signs, and daily weight.

■ Perform neurologic checks at least every 2 to 4 hours, depending on the patient's status. Look for and report early changes in LOC.

■ Observe for signs and symptoms of heart failure, which may occur as a result of fluid overload.

Thyroid storm

Also known as thyrotoxic crisis, thyroid storm is an acute manifestation of hyperthyroidism. It usually occurs in patients with preexisting (though typically unrecognized) thyrotoxicosis. If thyroid storm isn't promptly treated, the patient may experience hypotension, vascular collapse, coma, and death.

Causes

Onset is almost always abrupt, evoked by a stressful event, such as trauma, surgery, or infection. Less common causes include insulin-induced hypoglycemia or diabetic ketoacidosis, cerebrovascular accident, myocardial infarction, pulmonary embolism, sudden cessation of antithyroid medication, initiation of ^{131}I therapy, preeclampsia,

and subtotal thyroidectomy with excess intake of synthetic thyroid hormone.

Signs and symptoms

Initially, the patient may have marked tachycardia, vomiting, and stupor. Other findings include irritability and restlessness, visual disturbances such as diplopia, tremors and weakness, angina, shortness of breath, cough, and swollen extremities. Palpation may reveal warm, moist flushed skin and a high fever that begins insidiously and rapidly rises to a lethal level.

Treatment

Treatment of thyroid storm includes administration of an antithyroid drug I.V., propranolol to block sympathetic effects, a corticosteroid to inhibit conversion of thyroid hormone thyroxine (T_4) to triiodothyronine (T_3) and to replace depleted cortisol levels, and iodide to block release of thyroid hormone. Supportive measures include administration of nutrients, vitamins, fluids, and a sedative.

Nursing interventions

■ Monitor vital signs, electrocardiogram, and cardiopulmonary status continuously. Assess patient for changes in level of consciousness.

■ Expect to administer an antithyroid medication or a beta blocker to inhibit sympathetic effects. Monitor the patient's response to medications.

■ Administer a corticosteroid to inhibit conversion of T_4 and to replace depleted cortisol, as ordered. Anticipate administering iodide to block release of thyroid hormones.

■ Closely monitor the patient's temperature. Apply cooling measures, if indicated, and administer acetaminophen, as ordered. Never administer aspirin because it may further increase the patient's metabolic rate.

■ Institute safety measures, including seizure precautions, to protect the patient from injury.

■ Provide supportive care and administer vitamins, nutrients, fluids, and a sedative, as ordered.

Tracheal erosion

Tracheal erosion refers to damage to the tracheal lumen through mechanical or chemical irritation. Tissue destruction usually progresses from interior to exterior tracheal structures, but it also may be caused or abetted by external pressure, especially to the posterior tracheal wall.

Causes
Chemical injury to tracheal tissues occurs as epithelial cells and submucosal structures are destroyed by inhalation of toxic substances (such as smoke and corrosive gases) and by direct burn injury. Edema and inflammation also occur. Mechanical injury results from lodgment of a foreign body in the airway, which may be accompanied by inflammation.

In the clinical setting, tracheal erosion usually results from traumatic intubation with cuffed or uncuffed endotracheal or tracheal tube. High-pressure, low-volume cuffed tubes are most likely to cause damage.

Concomitant use of a nasogastric (NG) tube places additional friction on the tracheal muscle internally and externally, increasing the risk of tracheoesophageal fistula.

Signs and symptoms
Hemoptysis is the most common sign. Bleeding may be scant if only surface vessels are injured, or it may be severe and potentially result in death if erosion penetrates the adjacent neck vessels. In patients receiving mechanical ventilation, a persistent air leak may indicate tracheal dilation and possible erosion. Tracheal erosion should be suspected when the patient aspirates food or fluid, especially during prolonged tracheal and NG intubation.

Treatment
Treatment is primarily limited to allowing the affected area to heal spontaneously. For injury due to traumatic intubation, tube removal is most desirable. Otherwise, pressure on the erosion site can be reduced by cuff deflation, recannulation with a smaller airway, or replacement of a standard tracheostomy tube with a dual cuffed or longer tube. Removal of a nasogastric tube limits friction on the trachea. A gastric tube may be inserted to promote decompression or provide nutrition. An antibiotic may be given to treat infection and promote healing.

Nursing interventions
■ Make sure that the endotracheal or tracheal tube is the correct size to avoid placing unnecessary pressure on the tracheal wall.

■ Stabilize airway tubes to prevent irritation caused by movement.

■ Maintain lateral wall pressures for nonatmospheric tubes at less than 18 mm Hg.

■ Suction only as necessary, using a vacuum with less than 120 mm Hg of pressure. Never force a suction catheter against resistance.

■ Use small-bore NG or gastric tubes to prevent erosion.

■ If fistula is suspected, discontinue NG intubation and notify the doctor.

14 Alternative and complementary therapies
Enhancing and healing techniques

Aromatherapy

Aromatherapy refers to the inhalation or application of essential oils distilled from various plants. Those who use aromatherapy say it's effective in reducing stress, preventing disease, and even treating certain illnesses — both physical and psychological.

Aromatherapy is popular in Europe, where essential oils are inhaled, massaged into the skin, or placed in bathwater to create pleasant sensations, promote relaxation, or treat specific ailments. Aromatherapy can be used — either alone or with such therapies as massage or herbal therapy — to treat bacterial and viral infections, anxiety, pain, muscle disorders, arthritis, herpes simplex, herpes zoster, skin disorders, premenstrual syndrome, headaches, and indigestion. When absorbed by body tissues, these oils are thought to interact with hormones and enzymes to produce changes in blood pressure, pulse rate, and other physiologic functions. (See *Therapeutic effects of essential oils.*)

Aromatherapy may be administered by a trained aromatherapist or self-administered. In the United States, where interest has skyrocketed, several organizations train and certify people to self-administer and administer aromatherapy. These organizations can also provide information to interested laypeople and health care providers, referrals to aromatherapists, and sources for obtaining essential oils.

Although there's no scientific evidence indicating that aromatherapy prevents or cures disease, nurses trained in aromatherapy may recommend specific oils as adjuncts to conventional therapies, teach patients how to use them, and administer treatment themselves.

Implementation

■ In addition to the appropriate essential oil, aromatherapy may require other supplies, depending on how the oil is being administered (for example, massage, inhalation, bath, or diffusion).

■ Massage requires a carrier oil and, for a full body massage, a massage table. Massage involves diluting the essential oil in the appropriate carrier oil and applying it to the exposed body part or the entire body using massage techniques.

■ Inhalation requires a bowl of hot water and a large towel. The patient leans over a bowl of steaming water that contains a few drops of the essential oil. With the towel draped over his head and the bowl to concentrate the steam, the patient inhales the vapors for few minutes.

■ A bath requires a tub filled with warm water. The patient adds a few drops of essential oil to the surface of the bath water and then soaks in the tub for 10 to 20 minutes, inhaling the vapors as he soaks.

■ Diffusion requires a micromist or candle diffuser or a ceramic ring that can be placed on a light bulb. This method involves placing a few drops of the essential oil in the diffuser and turning on the heat source to diffuse microparticles of the oil into the air. The average treatment is 30 minutes.

Special considerations

■ Citrus oils shouldn't be applied before exposure to the sun. Advise patients to avoid applying cinnamon or clove oil on the skin. Be aware that certain oils — such as basil, fennel, lemon grass, rosemary, and verbena — may cause irritation if the patient has sensitive skin. If such irritation develops, advise him to stop using these oils. Also, high doses of certain oils —

Therapeutic effects of essential oils

This chart lists some popular essential oils and the traditional indications for which practitioners use them.

Essential oil	Traditional therapeutic uses
Chamomile (*Anthemis nobilis*)	■ Anti-inflammatory, antifungal, and antibacterial effects ■ Relieving mental or physical stress ■ Balancing body and mind
Eucalyptus (*Eucalyptus radiata*)	■ Antiviral and expectorant effects ■ Relieving nausea and motion sickness ■ Clearing the sinuses ■ Soothing irritable bowel ■ Stimulant effect
Geranium (*Pelargonium x asperum*)	■ Antiviral and antifungal effects ■ Stimulating metabolism in the skin ■ Improving cell regeneration ■ Improving circulation ■ Relieving pain ■ Improving vital organ function
Lavender (*Lavandula augustifolia*)	■ Anti-inflammatory and antibacterial effects ■ Treating burns, insect bites, and minor injuries ■ Soothing stomachache and colic ■ Relieving toothache and teething pain ■ Relieving mental or physical stress
Peppermint (*Mentha piperita*)	■ Antibacterial and antiviral effects ■ Decongestant and expectorant effects ■ Relieving nausea and motion sickness ■ Soothing irritable bowel ■ Stimulant effect
Rosemary (*Rosmarinus officinalis*)	■ Antibacterial, antifungal, and antiviral effects ■ Restoring energy and alleviating stress ■ Improving cell regeneration
Tea tree (*Melanleuca alternifolia*)	■ Anti-inflammatory, antibacterial, and antiviral effects ■ Treating burns, insect bites, and minor injuries ■ Providing calmness and sedation

such as wintergreen, sage, aniseed, thyme, lemon, fennel, clove, cinnamon, camphor, and cedar wood — can result in nonlethal poisoning.

■ Different administration methods require specific safety precautions. When using inhalation therapy, the patient should keep his face far enough from the water's surface to avoid a burn injury. When using the diffusion method, he should be at least 3′ (0.9 m) away from the diffuser.

■ Aromatherapy is contraindicated during pregnancy because it poses a toxic risk to the mother and fetus. It should be used with caution in infants and children younger than age 5 because many essential oils are toxic to patients in this age-group.

■ Caution patients to keep essential oils away from the eyes and mucous membranes to avoid irritation. If contact occurs, the patient should flush with plenty of water; if flushing doesn't relieve the pain, he should seek medical attention

Art therapy

Art therapy is the creative use of various expressive media to help a patient deal with thoughts, emotions, life changes, personal issues, and conflicts buried deep within his subconscious. The concept behind art therapy is that if the patient can externalize his feelings for examination and reflection, he can discover meaning and insight, which supports growth, change, healing, and integration of the whole person.

Creative activities include drawing, painting, sculpting, collaging, and puppetry. Mask making is another powerful and popular form of expression commonly used within groups and in individual healing rituals. Photography, videography, and computer-generated art are newer forms of art therapy.

Art therapy is useful in patients with posttraumatic stress disorder, substance abuse, addictions, catastrophic illness (for example, cancer or acquired immunodeficiency syndrome), chronic pain or disease, prolonged hospitalization or treatment, or extensive surgery. This therapy may also help patients who have lost their voice (through surgery, tracheostomy, or intubation), who are aging and experiencing a decrease in function, or who have chronic fatigue or immune dysfunction syndrome.

Implementation

■ Make sure the patient is physically capable of carrying out the artistic activity. Medications, a weakened condition, inflamed or painful joints in hands or fingers, or neurologic damage can impair the patient's ability.

■ Someone who is physically unable to manipulate media may still participate in collaging — for example, by choosing pictures, words, or materials for someone else to cut and paste or by indicating the position of cutouts and colors. Also, computer programs may be available to create art with adapted controls.

■ Explain the creative procedure to the patient, and make sure he's willing to participate.

■ Assess the patient's need for special equipment or other accommodations.

■ Collect and prepare all necessary materials.

■ Provide a quiet and comfortable environment and arrange a clean, flat surface on which the patient can work.

■ Reassure the patient that he needn't have any previous knowledge or training in art. For example, if drawing is the activity of choice, stick figures can get his message across effectively.

■ Allow the patient time to complete the project to his satisfaction. Sometimes it's important for the patient to attend to every small detail and search for just the right color.

■ When the project is complete, allow the patient to show it to you and tell you about it.

■ Be supportive of the patient's efforts, and summarize the experience for him.

■ If a patient is especially proud of his artwork, arrange to have it displayed so that others may admire it, thereby adding a source of acknowledgment for the patient.

Special considerations

■ Some patients may not be open to participating in art therapy, either because they're shy and self-conscious or because they just aren't interested. Don't insist: Instead, work on building a trusting therapeutic relationship. The patient may be willing to participate in the future.

■ Praise any and all efforts, and be careful not to make suggestions about colors or forms. Remain nonjudgmental and supportive.

■ If the patient has certain signs and symptoms of a disease, encourage him to draw a picture representing himself in relation to the disease. You may suggest that the patient draw himself before the disease, with the disease, and after treatment.

■ Listen attentively. There may be a healing story involved, or perhaps the patient will come up with new insights. You may want to point out certain details.

■ Repeat back to the patient what he has said to validate the meaning.

■ Notice how the patient represents his size in relation to other figures or objects. Is the entire body drawn? What are the dominant colors and shapes? Is there a smile or frown drawn on the face? What's the overall mood?

■ Strong emotions may surface as a patient explores and connects with underlying emotions. If the patient shows signs of agitation or uncontrolled emotion, end the session and reassure him that it's normal to have strong feelings and it's appropriate to express them. Refer the patient to other health care professionals as appropriate.

Biofeedback

A relatively new therapy, biofeedback refers to any modality that measures and immediately reports information about the patient's own physiologic processes. With biofeedback information, the patient can learn to consciously influence the measured body function, such as heart rate or blood pressure. The goal of biofeedback is to help him improve his overall health by consciously regulating bodily functions that are usually controlled unconsciously.

In this procedure, electrodes are attached to pertinent areas of the body to monitor such things as skeletal muscle activity, heart or brain wave activity, body temperature, or blood pressure. The electrodes feed information into a small monitoring box that reports the results by a sound or light that varies in pitch or brightness as the body function increases or decreases (the "feedback"). A biofeedback therapist leads the patient in mental exercises to help him regulate functions, such as body temperature, blood pressure, bladder control, or muscle tension, to reach the desired result. The patient eventually learns to control the body's inner mechanisms through mental processes.

The most common forms of biofeedback involve measuring muscle tension, skin temperature, electrical conductance or resistance within the skin, brain waves, and respiration. As advances in technology have made measurement devices more sophisticated, the applications of biofeedback have expanded. Sensors can now measure the activity of the internal and external rectal sphincters, the activity of the bladder's detrusor muscle, esophageal motility, and stomach acidity.

Some biofeedback treatments are accepted in traditional medicine. The American Medical Association, for instance, has endorsed electromyogram biofeedback training for the treatment of muscle contraction headaches.

Biofeedback has a vast range of preventive and restorative applications. It's most successful in cases where psychological factors play a role in the patient's health disturbance, such as sleep disorders and stress-related disorders. Patients with disorders arising from poor muscle control, such as incontinence, postural problems, back pain, and temporomandibular joint syndrome, also benefit. Biofeedback training has also been shown to benefit patients who have lost control of function due to brain or nerve damage or chronic pain disorders.

Improvement has also been seen in patients with heart dysfunctions, GI disorders, swallowing difficulties, esophageal dysfunction, tinnitus, eyelid twitching, fatigue, and cerebral palsy. Biofeedback isn't recommended for severe structural problems, such as broken bones or slipped discs.

Implementation

■ Provide the patient with a private environment that is free from noise or other distractions.
■ Gather the necessary equipment, and wash your hands.
■ Explain the procedure to the patient, and answer any questions he may have. If relaxation techniques or imagery will be used at the same time, review them with the patient.
■ Depending on the body function that will be monitored, clean and prepare the skin and attach the electrodes according to the manufacturer's instructions.
■ Set the monitor where both you and the patient can easily see the results.
■ Set a goal for the session with the patient, and review the information he'll be seeing on the monitor.

■ Turn on the monitor, and establish a baseline for the targeted body function.
■ If goggles will be used, help the patient place them comfortably over his eyes.
■ When the patient is ready, begin the session by starting the relaxation tapes or imagery sequence.
■ At the close of the session, disconnect the monitor and remove the electrodes.
■ Clean the patient's skin as needed.

Special considerations

■ You'll probably work with a trained biofeedback practitioner when conducting the session.
■ Reassure the patient that biofeedback isn't a test he has to pass, but a learning experience.
■ The patient may experience local skin irritation from the electrodes used in the biofeedback monitoring. Wash the skin well with soap and water to remove any leftover irritants, and pat it dry.

Dance therapy

Also known as dance movement therapy, dance therapy capitalizes on the direct relationship between body movement and the mind. Specific aspects of dance therapy, such as music, rhythm, and synchronous movement, alter mood states, reawaken old memories and feelings, and reduce isolation. Additionally, dance therapy organizes thoughts and actions and helps the patient establish relationships. Used in a group setting, dance therapy is believed to create the emotional intensity necessary for behavioral change.

Dance therapy is used for various purposes. It's used to help emotionally disturbed patients express their feelings, gain insight, and develop relationships. With physically disabled people, dance therapy increases movement and self-esteem while providing an enjoyable, creative outlet. In other groups of older people, dance therapy is used to maintain physical function, enhance self-worth, develop relationships, and help them express fear and grief.

A wide variety of disorders and disabilities can be treated using dance therapy. Typically, the target patient has social, emotional, cognitive, or physical problems. Dance therapy is even being used to prevent disease and promote health among healthy patients. Additionally, caregivers and patients with cancer, acquired immunodeficiency syndrome, and Alzheimer's disease use it to reduce stress. Dance therapy promotes flexibility, strengthens muscles, improves cardiovascular function, and improves pulmonary function. Also, it provides touch, socialization, and a sense of connectedness.

Group dance, probably the most common form of dance therapy, allows people of different physical abilities to participate. By simply tapping their toes or patting their thighs in time to the music, patients can feel a part of the session. Dance routines range from simple clapping and swaying to intricate aerobic sessions.

The music should be appropriate to the group, in both its pace and its aesthetic appeal. Fast-moving rock music is probably less enjoyable for a group of agile senior citizens than a fast polka would be. Use faster music to stimulate group members and slower music to calm them.

Implementation

■ Arrange the space so that participants can move freely.
■ Arrange chairs around the periphery for those who can't stand or who may become tired during the session.

■ Assess the group for risk factors. The presence of one or more risk factors doesn't preclude group members from participating but may influence the type of dance and the length of the session. Risk factors to consider include poor cardiovascular status, a history of chronic obstructive pulmonary disease, and degenerative musculoskeletal problems.
■ Explain the purpose of the session, and encourage everyone to participate to the degree they feel able.
■ When the group is ready, start the music and position yourself so you're facing the group.
■ If a structured routine is being used, demonstrate the movements you're seeking and encourage the group to mimic your movements.
■ If free expression is the goal, circulate through the group, providing encouragement and motivation to those who are hesitant.
■ Praise the participants' efforts, and encourage them to discuss the feelings they experienced while dancing.
■ After the session, document the type of activity and the group's response.

Special considerations

■ Because dancing is an aerobic activity, watch for signs of cardiovascular compromise, such as dizziness, flushing, profuse sweating, and disorientation.
■ Rapid motion may result in dizziness.
■ Help a patient who becomes dizzy to a seat as needed, and check his vital signs.

Imagery

Imagery is a mind-body technique in which patients use the imagination to promote relaxation, relieve symptoms (or better cope with them), and heal disease. It's successfully used to control pain and to enhance immune function as well as an adjunctive therapy for several diseases. Imagery is widely used in cancer patients to help mobilize the immune system, to alleviate the nausea and vomiting associated with chemotherapy, to relieve pain and stress, and to promote weight gain. It's also used in many cardiac rehabilitation programs and centers specializing in chronic pain. Imagery can also be effective in helping patients tolerate medical procedures.

According to imagery advocates, people with strong imaginations, those who can literally "worry themselves sick," are excellent candidates for using imagery to positively affect their health.

Two of the more popular imagery techniques are palming and guided imagery. In palming, the patient places his palms over his closed eyes and tries to fill his entire field of vision with only the color black. He then tries to picture the black changing to a color he associates with stress, such as red, and then mentally replaces that color with one he finds soothing, such as pale blue. In guided imagery, the patient is asked to visualize a goal he wants to achieve and then picture himself taking action to achieve it. This type of therapy is intended to complement traditional cancer treatments rather than replace them.

As an active means of relaxation, imagery is a central part of almost all stress-reduction techniques. Additionally, it's a useful self-care tool. With proper instruction, patients can use imagery to relieve stress, enhance immune function to fight a cold virus, and improve their sense of well-being.

Implementation

■ Provide the patient with a private, quiet environment that is free from distractions, and a comfortable place in which to lie down.
■ If using a taped imagery sequence, make sure the tape player is working and that the room has an electrical outlet.
■ Help the patient into a comfortable position and explain the exercise. Answer any questions the patient may have.
■ When the patient is comfortable, instruct him to close his eyes, and lower the lights if possible.
■ Use a steady, soothing, low voice throughout the exercise.
■ Instruct the patient to take a few deep breaths and to imagine that with each breath he's taking in calmness and peacefulness and releasing tension, discomfort, and worry. Tell him to let his breath find its own rate and rhythm, and to continue to breathe in calmness and peacefulness and breathe out tension and worry.
■ Help the patient relax his body. Instruct him to imagine that he's breathing calmness into his feet and legs and releasing tension with each exhalation. Continue this sequence moving from feet to head, having him breathe calmness into each successive body part.
■ As you complete this portion of the exercise, remind the patient to let his whole body sink into a peaceful, relaxed state.
■ Tell the patient to imagine himself in a place that is peaceful and beautiful, perhaps somewhere he has visited or a special place where he would like to be. Encourage him to notice the details in this place, such as colors, shapes, and living things found there. Have him think about the sounds and smells of the place and pay attention to

any feelings of peacefulness and relaxation.

■ While remaining quiet, allow the patient to spend as long as he wants in this place; tell him that when he's ready, he should allow the images to fade and slowly bring himself back to the outer world.

■ If the patient is willing, discuss the experience with him, concentrating on the positive feelings of relaxation and peace.

■ Document the length of the session, the imagery path used, and the patient's response.

Special considerations

■ To enhance the effects of imagery, consider adding a smell to trigger the image that the patient is trying to experience.

■ Occasionally, an imagery session may lead a person to remember an unpleasant period or event in his life. If this occurs, stop the session and encourage the patient to tell you what he was seeing and feeling. If the patient becomes upset, stay with him. When possible, notify the doctor.

■ Imagery is contraindicated in psychotic patients.

■ Be aware that patients with breathing problems may have difficulty controlling their breathing.

Magnetic field therapy

Magnetic field therapy (also called biomagnetic therapy, magnet therapy, or magnetotherapy) involves the use of magnetic fields to prevent and treat disease and to treat injuries. Its goal is to restore a person's internal bioelectromagnetic balance. With successful therapy, the patient should learn to maintain this internal balance without the need for continued external intervention.

One theory of magnetic therapy suggests that diseased cells have lost their magnetic equilibrium and that topically applied magnets work on a molecular level to restore this equilibrium within the cells. This, in turn, benefits surrounding cells and the entire organism. Another theory, based on the magnetic nature of red blood cells, supposes a magnetically induced increase in blood and oxygen supply to diseased tissues. This improved circulation helps adjust pH, increase nutrient availability, and relieve congestion and pain.

Practitioners of magnetic field therapy range from the self-healing layperson to licensed health care professionals, including massage therapists, nurses, physician assistants, acupuncturists, chiropractors, physical therapists, medical doctors, and dentists. The nurse's role is to be knowledgeable about magnetic field therapy as a possible health-enhancing therapy.

Practitioners claim that therapeutic magnets benefit a wide range of conditions from acute and chronic pain, strains, and swelling to systemic illness. Magnetic field therapy has been recognized in sports medicine for its effectiveness in relieving sprains and strains. It has also been used in conjunction with other therapies, such as nutrition, herbs, and acupuncture. Practitioners agree that biomagnetic therapy effectively relieves pain, swelling, and discomfort, but they disagree over whether therapeutic effects are best obtained using the bionorth (−) pole, the biosouth (+) pole, or both together. They also disagree about which gauss strengths are most appropriate.

Implementation

■ Magnets used for magnetic field therapy should be high-quality medical magnets. True bionorth and biosouth poles can be determined by using a simple compass. The bionorth pole is attracted to the biosouth, or positive, pole; the biosouth pole, to the bionorth, or negative, pole. Gauss meters are also available for measuring the external field strength of the magnet.

■ Handbooks of magnetic field therapy describe the best placement and magnet strength for self-treatment of various illnesses.

■ The simplest home remedy for pain involves applying a low- to medium-gauss (800-gauss or less) magnet to the area of discomfort and leaving it in place until well after the discomfort disappears. The longer the treatment, the quicker the healing and the greater the symptom relief. If the pain decreases with treatment, the magnet is correctly oriented; if the pain increases, even if the magnet's bionorth side is facing the patient, the magnet needs to be turned over.

■ Magnetic therapy may be of short duration (1 to 2 hours), or it may be used overnight or for 24 hours or more for maximum effect.

Special considerations

■ Positive (biosouth) magnetic energy should only be used under medical supervision because some investigators believe that the brain can become overstimulated, producing seizures, hallucinations, insomnia, hyperactivity, and magnetic addiction. It has also been claimed that positive magnetic energy may stimulate growth of tumors and microorganisms.

■ Recognize that magnets may alter magnetic instruments, such as pacemakers, battery-powered wristwatches, hearing aids, and other equipment in use around a patient. Keep magnets away from magnetic resonance imaging machines and away from patients who have metallic parts in their body. Post signs above a patient's bed to warn other staff and visitors.

■ Because of the complex range of symptoms that many elderly patients experience, you should encourage these patients to continue to seek conventional treatment and to report any alternative therapies they're using.

■ Because of the experimental nature of magnetic field therapy, it isn't recommended for children younger than age 5 or for pregnant women.

■ Patients with a pacemaker or defibrillator shouldn't use magnetic beds, and no magnets should be placed closer than 6″ (15 cm) to a pacemaker or defibrillator, to avoid interfering with their function.

■ Because magnet polarity is important in treatment, caution the patient to use a magnetometer or a compass to check the poles on the magnets he plans to use.

■ Inform patients to avoid using magnets on the abdomen for 60 to 90 minutes after meals to allow peristalsis to take place.

■ Monitor a patient who is undergoing magnetic field therapy for potential adverse effects and the subsequent need to decrease or discontinue use.

■ Inform patients that with magnetic field therapy, more and stronger magnets aren't necessarily better.

■ Warn patients to remove all magnets before undergoing surgery because they may cause life-threatening instrument malfunction.

■ If your patient is treating himself with magnets, teach him about safe magnet use: Inform him that magnets may alter magnetic instruments (such as pacemakers and hearing aids), that magnets shouldn't be banged or dropped, that they shouldn't be heated above 500° F (260° C) because doing so can decrease their strength, and that different-sized magnets shouldn't be kept together because doing so can alter their strength.

■ Magnets should be kept away from computer hard drives and any magnetic media — such as diskettes, recording tapes, credit or bank cards, videos, and compact disks — to prevent damage or erasure of contents.

Meditation

The ancient art of meditation — focusing one's attention on a single sound or image or on the rhythm of one's own breathing — has been found to have positive effects on health. By directing attention away from worries about the future or preoccupation with the past, meditation reduces stress, a major contributing factor in many health problems. Stress reduction in turn results in a wide range of physiologic and mental health benefits, from decreased oxygen consumption, heart rate, and respiratory rate to improved mood, spiritual calm, and heightened awareness.

Most meditation approaches fall into one of two techniques: concentrative meditation or mindful meditation. *Concentrative meditation* involves focusing on an image, a sound (called a mantra), or one's own breathing in order to achieve a state of calm and heightened awareness. Transcendental meditation is a form of concentrative meditation in which the individual repeats a mantra over and over again while sitting in a comfortable position. When other thoughts enter his mind, he's instructed to notice them and return to the mantra. Concentrating on the mantra prevents any distracting thoughts.

Mindful meditation takes the opposite approach, Instead of focusing on a single sensation or sound, the individual is aware of all sensations, feelings, images, thoughts, sounds, and smells that pass through his mind without actually thinking about them. The goal is a calmer, clearer, nonreactive state of mind.

Meditation has a wide variety of indications. It's used to enhance immune function in patients with cancer, acquired immunodeficiency syndrome, and autoimmune disorders and has been successful in treating drug and alcohol addiction as well as posttraumatic stress disorder. Anxiety disorders, pain, and stress are also commonly treated with meditation. Meditation can also be used with dietary and lifestyle changes for patients with hypertension or heart disease.

Implementation

■ To assist your patient with meditation, you'll need a private, quiet environment that's free from distractions and offers a comfortable place for your patient to sit or recline.

■ If you'll be helping a patient with meditation, begin by explaining the procedure and answer any questions. Tell the patient that he can stop the exercise if he becomes uncomfortable. Help him into a comfortable position. If he's in a sitting position, ask him to keep his back straight and let his shoulders droop.

■ Using a calm, soothing, low voice, instruct the patient to close his eyes, if doing so feels comfortable. Tell him to focus on his abdomen, feeling it rise each time he inhales and fall each time he exhales. Tell him to concentrate on his breathing. Explain that if his mind wanders off his breathing, he should simply bring it back, regardless of what the thought was.

■ Have the patient practice the exercise for 15 minutes every day for a week; then evaluate its benefits with him.

■ Document the session, the instructions you gave the patient, and his response.

Special considerations

■ Be aware that meditation may elicit negative emotions, disorientation, or memories of early childhood abuses or other traumas. If this occurs, try to find out what the feeling or memory concerns, and direct the patient to a safer, more pleasant thought or memory. If this isn't possible, stop the session, notify the doctor, and stay with the patient until he's calm and controlled.

■ Meditation should be used cautiously in schizophrenic patients and those with attention deficit hyperactivity disorder.

■ Remind the patient that meditation isn't a substitute for medical treatment. If he's taking a prescribed medication, such as an antihypertensive, tell him to keep taking it.

■ Be aware that patients with respiratory problems may have difficulty with meditation techniques that focus on breathing.

Music therapy

Music therapy uses the universal appeal of rhythmic sound to communicate, explore, and heal. It can take the form of creating music, singing, moving to music, or just listening to music.

Music therapy benefits patients with developmental disabilities, mental health disorders, substance addictions, and chronic pain. Studies have demonstrated the positive effects of music in reducing pain and procedural anxiety as well as in dental anesthesia.

Patients who listen to classical music before surgery and then again in the recovery room report minimal postoperative disorientation. Music has also been successfully used to communicate with Alzheimer's patients and head trauma victims when other approaches have failed. In a study on the effects of music on Alzheimer's patients, those who listened to big band music during their days were more alert and happier and had better long-term recollection than the control group. Throughout the illness, music can reorient confused patients. In the final stages of the disease, it provides psychological comfort.

Implementation

■ Arrange a comfortable environment.

■ Choose music that is appropriate to the patients and the session objectives. The music should be meaningful to the participants.

■ For sessions that involve making music, collect instruments appropriate for the group.

■ For sessions that involve singing, choose music that the group members are familiar with. Provide words for the songs, either in writing or by repeating them to the group.

■ Introduce the participants to one another. Explain the purpose of the session, and encourage everyone to participate as he feels able.

■ When the group is ready, start the music and position yourself so that you're facing the group.

■ If the group will be listening to music, watch the reactions of the participants. If they're making the music, circulate among the group members and offer individual support.

■ Encourage the participants to discuss the feelings they experienced while listening to or making the music. Praise their efforts.

■ After the session, document the type of activity and the group's response.

Special considerations

■ Music is especially effective as a means of reminiscence therapy for older people. For many of them, the music they enjoyed in their youth hasn't been part of their lives for decades.

Pet therapy

A pet can help an elderly patient combat loneliness and help bridge the gap between the patient and the health care provider. Commonly used in long-term care facilities, pet therapy helps the older patient break through apathy and depression and improves interaction with others. Some facilities adopt a pet as a mascot for the facility and let the residents share responsibility for caring for it, thus helping to build a sense of community.

Implementation

■ Select a pet that is well behaved and has a good temperament. Pets that have gone through obedience training are ideal.
■ Make sure the pet has been checked by a veterinarian and is up-to-date on his immunizations.
■ Allow the patient to play with and hold the pet. Encourage him to talk to the animal and reminisce about pets he once had. Provide as much time as the patient needs, if possible.

Special considerations

■ Make sure the environment is appropriate for pet therapy. The facility should have an area where the pet can retreat and be kept out of the way of patients who are allergic to animals,

have no interest in pets, or are afraid of them.
■ If the pet is chosen as a mascot for the facility, have a responsible person make a schedule for residents who are interested in caring for the animal.
■ If the pet isn't a permanent resident of the facility, arrange for a volunteer from an animal shelter to accompany the pet to ensure the safety of the animal and the patients.

Prayer and mental healing

Humans have used prayer and mental healing throughout the ages to seek assistance from a higher being for a wide range of problems. The underlying beliefs of those who use prayer for healing are the same for all religions. They include the belief that a higher power exists, that humans can communicate with this higher being through prayer, and that this deity can hear human prayers and intervene in human affairs, including healing the sick.

In prayer, the person communicates directly with the divine being, asking the being to intervene to heal the patient. In mental healing, the power of the divine being is channeled through a healer.

There are two main categories of mental healing. In type 1 healing, the healer enters into a spiritual level of consciousness where he views himself and the patient as a single being. No physical contact with the patient is necessary. Type 2 mental healing requires the healer to touch the patient in an attempt to transfer energy from the healer's hands to the diseased parts of the patient's body. Most people who use prayer for healing view it as an adjunct to conventional medical treatment.

Although the therapeutic uses of prayer and mental healing are limitless, the reliability of these practices still needs to be established. Proponents of prayer argue that even if prayer can't cure disease, it can at least relieve some of its effects, enhance the effectiveness of conventional medical treatments, and provide meaning and comfort to the patient.

Implementation

■ Provide the patient with privacy in a quiet, distraction-free environment.
■ Facilitate the use of prayer and mental healing by asking the patient such questions as "Is religion important to you?" and "Is it important in how you cope with your illness?"
■ If religion is important to the patient, explore his religious practices with him to identify ways to incorporate them into his present situation.
■ Determine whether the patient would like to discuss his faith with the facility chaplain or another clergy member.

Special considerations

■ One of the benefits of prayer and mental healing is the lack of complications. Patients who have attempted prayer and not seen the results they expected may express a sense of disappointment when the topic of spirituality is discussed. If this occurs and if it's possible, arrange for a clergy member to explore the patient's feelings with him.
■ Remain nonjudgmental when implementing the exercise.
■ Some prayer rituals may be more than your health care facility can handle. Rites involving incense, large groups, or loud music and dance can stress even the most tolerant facility. Although you should be sensitive to the patient's religious beliefs, sometimes a compromise is in order. For example, you could suggest that the patient be wheeled to an outside area of the facility if incense is involved or to a conference room off the unit during off-hours if noise is an issue or a prayer vigil involves a large number of people.
■ Be aware that ethical questions arise if prayer and mental healing are used without the patient's knowledge. Additionally, some are concerned that prayer and mental healing may be used to harm an individual instead of healing him.
■ Advise your patient to consider prayer a complementary therapy, not a substitute for conventional medical care. If you have a patient whose religion advocates the use of prayer as the sole form of treatment, make sure he understands the consequences of forgoing conventional medical treatment so he can make an informed decision.

Therapeutic massage

Massage, the process of stroking, rubbing, and kneading the body, has played an important role in traditional medical systems through the centuries. It's used primarily for stress reduction and relaxation, but it can serve as a complementary therapy for a wide range of conditions. These conditions include chronic pain, circulatory problems, digestive disorders, inflammation, intestinal disorders, joint mobility disorders, muscle tension, overstimulated or understimulated nervous system, skin conditions, and swelling.

The primary physiologic effect of therapeutic massage is improved blood circulation. As the muscles are kneaded and stretched, blood return to the heart increases and toxins, such as lactic acid, are carried out of the muscle tissue to be excreted from the body. Improved circulation results in increased perfusion and oxygenation of tissues. Improved oxygenation of the brain helps us think more clearly and feel more alive; improved perfusion and oxygenation of other organ systems leads to improved digestion and elimination as well as quicker wound healing. Massage also appears to trigger the release of endorphins, the body's natural pain relievers.

There are five basic techniques of massage. In *effeurage*, the therapist performs a long, gliding stroke using the whole hand or the thumb. This is a warm-up technique. The gliding stroke, which should always move toward the heart, improves circulation.

Petrissage is a kneading and compressing motion in which the muscles are grabbed and lifted. This motion relieves sore muscles by clearing away lactic acid and increasing circulation to the muscle tissue.

In *friction*, the therapist uses the thumbs and fingertips to work around the joints and the thickest part of the muscles. Circular motions break down adhesions and may also help make soft tissues and joints more flexible. For larger muscles, the palm or heel of the hand may be used.

In *tapotement*, the therapist uses the sides of the hands, fingertips, cupped palms, or slightly closed fists to make chopping, tapping, and beating motions. These motions invigorate and stimulate the muscles, resulting in a burst of energy. However, when the muscles are cramped, strained, or spastic, tapotement can exacerbate the problem if performed for a longer period.

In *vibration*, the therapist presses her fingers or flattened hands firmly into the muscle then "vibrates" (transmits a trembling motion) the area rapidly for a few seconds. This motion is repeated until the entire muscle has been vibrated. This helps stimulate the nervous system and may increase circulation and improve gland function.

Implementation

■ Massage therapy requires a sturdy massage table, lubricating oil, and a quiet room with relaxing music.

■ Have the patient undress in private and cover himself with a sheet or towel.

■ With the patient on the massage table, play soothing music to induce relaxation.

■ To respect the patient's modesty, the body is kept fully draped, exposing only the area being worked on at the moment.

■ A scented oil is usually used to prevent friction between the therapist's hands and the patient's skin while she kneads various muscle groups in a systematic way from head to toe.

Special considerations

■ A trained massage therapist pays close attention to body language as well as the patient's comments, to avoid causing pain or discomfort.

■ Be aware that massage is contraindicated for people with diabetes, varicose veins, or other blood vessel problems because it may dislodge a blood clot. Massage should also not be performed on patients with pitting edema.

■ The therapist performing the massage should take these precautions: Avoid massaging the abdomen of a patient with hypertension or gastric or duodenal ulcers, and massage at least 6″ (15 cm) away from bruises, cysts, broken bones, and breaks in skin integrity.

■ Advise your patients who are seeking a massage therapist to get recommendations from people who have been satisfied with their treatment. They should also make sure the therapist is properly trained and licensed and belongs to a professional organization.

Therapeutic Touch

Developed in the 1970s, Therapeutic Touch is a widely used complementary therapy developed by nurses for nurses in an attempt to bring a more humane and holistic approach to their practice. This technique focuses on "healing" rather than "curing" and is built on the belief that all healing is basically self-healing.

Central to Therapeutic Touch is the concept of a universal life force that practitioners believe permeates space and sustains all living organisms. Practitioners believe that in healthy people, this vital energy flows freely in and through the body in a balanced way that nourishes all body organs and that when people get sick it's because their energy field is out of equilibrium. By using their hands to manipulate the energy field above the patient's skin, practitioners say they can restore equilibrium, thereby reactivating the mind-body-spirit connection and empowering the patient to participate in his own healing. Although the existence of a human energy field hasn't been proven scientifically, nurses claim that they can actually feel something best described as energy when performing this technique.

Despite its name, Therapeutic Touch doesn't require actual physical contact during a treatment. In most case, the nurse's hands remain several inches above the patient's body.

Therapeutic Touch is widely used by practitioners of holistic nursing and other health professionals and is practiced in many hospitals, hospices, long-term care facilities, and other settings. Although most practitioners are nurses, other care professionals (massage therapists, physical therapists, dentists, and medical doctors) and nonprofessionals have incorporated this therapy in their practice. According to practitioners, anyone can study this technique and apply it to himself.

Therapeutic Touch is used as a complementary therapy for virtually all medical and nursing diagnoses as well as surgical procedures. Practitioners say it's especially helpful for patients with wounds or infections because it eases discomfort and speeds the healing process. However, the technique is best known for its ability to relieve pain and anxiety. Because of this characteristic, Therapeutic Touch is helpful in treating stress-related disorders, such as tension headaches, hypertension, ulcers, and emotional problems. It is also used in Lamaze classes and delivery rooms to induce relaxation and in neonatal intensive care units to help speed the growth of premature infants.

Implementation

■ Select an environment that will enable the patient to relax and the nurse to concentrate. This may include a comfortable chair, bed, or massage table for the patient and, possibly, soothing music to help create a relaxing atmosphere.

■ The nurse achieves a calm, meditative state that allows her to be sensitive to the patient's signs and symptoms. This heightened sensitivity is also necessary for perceiving subtle changes in the patient's energy field.

■ After becoming centered, the nurse begins her assessment by slowly moving her hands over the patient's body, 2″ to 4″ (5 to 10 cm) away from the skin surface, to detect any alterations in the energy field, such as feelings of cold or heat, vibration, or blockages.

■ Depending on the assessment findings, the nurse then performs interventions aimed at balancing the energy field and removing any obstructions.

Possible interventions include unruffling a chaotic and tangled field, eliminating "congestion," and acting as a conduit to direct the "life energy" from the environment into the patient.

■ Throughout the treatment, the patient remains quiet and relaxed. According to practitioners, it isn't necessary for the patient to consciously believe in the power of the procedure.

■ To be effective in channeling energy into the patient, the nurse must have "conscious intent" — that is, the intent to become a calm, focused instrument of healing, enabling the patient's body to ultimately heal itself.

Special considerations

■ Care must be taken to moderate the length and strength of the treatment for small children and elderly people because their bodies are more fragile. A common sign of overtreatment in these patients is restlessness during or after the treatment.

■ Other patients who warrant extra sensitivity and shorter treatment periods include pregnant women, patients with head injuries or psychosis, emaciated patients, and patients in shock.

■ Respect the personal preferences of those being treated. People have different tolerances for touch, and some regard energy work as an invasion of their personal space.

Yoga therapy

Among the oldest known health practices, yoga (meaning "union" in Sanskrit) is the integration of physical, mental, and spiritual energies to promote health and wellness. It can be practiced by the young and old alike, either individually or within groups, and can be started at any age.

Based on the idea that a chronically restless or agitated mind causes poor health and decreased mental strength and clarity, yoga outlines specific regimens for lifestyle, hygiene, detoxification, physical activity, and psychological practices. By integrating these practices, yoga aims to raise the individual's physical vitality and spiritual awareness.

There are several styles of yoga, the most common in the West being hatha yoga. It combines physical postures and exercises (called *asanas),* breathing techniques (called *pranayamas),* relaxation, diet, and "proper thinking."

Asanas fall into two categories, meditative and therapeutic. *Meditative asanas* promote proper blood flow through the body by bringing the spine and body into perfect alignment. The mind and body are brought into a state of relaxation and stillness, which facilitates concentration during meditation. These asanas also keep the heart, glands, and lungs properly energized. *Therapeutic asanas* are commonly prescribed for joint pain. The "cobra," "locust spinal twist," and "shoulder stand" are examples.

The goal of a properly executed asana is to create a balance between movement and stillness, which is the state of a healthy body. Very little movement is needed. Instead the mind provides discipline, awareness, and a relaxed openness to maintain the posture and properly execute the asana. Using these asanas, the individual learns to regulate such autonomic functions as heartbeat and respirations while relaxing physical tensions.

Pranayamas focus on disciplined breathing. Pranayama exercises regulate the flow of *prana* (breath and electromagnetic force), keeping the individual healthy. Pranayama has been shown to aid digestion, regulate cardiac function, and alleviate various physical ailments.

A simple pranayama exercise

The following pranayama exercise is called purification of the channels (*nadi shodhana*). You can easily teach it to a patient.

■ Have the patient sit upright on a cushion or in a firm chair with his head, neck, and body aligned.

■ Tell him to breathe from his diaphragm, in a relaxed fashion, taking care to keep his inhalation and exhalation even and slow.

■ Instruct him to begin by exhaling through his left nostril and inhaling through his right one. Have him use the thumb and forefinger of his right hand to alternately close one nostril. He should do three cycles, inhaling through the same nostril each time.

■ At the end of the third cycle, he should change the pattern to inhale through the left nostril and exhale through the right nostril. He should do three cycles.

■ Then have him place both hands on his knees and inhale and exhale through both nostrils for three cycles.

■ As the patient practices this technique, have him try to lengthen the duration of his inhalations and exhalations, always keeping them even.

■ Encourage him to practice nadi shodhana twice each day, in the morning and evening.

It can be especially effective at reducing the frequency of asthma attacks.

The goal of breathing in yoga is to make the process as smooth and regular as possible. The assumption is that the rhythm of the mind is mirrored in the rhythm of breathing. By keeping respirations steady and rhythmic, the mind will remain calm and focused.

Samadhi, or spiritual realization, is an additional component of Eastern yoga. Yoga practitioners compare samadhi to a fourth state of consciousness, separate from the normal states of waking, dream, and sleep. The technique called *HongSau* uses meditation to develop the powers of concentration. Thought and energy are withdrawn from outer distractions and focused on any goal or problem the individual chooses. The *Aum* technique expands the individual's awareness beyond the limitations of the body and mind, allowing the user to experience what is called the "Divine Consciousness," which is believed to underlie and uphold all life. *Aum* is the sound that exists with every inhaled breath. The sounds of inhalation are "a" through the mouth and "um" through the nose. Taken together, these sounds of attraction form the sound *Aum.* To achieve "Divine Consciousness" the user alters his breathing and focuses on sounding out the "a" and the "um" sounds.

Among yoga's measured benefits are improvement in the individual's health, vitality, and peace of mind. Yoga is successfully used to alleviate stress and anxiety, lower blood pressure, relieve pain, improve motor skills, treat addictions, increase auditory and visual perception, and improve metabolic and respiratory function. Yoga has also been effective in treating lung ailments because it can increase lung capacity and lower respiratory rates.

Yoga has been credited with decreasing serum cholesterol and increasing histamine levels to fight allergies. Its ability to help the user regulate blood flow is being studied in cancer therapy. Scientists are eager to see whether restricted blood flow to the tumor region will slow growth.

Implementation

■ Provide a private, quiet environment that is free from distractions.

■ Participants should have enough room to move without touching or distracting other members.

■ Each participant will need a small blanket or large towel to use in some of the postures.

■ Explain the purpose of the session, and describe the planned exercises and their benefits. (See *A simple pranayama exercise.*)

■ Answer any questions, and remind the participants that they don't have to engage in any posture that may be uncomfortable.

■ When the group is ready, talk them through the positions or breathing techniques, demonstrating each one.

■ After they've all assumed the position, begin the breathing pattern, and circulate among the students to assess and adjust their technique, as needed.

■ Praise all of their efforts.

■ After you've led them through all of the planned exercises, close the session by having everyone take slow, deep breaths.

■ Document the session, the techniques used, and the patients' responses.

Special considerations

■ Some of the more physical aspects of yoga can cause muscle injury if they aren't properly performed, or if an older adult tries to force his body into position.

■ Caution patients to attempt the various techniques and postures cautiously, and remind them that very few people are able to perform all of the techniques in the beginning.

■ There are yoga techniques to fit the needs of all people, regardless of their physical condition. Individuals who can't perform some of the more physically demanding postures can still benefit from the breathing or meditation techniques.

15

Documentation
Completing forms fully and concisely

General guidelines

Nursing documentation: What to cover

With a large number of health care professionals involved in each patient's care, nursing documentation must be complete, accurate, and timely to foster continuity of care. In effect, your documentation should cover:

■ initial assessment using the nursing process and applicable nursing diagnoses

■ nursing actions, particularly reports to the doctor

■ ongoing assessment, including the frequency of assessment

■ variations from the assessment and plan of care

■ accountability information, including forms that the patient signed, the location of the patient's valuables, and patient teaching

■ notation of care by staff in other disciplines, including doctor visits, if practical, and of health teaching, including content and response

■ procedures and diagnostic tests performed on the patient

■ patient's response to therapy, particularly to nursing interventions and diagnostic tests

■ statements that the patient made regarding his condition or care

■ patient comfort and safety measures

■ compliance to critical pathways or other plans of care.

Documentation timesavers

How can you document more accurately and quickly? The following suggestions will help.

Follow the nursing process

Your documentation can best substantiate quality care if it reflects this process. The resulting record will help other caregivers provide quality care.

Use nursing diagnoses

Using standardized diagnostic labels to identify the patient's actual or potential health problems will result in less confusion and better care. Depending on your facility's policy, you may be required to use nursing diagnoses.

Document frequently and immediately

If you chart during your shift — right after you make an observation or intervene — rather than at the end of your shift, you'll document more accurately because you'll remember more information. You'll also provide other team members with the most current information on the patient's care and progress.

Flow sheets help you keep your documentation current, as does bedside charting. A growing number of facilities are requiring immediate documentation. Check the facility policy on how often documentation is required.

Individualize your charting

Documenting the same information for all patients with the same diagnosis neither promotes accuracy nor demonstrates quality care. Make sure your charting demonstrates the particular care that each patient received.

Don't repeat information

Not only does repeating information waste time but it can also be misleading. If you record data on a flow sheet, don't repeat it in the progress notes. Instead, use the progress notes to clarify information on the flow sheet or to add data, such as psychosocial information or follow-up care, that you can't chart on a flow sheet.

Sign off with initials

If the policy at your facility allows, save time by signing your name, licensure, and initials on a flow sheet near the front of the chart, and then using only your initials thereafter.

Don't document for other caregivers

Doctors should regularly document their own progress notes, as should other health care team members. Documenting for others may be a favor to them, but it's a liability for you.

Use the Kardex effectively

A Kardex can be made more effective by tailoring the information to the needs of a particular setting. For instance, a home care Kardex should have information on family contacts, doctors, other services, and emergency referrals.

If the Kardex is included in the clinical record at your facility, you can save charting time because you won't need to repeat the information in another part of the record. Make sure you write in ink, revising information when the doctor writes new orders or when the patient's needs change. In some facilities, the Kardex has been eliminated and its information has been incorporated into the nursing plan of care. In other facilities, the plan of care is on a computerized chart. It's automatically updated as orders are input into the computerized order entry system.

Use computerized documentation

Although not widespread, computer documentation will become more common as costs decrease, equipment becomes easier to use, and better software programs are developed.

Use fax machines

Fax machines allow you to send and receive orders, documentation forms, patient records, and test results quickly. Machines in doctors' offices can save you from taking and documenting orders over the phone.

Documenting patient assessment

Standardized open-ended form

As shown below, the typical fill-in-the-blanks assessment form comes with preprinted headings and questions. The standardized open-ended form saves you time in two ways: First, information is categorized under specific headings, so you can easily record and retrieve it; second, the form can be completed using partial phrases and approved abbreviations.

Unfortunately, however, many open-ended forms don't provide the space or the instructions to encourage thorough descriptions. For example, a nurse may write that a patient performs a certain task "within normal limits." However, unless normal limits have been defined, this notation is neither clear nor legally sound.

Reason for hospitalization *"I've been having dizzy episodes and passing out."*

Expected outcomes *By discharge, pt. and family will understand the syncopal episodes, demonstrate understanding of pacemaker therapy, and adhere to self-care program.*

Last hospitalization
Date _____5/98_____ Reason _____FX right hip_____

Medical history _____hypertension_____

Medications and allergies

Drug	Dosage	Time of last dose	Patient's statement of drugs purpose
Cardizem CD	180 mg	9:00 am	"for BP "

Allergy	Reaction
penicillin	hives

Standardized close-ended form

As shown below, the standardized close-ended form provides preprinted checklists. It saves time, avoids illegible handwriting, makes checking documented information easy, and can be incorporated into most computerized systems. Although the form may use nonspecific terminology, guidelines clearly define responses. Accrediting agencies, such as the Joint Commission on Accreditation of Healthcare Organizations, may prefer the use of initials instead of check marks.

The form may also create some problems. It may provide no place to record information that doesn't fit the preprinted choices. Furthermore, it can be lengthy, especially when in-depth physical assessment data are required.

SELF-CARE ABILITY

Activity	1	2	3	4	5	6
Bathing			✓			
Cleaning				✓		
Climbing stairs		✓				
Cooking				✓		
Dressing and grooming			✓			
Drinking and eating	✓					
Moving in bed	✓					
Shopping				✓		
Toileting		✓				
Transferring		✓				
Walking		✓				
Other home functions			✓			

KEY
1 Independent
2 Requires assistive device
3 Requires personal assistance
4 Requires personal assistance and assistive device
5 Dependent
6 Experienced change in last week

ASSISTIVE DEVICES
☐ Bedside commode
☐ Brace or splint
☐ Cane
☑ Crutches
☐ Feeding device
☐ Trapeze
☐ Walker
☐ Wheelchair
☐ Other _____
☐ None

ACTIVITY TOLERANCE
☑ Normal
☐ Weakness
☐ Dizziness
☐ Exertional dyspnea
☐ Dyspnea at rest
☐ Angina
☐ Pain at rest
☐ Oxygen needed
☐ Intermittent claudication
☐ Unsteady gait
☐ Other _____

REST PATTERN
Sleep habits
☐ Less than 8 hours
☑ 8 hours
☐ More than 8 hours
☐ Morning nap
☐ Afternoon nap

Sleep difficulties
☐ Insomnia
☐ Early awakening
☐ Unrefreshing sleep
☐ Nightmares
☑ None

A medical model for nursing assessment

Many facilities still use a medical model to organize their nursing assessment forms. As shown below, the physical examination section of this form is organized according to a comprehensive review of body systems. Some facilities have adopted formats that more readily reflect the nursing process, organizing data according to either human response patterns, functional health care patterns, or published nursing theories.

SYSTEMS REVIEW

Admission date and time: ___2/11/01 2 p.m.___

Height ___5' 8"___   Weight ___150 lb___   TPR ___99°-82-20___

BP, right arm ___110/76___   BP, left arm ___110/76___

Check boxes or write descriptions as appropriate.

Mental status
- ☑ Alert
- ☑ Cooperative
- ☐ Calm
- ☐ Lethargic
- ☐ Withdrawn
- ☐ Depressed
- ☑ Agitated
- ☑ Anxious

Oriented to:
- ☑ Time
- ☑ Place
- ☑ Person

Speech
- ☑ Normal, clear
- ☐ Slurred
- ☐ Hesitant
- ☐ Hoarse
- ☐ Dysphasic

Neurologic system
- ☑ Normal
- ☑ Pupils: PERRLA
- ☐ Dizziness
- ☑ Headaches
- ☐ Numbness
- ☐ Paraplegia
- ☐ Hemiplegia, right
- ☐ Hemiplegia, left

Eyes
- ☐ Normal
- ☑ Glasses

- ☐ Contact lenses
- ☐ Implanted lenses
- ☐ Blind, right eye
- ☐ Blind, left eye
- ☐ Artificial prosthesis
- ☐ Discharge
- ☐ Diplopia
- ☐ Blurred vision
- ☐ Tearing
- ☐ Burning
- ☐ Itching
- ☐ Photophobia
- ☐ Pain
- ☐ Sclera color _____
- ☐ Cataract
- ☐ Glaucoma

Ears
- ☑ Normal
- ☐ Hearing loss
- ☐ Hearing aid
- ☐ Tinnitus
- ☐ Vertigo
- ☐ Discharge
- ☐ Pain

Nose
- ☑ Normal
- ☐ Sinusitis
- ☐ Rhinitis
- ☐ Discharge
- ☐ Obstruction
- ☐ Epistaxis

Mouth and throat
- ☐ Normal
- ☐ Dentures, upper
- ☐ Dentures, lower
- ☐ Partial plate
- ☑ Dental fillings
- ☐ Sores on tongue
- ☐ Gum swelling or bleeding
- ☐ Diminished taste
- ☐ Sore throat

Respiratory system
- ☐ Normal
- ☑ Dyspnea
- ☐ Cough
- ☐ Hemoptysis
- ☐ Pain
- ☐ Orthopnea
- ☑ Breath sounds
  ___clear___

Cardiovascular system
- ☑ Normal
- ☐ Edema
- ☐ Cyanosis
- ☐ Cold extremities
- ☐ Palpitations

Pulse:
- ☑ Regular
- ☐ Irregular
- ☐ Bounding
- ☐ Weak

(continued)

A medical model for nursing assessment *(continued)*

Cardiovascular system
(continued)
☐ Thready
☑ Pedal pulse, right
   palpable
☑ Pedal pulse, left
   palpable
☑ Heart sounds
   S₁, S₂ audible

GI system
☑ Normal
☐ Change in appetite
☐ Indigestion
☐ Flatulence
☐ Nausea
☐ Vomiting
☐ Bleeding
☐ Abdominal pain
☐ Abdominal distention
☐ Ascites
☐ Hemorrhoids
☐ Constipation
☐ Diarrhea
☑ Last bowel movement
   _2/9/01_
☑ Number of stools
per day _1_
Bowel sounds:
☑ Present
☐ Absent
☐ Hyperactive
☐ Other _____

Nutritional status
☑ Special diet _N/A_
☑ Recent weight gain
☐ Recent weight loss

GU system
☑ Normal
☐ Frequency
☐ Urgency
☐ Dysuria
☐ Nocturia
Number of times _____
☐ Bleeding
☐ Burning

Reproductive system — female
☑ Last menstrual period
   _2/11/01_
☐ Cramping
☐ Irregular bleeding
☐ Discharge
☐ Vaginal infections
☐ Pain or difficulty with intercourse
☐ Menopause
☐ Other _____

Reproductive system — male
☐ Prostate problems
☐ Lesions
☐ Impotence
☐ Other _____

Musculoskeletal system
☐ Normal
☐ Stiffness
☑ Pain
☐ Weakness
☐ Limited ROM
☐ Paralysis
☑ Tenderness

☐ Swelling
☐ Arthritis
☐ Prosthesis
☐ Other _____
Physical activity:
☑ No limitations
☐ Walks with help
☐ Uses cane
☐ Uses crutches
☐ Uses walker
☐ Bedridden

Skin
☐ Turgor_____
☑ Temperature _cool_
☑ Color _pale_
☑ Dry
☐ Moist
☐ Diaphoretic
☐ Rash
☐ Eczema
☐ Acne
☐ Bruises
☐ Burns
☐ Lumps
☐ Lacerations
☑ Abrasions
☐ Scars _____
☐ Other _____
Condition of:
☑ Hair _clean and neat_
☑ Nails _clean_
Pressure ulcers _none_
☐ Number _____
☐ Stage 1, 2, 3, 4
☐ Location _____
☐ Describe _____

Additional comments _____

Date and time completed _2/11/01 2:00 p.m._
RN signature _____Kathy Craig, RN_____

Assessment flow sheet

If you're developing a new assessment form or revising a current one, consider the following questions:

■ What data from the health history and physical examination are currently included?

■ Is this acceptable or is more information needed to ensure quality? Certain areas may need to be marked with an asterisk (*) indicating that they require a more detailed nurse's note, particularly if abnormalities or changes from the patient's baseline occur.

■ What problems exist with the current documentation system?

■ What types of changes would help correct these problems?

Most assessment flow sheets cover the categories of information shown below.

Assessment flow sheet

Date   1/10/01

DIET

Meal	Amount eaten
Breakfast	15 %
Lunch	50 %
Dinner	90 %

☐ By himself
☑ With help
☐ With NG tube

HYGIENE	7-3	3-11	11-7
By himself			
With some help	SS	PD	
With complete help			
Shower		PD	
Oral care	SS	PD	
P.M. care			
Catheter care	SS	PD	

ACTIVITY AND REST

On complete bed rest			
Turn q 2 hr			CG
OOB (chair)	SS	PD	
BRP			
Walking			

ELIMINATION

Normal voiding			
Has catheter	SS	PD	CG
Incontinent			
Bowel movement	SS		
Emesis			

PULSE	7-3	3-11	11-7
Regular			
Irregular	SS	PD	CG
Strong	SS	PD	CG
Weak			

MUSCULOSKELETAL

Moves all limbs			
Weak	SS	PD	CG
Paralyzed			
Parasthetic			

RESPIRATORY

Respirations			
Within normal limits	SS	PD	CG
Shallow			
Deep			
Labored			

Respiratory rate			
Within normal limits	SS	PD	CG
Slow			
Rapid			

Breath sounds			
Clear	SS		
Moist		PD	CG
Wheezing			
Coughing		PD	CG

SKIN

Temperature			
Cool			
Warm	SS	PD	CG
Hot			

(continued)

Assessment flow sheet *(continued)*

Turgor	7-3	3-11	11-7
Good			
Fair	SS	PD	CG
Poor			
Edematous			
Moisture			
Dry	SS	PD	CG
Moist			
Diaphoretic			
Color			
Within normal limits			
Pale	SS	PD	CG
Ashen			
Cyanotic			
Flushed			
Jaundiced			
MENTAL STATUS			
Alert			
Oriented × 3	SS	PD	CG
Disoriented			
Lethargic	SS	PD	CG
BEHAVIOR			
Cooperative	SS	PD	CG
Uncooperative			
Anxious			
Withdrawn			
Combative			
Depressed	SS	PD	CG
SPEECH			
Clear			
Slurred	SS	PD	CG
Rambling			
Aphasic			
Inappropriate			

SLEEP	7-3	3-11	11-7
Sleeps well			
Sleeps intermittently			CG
Awake most of time	SS	PD	
GENERAL INFORMATION			
In restraints			
Eggcratelike mattress	SS	PD	CG
Side rails up	SS	PD	CG
In traction			
Under isolation precautions			
Above not applicable			
WOUND			
Type			
Size			
Appearance			
Sutures and drains			
Treatments			
Not applicable	SS	PD	CG
TUBES			
Type			
Location			
Drainage			
Irrigation			
Not applicable	SS	PD	CG
I.V. THERAPY			
I.V. site	① wrist SS	① wrist PD	① wrist CG
Catheter size	#18G jelco SS	#18G jelco PD	#18G jelco CG
Tubing change	9 a.m. SS		
Site appearance	no redness or edema SS	no redness or edema PD	NO REDNESS OR EDEMA CG
Not applicable			

Signature and status	Initials
Steve Shaw, RN	SS
Pamela Davis, RN	PD
CINDY GATER, RN	CG

Developing a plan of care

Traditional plan of care

Also called the individually developed plan of care, the traditional plan of care is written from scratch for each patient. After analyzing the assessment data, you'll either write the plan or enter it into a computer.

The basic form can vary, depending on the needs of the facility or department. Most forms have three main columns: one for nursing diagnoses, another for patient outcomes, and a third for interventions.

What you must include on these forms also varies. Most facilities ask you

to write only short-term outcomes, which are those goals that the patient should reach by or before discharge. However, some facilities also want you to include long-term outcomes, which indicate the maximum functional level the patient can reach.

The sample here shows how a traditional plan of care organizes key information. Keep in mind that the plan of care you'll use will have wider columns to allow more room for your notes.

Date	Nursing diagnosis	Patient outcomes	Interventions	Resolution (initials and date)	Revision (initials and date)
1/3/01	Impaired gas exchange related to inadequate ventilation perfusion as evidenced by dyspnea and hypoxemia	Decrease in dyspnea, pulse oximetry > 92%, and normal ABG by 1/4/01	Auscultate chest sounds q 4 hr and monitor for signs and symptoms. Administer bronchodilators as prescribed. Administer oxygen therapy as prescribed. Monitor ABGs and pulse oximetry.		

Review dates

Date	Signature	Initials
1/3/01	Renee Thompson, RN	RT

Standardized plan of care

Developed to save documentation time and improve the quality of care, standardized plans of care list interventions for patients with similar diagnoses. Most plans also supply root outcome statements. Current versions allow you to tailor the plan to fit your patient's specific needs.

When a patient has more than one diagnosis, the resulting combination of standardized plans can be cumbersome. However, with computerized documentation, you can pull only what you need from each one and combine them to make one manageable plan. Some computer programs provide a checklist of interventions you can use to build your own plan.

The plan shown here concerns a patient with a nursing diagnosis of *decreased cardiac output.* To customize it to your patient, you would complete the diagnosis — including signs and symptoms — and fill in the patient outcomes. You would also modify, add, or delete interventions as necessary.

Date

1/25/01

Nursing diagnosis

Decreased cardiac output R/T

Accelerated heart rhythm as evidenced by hypotension, diaphoresis, and light-headedness

Target date

1/27/01

Expected outcomes

Adequate cardiac output as evidenced by:
Heart rate *≤ 100 beats/min*
Blood pressure *> 90/50 mm Hg and < 140/90 mm Hg*
Pedal pulse *palpable and regular*
Radial pulse *palpable and regular*
Cardiac rhythm *NSR*
Cardiac index *N/A*
Pulmonary artery wedge pressure (PAWP) *N/A*
Pulmonary artery pressure (PAP) *N/A*
Sv̄o$_2$ *N/A*
Urine output in ml/kg/hr *≥ 0.3 ml/kg/hr*

Date

1/27/01

Interventions

■ Monitor ECG results for rate and rhythm; note ectopic beats. If arrhythmias occur, note the patient's response. Document and report findings and follow the appropriate arrhythmia protocol.
■ Monitor S̶v̶o̶ $_2$, temperature, respirations, ~~and central pressures (including PAP) continuously.~~
■ ~~Monitor other hemodynamic pressures (such as PAWP) q 1 hr and p.r.n.~~ *N/A*
■ Auscultate heart sounds and palpate peripheral pulses q *4* hr and p.r.n.
■ Monitor I/O q *1* hr. Notify the doctor if urine output is less than 30 ml/hr × 2 hr.

Standardized plan of care *(continued)*

Interventions *(continued)*

■ Administer medications and fluids as ordered, noting their effectiveness and adverse reactions. Titrate vasoactive drugs as needed. Follow appropriate vasoactive drug protocol to wean the patient as tolerated.
■ Monitor O_2 therapy or other ventilatory support measures.
■ Decrease the patient's activity to reduce O_2 demands. Increase as tolerated.
■ Assess and document the patient's LOC. Assess for changes q __/__ hr and p.r.n.
■ Additional interventions: _____
_____
_____
_____
_____
_____
_____

Protocol format

Protocols provide specific sequential directions for treating patients with particular problems. They help ensure thorough, consistent care; teach inexperienced staff members; and save charting time. To use protocols effectively, follow these guidelines:

■ Use the protocols that best fit your patient, and make sure you have the current versions.

■ Tailor the protocol to fit your patient's needs. Cross out steps that don't apply, and modify or add material as needed.

■ To document properly, note in the interventions section of the plan of care that you'll follow the protocol or list the protocols you plan to use on a flow sheet. After you intervene, write in your progress notes that you followed the protocol or check the protocol off on your flow sheet and initial it. Include a copy of the protocol in the patient's record – especially if you've made changes to it.

As the sample here shows, protocols typically list staff requirements, patient outcomes, supportive information, and appropriate nursing actions.

Protocol

Title: *Imbalanced nutrition: Less than body requirements; Risk for deficient fluid volume*

Health care staff
■ Assessment: RN
■ Planning: RN
■ Intervention: RN, LPN, nursing assistant
■ Patient teaching: RN, LPN, dietitian
■ Evaluation: RN
■ Complications: RN, LPN, nursing assistant, dietitian
■ Documentation: RN, LPN

Caregiver qualifications
The caregiver must:
■ be able to identify patients at risk for imbalanced nutrition and deficient fluid volume
■ be able to assess patients at risk for imbalanced nutrition and deficient fluid volume
■ understand these problems and their treatments
■ be qualified to perform necessary interventions.

Patient outcomes
The patient will:
■ have less nausea, vomiting, and diarrhea
■ demonstrate knowledge of his nutritional needs
■ show signs of adequate hydration, including improved skin turgor, moist mucous membranes, and increased urine output
■ show signs of adequate caloric intake, including improved appetite, weight gain, and increased energy.

Supportive data
■ Risk factors:
– hyperthermia, anorexia, nausea and vomiting, and diarrhea
– infectious or inflammatory processes

Protocol format *(continued)*

■ Signs and symptoms of imbalanced nutrition and deficient fluid volume:
– dry mucous membranes
– poor skin turgor
– lethargy
■ Procedures for monitoring patients at risk for imbalanced nutrition and deficient fluid volume:
– measuring intake and output and weighing patient (I.V. equipment, total parenteral nutrition equipment, and scale may be used.)
– performing a neurologic assessment to provide early clues to a fluid volume deficit

Responsibilities	Nursing actions
Assessment	■ Assess general physical condition every 8 hours. ■ Assess neurologic status every 8 hours. Especially note subtle changes in behavior or level of consciousness. ■ Assess daily caloric and fluid intake, using these guidelines: – Good – Intake provides 50% or more of needed calories and fluids. – Fair – Intake provides more than 20% and less than 50% of needed calories and fluids. – Poor – Intake provides less than 20% of needed calories and fluids. – None – The patient's unable or refuses to eat or drink.
Planning	Collaborate with the doctor to decide when to perform interventions that will help the patient meet daily nutrition and fluid needs. Meet with the dietitian to ensure reinforcement of nutritional counseling in preparation for discharge.
Interventions	■ Monitor intake, output, and weight. ■ Monitor bowel function. ■ Monitor results of laboratory studies (serum albumin, total protein, urine protein, glucose, acetone, and nitrogen levels). ■ Observe the patient, and help him choose the amount and types of foods and liquids. ■ Provide smaller but more frequent meals. ■ Help the patient to a comfortable position at mealtimes. ■ Help the patient with meals; feed him, if necessary. ■ Arrange for the dietitian to assess the patient's caloric requirements. ■ Offer fluids every 4 hours between meals; try to ensure a total daily intake of 3 qt (2.8 L) unless contraindicated. ■ Provide parenteral fluids as ordered. ■ Provide nutritional supplements.

(continued)

Protocol format *(continued)*

Responsibilities	Nursing actions
Patient teaching	■ Explain the need to take in sufficient calories to maintain adequate nutrition and the need to maintain adequate fluid balance. ■ Instruct the patient and his family members about the patient's specific nutritional needs.
Evaluation	Evaluate the nutritional and fluid status of the patient every 8 hours and any time a significant change in patient status or regimen occurs.
Complications	■ Observe the patient for complications, including dehydration, anemia, malnutrition, and sepsis. ■ Notify the doctor, document appropriately, continue assessment and interventions, and carry out additional doctor's orders.
Documentation	Document: ■ ongoing nutritional and fluid assessment data on nurse's progress sheet ■ nutritional and fluid status of the patient on nurse's progress sheet ■ intake and output every 8 hours ■ vital signs as ordered by doctor but at least every 8 hours ■ patient teaching on nutritional and fluid needs ■ daily weights on graphic record ■ type and amount of nutritional therapy on patient care flow sheet ■ type and amount of fluid therapy on I.V. therapy sheet every 8 hours and at completion of infusion ■ complications and actions taken to correct them.

Critical pathway

A critical pathway is an abbreviated case management plan that covers only the key events that must occur for the patient to be discharged by the target date. Such events include consultations, diagnostic tests, physical activities the patient must perform, treatments, diet, drugs, discharge planning, and patient teaching. Critical pathways are multidisciplinary and are outcome oriented.

At shift report each day, review the critical pathway documents with the other nurses. Before you go off duty, note any changes in the expected length of stay and point out critical events scheduled for the next shift to the nurses coming on duty. Also, discuss any variances for the pathway that may have occurred during your shift. Other departments, such as physical, occupational, and respiratory therapy, should be encouraged to document on the critical pathway and individualize it to meet the patient's needs as appropriate.

The sample here shows selected portions of a typical critical pathway.

Diagnosis: Partial or total parotidectomy
DRG length of stay: 2.3 days
Actual length of stay: _____
Expected outcomes
By discharge, the patient will:
■ state possible complications, troubleshooting measures, and appropriate resources
■ perform suture line care
■ explain measures for managing his pain
■ explain how to maintain his nutritional status
■ demonstrate eye care measures (if applicable).

Nurse	Other health care providers	Patient and family members
PREOPERATIVE DAY		
■ Performs assessment ■ Explains case management model and recovery pathway to the patient ■ Completes contract with the patient and his family members ■ Performs preoperative teaching	*Primary doctor* ■ Performs physical examination ■ Orders special studies, including blood work, ECG, and chest X-rays ■ Orders anesthesia clearance assessment	*Patient and family members* ■ Sign contract ■ Visit immediate postoperative care unit

(continued)

Critical pathway *(continued)*

Nurse	Other health care providers	Patient and family members

■ Notifies the social worker, if appropriate, and explains assessment and possible discharge needs to her	*Social worker* ■ Consults with nurse (if appropriate)	

POSTOPERATIVE DAY (POD) 1

■ Provides morning care while the patient is on bed rest ■ Sets up heparin lock on I.V. line ■ Teaches suture line care ■ Teaches eye care (if applicable) ■ Encourages activity ■ Monitors diet	*Primary doctor* ■ Orders laboratory tests ■ Orders advance in diet as tolerated ■ Orders heparin lock on I.V. line ■ Consults with ophthalmologist, radiation therapist, and dentist (as applicable) *Ophthalmologist* ■ Consults with primary doctor (if applicable) *Radiation therapist* ■ Consults with primary doctor (if applicable) *Dentist* ■ Consults with primary doctor (if applicable)	*Patient* ■ Performs oral hygiene and incentive spirometry ■ Demonstrates suture line care and eye care (if applicable) ■ Ambulates q 4 hr p.r.n.

POD 2

■ Continues to teach suture line care and eye care ■ Continues to encourage activity and monitor diet	*Dietitian* ■ Performs nutrition assessment *Speech pathologist* ■ Performs nutrition assessment (if the patient has difficulty swallowing)	*Patient* ■ Performs morning self-care ■ Continues to perform oral hygiene and incentive spirometry ■ Demonstrates suture line care and eye care (if applicable) ■ Ambulates q 4 hr p.r.n.

Documenting interventions and evaluations

Flow sheet for routine care

For years, the Joint Commission on Accreditation of Healthcare Organizations has encouraged facilities to use flow sheets for documenting routine care measures. In response, many facilities have developed these forms for such measures as making basic assessments, giving wound care, and providing hygiene. In many facilities, you may also use flow sheets to document vital signs checks, I.V. monitoring, equipment checks, patient education, and discharge summaries.

As this sample shows, a patient care flow sheet allows you to quickly document your routine interventions. Note that the last page of this four-page form provides space for narrative notes.

PATIENT CARE FLOW SHEET

DATE	11 p.m. to 7 a.m.	7 a.m. to 3 p.m.	3 p.m. to 11 p.m.
Respiratory			
Breath sounds	crackles left lower base SK	CLEAR GD	clear BG
Treatments/results	chest PT q 2 hr SK	CHEST PT q 2 HR GD	chest PT q 2 hrs BG
Cough/results	small amt. of clear thin mucus SK	ō GD	ō BG
O₂ therapy nasal cannula @ 1 L/min	continuous SK	CONTINUOUS GD	continuous BG
Cardiac			
Chest pain	ō SK	ō GD	ō BG
Heart sounds	normal S₁ S₂ SK	NORMAL S₁ S₂ GD	normal S₁ S₂ BG
Telemetry	NSR SK	NSR GD	NSR BG
Pain			
Type and location	ō SK	DULL LOWER BACK PAIN GD	ō BG
Intervention	ō SK	DARVOCET-N 100 MG P.O. GD	ō BG
Response	ō SK	RELIEF IN 45 MIN GD	ō BG
Nutrition			
Type	n/a	1500 ADA GD	1500 ADA BG
Toleration %	n/a	100% GD	90% BG
Supplement	n/a	N/A	h.s. snack BG

(continued)

Flow sheet for routine care *(continued)*

DATE	11 p.m. to 7 a.m.	7 a.m. to 3 p.m.	3 p.m. to 11 p.m.
Elimination			
Stool appearance	ō SK	ō GD	ҭ soft light brown BG
Enema	n/a	N/A	n/a
Results	n/a	N/A	n/a
Bowel sounds	present all 4 quadrants SK	PRESENT ALL 4 QUADRANTS GD	present all 4 quadrants BG
Urine appearance	clear yellow x2 SK	CLEAR YELLOW X 2 GD	clear amber x 1 BG
Indwelling urinary catheter	n/a	N/A	n/a
Catheter irrigations	n/a	N/A	n/a
I.V. therapy			
Tubing change	n/a	8:00 A.M.	n/a
Dressing change	n/a	8:00 A.M.	n/a
Site appearance	no signs of redness or edema SK	NO SIGNS OF REDNESS OR EDEMA GD	no signs of redness or edema BG
Wound			
Type	n/a	N/A	n/a
Dressing change	n/a	N/A	n/a
Appearance	n/a	N/A	n/a
Tubes			
Type	n/a	N/A	n/a
Irrigation	n/a	N/A	n/a
Drainage appearance	n/a	N/A	n/a
Hygiene			
Self/partial/ complete	n/a	9:00 A.M. PARTIAL GD	9:00 pm BG
Oral care	n/a	9:00 A.M. GD	9:00 pm BG
Back care	n/a	9:00 A.M. GD	9:00 pm BG
Foot care	n/a	9:00 A.M. GD	9:00 pm BG

Flow sheet for routine care *(continued)*

DATE	11 p.m. to 7 a.m.	7 a.m. to 3 p.m.	3 p.m. to 11 p.m.
Activity			
Type	BRP SK	OOB AD LIB GD	OOB ad lib BG
Toleration	Turns self SK	TOLERATES ACTIVITY WELL GD	Tolerates activity well BG
Repositioned	n/a	N/A	n/a
ROM	n/a	N/A	n/a
Sleep			
Sleeps well	1:00 a.m. SK / 6:00 a.m. SK	N/A	n/a
Awake at intervals	n/a	N/A	n/a
Awake most of the time	n/a	N/A	n/a
Safety			
Side rails up	1:00 a.m. SK / 6:00 a.m. SK	9:00 A.M. GD / 1:00 P.M. GD	4:00 p.m. BG / 9:00 p.m. BG
Call light in reach	1:00 a.m. SK / 6:00 a.m. SK	9:00 A.M. GD / 1:00 P.M. GD	4:00 p.m. BG / 9:00 p.m. BG
Equipment			
Type Gemini pump	continuous SK	CONTINUOUS GD	continuous BG
Teaching			
Diabetic Protocol	n/a	GD	BG

(continued)

Flow sheet for routine care *(continued)*

PROGRESS SHEET

Time	Comments
9:00 A.M.	PT. ADMITS TO COMPLAINT OF DULL LOWER BACK PAIN, DENIES PAIN IN LEGS OR NUMBNESS OR TINGLING OF LOWER EXT. DR. JONES NOTIFIED OF PT.'S COMPLAINT OF LOWER BACK PAIN. ORDER RECEIVED DARVOCET-N 100 MG.————————————GRACE DARNEY, RN
9:45 A.M.	PT. DENIES COMPLAINT OF PAIN, DARVOCET EFFECTIVE. ———————————— GRACE DARNEY, RN
2:00 P.M.	REVIEWED S/S OF HYPO/HYPERGLYCEMIA WITH PT. AND FAMILY. PT. AND FAMILY RECEPTIVE TO INFORMATION. —————— GRACE DARNEY, RN
6:00 p.m.	Pt. ambulating in room. Offers no further complaint of lower back pain. Gait steady.——— Brooke Stevens, RN

Initials	Signature/title
SK	Sally Kendall, RN
GD	GRACE DARNEY, RN
BS	Brooke Stevens, RN

Code record

When documenting a patient emergency, follow standard guidelines, taking care to:
- be factual
- be specific about times and interventions
- include the name of the doctor you contacted, the time you contacted him, what you told him, and the outcome of the conversation
- indicate attempts to inform the patient's family or significant other of the changes in his situation.

Use a code record to keep the progress note concise and to ensure complete documentation. This specialized documentation form incorporates detailed information about a code, including observations, interventions, and medications administered. When signed by the doctor, the form is the order sheet for medications and treatments during the code. The sample here shows the typical features of a code record.

CODE RECORD

Name _Barry Craig_ **Body weight** _183 lbs_ **Date** _1/23/01_

Medical record # _12345678_

Vital signs				Bolus meds						Infused meds			Action			Blood			
Time a.m./p.m.	BP	Heart rate	Heart rhythm	Atropine (mg)	Calcium chloride (ampules)	Epinephrine (mg)	Lidocaine (mg)	Procainamide (mg)		Dopamine (mg/ml)	Isoproterenol (mg/ml)	Lidocaine (g/ml)	Defibrillation (joules)	CPR	Airway	PaO_2	$PacO_2$	HcO_3^-	pH
11:20	0	0												√	mask				
11:25	0	0	VT										200						
11:25			VT											√					
11:26			VF										300						
11:27													360						
11:29						1	100							√	ET				
11:30													360						
11:31														√					
11:31			▼									2 mg/min	360						
11:32	100/68	96	NSR																
11:32			NSR																
11:35	110/60	92	▼													64	45	23	7.35

(continued)

Code record *(continued)*

Time	Actions
11:20	Code called. CPR initiated by C. Krane, RN, and S. Walden, RN. Ambu-bagged by S. Walden, RN.
11:25	Connected to single-channel ECG, #20 jelco inserted via (L) antecubital by P. Downs, RN.
11:29	Intubation with #8 oral ET by M. Cress, anesthesiologist.
11:35	Converted to NSR, ABG via (R) femoral artery drawn by M. White, MD. Pressure applied x 5 min. Pt. remains unresponsive.

Time code called *11:20 p.m.*

☐ Arrest witnessed
☑ Arrest unwitnessed
☑ Intubation *11:29*

☑ Arrhythmia *pulseless VT*
☑ Informed family
☑ Informed attending doctor

Disposition

☐ SICU   ☑ CCU   ☐ Morgue
☐ MICU   ☐ OR   ☐ Other

Critical care nurse
Carol Krane, RN

Status after resuscitation
BP 110/60. Heart rate 92. Bagged with
100% O_2 and transported to CCU.

Code chief
M. White, MD

Patient teaching: Narrative notes

Listed here are the types of information you need to document, using a narrative format. Documentation methods may vary among facilities.

1. Date and time of each teaching session

2. Patient's name and number on every record page

3. Patient's health status and corresponding learning needs

4. Learning outcomes agreed on by health care team and patient

5. Identified learning enhancements

6. Actual teaching you carry out

7. Specific teaching techniques

8. Patient's characteristics as a learner

9. Precise description of exactly what occurred, avoiding broad statements, such as learned well and seems to understand

10. Your evaluation of patient's change or learning

11. Patient's response to teaching and learning experience, using his own words and behaviors

12. Specific teaching materials

13. Indications that patient or family member understands instructions

14. Identified learning barriers

15. Final progress notes with discharge teaching about diet, medications, activity, and follow-up care

16. Your signature

Charting progress notes

Narrative format

In this paragraph approach to charting, you document ongoing assessment data, nursing interventions, and patient responses in chronological order. You'll record this information in your progress notes. Flow sheets commonly supplement these narrative notes.

This sample shows how to write a progress note using the narrative format.

Nurse's progress notes

DATE	TIME	NOTES
1/22/01	9 a.m.	Pt. complains of ⒧ upper quadrant abd. pain. Reports pain is an 8 on a scale of 1 to 10. Color pale, skin cool and diaphoretic, BP 84/60, T-100.2° F (orally), P-124, RR-28, abd. drsg. saturated c̄ bright red blood. Reinforced abd. drsg. c̄ 2 abd. pads. Salem connected to low continuous drainage, bright red blood noted via Salem. #18 jelco intact via ⓡ hand, infusing c̄ no evidence of redness or infiltration. I.V. D5 1/2 NSS patent. Foley draining dark amber urine; total output 10 ml in past 3 hours. Dr. O'Brien notified of pt.'s condition. Orders noted; will continue to monitor closely. I.V. solution changed to LR @ 250 ml/hr. Dr. O'Brien to see pt. ——————————— J. Paul, RN
1/22/01	9:30 a.m.	VS remain unstable, BP 80/50, P-136, RR-32. Pt. anxious, trembling; color pale, skin cool and diaphoretic. 100 ml of bright red bleeding noted from Salem; 4 × 6 cm of bright red bleeding noted on abd. dressing. ————————————— J. Paul, RN

Problem-oriented format

The problem-oriented medical record (POMR) system of charting focuses on the patient's problems and provides a structure that's absent from narrative charting. Progress notes are organized according to the **SOAP** framework:

■ **S**ubjective data – information the patient tells you

■ **O**bjective data – information you gather by observation

■ **A**ssessment – your conclusions about the patient's problem, based on subjective and objective data

■ **P**lan – the proposed interventions to resolve the problem.

A modification, organized according to the **SOAPIE** framework, includes two more components:

■ **I**ntervention – the interventions you perform to resolve the problem

■ **E**valuation – your evaluation of the patient's response to interventions.

This sample shows how to write a progress note using the POMR system.

Nurse's progress notes

DATE	TIME	NOTES
1/22/01	2:00 p.m.	#1 Pain related to cholecystectomy surgical incision.
		S: "I'm having a lot of pain where they did my
		surgery."
		O: Pt. returned from postanesthesia care unit at
		1:30 p.m. Pt. reports pain of 6 on a scale of 1 to 10
		in abdominal RUQ. Color pale. Holding incisional area.
		BP 140/86. P-90. RR-20. T-99° orally. Abd.
		drsg. dry and intact. Received meperidine 50 mg
		I.M. at 10 a.m.
		A: Increased incisional pain related to wearing off
		of meperidine. BP and pulse increased over baseline.
		P: Administer meperidine 50 mg I.M. now as
		ordered. Reposition pt. from back to right side to
		promote comfort. Reassess pain level in 20 minutes.
		J. Paul, RN

FOCUS charting format

Developed by nurses who found the SOAP format awkward, FOCUS charting encourages you to organize your thoughts into patient-centered topics, or foci of concern, and then to document precisely and concisely. The format encourages you to use assessment data to evaluate these patient care concerns. It also helps you identify necessary revisions to the plan of care as you document each entry.

This sample shows how to write progress notes using the FOCUS charting format. "D" represents data, "A" indicates action, and "R" is the response.

Nurse's progress notes

DATE	TIME	FOCUS	NOTES
1/22/01	2:00 p.m.	Acute pain related to cholecys- tectomy surgical incision	D: Pt. reports pain at abdominal RUQ of 6 on a scale of 1 to 10. Color pale. Holding incisional area. BP 140/86. P-90. RR-20. T-99° orally. Abd. drsg. dry and intact. Received meperidine 50 mg I.M. at 10 a.m. A: meperidine 50 mg I.M. adminis- tered as ordered. Pt. repositioned from back to right side. Will reassess pain level and VS in 30 min and administer meperidine q 3 to 4 hr p.r.n. (see plan of care). J. Paul, RN
1/22/01	2:00 p.m.	Pt. teaching	D: Pt. states, "Every time I cough or move, my incision hurts." ——— A: Splinting of surgical incision reviewed with pt. to reduce discomfort during coughing, deep breathing, and movement. ——— R: Pt. demonstrates proper place- ment of hands over surgical incision site and verbalizes experiencing less incisional discomfort while coughing, deep breathing, and moving. ——— ————————— J. Paul, RN

PIE format

Developed to simplify the documentation process, problem-intervention-evaluation (PIE) charting organizes information based on patient problems. Documentation tools for this format include a daily patient assessment flow sheet and progress notes.

By integrating the plan of care into the progress notes, the PIE format eliminates the need for a separate plan of care. The intention is to provide a concise, efficient record of patient care that has a nursing — not a medical — focus.

This sample shows how to write progress notes using the PIE format. The letter "P" stands for "problem". Assign a number to P starting with one. Then add the corresponding intervention by adding an "I" or evaluation by adding an "E" to each "P." For example, P #1, IP #1, EP #1; P #2, IP #2, EP #2, and so on.

Progress notes

DATE	TIME	NOTES
1/22/01	2:00 p.m	P#1: Acute pain related to cholecystectomy surgical incision.
		IP#1: meperidine 50 mg I.M. administered as ordered. Pt. repositioned from back to right side. Splinting of surgical incision reviewed with pt., and pt. demonstrated proper technique.
		EP#1: Increased postoperative incisional pain due to wearing off of meperidine. BP and pulse increased over baseline. Reassess pain level and VS in 30 min. Will give meperidine q 3 to 4 hr p.r.n. ———— J. Paul, RN
1/22/01	2:00 p.m.	P#2: Risk for deficient fluid volume related to nausea.
		IP#2: prochlorperazine 10 mg I.M., administered as ordered.
		EP#2: Nausea possibly related to increased incisional pain and postanesthesia effects. Will reassess for nausea in 30 min. ———— J. Paul, RN

Charting-by-exception format

The charting-by-exception (CBE) format departs from traditional systems by requiring documentation of only significant or abnormal findings and uses the SOAP format for writing the nurse's notes. It also uses military time to help prevent misinterpretations.

To use the CBE format effectively, you must know and adhere to established guidelines for nursing assessments and interventions. The CBE nursing assessment format has printed guidelines for each body system. Guidelines for interventions are derived from standardized plans of care based on nursing diagnoses, protocols, doctor's orders, incidental orders, and standards of nursing practice.

Nurse's progress notes

DATE	TIME	NOTES
1/25/01	0900	*(Nursing entry)*
		S: "I can't remember how to use this glucose meter. I'll never be able to test my own blood sugar."
		O: Pt. unable to perform blood glucose test; difficulty remembering the steps in the procedure.
		A: Deficient knowledge related to use of glucose meter.
		P: Review step-by-step how to use glucose meter. Assist pt. in performing self glucose monitoring. Provide pt. with information to review; teach husband how to use glucose meter; reevaluate. — N. Jones, RN

Flow sheet for nursing-medical order

The nursing-medical order flow sheet is used to document assessments and interventions during a 24-hour period for one patient. To use the form, mark the appropriate category box with a check mark to indicate normal assessment findings, a completed intervention, or an expected patient response. Use an asterisk (*) to indicate abnormal or significant findings or responses, and write an ex-

planation in the comments section. Reference this note by nursing diagnosis number or doctor's order and time. If the patient's condition is unchanged, draw a horizontal arrow from the previous category box to the current one. Initial completed columns and all comments. Sign the form at the bottom of the page.

This sample shows the typical features of a nursing-medical order flow sheet.

Nursing-medical order flow sheet

Date ___1/20/01___

ND #/DO	Assessments and interventions				
ND 1	Cardiac assessment	8 am *	8:10 am *		
ND 2	Pain/comfort intervention	8:05 am *			
DO	12-lead ECG done	8:05 am			
Initials		CM	CM		

KEY
DO = doctor's orders
ND = nursing diagnosis
√ = normal findings

→ = no change in condition
* = abnormal or significant finding
(See "Comments" section.)

ND #/DO	Time	Comments	Initials
ND 1	8:00 am	Pt. complains of midsternal chest pain,	
		rates pain a 4 on a scale of 1 to 10. BP	
		140/86, P-74, RR-18. ———	CM
ND 2	8:05 am	Medicated c̄ NTG 1/200 gr sl. for	
		chest pain. Will reassess in 5 min. ———	CM
ND 1	8:10 am	Medication effective for the relief of	
		chest pain. ———	CM

Initials	Signature
CM	Carol Marker, RN

Flow sheet for graphic record

The graphic record is used to document trends in the patient's vital signs, weight, intake and output, stool, urine, appetite, and activity level. As with the nursing-medical flow sheet, use check marks and asterisks to indicate expected and abnormal findings, respectively. Note information on abnormalities in the progress notes or on the nursing-medical order flow sheet.

In the box labeled routine standards, initial that you've carried out established nursing care interventions such as providing hygiene. Don't rewrite these standards as orders on the nursing-medical flow sheet. Refer to the guidelines on the back of the graphic record for complete instructions.

This partial form shows how to use a typical graphic record.

Graphic record

Date	1/22/01						1/23/01									
Hour	2	6	10	14	18	22	6	10	14							
Temperature																

Temperature graph axis:

°F	°C
105°	40.6°
104°	40.0°
103°	39.4°
102°	38.9°
101°	38.3°
100°	37.8°
99°	37.2°
98.6°	37.0°
98°	36.7°
97°	36.1°
96°	35.6°

Pulse	76	70	78	100	84	88	76	72								
Respiratory rate	18	18	20	22	20	18	16	18								
BP	6 146/84	18 148/86				6 140/82										
	10 152/86					10 146/84										
	14 158/90															
Appetite		P	G													
Routine standards	CM	CM	CB	PT	CM											
Activity 11 to 7	sleeping			sleeping												
7 to 3	OOB to chair c̄ assist x 2			OOB to chair c̄ assist x 1												
3 to 7																

Key: P = Poor   G = Good

Documenting patient discharge

Discharge planning

How and where you document your discharge planning will depend on your facility's policy. Here's one of the more common ways of documenting this information — using a designated section of an initial assessment form (usually the last page).

Discharge planning needs

Occupation _____teacher_____ Language spoken _English_

Patient lives with ___wife___

Self-care capabilities _____independent_____

Assistance available
☐ Cooking   ☐ Cleaning   ☐ Shopping
☐ Dressing changes/treatments _____N/A_____

Medication administration routes
☑ P.O.   ☐ I.M.   ☐ Other _____
☐ I.V.   ☑ S.C.

Dwelling
☐ Apartment   ☑ Inside steps   ☑ Bathrooms
☑ Private home   (number) _10_   (number) _2_
☐ Single room   ☐ Kitchen   (location) 2nd floor
☐ Institution   (Gas stove)   1st floor (off kitchen)
☐ Elevator   Electric stove   ☑ Telephones
☑ Outside steps   Wood stove   (number) _2_
(number) _2_   Other _____   (location) _bedroom_
    kitchen

Transportation
☑ Drives own car   ☐ Takes public   ☐ Relies on family
    transportation   member or friend

After discharge, patient will be:
☐ Home alone   ☑ Home with family   ☐ Other _____

Patient has had help from:
☑ Visiting nurse   ☐ Housekeeper   ☑ Other _wife_
Anticipated needs _Patient will need help with insulin administration and_
follow-up diabetic education.

Social service requests _____visiting nurse_____
Date contacted _____1/30/01_____

Discharge summary and patient instructions

This sample form combines your discharge summary with your postdischarge instructions for the patient. You would give a copy of this form to the patient at discharge.

Discharge summary
Date _____1/14/01_____
Time _____11 a.m._____

Destination
☐ Home
☑ Nursing home
☐ Other _____

Mobility
☐ Ambulatory
☐ Wheelchair
☑ Stretcher

PATIENT STATUS
General
TPR _____98-84-18_____
BP _____128/76_____
☐ Eating regularly
Comments _____

Skin
☐ Good condition
☑ Wound _pressure ulcer Ⓛ leg_
☐ Other _____

Bowels
☐ Regular movement
☑ Irregular movement
☐ Ostomy

Bladder
☐ Continent
☐ Urinary frequency
☐ Incontinent
☑ Catheter
Type _____Foley #16_____
Date changed _____1/10/01_____

Compliance
☐ Understands physical condition
☐ Willing to comply with regimen
☐ States understanding of instructions
Comments _____
_____
_____

Medications
☐ Preadmission medications returned
_____
☐ Prescriptions given to patient
_____
☐ Medications given to patient
_____
☑ Patient or family knows of allergies
_____
Nurse's signature _Carol Brown, RN_

PATIENT INSTRUCTIONS
Diet
☐ Unrestricted
☑ Restricted _2 g._
low sodium–low cholesterol diet
_____

Activities
☑ Walking
☐ Climbing stairs
☐ Riding in car
☐ Driving car
☐ Showering
☐ Taking a tub bath
☐ Engaging in sexual intercourse
☐ Resuming regular activity
☐ Lifting
☐ Exercising
☐ Other _____
_____
_____
_____
_____
Comments_____Ambulates with_
walker; gradually resumes activity
_____
_____
_____
_____

(continued)

Discharge summary and patient instructions *(continued)*

Medications	**Dosage, route, and time**
Digoxin	0.125 mg P.O. q.d.
Lasix	40 mg P.O. b.i.d.
Darvocet-N	100 mg P.O. p.r.n. q 6 hrs for pain

Special instructions

Saline dressings to ℓ leg wound q shift

Referral

☐ Call Dr. _____ and schedule an appointment _____
☐ Home care agency _____
☐ Other _____

If you have questions, call Dr. *Wilson* _____ at ___ *251-1680* ___
I've read and understood these instructions, and I've received a copy of this form
Date __ */14/01* _____

Patient signature or significant other
_____ *Mildred Smith (daughter)* _____

Nurse and doctor
_____ *Dr. H. Wilson, MD* _____
_____ *Carol Brown, RN* _____

Discharge against medical advice

When a patient wants to leave the hospital against medical advice (AMA), you can encourage him to stay by explaining the risks involved in his decision. If he still wants to leave AMA, document a detailed description of the event in the progress notes, and ask him to sign a release form like the one shown below.

Responsibility release form

This is to certify that I, _____ *Karl Bird* _____

a patient in _____ *Weston Hospital* _____
.am being discharged against the advice of my doctor and the hospital administration. I acknowledge that I've been informed of the risks involved and hereby release my doctor and the hospital from all responsibility should I suffer any ill effects as a result of this discharge. I also understand that I may return to the hospital at any time and resume treatment.

_____ *Karl Bird* _____
(Patient's signature)

_____ *Janet Adamson, RN* _____
(Witness's signature)

_____ *3/8/01* _____
(Date)

_____ *432* _____
(Patient number)

Documenting special situations

Refusal-of-treatment release form

When a patient refuses treatment, first explain the risks involved in making this choice. Then, if he still refuses to have the treatment, ask him to sign a refusal-of-treatment release form like the one shown below.

Refusal-of-treatment release form

I, _____ *John Williams* _____
(patient's name)

refuse to allow anyone to

_____ *start an intravenous line* _____
(insert treatment)

The risks attendant to my refusal have been fully explained to me, and I fully understand the benefits of this treatment. I also understand that my refusal of treatment seriously reduces my chances for regaining normal health and may endanger my life.

I hearby release

_____ *Weston Hospital* _____
(name of hospital)

and its nurses and employees, together with all doctors in any way connected with me as a patient, from liability for respecting and following my express wishes and direction.

Kay Jackson, RN _____   *John Williams* _____
(Witness's signature)   (Patient's or legal guardian's signature)

3/24/01 _____   *32* _____
(Date)   (Patient's age)

Report for documenting incidents

The incident report (also called a CERF, a clinical event review form) is used to record certain events that are inconsistent with the facility's ordinary routine. These include patient injuries, patient complaints, medication errors, and injuries to employees and visitors.

An incident report serves two main purposes. First, it informs the facility's administrators of the incident so changes can be considered to help prevent similar incidents. This is known as *risk management.* Equipment, processes, and individuals are taken under consideration for review. Trends may be identified and also reviewed to prevent future problems. Second, the incident report alerts the administrators and the facility's insurance company to the possibility of a liability claim and the need for further investigation. This is known as *claims management.*

Filing an incident report

Only a person with firsthand knowledge of an incident should file a report, and only the person making the report should sign it. Never sign a report describing circumstances or events that you didn't witness personally. Each person with firsthand knowledge should fill out and sign a separate report.

Your report should:
- identify the person involved in the incident
- document accurately and truthfully any unusual occurrences that you witnessed
- record details of what happened and the consequences for the person (include sufficient information so the administrators can decide whether the matter requires further investigation)
- avoid opinions, judgments, conclusions, or assumptions about who or what caused the incident
- avoid making suggestions on how to prevent the incident from happening again.

The incident report isn't part of the patient's clinical record, but it may be used in litigation. In general, don't note in the clinical record that an incident report has been filed. Do, however, include the clinical details of the incident in your progress notes, making sure the descriptions on the incident report and the progress notes mirror each other.

Incident report forms vary among facilities, but most include the information shown in the sample on the following pages.

(continued)

Report for documenting incidents *(continued)*

Incident report

Name of person   *Robert Wilson*

Address   *643 Lincoln Street, Philadelphia, PA*

Date of report	Date of incident	Time of incident	If ED patient, give
1/9/01	*1/9/01*	*10:30 a.m.*	unit number

LOCATION OF INCIDENT
- ☑ Patient room
- ☐ Patient bathroom
- ☐ OR
- ☐ ED
- ☐ Facility grounds
- ☐ Nurses' station
- ☐ Other _____

IDENTIFICATION
- ☑ Inpatient
- ☐ ED patient
- ☐ Outpatient
- ☐ Employee
- ☐ Volunteer
- ☐ Visitor
- ☐ Other _____

Admitting diagnosis of patient *HF*

CONDITION BEFORE INCIDENT

Level of consciousness
(previous 4 hours)
- ☑ Alert
- ☐ Confused, disoriented
- ☐ Uncooperative
- ☐ Sedated (drug ____)
- ☐ Unconscious

Ambulation
- ☐ OOB
- ☑ OOB with assistance
- ☐ Bed rest with BRP
- ☐ Complete bed rest
- ☐ Not specified
- ☐ Other (specify) ____

Side rails
- ☐ Up
- ☑ Partially up
- ☐ Down

Restraints
Present ☐ yes ☑ no
Ordered ☐ yes ☑ no

Call system within reach
☑ yes   ☐ no

Bed height
- ☐ High
- ☑ Low

NATURE OF INCIDENT

Fall
- ☐ While ambulatory
- ☐ While sitting
    - ☐ Chair
    - ☐ Commode
- ☐ From bed
- ☐ Off table, stretcher, or equipment
- ☐ Found on floor
- ☐ Other _____

Medication
- ☐ Error in patient identification
- ☐ Incorrect drug
- ☐ Incorrect dosage
- ☑ Incorrect route
- ☐ Timing
- ☐ Duplication
- ☐ Omission

- ☐ Incorrect I.V. solution hung
- ☐ Incorrect I.V. rate
- ☐ Other _____

Report for documenting incidents *(continued)*

Surgical
☐ Consent problem
☐ Incorrect sponge and instrument count

☐ Foreign object left in patient
☐ Other _____

Burn
☐ Chemical
☐ Cigarette
☐ Treatment
☐ Hot liquid
☐ Other _____

EQUIPMENT

☐ Type _____
Control and serial number _____
_____
☐ Malfunction
☐ Shock
☐ Burn
☐ Other _____

Date of last maintenance
BioMed notified ☐ yes ☐ no
Risk Management notified
☐ yes   ☐ no

Personal property
☐ Damaged
☐ Lost
☐ Other _____
(Describe items)

Miscellaneous
☐ Treatment
☐ Needle stick
☐ Injuries in treatment
☐ Infection
☐ Discharge against medical advice
☐ Struck by door
☐ Other _____

Describe the incident.
Digoxin 0.25 mg P.O. ordered. Digoxin 0.25 mg administered intravenously.
_____

Witnesses ☐ yes   ☑ no
If yes, note names, addresses, and phone numbers, and indicate whether they're employees or visitors.
1. _____
2. _____

DISPOSITION
Seen by
☑ Attending doctor
☐ ED doctor
Name_____

Treatment
☑ Not indicated
☐ Treatment given
☐ Treatment refused
☐ X-ray ordered
☐ Admitted to facility
☐ Follow-up care indicated

Examination findings
NSR rate 80; BP 122/76
Doctor's signature
John B. Moyer, MD

Notification
(Include your name, the date, and the time.)
Attending doctor notified
☑ yes ☐ no

Roxanne Smith, RN   1/9/01 10:50 a.m.

(continued)

Report for documenting incidents *(continued)*

DISPOSITION *(continued)*

Supervisor notified
☑ yes ☐ no
Roxanne Smith, RN 1/9/01 10:50 a.m.

Noted in chart
☑ yes ☐ no
Roxanne Smith, RN 1/9/01 10:50 a.m.

Sick call request completed
☐ yes ☑ no

Patient or family notified
☐ yes ☑ no

☑ Documented in progress notes

GENERAL DATA

Attending doctor ___*John B. Moyer, MD*___

Room number   Bed number   Shift ☑ 1 ☐ 2 ☐ 3
305   *1*

Additional details of incident

Signature *Roxanne Smith*
Title ___*RN*___
Date ___*1/9/01*___

Nurse-manager's summary
(Detail follow-up to above incident and action taken.)

Signature _____
Title _____
Date _____

16

Home care
A caregiver's survival guide

Basic principles

What is home care?

Home care is a component of comprehensive health care in which services are provided to patients of all ages and their families in their homes to restore, maintain, or promote health and to minimize the effects of illness and disability. Based on the patient's needs, the appropriate care is planned, coordinated, and supplied by a home care agency.

With the speedy discharge of patients from hospitals (the "quicker and sicker" syndrome), the increasing number of elderly patients, and the availability of safe, easily operated health care equipment, home care has a bright future. Dramatic changes in home care regulation have occurred since the Balanced Budget Act of 1997. These legislative changes included prospective pay and the implementation of a standardized assessment tool when providing home care. In addition, the Health Care Financing Administration (HCFA) investigated billing practices and how care was being provided, which resulted in the closing of over 20% of home care agencies since 1996.

The home care industry may conceivably become one of the primary suppliers of health care in the United States. Currently, long-term care is the primary supplier of health care. Because skilled nursing service lies at the heart of any successful home care program, it's important for you to understand home care principles and practices.

Certification and accreditation

Home care agencies, except for hospices and home health aide (HHA) agencies, are regulated by the Medicare Conditions of Participation. Hospices are certified as Medicare providers under a separate federal standard.

Federal agencies ensure compliance with standards by providing audits by health surveyors employed and licensed by state department agencies. These health surveyors have moved from annual inspections to more frequent visits, commonly related to service complaints. Other federal compliances, such as Medicare, require certification that's critical to the success of a home care agency. For more information, see "Managing and improving care," page 686.

In addition to Medicare certification, agencies may opt for accreditation by the Joint Commission on Accreditation of Healthcare Organizations (JCAHO) or the National League for Nursing's Community Health Accreditation Program (CHAP). Although JCAHO and CHAP accreditation aren't required, many managed care insurance companies mandate this accreditation for their contracted agencies.

An agency applying for accreditation must demonstrate compliance with established standards. Every 3 years, the accrediting body reviews the agency's operations, policies, and procedures; interviews staff; and evaluates home visits and compliance with clinical practice standards.

Determining the patient's eligibility

The provider must recognize the patient as being homebound (able to leave the home infrequently, primarily for medical care) and requiring intermittent *skilled care* services (nursing, physical therapy, and speech therapy) for him to be eligible for home care. HHA services, occupational therapy, and medical social services are *ancillary* services that can only be provided under the auspices of skilled care services. Other services may be offered at home, such as dietary and respiratory services, but aren't considered skilled care.

Patients are referred for home care services primarily by facility discharge planners. They may also be referred by doctors, their families, community agencies, skilled nursing facilities, or insurance case managers. In any case, the home care agency must obtain a doctor's order before initiating service, and the doctor must review a progress report and recertify the need for continued service every 2 months (not more than 62 days).

Future developments

Several major trends are emerging as the home care industry continues to evolve:

■ *Accountability pressures* — Today, home care services are reimbursed by Medicare, Medicaid, and managed care private insurers. More and more private insurers are requiring that home care services be preauthorized. This cost-conscious environment confronts the nurse with challenges ranging from loss of control over patient care to ethical dilemmas and quality improvement issues.

■ *Emphasis on outcomes* — Disease-specific management programs — such as those now in place for diabetes and heart failure — will require home care agencies to develop critical pathways that incorporate patient outcome analysis. In the future, an agency's quality will be measured by outcome data.

■ *Computerizing care* — Increasingly, home care nurses are coping with an expanding paperwork load by using laptop computers. These are equipped with software that speeds clinical documentation to develop the plan of care, formulate goals, monitor patient progress, update medications, and generate visit notes. The new technology also expedites the exchange of current clinical data and other information among

doctors, other care providers, and reimbursers.

■ *Financial stability* — As reimbursement moves from cost-based to prospective pay, greater emphasis will be placed on streamlining care, triaging admissions, and improving efficiency.

■ *Client satisfaction* — Home care agencies have always focused on client satisfaction. However, given the potential that a single complaint can turn into a full agency survey, many home care agencies are extending their response to service complaints.

Ethical and legal aspects of home care

The Code for Nurses of the American Nurses Association (ANA) includes standards of ethical conduct and practice that are relevant to home care. As in any other health care setting, you're expected to provide services while respecting the patient's human dignity and uniqueness without regard to his socioeconomic status, personal attributes, or nature of the health problem. Specific ethical principles include autonomy, beneficence, veracity, fidelity, justice, and respect for others. Each of these principles helps to define the quality and adequacy of health care delivered in the home setting. (See *Applying ethical principles in home health nursing,* page 676.)

Many factors can complicate ethical decisions, such as the legal right of a competent adult to refuse care, increasing patient sophistication, living wills, confidentiality issues, and limited financial resources.

You should be aware that ethical concerns are strongly emphasized in the home care field. In its accreditation process, JCAHO directs agencies to establish committees that handle ethical issues arising in the home.

Applying ethical principles in home health nursing

Principle	Meaning	Example of nursing application
Autonomy	Personal freedom	Allowing the patient to decide when to implement care or to refuse treatment
Beneficence	Duty to promote good	Allowing the patient to die without life-sustaining treatment if that's what he desires
Veracity	Being truthful	Providing the patient with enough information to allow him to make informed choices about care
Fidelity	Keeping one's promise	Refraining from promising the patient that you or another health care worker will be at the bedside when death comes (It may not be possible to keep such a promise.)
Justice	Treating others fairly	Ensuring that you'll provide the care that the patient needs even if there are other, more seriously ill patients that you need to see
Respect for others	Right of individuals to be treated equally	Treating all patients with the same level of empathy and competent care, even when they're noncompliant or of another culture or race

Ethical guidelines are supported by a network of federal and state laws relating to home nursing care. For example, you won't lose your nursing license if you fail to abide by the ANA's Code for Nurses — a voluntary guide document. However, you will lose your license if you violate your state's nurse practice act, which sets legal practice standards in your state. Federal and state laws relevant to home care are briefly reviewed here.

Federal legislation

Federal legislation sets requirements for all home health care nurses. The Omnibus Budget Reconciliation Act (OBRA), as amended in 1987, substantially changed the law relating to participating Medicare agencies. The law requires that patients be screened for eligibility, that they be informed of their legal rights before signing the home care contract, and that they be fully informed in advance about the agency's plan of care and about changes in care or treatment that may affect their well-being. Also, the law gives the patient a voice in planning his care and treatment and addresses confidentiality and grievance issues.

A separate OBRA provision sets strict criteria for home health care aides, who typically provide a large share of hands-on patient care. An agency may not use any individual who isn't a licensed health care professional unless that professional has successfully completed a training program that meets minimum federal standards and is deemed competent to provide assigned services. For more information, see "Working with home health aides," page 681.

The Older Americans Act was amended in 1987 to strengthen home care consumer protections such as the rights of developmentally disabled persons.

The Patient Self-Determination Act of 1991 requires federally funded home care agencies to abide by the terms of a patient's living will or other special directive such as a durable power of attorney. If a patient lacks such an instrument but wants to obtain it, the agency must instruct the patient how to do so.

Since 1999, home care agencies have been required to collect specific information on each patient who is older than age 18 and not receiving services related to childbirth. An Outcome and Assessment Information Set (OASIS), made up of 79 data elements, helps this process by allowing the agency to submit completed information electronically to the HCFA. In addition to the initial OASIS assessment, a repeat assessment is done if the patient is admitted to a health care facility, has a significant change in his condition, is recertified, or is discharged. OASIS helps home care agencies determine patient needs, plans care, assesses care over the course of treatment, and learns how to improve the quality of that care. It incorporates all information regarding the patient's health, functional status, health service use, living conditions, and social supports. It allows quality to be monitored and is essential for accurate payment under the new home health prospective payment system (PPS) instituted on October 1, 2000. Timely and accurate completion of the OASIS is essential so that the employer can review the guidelines and identify the specifications of the OASIS. The PPS sets an amount of money per patient, and care is reviewed per episode rather than per number of visits. Patients who don't have a caregiver may not be admitted as the care

needs are generally expected to exceed the government reimbursement rate. Although the exact impact of the PPS is unknown, it's generally agreed that home care will offer less care for the majority of patients.

State legislation

As you might expect, your state's nurse practice act governs the standards of practice and standards of care in the patient's home as in other health care settings. You should also be aware of your state's laws in such areas as tenants' rights, protection of uninsured persons, and abused or homeless persons. For example, you should know how and when to report cases of suspected abuse. Also, familiarize yourself with family law issues, such as guardians' rights, durable power of attorney, and consent to perform procedures on minors or incompetent persons.

Common legal issues
Verbal orders

If you obtain a verbal order, document it, have the doctor co-sign it as soon as possible, and insert it in the patient's record. If a patient is injured while you were relying on a verbal order and no documentation of the order can be found, you may have trouble proving that you accurately implemented the doctor's order. Also, be sure you've obtained the verbal order and had it approved *before* the approved plan of care expires. Medicare won't cover care that the patient's doctor hasn't fully described and authorized. Because home care is reimbursed through prospective pay, all reimbursement for each episode, rather than for each visit, is jeopardized by irregularities in authorization.

Contracts

Home health nurses must honor contracts made with patients. Contracts include written and oral agreements of understanding made between the agency and the prospective patient. Be aware that the services offered in the agency's brochures and other advertisements can also be construed as part of the formal contract.

A home care plan of care contract, generally referred to as the "HCFA-485," should specify the following elements: the provider's and patient's respective roles and responsibilities; the duration, type, frequency, and limitations of services; discharge planning, cost, and payment schedules; and provisions for obtaining informed consent from the patient or patient's surrogate for specific interventions.

Before the contract is signed, the patient should be informed about the availability of 24-hour staffing, the way to contact staff during off-hours, and the reasons this service may be needed.

If necessary, a patient may be transferred to another site by the agency after the contract has been signed. All aspects of a transfer (physical, psychological, and financial) should be discussed with the patient beforehand.

The agency must develop and implement a satisfactory discharge plan to avoid liability in the event of perceived patient "abandonment" or "dumping" at termination or discharge. Discharge planning should be started with the initial patient evaluation, and the patient should be involved in the plan throughout the care period.

When a patient is to be discharged, he must be given reasonable notice and adequate health care services up to the discharge date. The final OASIS form is completed during the last visit. However, the agency isn't obligated to provide ongoing services without due compensation. Nor must the agency continue to care for a patient who is a threat to the physical safety of the staff.

Confidentiality

As a general rule, you must protect the confidentiality of the patient's medical record. In most states, all health care records — including clinical data obtained from examinations, treatments, observations, and conversations — are considered confidential. Specific state laws may restrict disclosure of this information. The implementation of OASIS has brought issues of confidentiality to the forefront of home care. At the center of the controversy is the government's right to the data from OASIS assessments that are for patients whose insurance carrier isn't the federal government.

Nevertheless, you may have to share the patient's record with other members of the home care team and with third-party payers. You may also be legally required to disclose confidential information in exceptional instances, such as child abuse cases, matters of public health and safety, and criminal cases. To address these issues, obtain written consent from your patient beforehand, preferably at contract signing. If no provision was made for sharing of information, have the patient sign a release form. This form should specify what information is to be released, to whom it will be given, and the time period during which the release is valid.

Because the patient may also request information from the record, the agency should have a written policy concerning release of information to the patient or patient's surrogate. Although the original record is the property of the agency, a copy may be given to the patient for his records.

More common confidentiality issues may also include:

■ listening to voice messages on the office speaker phone when other staff is present

■ leaving patient files where they may be viewed by others, such as in a car

■ talking to neighbors about the location of the patient.

Refusal of care

An issue of growing concern is the patient's right to refuse treatment. Even if the patient has previously consented to treatment, a mentally competent patient can later withdraw consent if the patient has been fully informed about his medical condition and the likely consequences of refusal. Verbal withdrawal of consent is adequate, and this should be immediately communicated to other members of the home care team. The patient's refusal or withdrawal of consent must be documented, along with any patient education measures, and placed in the patient's medical record.

Implementation

Ensuring safe home care visits

When providing patient care in the home, you're faced with two challenges that don't normally arise in a hospital setting: first, making sure you aren't harmed before, during, and after the home visit; and second, making sure the patient can receive care in a safe home environment. This section will help you meet these challenges.

Personal safety guidelines

Most home care agencies have specific policies and procedures to ensure staff safety. You should discuss any safety concerns with your supervisor as soon as they arise so that the appropriate corrective action can be taken. The chart on the next page summarizes what you can do to protect yourself. (See *Personal safety pointers*, page 680.)

Assessing the home environment

You're legally responsible for ensuring that the home is indeed the best place for your patient to receive his prescribed care and treatment. Begin checking the patient's home environment for actual and potential safety problems at your first visit. Document your findings regarding room layout, accessibility, bathroom facilities, storage areas, provision for medical waste disposal, and availability of support persons. You'll be assessing and correcting safety concerns for the duration of the contract period. You'll also be teaching the patient and his family about specific safety measures to implement in your absence. The information below will help you assess possible safety hazards and provide appropriate teaching.

General safety

■ Make sure stairs have secure railings and nonslip tread surfaces.

■ Provide good lighting in halls and stairways.

■ Install a bedside telephone. Provide phone numbers of emergency contact persons, the doctor, 911 (local fire and police), and the agency (agencies must be accessible 24 hours a day). If necessary, install a telephone alert system.

■ Make sure pathways are clear and unobstructed; rugs, if used, should have nonslip backings. Avoid using rugs in high-traffic areas.

■ Provide nonskid slippers or shoes for the patient to use when out of bed.

■ Have a plan for natural disasters, such as earthquakes, tornadoes, and hurricanes.

Bathroom safety

■ Adjust water heater temperature to below 120° F (48.9° C); instruct the patient or family member to check water temperature before getting into the tub or shower.

Personal safety pointers

As a home health care nurse, you'll serve many patients who may be scattered over a wide area in various settings. The suggestions here will help you to avoid potential problems.

Before you go

- Know your agency's safety protocols.
- Verify where the patient lives; call the family or use a map. Use a public telephone or mobile telephone so that your home address can't be tracked by the patient.
- Leave a copy of your itinerary at the office.
- If the patient lives in an unsafe area, try planning your visit early in the day; if possible, bring a nurse "buddy" along.
- If you don't wear a uniform, dress in business clothes, wear a name tag, and carry agency identification; make it easy for the patient to identify you.
- Carry an extra set of keys with you (in case you lock yourself out of your car), bring just enough money for emergency calls and transportation, and have a list of important phone numbers (agency, police, fire).

On the road

- Make sure your car runs well, and fill the gas tank before a visit. Consider joining an automobile club for quick access to road service.
- Always use your seat belt; practice defensive driving.
- If you're taking public transportation, make sure you know the route; if you must walk, don't accept rides from strangers.
- Be prepared for poor weather and delays on the road. Have a flashlight, blanket, and extra snacks handy.

When you arrive

- Don't park your car near the patient's home if it's in an unsafe area. Instead, park in a public area and walk to the home along well-lit streets. If you must visit in the evening, park in an open, well-lit area.
- Before you get out of your car, look around. If you feel unsafe, drive to a safe place to phone the agency about your concern.
- If you have doubts about the safety of entering the patient's home or building, don't enter. Immediately contact the agency.
- If the patient doesn't answer the door, call the patient from a pay phone or mobile phone or have the agency contact the patient.
- When entering the home, observe all the exits. If you're uneasy or if you suspect anyone in the home is using alcohol or drugs, do what is necessary for the patient and leave. If this isn't possible, leave immediately.
- If a pet is obnoxious or hostile, politely ask that it be moved to another room. Always be respectful of the patient's attachment to the pet. After your visit, document the animal's presence in the home to warn other caregivers.

■ Advise the patient and his family to install rubber mats or nonslip strips in the tub and shower.

■ Advise the patient and his family to install grab bars in the tub and shower.

Patient care safety
■ Determine availability of a support person.

■ Demonstrate storage of medications in a safe place, out of the reach of children, and disposal of old or expired medication.

■ Instruct the patient to use bed rails when in bed; use seat belts, if necessary, when in a chair; and keep wheelchair brakes locked and footrests out of the way when transferring to a wheelchair.

■ If ordered, apply patient restraints properly.

■ Advise the patient to set electrical heating pads on low to medium and to keep them covered.

■ Place bedside items within the patient's reach.

■ Institute and teach infection-control measures.

Fire safety
■ Warn the patient against smoking in bed or during oxygen use, and tell him to make sure all cigarettes and matches are out before throwing them away.

■ Advise installation of smoke or heat detectors on each level of the home.

■ Place portable heaters in well-ventilated areas.

■ Make sure appliances' electrical cords are intact, not frayed or split, and have straight plug prongs.

Medical equipment
■ Instruct the patient or family regarding the function and proper use of prescribed equipment and the reporting of malfunctions.

■ Explain possible hazards related to electrical, mechanical, and fire safety aspects of equipment.

■ Store medical gases, supplies, and drugs in a safe, protected area.

Medical waste disposal
■ Make sure appropriate containers are available for disposal of needles, syringes, and other contaminated medical supplies.

■ Teach proper handling of medical waste.

Document your actions
Document your home care safety recommendations. Enclose a statement in the patient's record listing what was taught or recommended, and record instances of the patient's or family's refusal or failure to follow your recommendations. For example, they may balk at the extra expense of installing smoke detectors or a tub rail. Or the patient may continue to smoke when oxygen is being used. Carefully documenting noncompliance will help protect you and your agency from possible liability.

Working with home health aides

If the patient's condition and situation warrant it, you may assign a paraprofessional HHA to assist the patient intermittently with personal care and activities of daily living. The HHA's role is crucial because she may spend more time with the patient and family than any other member of the health care team. Typically, you'll determine the need for HHA services during the initial home visit.

Criteria for HHA services
For planning and reimbursement purposes, the use of HHAs is considered an ancillary (not a skilled care) service. The National Association for Home

Care has identified three levels of HHA services. An HHA I performs housekeeping services only; an HHA II performs nonmedical personal care as well as level I tasks; and an HHA III performs medically supervised tasks, such as providing nonsterile wound care, assisting with prescribed rehabilitation therapy, and assisting with self-administered medications, in addition to performing levels I and II tasks.

Depending on the patient's situation, you may elect to use HHA services at levels I, II, or III. However, Medicare will reimburse a home care agency only for care provided by a certified level III HHA. An HHA III may become certified after completing a training program of at least 75 hours, 16 of which must be in laboratory and clinical settings. To justify HHA III services, you must be able to demonstrate that skilled care is being provided on an intermittent basis, thereby creating a need for hands-on personal care and assistance with the patient's treatment.

In any case, the continued need for HHA services must be documented at least every 2 weeks. The doctor must confirm the type and frequency of HHA service in the plan of care and must also recertify the order for HHA service every 2 months.

Explain to the patient and family that HHA services will only be reimbursed if the above criteria are met. Patients and their families can become dependent on the HHA and have difficulty adjusting when HHA services are discontinued.

What home health aides do
Most of an HHA's tasks are related to the patient's personal care. This includes assisting with bathing, dressing, grooming, oral hygiene, shaving, skin care, and routine foot care and changing bed linens of an incontinent patient.

The HHA may also help with feeding and elimination; she may administer an enema or give routine catheter and colostomy care, unless the patient's condition requires skilled care (for example, if the patient has a heart disorder). The HHA also can assist the patient with ambulation, changing position in bed, and transfers.

Examples of reimbursable HHA services include:
■ a dressing change that doesn't require skilled care, such as a dry, nonsterile dressing change
■ helping to give medications that the patient would normally take unaided and that don't require a nurse's skills to achieve safe, accurate administration
■ helping with activities related to skilled therapy services that don't require the therapist to be present, such as maintenance exercises and speech exercises
■ performing routine care of prosthetic and orthotic devices.

The HHA may perform other activities during a home visit, but these aren't reimbursable unless they're performed during that same visit. Such activities, labeled by Medicare as "incidental," may include light housekeeping, light cleaning of the patient's immediate area, meal preparation and cleanup, laundry related to the patient's care, essential grocery shopping and errands, and taking out the trash.

Supervising HHAs
When HHA services are ordered, plan to meet with the aide during one of your home care visits. This allows the aide and the patient to get acquainted and discuss the plan of care together. The plan of care will specify the HHA's duties. At the end of the visit, you'll leave a copy with the patient.

Typically, you're responsible for communicating with the HHA about any changes in the patient's condition or care and communicating with the patient and family about the care provided. However, if another skilled service (such as physical or speech therapy) is involved and skilled nursing isn't, you can delegate supervisory responsibility to the therapist.

You can monitor the HHA's performance during a home visit while the aide is present to directly observe, to instruct the HHA, and to make recommendations and suggestions for care. Also, plan a visit when the HHA isn't present so that you can get additional feedback. The patient may be reluctant to say anything about the HHA while she is present.

Managed care organizations and private insurers have reimbursement and supervisory criteria for HHA services similar to Medicare's. Consult your case manager about specific requirements.

Documenting HHA services

Most home care agencies use a standardized form for documenting HHA supervision. These data should also be entered in the patient's care record. Include information relating to assessment of the patient's health status, rapport of the patient and HHA, and determination of goal achievement. Include any recommendations and suggestions. If teaching is involved, document what was taught and the HHA's response to the teaching, including a return demonstration, if appropriate.

Ensuring reimbursement

In no other health care setting are you as responsible for ensuring reimbursement payments as you are in the home care setting. Your success or failure largely depends on your documentation skills. For this reason, home care agencies have a highly structured documentation system.

The HCFA, which monitors Medicare and Medicaid disbursements, requires home care agencies to standardize their documentation. Required data for each certified patient are collected using a Home Health Certification and Plan of Treatment form (HCFA-485) and a Medical Update and Patient Information form (HCFA-486). These forms allow Medicare reviewers to evaluate each claim in accordance with the established criteria for coverage. Medicare won't provide payment unless these forms are properly completed, signed by the nurse and the attending doctor, and submitted.

Developing the plan of care

Many home care agencies use HCFA-485 as the patient's official plan of care. Be aware that because the patient's care occurs in the home — usually with the family participating — you have less control than you would in an institutional setting. The patient and his family become the decision makers in many aspects and have greater control of the situation. These factors must be addressed realistically when developing the plan of care, and you may need to readjust your interventions, patient goals, and teaching accordingly.

To justify reimbursement, to support the patient's need for services and supplies, and to justify any change in the plan of care, your documentation must be clear, thorough, and accurate. Good documentation also facilitates medical review and continuity of care and helps protect you legally.

The initial home visit

During the initial home visit, you'll evaluate the patient's eligibility for home care based on Medicare guidelines and a completed OASIS form. You'll also obtain a complete health history and assess the patient's psychosocial and physiologic status in the context of his environment.

The history and assessment should focus primarily on acute medical instabilities (especially those that influence the patient's homebound status). Be sure to document all functional limitations of the patient and caregiver, including mobility, dexterity, vision, hearing, and strength. Also, assess and document home safety needs.

When documenting the patient's psychosocial status, include data on living conditions, economic situation, culture, primary language of the patient and caregiver, ability of the patient and caregiver to learn, availability of the caregiver, coping styles, support systems, and availability of transportation.

Also, obtain a medication history. Because Medicare reimburses for teaching related to new medications (and, in some instances, for old and changed medications as well), the plan of care must indicate whether each medication (prescription and over-the-counter) is new, old, or changed.

Obtaining a doctor's order

The plan of care that results from the initial visit must be signed by the attending doctor to become a valid order. This signature must be obtained before the claim is submitted for payment. The doctor's order must specify the type of skilled and unskilled services required and the frequency of those services. Amended orders must clearly indicate what is to be changed and the reason for the changes.

A verbal order for skilled services must be documented in the patient's record to cover the services rendered from the initial visit (start of certification period) to the time the plan of care is signed by the doctor. Amendments to the plan of care must also be signed and placed in the patient's record within 10 days of receiving verbal orders.

Documenting the plan of care

The number of home visits per week is specified during the initial home visit. Daily or multiple daily visits (five or more visits per week) are allowed only when the visits won't be required for an indefinite period of time. Visits are usually less frequent as the patient's condition improves. Typically, a range of visit frequency is specified in the plan of care to provide some flexibility and to ensure that the most appropriate level of care is being provided. Since the implementation of the PPS, the focus is now on episodes of care; however, visit frequency must still be documented.

When documenting each home visit, you'll need to clearly explain to the payer why the provided service is reasonable and necessary. Do this by charting the "negative" (the illness or disability), thereby focusing on the patient's problems and the skilled care needed to deal with them. For example, include detailed information about why the patient or caregiver can't or won't learn to perform a skilled procedure or comply with a medication regimen. Because of the PPS, the focus is always on progress toward goals. Eliminating barriers to goal achievement is key to the patient outcome.

Documenting ancillary services

If ancillary services (occupational therapy, nutritional therapy, respiratory care, medical social services, or home health aides) are needed and ordered, a referral for the appropriate service must be completed. It should outline the type of ancillary service required and explain why it's needed. The patient's rehabilitation potential must be judged as at least "fair" to qualify for reimbursement. (See *Understanding skilled and ancillary home care services.*)

Understanding skilled and ancillary home care services

This chart gives examples of skilled and ancillary services used in home health care and how they may be reimbursed.

Services	Indications and examples	Notes
Physical therapy (skilled service)	Indicated for functional limitations and deficits in safety, mobility, strength, and range of motion; examples: gait training, strengthening exercises	Some states allow trained physical therapists to perform wound debridement. A physical therapist may be the sole professional on a home care case and may complete all OASIS tools.
Speech therapy (skilled service)	Indicated for dysphasia and dysphagia; examples: assessment and evaluation, diagnostic testing, teaching and training, aural rehabilitation, maintenance therapy	Medicare won't reimburse for repetition and reinforcement, work-related therapy, or a nondiagnostic or nontherapeutic routine. Speech therapists may also complete OASIS data.
Occupational therapy (not considered a skilled service)	Indicated for functional limitation of activities of daily living that relates to the primary or secondary diagnosis; examples: therapeutic activities, energy-conservation methods, task simplification	Skilled nursing, physical therapy, or speech therapy must be ordered and provided for occupational therapy services to be reimbursed. The occupational therapist can complete the discharge OASIS tool.
Medical social service (not considered a skilled service)	Indicated for social or emotional difficulties of the patient or caregiver that affect treatment or rate of recovery; examples: referrals, counseling, long-term care planning	Skilled nursing, physical therapy, or speech therapy must be ordered and provided for medical social service to be reimbursed. OASIS forms may not be completed by medical social service representatives.
Home health aide (HHA) care (not considered a skilled service)	Determined by the home care nurse, usually at the initial visit; HHA assistance with personal hygiene, patient transfers, light meal preparation, light housekeeping and, possibly, medications (for medications, check state laws)	Skilled nursing, physical therapy, or speech therapy must be ordered and provided for HHA care services to be reimbursed.

Documenting patient teaching

Medicare reimburses for teaching as a skilled service within the PPS plan of care. Certain guidelines must be followed and documented:

■ Identify precisely what was taught and to whom it was taught (patient or caregiver).

■ Document the patient or caregiver's ability to learn, especially if he's slow or overwhelmed.

■ Describe the teaching outcome. What was the level of understanding? Evaluate and document the patient's or caregiver's return demonstration performance.

Obtaining recertification

Documentation requesting recertification must clearly support the need for continued care within Medicare guidelines. Every 2 months, a progress report summarizing the patient's condition and stating any proposed changes in the plan of care must be sent to the doctor for review. At this point, a new HCFA-485 is completed and signed by the doctor.

Discharge notification

If the patient is deemed ready for discharge from home care services, the doctor is consulted, appropriate orders are obtained, and a discharge OASIS and a summary are completed. The summary should state the patient's condition at discharge, the reason for discharge, the extent to which the goals of care were met, and any instructions for patient follow-up with the doctor.

Managing and improving care

Case management and quality improvement are concepts central to providing professional home care services. They are intended to provide a structure for providing care according to standards established by government regulation, voluntary accreditation agencies, professional organizations, third-party payers, and individual agencies. This section will examine the two concepts in turn.

Case management

Case management involves prioritizing care among the patients in a caseload and delivering that care according to procedural steps that ensure successful patient outcomes. These steps are based on the nursing process and include information gathering and assessment, establishing a multidisciplinary plan of care, and implementing and evaluating the plan of care.

You may feel that a managed care environment impairs your agency's flexibility in responding to changing patient needs or that much of the decision making you were accustomed to is curtailed. Also, you may have to deal with several case managers from different managed care organizations with different policies and procedures. Case managers, for their part, may be frustrated by the need to constantly explain and justify their role when they feel they should be treated as valued customers. Effective communication can reduce the level of mutual distrust and frustration. At its best, external case management matches the home care nurse's strengths — knowledge of the patient and the community resources available — with the case manager's strengths — knowledge of reimbursement procedures and efficient use of available resources.

Suggestions for working with managed care providers

These pointers will help you work well with managed care providers and maintain quality care for patients:

■ Learn as much as possible about trends in reimbursement for home care, the various types of managed care organizations, and the ways your agency has adapted to this new type of health care.

■ Work with an understanding of the managed care organization's interest in finding the most efficient way of meeting patient needs. Know the most current treatment strategies and patient-teaching methods, and be aware of the cost of various treatment alternatives.

■ Redouble your efforts to be familiar with community resources that can help patients become more independent. Services coordinated by area agencies on aging usually can help a patient make the transition to home care service. Churches are a largely untapped resource for help in meeting patient needs.

■ Be aware of the need to document successful patient outcomes. Present the patient's needs with a clear explanation of the specific actions you have requested and the specific outcomes you believe will result. Support this with evidence that the outcome will prevent a complication or a recurring problem.

Quality improvement
Health care agencies' quality control efforts have advanced from static reviews of patient care documentation to ongoing integration of quality improvement measures into all procedures. The term *quality assurance* has given way to total quality management, followed by total quality improvement and, finally, continuous quality improvement (CQI).

The CQI process can be seen as yet another variation of the nursing process. Data is gathered; problems are defined; goals are set; actions are selected; evaluations are made using structure, process, and outcome indicators; and variances are identified. This, in turn, cues a new round of the CQI process. Nurses have multiple opportunities to become in-

volved in the CQI process. If chosen to participate on a quality improvement committee, you would work with other caregivers to set the course for the CQI program for a significant time period. Many agencies have a quality improvement coordinator or director who chairs the committee.

On another quality front, many health care providers are developing sets of standard interventions, based on medical diagnoses or surgical procedures, to ensure that patients receive care that's normative for the specific condition. These standard interventions are known as clinical paths, critical paths, care tracks, and coordinated care guides.

Clinical paths resemble standardized nursing plans of care in some respects. They're multidisciplinary tools that need to be accepted by all involved in the patient's care, particularly the doctor. Clinical paths can reduce documentation requirements and streamline the quality improvement process.

Medicare site visits
When home care agencies are reviewed to certify them for Medicare reimbursement, the aspects of care that are examined are determined by the conditions of participation in the Medicare program documented in the Home Health Agency Health Insurance Manual. To prepare for a Medicare site visit, you should review your practices to make sure Medicare guidelines are followed for every Medicare-reimbursed case:

■ Check admission practices to ensure that the patient and family understand the conditions of Medicare eligibility, their rights with regard to Medicare service, and the way to access information about these rights.

■ Document that a copy of the patient's bill of rights was given to the patient, and place a copy in the patient's record.

■ Document that the patient's wishes with regard to advance medical directives were discussed.

■ Review the patient's record for adherence to standards of timeliness of documentation, for visit frequency, and for completion of all necessary forms, particularly doctor's orders (HCFA-485).

■ Ensure that visit records reflect the skilled care given, the homebound status of the patient, and the coordination of all services provided by the agency.

■ Perform supervision of HHAs according to your agency's policy. Documentation always includes the patient's or caregiver's satisfaction with the service, the rationale for continued HHA service, and the nurse's recommendation to continue or modify the service.

- **Appendices**
- **Selected references**
- **Index**

Appendix A
Cultural considerations in patient care

Regardless of the particular setting in which you work, as a health care professional you'll typically interact with a diverse, multicultural patient population. Each culture has its own unique set of beliefs about health and illness, dietary practices, and other matters that you should consider when providing care.

Cultural group	Health and illness philosophy
African Americans	■ May believe illness is related to supernatural causes such as punishment from God or an evil spell ■ Believe health is a feeling of well-being ■ May seek advice and remedies from faith or folk healers
Arab Americans	■ Believe health is a gift from God and that one should care for oneself by eating right and minimizing stressors ■ May believe illness is caused by the evil eye, bad luck, stress, or an imbalance between hot and cold or moist and dry ■ May assume a passive role as a patient ■ May use amulets to ward off the evil eye during illness ■ Believe in complete rest and relieving oneself of responsibilities during an illness ■ Tend to express pain vocally and may have a low pain threshold
Chinese Americans	■ Believe health is a balance of Yin and Yang and that illness stems from an imbalance of these elements; believe good health requires harmony between body, mind, and spirit ■ May use herbalists or acupuncturists before seeking medical help; ginseng root also common as a home remedy ■ May use good luck objects, such as jade or a rope tied around the waist ■ Expect family to take care of patient (who assumes a passive role) ■ Tend not to readily express pain; may be stoic by nature
Iranian Americans	■ Believe illness stems from an imbalance of hot and cold foods; proper food combinations important in daily life ■ May use home or humoral cures before seeing a doctor ■ Show great respect for health care providers ■ May seek alternative therapies and advice ■ Express pain with grimaces and moans
Japanese Americans	■ Believe that health is a balance of oneself, society, and the universe ■ May believe illness is karma, resulting from behavior in present or past life ■ May believe certain food combinations cause illness ■ May use prayer beads if Buddhist ■ May use tea to treat stomach ailments and constipation ■ May not complain of symptoms until severe
Mexican Americans	■ Believe that health is influenced by environment, fate, and God's will ■ May believe in Galen's theory that the four humors in the body — blood, phlegm, yellow bile, and black bile — must be kept in balance ■ May use herbal teas and soup to aid in recuperation ■ May self-medicate (prescription drug sales aren't controlled in Mexico) ■ May have family request to keep seriousness of illness from patient ■ May express pain by nonverbal cues

This appendix summarizes the beliefs and customs of six cultures common in the United States, including African Americans, Arab Americans, Chinese Americans, Iranian Americans, Japanese Americans, and Mexican Americans. Understanding these cultures will help you provide appropriate interventions without compromising your patients' cultural integrity.

Dietary practices	Other considerations
■ May have food restrictions based on religious beliefs such as not eating pork if Muslim ■ May view cooked greens as good for health	■ Tend to be affectionate, as shown by touching and hugging friends and loved ones ■ Must have head covered at all times if Muslim ■ Respect elders, especially for their wisdom ■ Primary religions: Baptist, other Protestant denominations, Muslim
■ Don't mix milk and fish, sweet and sour, or hot and cold ■ Don't use ice in drinks; believe hot soup can help recovery ■ Prohibited from drinking alcohol and eating pork or ham if Muslim	■ Respect elders and professionals ■ May avoid contact with male strangers (traditional women) ■ Use same-sex family members as interpreters ■ Primary religions: Muslim, Christian (Greek Orthodox, Protestant)
■ Select rice, noodles, and vegetables as staples; tend to use chopsticks ■ Choose foods to help balance the Yin (cold) and Yang (hot) ■ Drink hot liquids, especially when sick	■ Prefer a comfortable distance between patient and health care provider ■ Address elders by surname (addressing by first name is a sign of disrespect) ■ May show respect by lack of eye contact ■ Tend to be very modest; prefer same-sex clinicians ■ Primary religions: Buddhist, Catholic, Protestant
■ Choose foods based on humoral theory of balancing hot and cold ■ Prefer dairy products, rice, and wheat breads ■ May avoid pork and alcohol	■ Greet elders first as a sign of respect ■ May feel shame from full disclosure of an illness ■ Tend to be modest and reserved; prefer same-sex clinicians ■ Primary religion: Shiite Muslim
■ Eat rice with most meals; may use chopsticks ■ Eat a diet high in salt and low in sugar, fat, animal protein, and cholesterol	■ Usually quiet and polite; may ask few questions about care, deferring to health care providers ■ May nod, especially elderly patients, but not necessarily understand ■ May be very modest; tend to avoid touching; prefer same-sex clinicians ■ Primary religions: Buddhist, Shinto, Christian
■ Select beans and tortillas as staples ■ Eat a lot of fresh fruits and vegetables	■ May be modest (especially women) ■ Use same-sex family members as interpreters ■ Primary religion: Roman Catholic

Appendix B
Abbreviations and terms

ā	before	ALT	alanine aminotransferase
āā	of each	a.m., A.M.	morning
AAA	abdominal aortic aneurysm	AMA	against medical advice
Ab	antibody	AMI	acute myocardial infarction
ABC	airway, breathing, and circulation	AML	acute myelocytic leukemia
ABG	arterial blood gas	ANA	antinuclear antibody
a.c.	before meals	AP	anteroposterior apical pulse
ACE	angiotensin-converting enzyme	APTT	activated partial thromboplastin time
ACh	acetylcholine	aq	aqueous (watery)
ACLS	advanced cardiac life support	ara-A	adenine arabinoside (vidarabine)
a.d., AD	auris dextra (right ear)	ara-C	arabinosylcytosine cytosine arabinoside (cytarabine)
AD	Alzheimer's disease		
ADH	antidiuretic hormone	ARDS	acute respiratory distress syndrome adult respiratory distress syndrome
ADL	activities of daily living		
AER	aldosterone excretion rate		
AFIB	atrial fibrillation	ARF	acute renal failure acute respiratory failure acute rheumatic fever
AFL	atrial flutter		
AFP	alpha-fetoprotein		
Ag	antigen	a.s., AS	auris sinistra (left ear)
A-G	albumin-globulin (ratio)	AS	aortic sounds aqueous solution astigmatism
AGA	appropriate for gestational age		
AHD	arteriosclerotic heart disease autoimmune hemolytic disease	ASA	acetylsalicylic acid (aspirin)
		ASD	atrial septal defect
		ASO	antistreptolysin-O
AHF	antihemophilic factor (factor VIII)	AST	aspartate aminotransferase
		ATP	adenosine triphosphate
AIDS	acquired immunodeficiency syndrome	A.U.	auris utraque (each ear)
		AV	arteriovenous atrioventricular
ALL	acute lymphocytic leukemia		
ALS	amyotrophic lateral sclerosis	AVM	arteriovenous malformation

BBB	bundle-branch block	**cc**	cubic centimeter
BCG	bacille Calmette-Guérin	**CCNU**	lomustine
BCNU	carmustine	**CCU**	cardiac care unit
BE	barium enema		critical care unit
	base excess	**CDC**	Centers for Disease Control
b.i.d.	twice daily		and Prevention
BJ	Bence Jones	**CEA**	carcinoembryonic antigen
BLS	basic life support	**CF**	cardiac failure
BMR	basal metabolic rate		cystic fibrosis
BP	blood pressure	**CFS**	chronic fatigue syndrome
BPH	benign prostatic hyperplasia	**CGL**	chronic granulocytic
	benign prostatic hypertrophy		leukemia
BPM	beats per minute	**CHB**	complete heart block
BSA	body surface area	**CHD**	childhood disease
BUN	blood urea nitrogen		congenital heart disease
C	Celsius		congenital hip disease
	centigrade	**CK**	creatine kinase
	certified	**CK-BB**	creatine kinase, brain
	cervical	**CK-MB**	creatine kinase, heart
c̄	with	**CK-MM**	creatine kinase, skeletal
CA	cardiac arrest		muscle
Ca	calcium	**cm**	centimeter
CABG	coronary artery bypass	**CML**	chronic myelogenous
	grafting		leukemia
CAD	coronary artery disease	**CMV**	continuous mandatory venti-
cAMP	cyclic adenosine monophos-		lation
	phate		cytomegalovirus
CAPD	continuous ambulatory	**CNS**	central nervous system
	peritoneal dialysis	**CO**	carbon monoxide
caps	capsules		cardiac output
CBC	complete blood count	**CO₂**	carbon dioxide
CC	Caucasian child	**COEPS**	cortically originating
	chief complaint		extrapyramidal system
	common cold	**COLD**	chronic obstructive lung
	creatinine clearance		disease
	critical care	**comp**	compound
	critical condition		

COPD	chronic obstructive pulmonary disease	**DJD**	degenerative joint disease
CP	capillary pressure	**DKA**	diabetic ketoacidosis
	cerebral palsy	**dl**	deciliter
	cor pulmonale	**DNA**	deoxyribonucleic acid
	creatine phosphate	**DNR**	do not resuscitate
CPAP	continuous positive airway pressure	**DOA**	date of admission
			dead on arrival
cpm	counts per minute	**DS**	double strength
	cycles per minute	**DSA**	digital subtraction angiography
CPR	cardiopulmonary resuscitation	***DSM-IV***	*Diagnostic and Statistical Manual of Mental Disorders,* 4th ed.
CSF	cerebrospinal fluid		
CT	clotting time	**DTP**	diphtheria and tetanus toxoids and pertussis vaccine
	coated tablet		
	compressed tablet	**DVT**	deep vein thrombosis
	computed tomography	**D₅W**	5% dextrose in water
	corneal transplant	**EBV**	Epstein-Barr virus
CV	cardiovascular	**EC**	enteric-coated
	central venous	**ECF**	extended care facility
CVA	cerebrovascular accident		extracellular fluid
	costovertebral angle	**ECG**	electrocardiogram
CVP	central venous pressure	**ECHO**	echocardiography
d	day	**ECMO**	extracorporeal membrane oxygenator
/d	per day		
D	dextrose	**ECT**	electroconvulsive therapy
dB	decibel	**ED**	emergency department
D/C	discharge	**EDTA**	ethylenediaminetetra-acetic acid
	discontinue		
D&C	dilatation and curettage	**EEG**	electroencephalogram
DD	differential diagnosis	**EENT**	eyes, ears, nose, and throat
	discharge diagnosis	**EF**	ejection fraction
	dry dressing	**ELISA**	enzyme-linked immunosorbent assay
D&E	dilatation and evacuation		
DES	diethylstilbestrol	**elix**	elixir
DIC	disseminated intravascular coagulation	**EMG**	electromyography
dil	dilute		
disp	dispense		

EMIT	enzyme-multiplied immunoassay technique
ENG	electrostagmography
EOM	extraocular movement
ER	emergency room expiratory reserve
ERCP	endoscopic retrograde cholangiopancreatography
ERV	expiratory reserve volume
ESR	erythrocyte sedimentation rate
ESWL	extracorpeal shock-wave lithotripsy
et	and
ext.	extract
F	Fahrenheit
FDA	Food and Drug Administration
FEF	forced expiratory flow
FEV	forced expiratory volume
FFP	fresh frozen plasma
FHR	fetal heart rate
fl, fld	fluid
FRC	functional residential capacity
FSH	follicle-stimulating hormone
FSP	fibrogen-split products
FT$_3$	free triiodothyronine
FT$_4$	free thyroxine
FTA	fluorescent treponemal antibody (test)
FTA-ABS	fluorescent treponemal antibody absorption (test)
FUO	fever of undermined origin
FVC	forced vital capacity
G	gauge
g, gm, GM	gram
GFR	glomerular filtration rate
GI	gastrointestinal
G6PD	glucose-6-phosphate dehydrogenase
gr	grain
gtt	drop
GU	genitourinary
GVHD	graft-versus-host disease
GYN	gynecologic
h, hr	hour
Ⓗ	hypodermic injection
HAV	hepatitis A virus
Hb	hemoglobin
HBD	α-hydroxybutyrate dehydrogenase
HBIG	hepatitis B immunoglobulin
HbsAg	hepatitis B surface antigen
HBV	hepatitis B virus
hCG	human chorionic gonadotropin
Hct	hematocrit
HDL	high-density lipoprotein
HDN	hemolytic disease of the newborn
HF	heart failure
hGH	human growth hormone
HHNK	hyperosmolar hyperglycemic nonketotic syndrome
HIV	human immunodeficiency virus
HLA	human leukocyte antigen
HMO	health maintenance organization
hPL	human placental lactogen

h.s.	at bedtime	**IRV**	inspiratory reserve volume
HS	half strength hour of sleep house surgeon	**IU**	International Unit
		IUD	intrauterine device
HSV	herpes simplex virus	**I.V.**	intravenous
HVA	homovanillic acid	**IVGTT**	intravenous glucose tolerance test
Hz	hertz	**IVH**	intravenous hyperalimentation (now called total parenteral nutrition)
HZV	herpes zoster virus		
IA	internal auditory intra-arterial intra-articular	**IVP**	intravenous pyelogram
		IVPB	intravenous piggyback
IABP	intra-aortic balloon pump	**J**	joule
IC	inspiratory capacity	**JCAHO**	Joint Commission on Accreditation of Healthcare Organizations
ICD	implantable cardioverter-defibrillator		
ICF	intracellular fluid	**JVD**	jugular venous distention
ICHD	Inter-Society Commission for Heart Disease	**JVP**	jugular venous pressure
		kg	kilogram
ICP	intracranial pressure	**17-KGS**	17-ketogenic steroids
ICU	intensive care unit	**17-KS**	17-ketosteroids
ID	identification initial dose inside diameter intradermal	**KUB**	kidneys-ureters-bladder
		KVO	keep vein open
		L	liter lumbar
I&D	incision and drainage	Ⓛ	left
IDDM	insulin-dependent diabetes mellitus	**LA**	left atrium long-acting
Ig	immunoglobulin	**LAP**	left atrial pressure leucine aminopeptidase
IM	infectious mononucleosis		
I.M.	intramuscular	**lb., #**	pound
IMV	intermittent mandatory ventilation	**LD**	lactate dehydrogenase
		LDL	low-density lipoproteins
in., ″	inch	**LE**	lupus erythematosus
IND	investigational new drug	**LES**	lower esophageal sphincter
IPPB	intermittent positive-pressure breathing	**LGL**	Lown-Ganong-Levine variant syndrome
IQ	intelligence quotient		

LH	luteinizing hormone
LLQ	left lower quadrant
LOC	level of consciousness
LR	lactated Ringer's solution
LSB	left scapular border left sternal border
LTC	long-term care
LUQ	left upper quadrant
LV	left ventricle
LVEDP	left ventricular end-diastolic pressure
LVET	left ventricular ejection time
LVF	left ventricular failure
m	meter
M	molar (solution)
m²	square meter
mm³	cubic millimeter
MAO	maximal acid output monamine oxidase
MAST	medical antishock trousers (pneumatic antishock garment)
mcg, µg	microgram
MCH	mean corpuscular hemoglobin
MCHC	mean corpuscular hemoglobin concentration
MCV	mean corpuscular volume
MD	manic depressive medical doctor muscular dystrophy
mEq	milliequivalent
mg	milligram
mgtt	microdrip minidrip

MI	mental illness mitral insufficiency myocardial infarction myocardial ischemia
ml	milliliter
µL	microliter
MLC	mixed lymphocytic culture
mm	millimeter
MMEF	maximal midexpiratory flow
mmol	millimole
MRI	magnetic resonance imaging
M.R. × 1	may repeat once
MS	mitral sounds mitral stenosis morphine sulfate multiple sclerosis musculoskeletal
MUGA	multiple-gated acquisition scanning
MVI	multivitamin infusion
MVP	mitral valve prolapse
MVV	maximal voluntary ventilation
Na	sodium
NaCl	sodium chloride
NCV	nerve conduction velocity
ng	nanogram
NG	nasogastric
NICU	neonatal intensive care unit
NIDDM	non–insulin-dependent diabetes mellitus (type 2 diabetes)
NKA	no known allergies
NMR	nuclear magnetic resonance
Noct.	night

NP	nasopharynx
	nerve palsy
	new patient
	not palpable
NPN	nonprotein nitrogen
NPO	nothing by mouth
NR	nerve root
	nonreactive
	no refills
	no report
	no respirations
N/R	not remarkable
NS, NSS	normal saline solution (0.9% sodium chloride)
¼ NS	¼ normal saline solution (0.225% sodium chloride)
½ NS	½ normal saline solution (0.45% sodium chloride)
NSAID	nonsteroidal anti-inflammatory drug
O$_2$	oxygen
OB	obstetric
OD	occupational disease
	overdose
	right eye
OGTT	oral glucose tolerance test
OR	operating room
OS	left eye
O$_2$ sat.	oxygen saturation
OTC	over-the-counter
OU	each eye
oz	ounce
p̄	after
PA	pernicious anemia
	posteroanterior
	pulmonary artery
PABA	para-aminobenzoic acid
PAC	premature atrial contraction

Paco$_2$	partial pressure of carbon dioxide in arterial blood
Pao$_2$	partial pressure of oxygen in arterial blood
PAP	Papanicolaou
	passive-aggressive personality
	primary atypical pneumonia
	pulmonary artery pressure
PAT	paroxysmal atrial tachycardia
PAWP	pulmonary artery wedge pressure
p.c.	after meals
PCA	patient-controlled analgesia
PDA	patent ductus arteriosus
PE	pelvic examination
	physical examination
	pulmonary embolism
PEEP	positive end-expiratory pressure
PEFR	peak expiratory flow rate
PEP	pre-ejection period
per	by or through
PET	positron-emission tomography
pg	picogram
PID	pelvic inflammatory disease
PKU	phenylketonuria
p.m., P.M.	afternoon
PMI	point of maximum impulse
PML	progressive multifocal leukoencephalopathy
PMS	premenstrual syndrome
PND	paroxysmal nocturnal dyspnea
	postnasal drip
P.O.	by mouth
	postoperative

PP	partial pressure
	peripheral pulses
	postpartum
	postprandial
	presenting problem
p.r.n.	as needed
PROM	passive range of motion
	premature rupture of the membranes
pt.	pint
PT	prothrombin time
PTCA	percutaneous transluminal coronary angioplasty
PTH	parathyroid hormone
PTT	partial thromboplastin time
PUD	peptic ulcer disease
	pulmonary disease
PVC	premature ventricular contraction
	polyvinyl chloride
q	every
QA	quality assurance
q.a.m.	every morning
q.d.	every day
q.h.	every hour
q.i.d.	four times daily
q.n.	every night
QNS	quantity not sufficient
q.o.d.	every other day
QS	quantity sufficient
qt.	quart
R, PR	by rectum
Ⓡ	right
RA	renal artery
	rheumatoid arthritis
	right arm
	right atrium

RAF	rheumatoid arthritis factor
RAP	right atrial pressure
RAST	radioallergosorbent test
RBB	right bundle branch
RBC	red blood cell
RDA	recommended daily allowance
RE	rectal examination
	right ear
REM	rapid eye movement
RES	reticuloendothelial system
Rh	rhesus blood factor
RHD	relative hepatic dullness
	rheumatic heart disease
RIA	radioimmunoassay
RL	right lateral
	right leg
	Ringer's lactate (lactated Ringer's solution)
RLQ	right lower quadrant
RNA	ribonucleic acid
ROM	range of motion
	right otitis media
RSV	respiratory syncytial virus
	right subclavian vein
	Rous sarcom virus
RUQ	right upper quadrant
RV	residual volume
	right ventricle
RVEDP	right ventricle end-diastolic pressure
RVEDV	right ventricular end-diastolic volume
RVP	right ventricular pressure
Rx	prescription
s̄	without
SA	sinoatrial

sat.	saturated
S.C., SQ	subcutaneous
SCID	severe combined immuno-deficiency syndrome
sec	second
SHBG	sex hormone-binding globulin
SI	Système International d'Unités
SIADH	syndrome of inappropriate antidiuretic hormone
SIDS	sudden infant death syndrome
Sig	write on label
SIMV	synchronized intermittent mandatory ventilation
S.L., sl.	sublingual
SLE	systemic lupus erythematosus
SOB	shortness of breath
sol., soln.	solution
sp.	spirit
SR	sustained release
SRS-A	slow-reacting substance of anaphylaxis
s̄s̄	one-half
stat.	immediately
STD	sexually transmitted disease
supp.	suppository
susp.	suspension
Sv̄o₂	mixed venous oxygen saturation
syr.	syrup
T, Tbs., tbsp.	tablespoon
t, tsp.	teaspoon

tab.	tablet
TBG	thyroxine-binding globulin
TCA	tricyclic antidepressant
TENS	transcutaneous electrical nerve stimulation
TIA	transient ischemic attack
t.i.d.	three times daily
TIL	tumor-infiltrating lymphocytes
tinct., tr.	tincture
TLC	total lung capacity
TM	temporomandibular tympanic membrane
TMJ	temporomandibular joint
TNF	tumor necrosis factor
tPA	tissue plasminogen activator
TPN	total parenteral nutrition
TRH	thyrotropin-releasing hormone
TSH	thyroid-stimulating hormone
UCE	urea cycle enzymopathy
USP	United States Pharmacopeia
UTI	urinary tract infection
UV	ultraviolet
VAD	vascular access device ventricular assist device
vag., V, PV	vaginal
VDRL	Venereal Disease Research Laboratory (test)
VLDL	very low-density lipoprotein
VMA	vanillylmandelic acid
VO	verbal order
V̇/Q̇	ventilation-perfusion ratio
VSD	ventricular septal defect
V$_T$	tidal volume

WBC	white blood cell
WPW	Wolff-Parkinson-White Syndrome
Z/G, ZIG	zoster immune globulin
×	times, multiply
℈	dram
z or ℥	ounce
>	greater than
<	less than
↑	increase
↓	decrease
≈	approximately equal

Appendix C
NANDA Taxonomy II codes

The North American Nursing Diagnosis Association (NANDA) endorsed its first nursing diagnosis taxonomic structure, NANDA Taxonomy I, in 1986. This taxonomy has been revised several times, most recently in 2000. The new Taxonomy II has a code structure that's compliant with recommendations from the National Library of Medicine concerning health care terminology codes. The taxonomy that appears here represents the currently accepted classification system for nursing diagnosis.

Nursing diagnosis	Taxonomy II code
Imbalanced nutrition: More than body requirements	00001
Imbalanced nutrition: Less than body requirements	00002
Risk for imbalanced nutrition: More than body requirements	00003
Risk for infection	00004
Risk for imbalanced body temperature	00005
Hypothermia	00006
Hyperthermia	00007
Ineffective thermoregulation	00008
Autonomic dysreflexia	00009
Risk for autonomic dysreflexia	00010
Constipation	00011
Perceived constipation	00012
Diarrhea	00013
Bowel incontinence	00014
Risk for constipation	00015
Impaired urinary elimination	00016
Stress urinary incontinence	00017
Reflex urinary incontinence	00018
Urge urinary incontinence	00019
Functional urinary incontinence	00020
Total urinary incontinence	00021
Risk for urge urinary incontinence	00022
Urinary retention	00023

Nursing diagnosis	Taxonomy II code
Ineffective tissue perfusion (specify type: renal, cerebral, cardiopulmonary, gastrointestinal, peripheral)	00024
Risk for imbalanced fluid volume	00025
Excess fluid volume	00026
Deficient fluid volume	00027
Risk for deficient fluid volume	00028
Decreased cardiac output	00029
Impaired gas exchange	00030
Ineffective airway clearance	00031
Ineffective breathing pattern	00032
Impaired spontaneous ventilation	00033
Dysfunctional ventilatory weaning response	00034
Risk for injury	00035
Risk for suffocation	00036
Risk for poisoning	00037
Risk for trauma	00038
Risk for aspiration	00039
Risk for disuse syndrome	00040
Latex allergy response	00041
Risk for latex allergy response	00042
Ineffective protection	00043
Impaired tissue integrity	00044
Impaired oral mucous membrane	00045
Impaired skin integrity	00046
Risk for impaired skin integrity	00047

Nursing diagnosis	Taxonomy II code	Nursing diagnosis	Taxonomy II code
Impaired dentition	00048	Noncompliance (specify)	00079
Decreased intracranial adaptive capacity	00049	Ineffective family therapeutic regimen management	00080
Disturbed energy field	00050	Ineffective community therapeutic regimen management	00081
Impaired verbal communication	00051	Effective therapeutic regimen management	00082
Impaired social interaction	00052	Decisional conflict (specify)	00083
Social isolation	00053	Health-seeking behaviors (specify)	00084
Risk for loneliness	00054		
Ineffective role performance	00055	Impaired physical mobility	00085
Impaired parenting	00056	Risk for peripheral neurovascular dysfunction	00086
Risk for impaired parenting	00057	Risk for perioperative-positioning injury	00087
Risk for impaired parent/infant/child attachment	00058	Impaired walking	00088
Sexual dysfunction	00059	Impaired wheelchair mobility	00089
Interrupted family processes	00060	Impaired transfer ability	00090
Caregiver role strain	00061	Impaired bed mobility	00091
Risk for caregiver role strain	00062	Activity intolerance	00092
Dysfunctional family processes: Alcoholism	00063	Fatigue	00093
Parental role conflict	00064	Risk for activity intolerance	00094
Ineffective sexuality patterns	00065	Disturbed sleep pattern	00095
Spiritual distress	00066	Sleep deprivation	00096
Risk for spiritual distress	00067	Deficient diversional activity	00097
Readiness for enhanced spiritual well-being	00068	Impaired home maintenance	00098
Ineffective coping	00069	Ineffective health maintenance	00099
Impaired adjustment	00070	Delayed surgical recovery	00100
Defensive coping	00071	Adult failure to thrive	00101
Ineffective denial	00072	Feeding self-care deficit	00102
Disabled family coping	00073	Impaired swallowing	00103
Compromised family coping	00074	Ineffective breast-feeding	00104
Readiness for enhanced family coping	00075	Interrupted breast-feeding	00105
Readiness for enhanced community coping	00076	Effective breast-feeding	00106
Ineffective community coping	00077	Ineffective infant feeding pattern	00107
Ineffective therapeutic regimen management	00078	Bathing or hygiene self-care deficit	00108

Nursing diagnosis	Taxonomy II code
Dressing or grooming self-care deficit	00109
Toileting self-care deficit	00110
Delayed growth and development	00111
Risk for delayed development	00112
Risk for disproportionate growth	00113
Relocation stress syndrome	00114
Risk for disorganized infant behavior	00115
Disorganized infant behavior	00116
Readiness for enhanced organized infant behavior	00117
Disturbed body image	00118
Chronic low self-esteem	00119
Situational low self-esteem	00120
Disturbed personal identity	00121
Disturbed sensory perception (specify: visual, auditory, kinesthetic, gustatory, tactile, olfactory)	00122
Unilateral neglect	00123
Hopelessness	00124
Powerlessness	00125
Deficient knowledge (specify)	00126
Impaired environmental interpretation syndrome	00127
Acute confusion	00128
Chronic confusion	00129
Disturbed thought processes	00130
Impaired memory	00131
Acute pain	00132
Chronic pain	00133
Nausea	00134
Dysfunctional grieving	00135
Anticipatory grieving	00136
Chronic sorrow	00137

Nursing diagnosis	Taxonomy II code
Risk for other-directed violence	00138
Risk for self-mutilation	00139
Risk for self-directed violence	00140
Posttrauma syndrome	00141
Rape-trauma syndrome	00142
Rape-trauma syndrome: Compound reaction	00143
Rape-trauma syndrome: Silent reaction	00144
Risk for posttrauma syndrome	00145
Anxiety	00146
Death anxiety	00147
Fear	00148

NEW NURSING DIAGNOSES: EFFECTIVE APRIL 2000

Risk for relocation stress syndrome	00149
Risk for suicide	00150
Self-mutilation	00151
Risk for powerlessness	00152
Risk for situational low self-esteem	00153
Wandering	00154
Risk for falls	00155

Appendix D
Herb-drug interactions

Herb	Drug	Possible effects
Aloe	Cardiac glycosides, antiarrhythmics	May lead to hypokalemia, which may potentiate cardiac glycosides and antiarrhythmics
	Thiazide diuretics, licorice, and other potassium-wasting drugs	Increases effects of potassium wasting with thiazide diuretics and other potassium-wasting drugs
	Orally administered drugs	Causes potential for decreased absorption of drugs because of more rapid GI transit time
Bilberry	Antiplatelets, anticoagulants	Decreases platelet aggregation
	Insulin, hypoglycemics	May increase serum insulin levels, causing hypoglycemia; increases effects with diabetes drugs
Capsicum	Antiplatelets, anticoagulants	Decreases platelet aggregation and increases fibrinolytic activity, prolonging bleeding time
	NSAIDs	Stimulates GI secretions to help protect against NSAID-induced GI irritation
	ACE inhibitors	May cause cough
	theophylline	Increases absorption of theophylline, possibly leading to higher serum levels or toxicity
	MAO inhibitors	Decreases effects of MAO inhibitors resulting from the increased catecholamine secretion
	CNS depressants (such as opioids, benzodiazepines, barbiturates)	Increases sedative effect
	H_2 blockers, proton pump inhibitors	Causes potential for decreased effectiveness because of increased acid secretion
Chamomile	Drugs requiring GI absorption	May delay drug absorption
	Anticoagulants	May enhance anticoagulant therapy and prolong bleeding time (if warfarin constituents)
	Iron	May reduce iron absorption because of tannic acid content
Echinacea	Immunosuppressants	May counteract immunosuppressant drugs
	Hepatotoxics	May increase hepatotoxicity with drugs known to elevate liver enzyme levels

(continued)

Herb	Drug	Possible effects
Echinacea *(continued)*	warfarin	Increases bleeding time without an increased INR
Evening primrose	Anticonvulsants	Lowers seizure threshold
Feverfew	Antiplatelets, anticoagulants	May decrease platelet aggregation and increase fibrinolytic activity
	methysergide	May potentiate methysergide
Garlic	Antiplatelets, anticoagulants	Enhances platelet inhibition, leading to increased anticoagulation
	Insulin, other drugs causing hypoglycemia	May increase serum insulin levels, causing hypoglycemia, an additive effect with antidiabetics
	Antihypertensives	Causes potential for additive hypotension
	Antihyperlipidemics	May have additive lipid-lowering properties
Ginger	Chemotherapeutic drugs	May reduce nausea associated with chemotherapy
	H_2 blockers, proton pump inhibitors	Causes potential for decreased effectiveness because of increased acid secretion by ginger
	Antiplatelets, anticoagulants	Inhibits platelet aggregation by antagonizing thromboxane synthase and enhancing prostacyclin, leading to prolonged bleeding time
	Calcium channel blockers	May increase calcium uptake by myocardium, leading to altered drug effects
	Antihypertensives	May antagonize antihypertensive effect
Ginkgo	Antiplatelets, anticoagulants	May enhance platelet inhibition, leading to increased anticoagulation
	Anticonvulsants	May decrease effectiveness of anticonvulsants
	Drugs known to lower seizure threshold	May further reduce seizure threshold
Ginseng	Stimulants	May potentiate stimulant effects
	warfarin	May antagonize warfarin, resulting in a decreased INR
	Antibiotics	May enhance the effects of some antibiotics (Siberian ginseng)
	Anticoagulants, antiplatelets	Decreases platelet adhesiveness
	digoxin	May falsely elevate digoxin levels
	MAO inhibitors	Potentiates the action of MAO inhibitors

Herb	Drug	Possible effects
Ginseng *(continued)*	Hormones, anabolic steroids	May potentiate the effects of hormone and anabolic steroid therapies (estrogenic effects of ginseng may cause vaginal bleeding and breast nodules)
	Alcohol	Increases alcohol clearance, possibly by increasing activity of alcohol dehydrogenase
	furosemide	May decrease diuretic effect of furosemide
	Antipsychotics	May stimulate CNS activity
Goldenseal	heparin	May counteract the anticoagulant effect of heparin
	Diuretics	Increases diuretic effect
	H_2 blockers, proton pump inhibitors	Causes potential for decreased effectiveness because of increased acid secretion by goldenseal
	General anesthetics	May potentiate hypotensive action of general anesthetics
	CNS depressants (such as opioids, barbiturates, benzodiazepines)	Increases sedative effect
Grapeseed	warfarin	Increases effects and INR caused by tocopherol content of grapeseed
Green tea	warfarin	Decreases effectiveness resulting from vitamin content of green tea
Hawthorn berry	Digoxin	Causes additive positive inotropic effect, with potential for digoxin toxicity
Kava	CNS stimulants or depressants	May hinder therapy with CNS stimulants
	Benzodiazepines	May result in comalike states
	Alcohol, other CNS depressants	Potentiates the depressant effect of alcohol and other CNS depressants
	levodopa	Decreases effectiveness of levodopa
Licorice	digoxin	Causes hypokalemia, which predisposes the patient to digoxin toxicity
	Oral contraceptives	Increases fluid retention and potential for increased blood pressure resulting from fluid overload
	Corticosteroids	Causes additive and enhanced effects of corticosteroids

(continued)

Herb	Drug	Possible effects
Licorice *(continued)*	spironolactone	Decreases the effects of spironolactone
Ma huang	MAO inhibitors	Potentiates MAO inhibitors
	CNS stimulants, caffeine, theophylline	Causes CNS stimulation
	digoxin	Increases risk of arrhythmias
	Hypoglycemics	Decreases hypoglycemic effect because of hyperglycemia caused by ma huang
Melatonin	CNS depressants (such as opioids, barbiturates, benzodiazepines)	Increases sedative effect
Milk thistle	Drugs causing diarrhea	Increases bile secretion and commonly causes loose stools; may increase the effects of other drugs commonly causing diarrhea; also causes liver membrane-stabilization and antioxidant effects, leading to protection from liver damage from various hepatotoxic drugs, such as acetaminophen, phenytoin, ethanol, phenothiazines, butyrophenones
Nettle	Anticonvulsants	May increase sedative adverse effects and the risk of seizure
	Narcotics, anxiolytics, hypnotics	May increase sedative adverse effects
	warfarin	Decreases effectiveness resulting from vitamin K content of aerial parts of nettle
	iron	May reduce iron absorption because of tannic acid content
Passion flower	CNS depressants (such as opioids, barbiturates, benzodiazepines)	Increases sedative effect
St. John's wort	SSRIs, MAO inhibitors, nefazodone, trazodone	Causes additive effects with SSRIs, MAO inhibitors, and other antidepressants, potentially leading to serotonin syndrome, especially when combined with SSRIs
	indinavir; HIV protease inhibitors (PIs); nonnucleoside reverse transcriptase inhibitors (NNRTIs)	Induces cytochrome P450 metabolic pathway, which may decrease the therapeutic effects of drugs using this pathway for metabolism (use of St. John's wort and PIs or NNRTIs should be avoided because of the potential for subtherapeutic antiretroviral levels and insufficient virologic response that could lead to resistance or class cross-resistance)

Herb	Drug	Possible effects
St. John's wort *(continued)*	Narcotics, alcohol	Enhances the sedative effects of narcotics and alcohol
	Photosensitizing drugs	Increases photosensitivity
	Sympathomimetic amines (such as pseudoephedrine)	Causes additive effects
	digoxin	May reduce serum digoxin concentrations, decreasing therapeutic effects
	reserpine	Antagonizes the effects of reserpine
	Oral contraceptives	Increases breakthrough bleeding when taken with oral contraceptives; also decreases the contraceptive's effectiveness
	theophylline	May decrease serum theophylline levels, making the drug less effective
	Anesthetics	May prolong the effect of anesthetic drugs
	cyclosporine	Decreases cyclosporine levels below therapeutic levels, threatening transplanted organ rejection
	Iron	May reduce iron absorption because of tannic acid content
	warfarin	Has potential to alter INR; reduces the effectiveness of anticoagulant, requiring increased dosage of drug
Valerian	Sedative hypnotics, CNS depressants	Enhances the effects of sedative hypnotic drugs
	Alcohol	Increases sedation with alcohol (although this is debated)
	Iron	May reduce iron absorption because of tannic acid content

Appendix E
Monitoring patients using herbs

Altered laboratory values and changes in a patient's condition can help target your assessments and better meet the needs of your patient who uses herbs.

Herb	What to monitor	Explanation
Aloe	■ Serum electrolyte level ■ Weight pattern ■ BUN and creatinine levels ■ Heart rate ■ Blood pressure ■ Urinalysis	Aloe possesses cathartic properties that inhibit water and electrolyte reabsorption, which may lead to potassium depletion, weight loss, and diarrhea. Long-term use may lead to nephritis, albuminuria, hematuria, and cardiac disturbances.
Bilberry	■ Weight pattern ■ CBC ■ Blood glucose level ■ Triglyceride level ■ Liver function	Bilberry contains flavonoids and chromium, which are thought to have blood glucose- and triglyceride-lowering effects. Continued intoxication may lead to wasting, anemia, and jaundice.
Capsicum	■ Liver function ■ BUN and creatinine levels	Oral administration of capsicum can lead to gastroenteritis and hepatic or renal damage.
Cat's claw	■ Blood pressure ■ Lipid panel ■ Serum electrolyte level	Cat's claw can potentially cause hypotension through inhibition of the sympathetic nervous system and its diuretic properties. It may also lower cholesterol level.
Chamomile (German, Roman)	■ Menstrual changes ■ Pregnancy	Chamomile has been reported to cause changes in menstrual cycle and is a known teratogen in animals.
Echinacea	■ Temperature	When echinacea is used parenterally, dose-dependent, short-term fever, nausea, and vomiting can occur.
Ephedra	■ Blood pressure ■ Heart rate ■ BUN and creatinine levels ■ Weight pattern	Ephedra's active ingredient, ephedrine, stimulates the CNS in a manner similar to that of amphetamines. Adverse effects include hypertension, tachycardia, and kidney damage.
Evening primrose	■ Pregnancy ■ CBC ■ Lipid profile	Evening primrose elevates plasma lipid levels and reduces platelet aggregation. It may increase the risk of pregnancy complications, including rupture of membranes, oxytocin augmentation, arrest of descent, and vacuum extraction.

Herb	What to monitor	Explanation
Fennel	■ Liver function ■ Blood pressure ■ Serum calcium level ■ Blood glucose level	Fennel contains trans-anethole and estrogole. Trans-anethole has estrogenic activity, whereas estrogole is a procarcinogen with the potential to cause liver damage. Adverse effects include photodermatitis and allergic reactions, particularly in those sensitive to carrots, celery, and mugwort.
Feverfew	■ CBC ■ Pregnancy ■ Sleep pattern	Feverfew may inhibit blood platelet aggregation and decrease neutrophil and platelet secretory activity. It can cause uterine contractions in full-term, pregnant women. Adverse effects include mouth ulceration, tongue irritation and inflammation, abdominal pain, indigestion, diarrhea, flatulence, nausea, and vomiting. Postfeverfew syndrome includes nervousness, headache, insomnia, joint pain, stiffness, and fatigue.
Flaxseed	■ Lipid panel ■ Blood pressure ■ Serum calcium level ■ Blood glucose level ■ Liver function	Flaxseed possesses weak estrogenic and antiestrogenic activity. It may cause a reduction in platelet aggregation and serum cholesterol level. Oral administration with inadequate fluid intake can cause intestinal blockage.
Garlic	■ Blood pressure ■ Lipid panel ■ Blood glucose level ■ CBC ■ PT and PTT	Garlic is associated with hypotension, leukocytosis, inhibition of platelet aggregation, and decreased blood glucose and cholesterol levels. Postoperative bleeding and prolonged bleeding time can occur.
Ginger	■ Blood glucose level ■ Blood pressure ■ Heart rate ■ Respiratory rate ■ Lipid panel ■ Electrocardiogram	Ginger contains gingerols, which have positive inotropic properties. Adverse effects include platelet inhibition, hypoglycemia, hypotension, hypertension, and stimulation of respiratory centers. Overdoses cause CNS depression and arrhythmias.
Ginkgo	■ Respiratory rate ■ Heart rate ■ PT and PTT	Consumption of ginkgo seed may cause difficulty breathing, weak pulse, seizures, loss of consciousness, and shock. Ginkgo leaf is associated with infertility as well as GI upset, headache, dizziness, palpitations, restlessness, lack of muscle tone, weakness, bleeding, subdural hematoma, subarachnoid hemorrhage, and a bleeding iris.

(continued)

Herb	What to monitor	Explanation
Ginseng (American, Panax, Siberian)	■ BUN and creatinine levels ■ Blood pressure ■ Serum electrolyte levels ■ Liver function ■ Serum calcium level ■ Blood glucose level ■ Heart rate ■ Sleep pattern ■ Menstrual changes ■ Weight pattern ■ PT, PTT, and INR	Ginseng contains ginsenosides and eleutherosides that can affect blood pressure, CNS activity, platelet aggregation, and coagulation. A reduction in glucose and hemoglobin A_{1C} levels has also been reported. Adverse effects include drowsiness, mastalgia, vaginal bleeding, tachycardia, mania, cerebral arteritis, Stevens-Johnson syndrome, cholestatic hepatitis, amenorrhea, decreased appetite, diarrhea, edema, hyperpyrexia, pruritus, hypotension, palpitations, headache, vertigo, euphoria, and neonatal death.
Goldenseal	■ Respiratory rate ■ Heart rate ■ Blood pressure ■ Liver function ■ Mood pattern	Goldenseal contains berberine and hydrastine. Berberine improves bile secretion and bilirubin level, increases coronary blood flow, and stimulates or inhibits cardiac activity. Hydrastine causes hypotension, hypertension, increased cardiac output, exaggerated reflexes, seizures, paralysis, and death from respiratory failure. Other adverse effects include digestive disorders, constipation, excitatory states, hallucinations, delirium, GI upset, nervousness, depression, dyspnea, and bradycardia.
Kava	■ Weight pattern ■ Lipid panel ■ CBC ■ Blood pressure ■ Liver function ■ Urinalysis ■ Mood changes	Kava contains arylethylene pyrone constituents that have CNS activity. It also has antianxiety effects. Long-term use may lead to weight loss, increased HDL cholesterol levels, hematuria, increased RBCs, decreased platelet count, decreased lymphocyte levels, reduced protein levels, and pulmonary hypertension.
Milk thistle	■ Liver function	Milk thistle contains flavono-lignans, which have liver-protective and antioxidant effects.
Nettle	■ Blood glucose level ■ Blood pressure ■ Weight pattern ■ BUN and creatinine levels ■ Serum electrolyte level ■ Heart rate ■ PT and INR	Nettle contains significant amounts of vitamin C, vitamin K, potassium, and calcium. Nettle may cause hyperglycemia, decreased blood pressure, decreased heart rate, weight loss, and diuretic effects.
Passion flower	■ Liver function ■ Amylase level ■ Lipase level	Passion flower may contain cyanogenic glycosides, which can cause liver and pancreas toxicity.

Herb	What to monitor	Explanation
St. John's wort	■ Vision ■ Menstrual changes	Changes in menstrual bleeding and a reduction in fertility may be caused by St. John's wort. Other adverse effects include GI upset, fatigue, dry mouth, dizziness, headache, delayed hypersensitivity, phototoxicity, and neuropathy. St. John's wort may also increase the risk of cataracts.
SAM-e	■ Blood pressure ■ Heart rate ■ BUN and creatinine levels	SAM-e contains homocysteine, which requires folate, cyanocobalamin, and pyridoxine for metabolism. Increased levels of homocysteine are associated with CV and renal disease.
Saw palmetto	■ Liver function	Saw palmetto inhibits conversion of testosterone to dihydrotestosterone and may cause inhibition of growth factors. Adverse effects include cholestatic hepatitis, erectile or ejaculatory dysfunction, and altered libido.
Valerian	■ Blood pressure ■ Heart rate ■ Sleep pattern ■ Liver function	Valerian contains valerenic acid, which increases gamma-butyric acid and decreases CNS activity. Adverse effects include cardiac disturbances, insomnia, chest tightness, and hepatotoxicity.

Selected references

American Association of Critical-Care Nurses, Lynn-McHale, D.J. Carlson, K.K. eds. *AACN Procedure Manual for Critical Care,* 4th ed. Philadelphia: W.B. Saunders Co., 2001.

Bickley, L.S., and Hoekelman, R.A. *Bates' Pocket Guide to Physical Examination and History Taking,* 3rd ed. Philadelphia: Lippincott Williams & Wilkins, 2000.

Bickley, L.S., and Hoekelman, R.A. *Bates' Guide to Physical Examination and History Taking,* 7th ed. Philadelphia: Lippincott Williams & Wilkins, 1999.

Braunwald, E., et al., eds. *Heart Disease: A Textbook of Cardiovascular Medicine,* 6th ed. Philadelphia: W.B. Saunders Co., 2001.

Craven, R.F., and Hirnle, C.J. *Fundamentals of Nursing: Human Health and Function,* 3rd ed. Philadelphia: Lippincott Williams & Wilkins, 2000.

Curren, A.M., and Munday, L.D. *Math for Meds: Dosages and Solutions,* 8th ed. San Diego: W.I. Publications, 2000.

Diagnostics: An A-to-Z Guide to Laboratory Tests & Diagnostic Procedures. Springhouse, Pa.: Springhouse Corp., 2001.

Diseases, 3rd ed., Springhouse, Pa.: Springhouse Corp., 2001.

ECG Cards, 3rd ed., Springhouse, Pa.: Springhouse Corp., 2000.

Elkin, M.K., et al. *Nursing Interventions and Clinical Skills,* 2nd ed. St. Louis: Mosby–Year Book, Inc., 2000.

Fauci, A.S., et al. *Harrison's Principles of Internal Medicine,* 15th ed., New York: McGraw-Hill Book Co., 2001.

Fischbach, F.T. *A Manual of Laboratory and Diagnostic Tests,* 6th ed. Philadelphia: Lippincott Williams & Wilkins, 2000.

Fortunato, N.H. *Berry and Kohn's Operating Room Technique,* 9th ed. St. Louis: Mosby–Year Book, Inc., 2000.

Goldman, L., and Bennett, J.C. *Cecil Textbook of Medicine,* 21st ed. Philadelphia: W.B. Saunders Co., 2000.

Hadaway, L.C. "I.V. Infiltration: Not Just a Peripheral Problem," *Nursing99* 29(9):41-47, September 1999.

Holt-Ashley, M. "Nurses Pray: Use of Prayer and Spirituality as a Complementary Therapy in the Intensive Care Setting," *American Association of Critical-Care Nurses Clinical Issues* 11(1):60-67, February 2000.

Horne, C., and Derrico, D. "Mastering ABGs. The Art of Arterial Blood Gas Measurement," *AJN* 99(8):26-33, August 1999.

Kreitzer, M.J., and Jensen, D. "Healing Practices: Trends, Challenges, and Opportunities for Nurses in Acute and Critical Care," *American Association of Critical-Care Clinical Issues* 11(1):7-16, February 2000.

Ignatavicius, D.D., et al. *Medical-Surgical Nursing Across the Health Care Continuum,* 3rd ed. Philadelphia: W.B. Saunders Co., 1999.

Jagger, J., and Perry, J. "Power in Numbers: Reducing your Risk of Bloodborne Exposures," *Nursing99* 29(1):51-52, January 1999.

Jarvis, C. *Pocket Companion for Physical Examination and Health,* 3rd ed. Philadelphia: W.B. Saunders Co., 2000.

Joint Commission on Accreditation of Healthcare Organizations. *Comprehensive Accreditation Manual for Hospitals,* Oakbrook Terrace, Ill., 2001.

Kost, M. "Conscious Sedation: Guarding your Patient Against Complications," *Nursing99* 29(4):34-39, April 1999.

Kozier, B., et al. *Fundamentals of Nursing: Concepts, Process, and Practice,* 6th ed. Upper Saddle River, N.J.: Prentice Hall Health, 2000.

Marriott, H.J., and Conover, M.B. *Advanced Concepts in Arrhythmias,* 3rd ed. St. Louis: Mosby–Year Book, Inc., 1999.

Nicol, M., et al. *Essential Nursing Skills.* St. Louis: Mosby–Year Book, Inc., 2000.

Nursing Diagnoses: Definitions and Classification 2001-2002. Philadelphia: North American Nursing Diagnosis Association, 2001.

Nursing Procedures, 3rd ed., Springhouse, Pa.: Springhouse Corp., 2000.

Pierson, F.M. *Principles and Techniques of Patient Care*, 2nd ed. Philadelphia: W.B. Saunders Co., 1999.

Phillips, L.D. *Manual of I.V. Therapeutics*, 3rd ed. Philadelphia: F.A. Davis Co., 2001.

Phippen, M.L., and Wells, M.P. *Patient Care During Operative and Invasive Procedures.* Philadelphia: W.B. Saunders Co., 2000.

Professional Guide to Signs & Symptoms, 3rd ed. Springhouse, Pa.: Springhouse Corp., 2001.

Rakel, R.E., and Bope, E.T., eds. *Conn's Current Therapy.* Philadelphia: W.B. Saunders Co., 2001.

Rodts, M.F. "Alternative or Complementary Therapies: Hocus Pocus or In-between?," *Orthopaedic Nursing* 19(1):15, January 2000.

Shoemaker, W.C., and Grenvik, A., et al. *Textbook of Critical Care*, 4th ed. Philadelphia: W.B. Saunders Co., 2000.

Smeltzer, S.C., and Bare, B.G. *Brunner and Suddarth's Textbook of Medical-Surgical Nursing*, 9th ed. Philadelphia: Lippincott Williams & Wilkins, 2000.

Sole, M.L., et al., eds. *Introduction to Critical Care Nursing*, 3rd ed. Philadelphia: W.B. Saunders Co., 2001.

Turjanica, M.A. "Anatomy of a Code: How Do You Feel at the Start of a Code Blue?," *Nursing Management* 30(11):44-49, November 1999.

Index

i refers to an illustration; t refers to a table.

i refers to an illustration; t refers to a table.

i refers to an illustration; t refers to a table.

i refers to an illustration; t refers to a table.

i refers to an illustration; t refers to a table.

Crisis values of laboratory tests

The abnormal laboratory test values listed below have immediate life-and-death significance to the patient. Report such values to the patient's doctor immediately.

Test	Low value	Common causes and effects	High value	Common causes and effects
Ammonia	< 15 µg/dl	Renal failure	> 50 µg/dl	Severe hepatic disease: hepatic coma, Reye's syndrome, GI hemorrhage, heart failure
Calcium, serum	< 7 mg/dl	Vitamin D or parathyroid hormone deficiency: tetany, seizures	> 12 mg/dl	Hyperparathyroidism: coma
Carbon dioxide and bicarbonate, blood	< 10 mEq/L	Complex pattern of metabolic and respiratory factors	> 40 mEq/L	Complex pattern of metabolic and respiratory factors
Creatine kinase isoenzymes			> 5%	Acute myocardial infarction (MI)
Creatinine, serum			> 4 mg/dl	Renal failure: coma
D-dimer, serum or cerebrospinal fluid (CSF)			> 250 µg/ml	Disseminated intravascular coagulation (DIC), pulmonary embolism, arterial or venous thrombosis, subarachnoid hemorrhage (CSF only), secondary fibrinolysis
Glucose, blood	< 40 mg/dl	Excess insulin administration: brain damage	> 300 mg/dl (with ketonemia and electrolyte imbalance)	Diabetes: diabetic coma
Gram stain, CSF			Gram-positive or gram-negative	Bacterial meningitis
Hemoglobin	< 8 g/dl	Hemorrhage, vitamin B_{12} or iron deficiency: heart failure	> 18 g/dl	Chronic obstructive pulmonary disease: thrombosis, polycythemia vera
International Normalized Ratio			> 3.0	DIC, uncontrolled oral anticoagulation
Partial pressure of carbon dioxide, in arterial blood	< 20 mm Hg	Complex pattern of metabolic and respiratory factors	> 70 mm Hg	Complex pattern of metabolic and respiratory factors
Partial pressure of oxygen, in arterial blood	< 50 mm Hg	Complex pattern of metabolic and respiratory factors		
Partial thromboplastin time			> 40 sec (> 70 sec for patient on heparin)	Anticoagulation factor deficiency: hemorrhage
pH, arterial blood	< 7.2	Complex pattern of metabolic and respiratory factors	> 7.6	Complex pattern of metabolic and respiratory factors
Platelet count	< 50,000/µl	Bone marrow suppression: hemorrhage	> 500,000/µl	Leukemia, reaction to acute bleeding: hemorrhage
Potassium, serum	< 3 mEq/L	Vomiting and diarrhea, diuretic therapy: cardiotoxicity, arrhythmia, cardiac arrest	> 6 mEq/L	Renal disease, diuretic therapy: cardiotoxicity, arrhythmia
Prothrombin time			> 14 sec (> 20 sec for patient on warfarin)	Anticoagulant therapy, anticoagulation factor deficiency: hemorrhage
Sodium, serum	< 120 mEq/L	Diuretic therapy: cardiac failure	> 160 mEq/L	Dehydration: vascular collapse
Troponin I			> 2 µg/ml	Acute MI
White blood cell (WBC) count	< 2,000/µl	Bone marrow suppression: infection	> 20,000/µl	Leukemia: infection
WBC count, CSF			> 10/µl	Meningitis, encephalitis: infection